THE HARRIET LANE HANDBOOK

A Manual for Pediatric House Officers

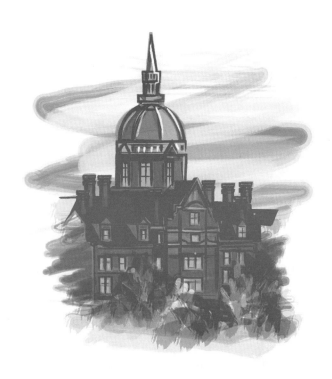

sixteenth
EDITION

THE
HARRIET LANE
HANDBOOK

A Manual for Pediatric House Officers

The Harriet Lane Service
Children's Medical and Surgical Center of
The Johns Hopkins Hospital

EDITORS

Veronica L. Gunn, MD, MPH
Christian Nechyba, MD

with 145 illustrations and 44 color plates

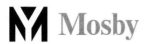

An Imprint of Elsevier Science

Philadelphia   St. Louis   London   Sydney   Toronto

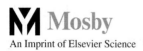
Mosby

An Imprint of Elsevier Science

The Curtis Center
Independence Square West
Philadelphia, Pennsylvania 19106

The Harriet Lane Handbook: A Manual for Pediatric House Officers

0-323-01486-0

NOTICE

Pediatrics is an ever-changing field. Standard safety precautions must be
followed, but as new research and clinical experience broaden our
knowledge, changes in treatment and drug therapy may become necessary or appropriate. Readers are advised to check the most current
product information provided by the manufacturer of each drug to be
administered to verify the recommended dose, the method and duration
of administration, and contraindications. It is the responsibility of the
licensed prescriber, relying on experience and knowledge of the patient,
to determine dosages and the best treatment for each individual patient.
Neither the publisher nor the editor assumes any liability for any injury
and/or damage to persons or property arising from this publication.

Previous edition copyrighted 2000.

International Standard Book Number 0-323-01486-0

Acquisitions Editor: Dolores Meloni
Publishing Services Manager: Pat Joiner
Senior Project Manager: Karen M. Rehwinkel
Senior Designer: Mark A. Oberkrom

GW/WC

Printed in Canada

Last digit is the print number: 9   8   7   6   5   4   3   2   1

To our parents

James and Judith Lawson, and extended family,
whose support and encouragement have made my aspirations possible

Ludwig and Ingrid Nechyba,
for their nurturing and their guidance, which have taught me the value of children

Our families

Peter Gunn,
loving supporter, excellent role model, and best friend

Lyana Nechyba,
whose unconditional love and devotion fills my life
and makes me thankful for each day,
Alexander Nechyba,
who makes every day special

Our role model, teacher, and friend

Julia McMillan

And to

George Dover
Chairman of Pediatrics
The Johns Hopkins Hospital
Devoted advocate for residents, children, and their families

PREFACE

Sir William Osler, probably one of the most notable physicians in the history of the Johns Hopkins Hospital, once described our intellectual maturation thus; we are, he said, "sane morally at 30, rich mentally at 40, and wise spiritually at 50—or never." The Harriet Lane Handbook, in its sixteenth edition, turns 52 this year. It is a credit to all of its past editors that it, too, has passed through such a process of maturation, and we sincerely hope that you may find within it not only facts or figures, but perhaps the occasional pearl of wisdom.

From the time Dr. Harrison Spencer proposed the idea of a practical bedside manual for pediatric house officers to be written not by their professors, but by the residents themselves, the Harriet Lane Handbook has grown and flourished. The credit for nursing the handbook from a collection of loose pages in a pocket binder in 1950 to the globally available pediatric reference manual it is today must go to all of its former editors since the time of Dr. Spencer: Drs. Henry Seidel, Herbert Swick, William Friedman, Robert Haslam, Jerry Winkelstein, Dennis Headings, Kenneth Schuberth, Basil Zittelli, Jeffrey Biller, Andrew Yeager, Cynthia Cole, Mary Greene, Peter Rowe, Kevin Johnson, Michael Barone, George Siberry, and Rob Iannone. We feel especially indebted to Drs. Siberry and Iannone, who were there to guide us through the preparation of the sixteenth edition from its inception.

As in editions past, the senior residents on the Harriet Lane Service have worked long hours above and beyond the already rigorous schedule of a resident to revise and update the various chapters of this handbook, with expert guidance from their faculty advisors. They are truly a remarkable group of individuals and we have felt honored to know and work with them over the past few years. To each of them, and to their faculty advisors, we extend our heartfelt gratitude:

Resident	Chapter Title	Faculty Advisor
Monique Soileau-Burke, MD	Emergency Management	Allen R. Walker, MD
Julie Yeh, MD	Poisonings	Erica Liebelt, MD Cecilia Davoli, MD
Matthew Grady, MD	Procedures	Allen R. Walker, MD
Karyn Kassis, MD, MPH Matthew Grady, MD	Trauma and Burns	Allen R. Walker, MD
Dominique Foulkes, MD Karyn Kassis, MD, MPH	Adolescent Medicine	Alain Joffe, MD, MPH
Brett H. Siegfried, MD Tara O. Henderson, MD	Cardiology	Reid Thompson, MD Jean Kan, MD
Monique Soileau-Burke, MD	Dermatology	Bernard Cohen, MD
Lori Chaffin Jordan, MD	Development and Behavior	Mary Leppert, MD

cont'd

Continued

Resident	Chapter Title	Faculty Advisor
Irene Moff, MD	Endocrinology	David Cooke, MD
Renu Peterson, MD		
Dominique Foulkes, MD	Fluids and Electrolytes	Michael Barone, MD
Samina H. Taha, MD	Gastroenterology	Jose Saavedra, MD
Vivian V. Pearson, MD	Genetics	Ada Hamosh, MD
Michelle Hudspeth, MD	Hematology	James F. Casella, MD
Heather Symons, MD		
Michelle Hudspeth, MD	Immunology	Jerry Winkelstein, MD
Heather Symons, MD		
Irene Moff, MD	Immunoprophylaxis	Neal A. Halsey, MD
Laurel Bell, MD	Microbiology and Infectious Disease	George Siberry, MD
Shilpa Hattangadi, MD		James Dick, MD
Lisa A. Irvine, MD, PhD	Neonatology	Sue Aucott, MD
Melissa M. Sparrow, MD	Nephrology	Alicia Neu, MD
H. Scott Cameron, MD	Neurology	Thomas Crawford, MD
		Tyler Reimschisel, MD
Jeanne Cox, MS, RD	Nutrition and Growth	
Lori Chaffin Jordan, MD		
Michelle Hudspeth, MD	Oncology	Ken Cohen, MD
Heather Symons, MD		
Melissa M. Greenfield, MD	Pulmonology	Gerald Loughlin, MD
Chicky Dadlani, MD	Radiology	Jane Benson, MD
Shalloo Sachdev, MD		
Christian Nechyba, MD	Blood Chemistries and Body Fluids	
Veronica L. Gunn, MD, MPH	Biostatistics and Evidence-Based Medicine	Harold Lehmann, MD, MPH
Christian Nechyba, MD	Drug Doses	Carlton Lee, PharmD, MPH
Veronica L. Gunn, MD, MPH		
Javier Tejedor-Sojo, MD	Analgesia and Sedation	Myron Yaster, MD
Shalloo Sachdev, MD	Formulary Adjunct	Carlton Lee, PharmD, MPH
Christian Nechyba, MD	Drugs in Renal Failure	Carlton Lee, PharmD, MPH
Veronica L. Gunn, MD, MPH		

The reader will note several important changes in the contents of this edition. A chapter on dermatology has been added and includes color plates of representative skin findings, as well as algorithms describing diagnostic approaches to various types of rashes. In an era in which physicians are increasingly encouraged to base their clinical practice on established medical literature, we have included a new chapter on evidence-based medicine. An attempt has also been made to include internet-based resources at the beginning of chapters whenever applicable to facilitate the reader's search for updated and in-depth clinical information. Several previous chapters have been consolidated into a reference chapter, including common unit conversions, laboratory reference ranges, and body fluid chemistries. The section on growth charts has been consolidated with the nutrition chapter, and microbiology and infectious diseases have been combined into a single chapter. Finally, it is inevitable that the size of this handbook has a tendency to increase as we broaden our knowledge of new diagnoses and therapeutic approaches with each edition. Therefore we have cut two chapters from the fifteenth edition (Surgery and Psychiatry) from this edition in an attempt to maintain the handbook's "pocketable" qualities. Although we recognize the vital importance of these subspecialties to pediatrics, and are thankful to their many dedicated practicioners, we believe that we cannot adequately summarize these topics and meet our goal of maintaining a succinct and portable reference handbook.

As with past editions, the creation of this handbook is a quintessential team effort, and we owe a debt of gratitude to more individuals than we can name here. Credit for the formulary, consistently the most utilized section of this book, goes in large part to Carlton Lee, PharmD, MPH. We also thank all those who have volunteered their time and talents to make this edition possible: Jeanne Cox, MS, RD for her ongoing work on the nutrition chapter; Dr. William Zinkham for providing the hematology color plates; Josie Pirro, RN, for providing illustrations for common procedures; the medical staff of the Johns Hopkins laboratories for their assistance in preparing the Reference section; and Wayne Reisig for his countless internet searches and trips to the Welch medical library on our behalf. The artwork at the section headings is the work of the late Aaron Sopher, whose timeless illustrations of the Harriet Lane Home were created over three decades ago. We also thank the staff of the Department of Pediatrics at Johns Hopkins, including Kenneth Judd, Kathy Miller, Francine Cheese, and Leslie Burke. Their support has been unwavering, and they have truly made it a joy to come to work each day.

Our role model, and the role model for all of our residents, has been Dr. Julia McMillan. She has been a tireless advocate for our house staff, and she reminds us daily, in her actions and in her words, to be advocates for the children and families in our care. A special thanks goes to Dr. George Dover, Chairman of the Department of Pediatrics at Johns Hopkins, a visionary who settles for nothing short of excellence from each of us. He has been a constant support to us as chief residents and continues to work tirelessly to maintain excellent patient care, teaching, and research throughout the Johns Hopkins Children's Center.

Finally, our thanks and greatest appreciation to all of the Harriet Lane residents. It has been an honor to teach and be taught by you. Each of you has even greater contributions yet to make, and we are certain that you will make them.

CONTENTS

sixteenth
EDITION

THE HARRIET LANE HANDBOOK

A Manual for Pediatric House Officers

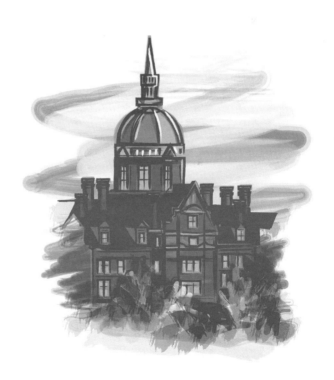

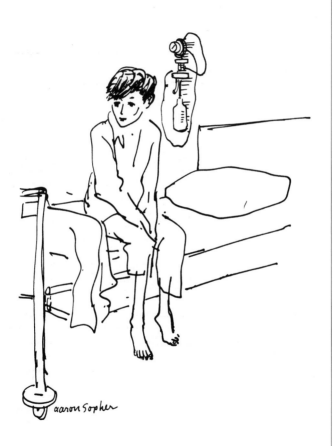

PART I

EMERGENCY MANAGEMENT

Monique Soileau-Burke, MD

I. WEBSITES

www.aaem.org (American Academy of Emergency Medicine)
www.ems-c.org (Emergency Medical Services for Children)

II. AIRWAY[1]

A. ASSESSMENT

1. **Open airway:** Establish an open airway with the head-tilt/chin-lift maneuver. If neck injury is suspected, jaw thrust with cervical-spine (C-spine) immobilization should be used.
2. **Obstruction:** Rule out foreign body, anatomic, or other obstruction.

B. MANAGEMENT

1. **Equipment**
a. Oral airway
   (1) Poorly tolerated in conscious patient.
   (2) Size: With flange at teeth, tip reaches angle of jaw.
   (3) Length ranges from 4 to 10 cm.
b. Nasopharyngeal airway
   (1) Relatively well tolerated in conscious patient. Rarely provokes vomiting or laryngospasm.
   (2) Size: Length equals tip of nose to angle of jaw.
   (3) Diameter: 12 to 36 French (F).
c. Laryngeal mask airway is an option for a secure airway that does not require laryngoscopy or tracheal intubation. It allows spontaneous or assisted respiration, but does not prevent aspiration.
2. **Intubation:** Sedation and paralysis are recommended for intubation unless the patient is unconscious or is a newborn.
a. Indications: Obstruction (functional or anatomic), prolonged ventilatory assistance or control, respiratory insufficiency, loss of protective airway reflexes, or route for approved medications.
b. Equipment (see table on inside front cover).
   (1) Endotracheal tube (ETT): The following equation should be used to determine the size of the ETT to be used:

$$(Age + 16)/4 = \text{Internal diameter of ETT tube.}$$

   An uncuffed ETT should be used in patients <8 years old. The depth of insertion (in cm; at the teeth or lips) is approximately three times the ETT size.
   (2) Laryngoscope blade: Generally, a straight blade can be used in all patients. A curved blade may be easier to use in patients >2 years old.
   (3) Bag and mask should be attached to 100% oxygen.
   (4) ETT stylets should not extend beyond the distal end of the ETT.

TABLE 1-1

RAPID SEQUENCE INTUBATION MEDICATIONS

Drug	Dose (IV) (mg/kg)	Comments
ADJUNCTS (FIRST)		
Atropine *(vagolytic)*	0.01-0.02 Min. 0.1 mg Max. 1 mg	Vagolytic, prevents bradycardia and reduces oral secretions, may increase HR
Lidocaine (optional anesthetic)	1-2	Blunts ICP spike, cough reflex, and CV effects of intubation; controls ventricular dysrhythmias
SEDATIVE/HYPNOTIC (SECOND)		
Thiopental	1-7	May cause hypotension; myocardial depression (barbiturate); decreases ICP and cerebral blood flow; use low dose in hypovolemia (1-2 mg/kg); may increase oral secretions, cause bronchospasm and laryngospasm; contraindicated in status asthmaticus
OR		
Ketamine	1-4	May increase ICP, BP, HR, and oral secretions; (general anesthetic); causes bronchodilation, emergence delirium; give with atropine; contraindicated in eye injuries
OR		
Midazolam (benzodiazepine)	0.05-0.1	May cause decreased BP and HR and respiratory depression; amnestic properties; benzodiazepines reversible with flumazenil (seizure warning applies)
OR		
Fentanyl (opiate)	2-5 mcg/kg	Fewest hemodynamic effects of all opiates; chest-wall rigidity with high dose or rapid administration; opiates reversible with naloxone (seizure warning applies); don't use with MAO inhibitors

BP, Blood pressure; *CV,* cardiovascular; *HR,* heart rate; *ICP,* intracranial pressure; *MAO,* monoamine oxidase.

    (5) Suction: Use a large-bore (Yankauer) suction catheter or 14 to 18F suction catheter.

    (6) Nasogastric (or orogastric) tube: Size from nose to angle of jaw to xyphoid process.

    (7) Monitoring equipment: Electrocardiography (ECG), pulse oximetry, blood pressure (BP) monitoring, capnometry (end-tidal CO_2 monitoring).

  c. Procedure

    (1) Preoxygenate with 100% O_2 via bag and mask.

    (2) Administer intubation medications (Table 1-1 and Fig. 1-1).

    (3) Apply cricoid pressure to prevent aspiration (Sellick maneuver).

    (4) With patient lying supine on a firm surface, head midline and slightly extended, open mouth with right thumb and index finger.

TABLE 1-1

RAPID SEQUENCE INTUBATION MEDICATIONS—cont'd

Drug	Dose (IV) (mg/kg)	Comments
PARALYTICS (THIRD)*		
Rocuronium	0.6-1.2	Onset 30-60 sec, duration 30-60 min; coadministration with sedative; may reverse in 30 min with atropine and neostigmine; minimal effect on HR or BP; precipitates when in contact with other drugs, so flush line before and after use
OR		
Pancuronium	0.1-0.2	Onset 70-120 sec, duration 45-90 min; contraindicated in renal failure, tricyclic antidepressant use; may reverse in 45 min with atropine and neostigmine
OR		
Vecuronium	0.1-0.2	Onset 70-120 sec, duration 30-90 min; minimal effect on BP or HR; may reverse in 30-45 min with atropine and edrophonium
OR		
Succinylcholine	1-2	Onset 30-60 sec, duration 3-10 min; increases ICP, irreversible; contraindicated in burns, massive trauma, neuromuscular disease, eye injuries, malignant hyperthermia, and pseudocholinesterase deficiency. *Risk:* Lethal hyperkalemia in undiagnosed muscular dystrophy

*Nondepolarizing neuromuscular blockers, except succinylcholine, which is depolarizing.

1

EMERGENCY MANAGEMENT

(5) Hold laryngoscope blade in left hand. Insert blade into right side of mouth, sweeping tongue to the left out of line of vision.

(6) Advance blade to epiglottis. With straight blade, lift laryngoscope straight up, directly lifting the epiglottis until vocal cords are visible. With curved blade, the tip of blade rests in the vallecula (between the base of the tongue and epiglottis). Lift straight up to elevate the epiglottis and visualize the vocal cords.

(7) While maintaining direct visualization, pass the ETT from the right corner of the mouth through the cords.

(8) Verify ETT placement by end-tidal CO_2 detection (there will be a false negative if there is no effective pulmonary circulation), auscultation in both axillae and epigastrium, chest rise, and chest radiograph.

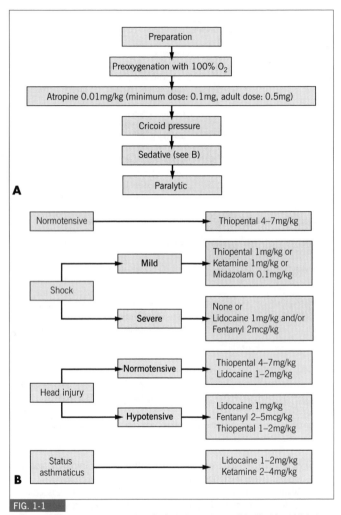

FIG. 1-1

A, Treatment algorithm for intubation. B, Sedation options. *(Modified from Nichols DG et al, editors. Golden hour: the handbook of advanced pediatric life support. St Louis: Mosby; 1996.)*

(9) Securely tape ETT in place, noting depth of insertion (cm) at teeth or lips.

C. RAPID SEQUENCE INTUBATION MEDICATIONS

NOTE: Titrate drug doses to achieve desired effect (see Fig. 1-1 and Table 1-1).

III. BREATHING[1]

A. ASSESSMENT

Once the airway is established, evaluate air exchange. Examine for evidence of abnormal chest-wall dynamics, such as tension pneumothorax, or central problems such as apnea.

B. MANAGEMENT

Positive pressure ventilation (application of 100% oxygen is never contraindicated in resuscitation situations).

1. **Mouth-to-mouth or nose-to-mouth breathing** is used in situations in which no supplies are available. Provide two slow breaths (1 to 1.5 sec/breath) initially, then 20 breaths/min (30 breaths/min in infants). Provide one breath every fifth chest compression in cardiopulmonary resuscitation (CPR).
2. **Bag-mask ventilation** is used at a rate of 20 breaths/min (30 breaths/min in infants). Assess chest expansion and breath sounds. Decompress stomach with orogastric (OG) or nasogastric (NG) tube with prolonged bag mask ventilation (BMV).
3. Endotracheal intubation: See pp. 3-7.

IV. CIRCULATION[1]

A. ASSESSMENT

1. **Rate:** Assess for bradycardia, tachycardia, or absent heart rate. Generally, bradycardia is <100 beats/min in a newborn and <60 beats/min in an infant or child; tachycardia of >240 beats/min suggests primary cardiac disease.
2. **Assess pulse (central and peripheral) and capillary refill (assuming extremity is warm):** <2 sec is normal, 2 to 5 sec is delayed, and >5 sec is markedly delayed, suggesting shock. Decreased or altered mental status may be a sign of inadequate perfusion.
3. **Blood pressure (BP):** Measuring blood pressure is one of the least sensitive measures of adequate circulation in children.

$$\text{Hypotension} = \text{Systolic BP} < [70 + (2 \times \text{Age in years})]$$

B. MANAGEMENT (Table 1-2)

1. Chest compressions
2. Fluid resuscitation

a. If peripheral intravenous (IV) access is not obtained in 90 sec or three attempts, and the patient is <8 years old, then place an intraosseous (IO) needle (see pp. 57-59). If still unsuccessful, consider central venous access.

EMERGENCY MANAGEMENT

1

TABLE 1-2

MANAGEMENT OF CIRCULATION

	Location*	Rate (per min)	Compressions: Ventilation
Infants	1 finger-breadth below intermammary line	>100	5:1
Children (<8 yr)	2 finger-breadths below intermammary line	100	5:1
Older children (>8 yr)	Lower half of sternum	100	15:2

*Depth of compressions should be one third to one half anteroposterior (AP) diameter of the chest and should produce palpable pulses.

b. Initial fluid should be lactated Ringer's (LR) or normal saline (NS). Administer a bolus with 20 mL/kg over 5 to 15 minutes. Reassess. If there is no improvement, consider a repeat bolus with 20 mL/kg of the same fluid. Reassess. If replacement requires more than 40 mL/kg, or if there is acute blood loss, consider 5% albumin, plasma, or packed red blood cells (RBCs) at 10 mL/kg.

c. If cardiogenic etiology is suspected, fluid resuscitation may worsen clinical status.

3. **Pharmacotherapy:** See inside front and back covers for guidelines for drugs to be considered in cardiac arrest.

NOTE: Consider early administration of antibiotics or corticosteroids if clinically indicated.

V. ALLERGIC EMERGENCIES (ANAPHYLAXIS)

A. DEFINITION

Anaphylaxis is the clinical syndrome of immediate hypersensitivity. It is characterized by cardiovascular collapse, respiratory compromise, and cutaneous and gastrointestinal (GI) symptoms (e.g., urticaria, emesis).

B. INITIAL MANAGEMENT

1. **ABCs:** Establish airway (A) if necessary. Supply with 100% oxygen with respiratory support (B) as needed. Assess circulation (C) and establish IV access. Place patient on cardiac monitor.

2. **Epinephrine:** Give epinephrine 0.01 mL/kg (1:1000) subcutaneously (SC) (maximum dose 0.5 mL). Repeat every 15 min as needed.

3. **Albuterol:** Give nebulized albuterol 0.05 to 0.15 mg/kg in 3 mL NS (quick estimate: 2.5 mg for <30 kg, 5 mg for >30 kg) every 15 min as needed.

4. **Administer an H_1-receptor antihistamine,** such as diphenhydramine 1 to 2 mg/kg via intramuscular (IM), IV, or oral (PO) routes (maximum dose 50 mg). Also, consider an H_2-receptor antagonist.

5. **Corticosteroids** help prevent the late phase of the allergic response. Administer methylprednisolone in a 2-mg/kg IV bolus, then 2 mg/kg per day IV or IM divided every 6 hr, or prednisone 2 mg/kg PO in a bolus once daily. Observe for 6 to 24 hours for late-phase symptoms.

6. **Patient should be discharged with an Epi-Pen** (>30 kg), Epi-Pen Junior (<30 kg), or comparable injectable epinephrine product with specific instructions on appropriate usage.

C. HYPOTENSION

1. **Trendelenburg position:** Put patient's head at 30-degree angle below feet.
2. **Normal saline:** Administer 20 mL/kg IV NS rapidly. Repeat bolus as necessary.
3. **Epinephrine:** Epinephrine 0.1 mL/kg (1:10,000) may be given IV over 2 to 5 minutes while an epinephrine or dopamine infusion is being prepared. (See infusion table inside front cover for details of preparation and dosages.)

1

VI. RESPIRATORY EMERGENCIES

The hallmark of upper-airway obstruction is inspiratory stridor, whereas lower-airway obstruction is characterized by cough, wheeze, and a prolonged expiratory phase.

A. ASTHMA

1. **Assessment:** Assess heart rate (HR), respiratory rate (RR), O_2 saturation, peak expiratory flow rate, use of accessory muscles, pulsus paradoxus (>20 mmHg difference in systolic BP for inspiratory versus expiratory phase), dyspnea, alertness, color.
2. **Initial management**
   a. Oxygen to keep saturation >95%.
   b. Inhaled β-agonists: Nebulized albuterol 0.05 to 0.15 mg/kg/dose every 20 minutes to effect.
   c. Additional nebulized bronchodilators include ipratropium bromide 0.25 to 0.5 mg nebulized with albuterol (as above). Benefit has only been demonstrated for moderate to severe exacerbations.
   d. If there is very poor air movement, or the patient is unable to cooperate with a nebulizer, give epinephrine 0.01 mL/kg SC (1:1000; maximum dose 0.3 mL) every 15 min up to three doses, or terbutaline 0.01 mg/kg SC (maximum dose 0.4 mg) every 15 minutes up to three doses.
   e. Start corticosteroids if there is no response after one nebulized treatment or if patient is steroid dependent. Prednisone or prednisolone 2 mg/kg PO every 24 hr; or (if severe) methylprednisolone 2 mg/kg IV/IM then 2 mg/kg/day divided every 6 hr. Parenteral steroids have not been proven to routinely provide more rapid onset of action or greater clinical effect than oral steroids in children with mild to moderate asthma.
3. **Further management if incomplete or poor response**
   a. Continue nebulization therapy every 20 to 30 minutes and space interval as tolerated.
   b. Administer magnesium 25 to 75 mg/kg/dose IV/IM (2 g max.) infused over 20 minutes every 4 to 6 hr up to three to four doses. Many clinicians suggest the higher end of this dosing range (75 mg/kg/dose), although further dosing studies are needed.

EMERGENCY MANAGEMENT

c. Administer terbutaline 2 to 10 mcg/kg IV load followed by continuous infusion at 0.1 to 0.4 mcg/kg/min titrated to effect (see inside front cover).

d. A helium (>70%)-oxygen mixture may be of some benefit in the critically ill patient, but is more useful in upper-airway edema. Avoid use in the severely hypoxic patient.

e. Although aminophylline may be considered, it is no longer considered a preferred mode of therapy for status asthmaticus (see Formulary for dosage information).

4. **Intubation:** Intubation of those with acute asthma is dangerous and should be reserved for impending respiratory arrest. Premedicate with lidocaine and ketamine (see Fig. 1-1 and Table 1-1).

B. UPPER AIRWAY OBSTRUCTION

Upper airway obstruction is most commonly caused by foreign-body aspiration or infection.

1. **Epiglottitis** is a true emergency. Any manipulation, including aggressive physical examination, attempt to visualize the epiglottis, venipuncture, or IV placement, may precipitate complete obstruction. If epiglottitis is suspected, definitive airway placement should precede all diagnostic procedures. A prototypic "epiglottitis protocol" may include the following:

a. Unobtrusively give O_2 (blow-by). Place patient on NPO status.

b. Have parent accompany child to allay anxiety.

c. Have physician accompany patient at all times.

d. Summon "epiglottitis team" (most senior pediatrician, anesthesiologist, and otolaryngologist in hospital).

e. Management options
   (1) If patient is unstable (unresponsive, cyanotic, bradycardic), emergently intubate.
   (2) If patient is stable with high suspicion, escort patient with team to operating room for endoscopy and intubation under general anesthesia.
   (3) If patient is stable with moderate or low suspicion, obtain lateral neck radiographic examination to confirm. An epiglottitis team must accompany the patient at all times.

f. After airway is secured, obtain cultures of blood and epiglottic surface. Begin antibiotics to cover *Haemophilus influenzae* type B, *Streptococcus pneumoniae,* and group A streptococci.

2. **Croup**

a. Mild (no stridor at rest): Treat with cool mist therapy, minimal disturbance, hydration, and antipyretics. Consider steroids (see below).

b. Moderate to severe
   (1) Mist or humidified oxygen mask near child's face may be used, although the efficacy of mist therapy is not established. A mist tent may increase a child's anxiety and decrease the physician's ability to observe the patient.

(2) Administer racemic epinephrine (2.25%) 0.05 mL/kg/dose (maximum dose is 0.5 mL) in 3 mL NS, no more than every 1 to 2 hr, or nebulized epinephrine 0.5 mL/kg of 1:1000 (1 mg/mL) in 3 mL NS (maximum dose is 2.5 mL for ≤4 years old, 5 mL for > 4 years old). Hospitalize if more than one nebulization is required. Observe for a minimum of 2 to 4 hours if discharge is planned after administering nebulized epinephrine.

(3) Administer dexamethasone 0.6 mg/kg IM or PO once. Prednisolone or prednisone may be adequate but should be administered for several days because of the shorter half-life of these steroid preparations.

(4) Nebulized budesonide (2 mg) has been shown to be effective in mild to moderate croup.

(5) A helium-oxygen mixture may decrease the work of breathing by decreasing resistance to turbulent gas flow through a narrowed airway. Inspired helium concentration must be >70% to be effective.

c. If a child fails to respond as expected to therapy, consider airway radiography, computed tomography (CT), or evaluation by otolaryngology or anesthesiology. Consider retropharyngeal abscess, bacterial tracheitis, subglottic stenosis, epiglottitis, or foreign body.

3. Foreign body aspiration occurs most often in children <5 years old. It frequently involves hot dogs, candy, peanuts, grapes, balloons, and other small objects.

a. If the patient is stable (i.e., forcefully coughing, well-oxygenated), removal of the foreign body by bronchoscopy or laryngoscopy should be attempted in a controlled environment.

b. If the patient is unable to speak, moves air poorly, or is cyanotic, intervene immediately.

(1) Infant: Place infant over arm or rest on lap. Give five back blows between the scapulae. If unsuccessful, turn infant over and give five chest thrusts (in the same location as external chest compressions). Use tongue-jaw lift to open mouth. Remove object only if visualized. Attempt to ventilate if unconscious. Repeat sequence as often as necessary.

(2) Child: Perform five abdominal thrusts (Heimlich maneuver) from behind a sitting or standing child or straddled over a child lying supine. Direct thrusts upward in the midline and not to either side of the abdomen.

(3) After back, chest, and/or abdominal thrusts, open mouth and remove foreign body if visualized. Blind finger sweeps are not recommended. Magill forceps may allow removal of foreign bodies in the posterior pharynx.

(4) If the patient is unconscious, remove the foreign body using Magill forceps if needed after direct visualization or laryngoscopy. If there is complete airway obstruction, consider percutaneous (needle)

1

EMERGENCY MANAGEMENT

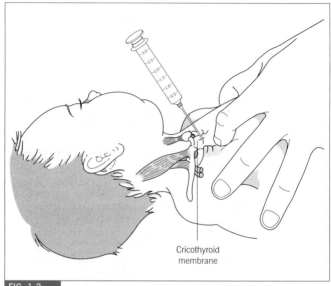

FIG. 1-2

Percutaneous (needle) cricothyrotomy. Extend neck, attach a 3-mL syringe to a 14- to 18-gauge IV catheter and introduce catheter through the cricothyroid membrane (inferior to the thyroid cartilage, superior to the cricoid cartilage). Aspirate air to confirm position. Remove the syringe and needle, attach the catheter to an adaptor from a 3.0-mm ETT, which can then be used for positive-pressure oxygenation. *(Modified from Dieckmann RA, Fiser DH, Selbst SM. Illustrated textbook of pediatric emergency & critical care procedures. St Louis: Mosby; 1997.)*

cricothyrotomy (Fig. 1-2)[2] if attempts to ventilate via bag-valve mask or ETT are unsuccessful.

VII. CARDIOVASCULAR EMERGENCIES[1]

See inside back cover for algorithms for asystole and pulseless arrest, bradycardia, and tachycardia.

A. ACUTE HYPERTENSION

1. Assessment
a. The width of the bladder in the BP cuff should be at least two thirds the length of the upper arm and completely encircle the upper arm. Inadequate bladder size can result in a falsely elevated reading.

b. Patients with BP over the 95th percentile require further evaluation.
c. Hypertensive urgency, much more common in children, is significant elevation in BP without accompanying end-organ damage. Symptoms include headache, blurred vision, and nausea. Hypertensive emergency is defined as elevation of both systolic and diastolic BP with acute end-organ damage (e.g., cerebral infarction, pulmonary edema, hypertensive encephalopathy, and cerebral hemorrhage). It is important to note that the clinical differentiation between hypertensive urgencies and hypertensive emergencies depends on end-organ damage rather than BP measurement.
d. Evaluate for underlying etiology: Medication/ingestion, cardiovascular, renovascular, renal parenchymal, endocrine, or CNS. Rule out hypertension secondary to elevated intracranial pressure (ICP) before lowering BP.
e. A physical examination should include measurement of four-extremity BP, funduscopy (papilledema, hemorrhage, exudate), visual acuity, thyroid examination, evidence for congestive heart failure (tachycardia, gallop rhythm, hepatomegaly, edema), abdominal examination (mass, bruit), thorough neurologic examination, evidence of virilization, or cushingoid effect.
f. Initial diagnostic evaluation should include urinalysis, blood urea nitrogen (BUN), creatinine, electrolytes, chest radiograph, and ECG. Consider obtaining renin level before beginning antihypertensive therapy. Consider a toxicology screen, thyroid/adrenal testing, urine catecholamines, renal Doppler ultrasound, and computed tomography (CT) of the head as indicated.

2. Management

a. Hypertensive emergency: IV line, monitor, possible arterial line for continuous BP monitoring. Seek consultation with a nephrologist or cardiologist. The goal is to lower BP promptly but gradually to preserve cerebral autoregulation. The mean arterial pressure (MAP) (where MAP = 1/3 SBP + 2/3 DBP) should be lowered by one third of the planned reduction over 6 hours, an additional third over the next 24 to 36 hours, and the final third over the next 48 hours. After elevated ICP is ruled out, do not delay treatment because of diagnostic evaluation (Table 1-3). Note that the use of IV hydralazine may result in severe, prolonged, and uncontrollable hypotension and is not recommended.
b. Hypertensive urgency: Aim to lower MAP by 20% over 1 hour and return to baseline levels over 24 to 48 hours. An oral route may be adequate. Observe in the emergency department for 4 to 6 hours. Close follow-up is mandatory. Many other medications are available; the two listed in Table 1-4 have been used with success. Note that use of sublingual nifedipine is not recommended because this agent can result in a precipitous, uncontrolled fall in BP.

1

EMERGENCY MANAGEMENT

TABLE 1-3

MEDICATIONS FOR HYPERTENSIVE EMERGENCY*

Drug	Onset (Route)	Duration	Interval to Repeat or Increase Dose	Comments
Diazoxide (arteriole vasodilator)	1-5 min (IV)	Variable (2-12 hr)	15-30 min	May cause edema, hyperglycemia
INFUSIONS				
Nitroprusside (arteriole and venous vasodilator)	<30 sec (IV)	Very short	30-60 min	Requires ICU setting; follow thiocyanate level
Labetalol (α-, β-blocker)	1-5 min (IV)	Variable, about 6 hr	10 min	May require ICU setting
Nicardipine (calcium channel blocker)	1 min (IV)	3 hr	15 min	May cause edema, headache, nausea/vomiting

ICU, Intensive care unit.
*See Formulary for dosing.

TABLE 1-4

MEDICATIONS FOR HYPERTENSIVE URGENCY*

Drug	Onset (Route)	Duration	Interval to Repeat	Comments
Enalaprilat	15 min (IV)	12-24 hr	8-24 hr	May cause hyperkalemia, hypoglycemia
Minoxidil	30 min (PO)	2-5 days	4-8 hr	Contraindicated in pheochromocytoma

PO, Per os.
*See Formulary for dosing.

VIII. NEUROLOGIC EMERGENCIES

A. INCREASED INTRACRANIAL PRESSURE[3,4]

See Chapter 19 for evaluation and management of hydrocephalus.

1. **Assessment**

a. History: Obtain history regarding trauma, vomiting, fever, headache, neck pain, unsteadiness, seizure or other neurologic conditions, visual change, gaze preference, and change in mental status. In infants, look for irritability, poor feeding, lethargy, and bulging fontanel.

b. Examination: Assess for Cushing's response (hypertension, bradycardia, abnormal respiratory pattern), neck stiffness, photophobia, pupillary response, cranial nerve dysfunction (especially paralysis of upward gaze or of abduction), papilledema, absence of venous pulsations on eye grounds, neurologic deficit, abnormal posturing, and abnormal mental status examination.

2. **Management:** Do not lower BP if elevated ICP is suspected. C-spine immobilization is necessary if trauma is suspected.

a. Stable child (not comatose, stable vital signs, no focal findings): Apply cardiac monitor. Elevate head of the bed 30 degrees. Obtain complete blood count (CBC), electrolyte and glucose levels, and blood culture as indicated. Request an urgent head CT scan and emergent neurosurgical consultation/management. Give antibiotics early if meningitis is suspected.

b. Unstable child: Request emergent neurosurgical consultation and management.

   (1) Elevate head of the bed 30 degrees.
   (2) Avoid hypoosmolar IV solutions.
   (3) Mannitol 0.25 to 1 g/kg IV and/or furosemide 1 mg/kg IV for temporary reduction of ICP. A lower dose of mannitol is generally recommended because high-dose mannitol can produce significant hypotension.
   (4) Reserve hyperventilation for acute management; keep P_{CO_2} at 30 to 35 mmHg. Provide controlled intubation as outlined in Fig. 1-1 and Table 1-1 (consider lidocaine, atropine, thiopental, pancuronium; avoid ketamine). Continue paralysis and sedation.
   (5) Request emergent head CT scan and a shunt series of radiographs if patient has a ventriculoperitoneal (VP) shunt (see Chapter 19). Lumbar puncture (LP) is contraindicated because of herniation risk. Do not delay antibiotics if meningitis is suspected. Consider dexamethasone to reduce cerebral edema in consultation with neurosurgeon.
   (6) Treat hyperthermia.
   (7) Avoid hypotension or hypovolemia.

B. COMA[3]

1. **Assessment**

a. History: Obtain history of trauma, ingestion, infection, fasting, drug use, diabetes, seizure, or other neurologic disorder.

b. Examination: Assess HR, BP, respiratory pattern, temperature, pupillary response, funduscopy, rash, abnormal posturing, and focal neurologic signs.

2. **Management:** "ABC DON'T"

a. **A**irway (with C-spine immobilization), **B**reathing, **C**irculation, **D**extrostick, **O**xygen, **N**aloxone, **T**hiamine.

   (1) Naloxone 0.1 mg/kg IV/IM/SC/ETT (maximum dose 2 mg). Repeat as necessary.
   (2) Thiamine 50 mg IV (before starting glucose). Consider in adolescents for deficiencies secondary to alcoholism or eating disorders.

TABLE 1-5			
COMA SCALES			
Glasgow Coma Scale		Modified Coma Scale for Infants	
Activity	Best Response	Activity	Best Response
EYE OPENING			
Spontaneous	4	Spontaneous	4
To speech	3	To speech	3
To pain	2	To pain	2
None	1	None	1
VERBAL			
Oriented	5	Coos, babbles	5
Confused	4	Irritable	4
Inappropriate words	3	Cries to pain	3
Nonspecific sounds	2	Moans to pain	2
None	1	None	1
MOTOR			
Follows commands	6	Normal spontaneous movements	6
Localizes pain	5	Withdraws to touch	5
Withdraws to pain	4	Withdraws to pain	4
Abnormal flexion	3	Abnormal flexion	3
Abnormal extension	2	Abnormal extension	2
None	1	None	1

From Jennet B, Teasdale G. Lancet 1977; 1:878 and James HE. Pediatr Ann 1986; 15:16.

(3) $D_{25}W$ 2 to 4 mL/kg IV bolus if hypoglycemia is present.
b. Laboratory tests: Consider CBC, electrolytes, liver function tests (LFTs), NH_3, lactate, toxicology screen (serum and urine), blood gas, and blood and urine culture. If patient is an infant or toddler, consider assessment of plasma amino acids, urine organic acids, and other appropriate metabolic workup.
c. If meningitis or encephalitis is suspected, consider LP and start antibiotics. Consider acyclovir.
d. Request emergent head CT scan; consider neurosurgical consultation and electroencephalogram (EEG) if indicated.
e. If ingestion is suspected, airway must be protected before gastrointestinal (GI) decontamination (see Chapter 3).
f. Monitor Glasgow Coma Scale (Table 1-5).

C. STATUS EPILEPTICUS[5]

See Chapter 19 for nonacute evaluation and management of seizures.
1. **Assessment:** Common causes of childhood seizures include fever, subtherapeutic anticonvulsant levels, CNS infections, trauma, toxic ingestion, and metabolic abnormalities. Less common causes include vascular, neoplastic, and endocrine diseases.
2. **Acute management of seizures** (Table 1-6)
3. **Diagnostic workup:** When stable, workup may include CT or magnetic resonance imaging (MRI), EEG, and LP.

TABLE 1-6

ACUTE MANAGEMENT OF SEIZURES

Time (min)	Intervention
0-5	Stabilize the patient
	Assess airway, breathing, circulation, and vital signs
	Administer oxygen
	Obtain intravenous access or intraosseous access
	Correct hypoglycemia if present
	Obtain laboratory studies: Consider glucose, electrolytes, calcium, magnesium, BUN, creatinine, and LFTs, CBC, toxicology screen, anticonvulsant levels, blood culture (if infection is suspected)
	Initial screening history and physical examination
5-15	Begin pharmacotherapy
	Lorazepam (Ativan), 0.05-0.1 mg/kg IV, up to 4-6 mg
	OR
	Diazepam (Valium), 0.2-0.5 mg/kg IV (0.5 mg/kg rectally) up to 6-10 mg
	May repeat lorazepam or diazepam 5-10 min after initial dose
15-35	If seizure persists, load with:
	Phenytoin* 15-20 mg/kg IV at rate not to exceed 1 mg/kg/min
	OR
	Fosphenytoin† 15-20 mg PE/kg IV/IM at 3 mg PE/kg/min (maximum 150 mg PE/min). If given IM, may require multiple dosing sites
	OR
	Phenobarbital 15-20 mg/kg IV at rate not to exceed 1 mg/kg/min
45	If seizure persists:
	Load with phenobarbital if phenytoin was previously used
	Additional phenytoin or fosphenytoin 5 mg/kg over 12 hr for goal serum level of 20 mg/L
	Additional phenobarbital 5 mg/kg/dose Q15-30 min (maximum total dose of 30 mg/kg; be prepared to support respirations)
	Consider IV valproate, especially for partial status epilepticus
60	If seizure persists,‡ consider pentobarbital, midazolam, or general anesthesia in intensive care unit

Modified from Fischer P. Child Adol Psychiatr Clin North Am 1995; 4:461.

BUN, Blood urea nitrogen; *CBC,* complete blood count; *CT,* computed tomography; *EEG,* electroencephalogram.

*Phenytoin may be contraindicated for seizures secondary to alcohol withdrawal or most ingestions (see Chapter 2).

†Fosphenytoin dosed as phenytoin equivalent (PE).

‡Pyridoxine 100 mg IV in infant with persistent initial seizure.

1

EMERGENCY MANAGEMENT

REFERENCES

1. Nichols DG et al, editors. Golden hour: the handbook of advanced pediatric life support. St Louis: Mosby; 1996.
2. Dieckmann RA, Fiser DH, Selbst SM. Illustrated textbook of pediatric emergency & critical care procedures. St Louis: Mosby; 1997.
3. Jennet B, Teasdale G. Aspects of coma after severe head injury. Lancet 1977; 1:878.
4. James HE. Neurologic evaluation and support in the child with an acute brain insult. Pediatr Ann 1986; 15:16.
5. Fischer P. Seizure disorders. Child Adol Psychiatr Clin North Am 1995; 4:461.

POISONINGS

Julie Yeh, MD

The importance of local poison control centers must be emphasized. Early consultation with these centers allows physicians access to resources not normally found in emergency departments, as well as guidance from expert personnel trained in the management of toxic exposure.

I. HISTORY[1]

1. **Corroboration:** Obtain histories from different family members to help confirm the type and dose of exposure.
2. **High suspicion for toxic exposure:** (1) Abrupt onset of symptoms, (2) inconsistent history, (3) previous history of ingestion.
3. **Identification of toxin:** (1) Obtain the bottle or container of the ingestant; request the assistance of the police if necessary. (2) Obtain all medicines from the household if there is any doubt as to which agents have been ingested. (3) Ask specifically about herbal or folk remedies, medications that the patient is taking, any medication that is present in the home, including over-the-counter (OTC) medications.
4. **The following details should be obtained:** (1) Exact name of the drug or chemical exposure, (2) preparation and concentration of the drug or chemical exposure, (3) probable dose (by history) of drug ingested in milligrams per kilogram, as well as the maximum possible dose, (4) time since ingestion/exposure.

II. SIGNS AND SYMPTOMS OF POISONING[1]

A. VITAL SIGNS

1. **Pulse**
a. Bradycardia: β-blockers, calcium channel blockers (diltiazem, verapamil), carbamates, clonidine, digoxin, opiates, organophosphates, plants (lily of the valley, foxglove, oleander).
b. Tachycardia: Sympathomimetics (amphetamine, cocaine, OTC cough and cold medications), phencyclidine, Synthroid, theophylline, tricyclic antidepressants, anticholinergics, antihistamines, ethanol withdrawal.

2. **Respiration**
a. Bradypnea: Alcohols and ethanol, barbiturates (late), clonidine, opiates, sedative/hypnotics.
b. Tachypnea: Amphetamines, barbiturates (early), caffeine, cocaine, ethylene glycol, methanol, salicylates.

3. **Blood pressure**
a. Hypotension: Antihypertensives, barbiturates, β-blockers and calcium channel blockers, clonidine, cyanide, methemoglobinemia (nitrates, nitrites), opiates, phenothiazines, tricyclic antidepressants (late).
b. Hypertension: Amphetamines/sympathomimetics (especially pseudoephedrine in OTC cold remedies, diet pills), antihistamines,

anticholinergics, clonidine (short-term effect at high doses), ethanol withdrawal, marijuana, phencyclidine.

4. **Temperature**
a. Hypothermia: Barbiturates, clonidine, ethanol, hypoglycemic agents, opiates, phenothiazines, sedative/hypnotics.
b. Hyperthermia: Amphetamines, anticholinergic agents, antipsychotic agents, cocaine, monoamine oxidase inhibitors, phenothiazines, salicylates, theophylline.

B. NEUROMUSCULAR
1. **Ataxia:** Alcohol, barbiturates, phenytoin, sedatives/hypnotics (including benzodiazepines), carbon monoxide, heavy metals, organic solvents.
2. **Delirium/psychosis:** Antihistamines, drugs of abuse (phencyclidine, lysergic acid diethylamide [LSD], peyote, mescaline, marijuana, cocaine), ethanol, heavy metals (lead), phenothiazines, steroids, sympathomimetics and anticholinergics (including prescription and OTC cold remedies), theophylline.
3. **Convulsions:** Amphetamines, antihistamines, caffeine, camphor, carbamazepine, cocaine, ethanol withdrawal, isoniazid, lead, lidocaine, lindane, nicotine, organophosphates, phenothiazines, phencyclidine, plants (water hemlock), salicylates, strychnine, theophylline, tricyclic antidepressants.
4. **Paralysis:** Botulinum toxin, heavy metals, organophosphates, plants (poison hemlock).
5. **Coma:** Alcohols, anticholinergics, anticonvulsants, antihistamines, barbiturates, carbon monoxide, clonidine, opiates, organophosphate insecticides, OTC sleep preparations, phencyclidine hydrochloride (PCP), phenothiazines, salicylates, sedatives/hypnotics, sulfonylureas, tricyclic antidepressants, gamma hydroxybutyrate (GHB).

C. OPHTHALMOLOGIC
1. **Pupils**
a. Miosis (constricted pupils): barbiturates, clonidine, ethanol, mushrooms of the muscarinic type, nicotine, opiates, organophosphates, phencyclidine, phenothiazines.
b. Mydriasis (dilated pupils): Amphetamines, anticholinergics, carbamazepine, cocaine, diphenhydramine, LSD, marijuana, sympathomimetics.
2. **Nystagmus:** Barbiturates, carbamazepine, phencyclidine (both vertical and horizontal), phenytoin, sedatives/hypnotics.

D. SKIN
1. **Jaundice:** Acetaminophen, carbon tetrachloride, cyclopeptide mushrooms, fava beans, heavy metals (phosphorus, arsenic), naphthalene.
2. **Cyanosis** (unresponsive to oxygen as a result of methemoglobinemia): Aniline dyes, benzocaine, dapsone, nitrates, nitrites, nitrobenzene, phenacetin, phenazopyridine, Pyridium.

3. **Dry:** Anticholinergics, antihistamines.
4. **Needle tracks:** Substance abuse.

E. ODORS

1. **Acetone:** Acetone, isopropyl alcohol, salicylates.
2. **Alcohol:** Ethanol, isopropyl alcohol.
3. **Bitter almond:** Cyanide.
4. **Garlic:** Heavy metals (arsenic, phosphorus, and thallium), organophosphates.
5. **Oil of wintergreen:** Methyl salicylates.
6. **Pears:** Chloral hydrate.
7. **Carrots:** Water hemlock.

III. MANAGEMENT OF ACUTE POISONING

2

POISONINGS

Initial support of acute poisoning must always include the ABCs: ensuring adequate airway, ventilation, circulation, and assessing need for intravenous (IV) access.

A. GASTROINTESTINAL DECONTAMINATION[2]

NOTE: Airway protection is the major concern with gastrointestinal (GI) decontamination procedures because aspiration of charcoal may cause a severe and potentially fatal pneumonitis. Insertion of an endotracheal tube (ETT) is important in patients who have a depressed gag reflex or altered mental status, especially in those undergoing gastric lavage.

1. **Activated charcoal:** Activated charcoal is the treatment of choice for GI decontamination in the emergency department for substances that can adsorb onto charcoal. Numerous studies fail to show a clear benefit of treatment with ipecac or lavage plus activated charcoal over treatment with charcoal administered alone.

a. Mechanism of action: Effectively adsorbs toxins and prevents their systemic absorption.

b. Initial dose (if patient vomits dose within 1 hour, it should be repeated): Premixed charcoal with sorbitol may be used for initial dose.
   (1) Children: 1 g/kg body weight activated charcoal by mouth (PO) or nasogastric (NG) tube, or more ideally 10 g charcoal/g ingested drug.
   (2) Adults: 50 to 60 g PO or NG.

c. Contraindications
   (1) Increased risk of aspiration: Ileus, intestinal obstruction, hydrocarbons, absent gag reflex.
   (2) Ingestion of alcohols, iron, boric acid, caustics, lithium, electrolyte solutions.

d. Multiple-dose activated charcoal
   (1) Consider a multiple-dose charcoal regimen (cathartic only in first dose) for severe intoxication with salicylates, theophylline, phenobarbital, carbamazepine, or sustained-release preparations.
   (2) Give half of the initial dose every 2 to 4 hours. End point is non-toxic blood levels or lack of signs or symptoms of clinical toxicity

after 12 to 24 hours. Check for bowel sounds and abdominal distention.

(3) Tolerance can be improved using metoclopramide or ondansetron.

2. Cathartics: No longer recommended as a method of gut decontamination.

3. Gastric lavage

a. Indications: Orogastric lavage with a large-bore tube may still be useful in patients who arrive soon (within 1 hour) after a life-threatening ingestion and/or those who are obtunded. The decision to lavage should be made in consultation with a toxicologist or poison control center.

b. Contraindications: Caustic or hydrocarbon ingestions, co-ingestion of sharp objects.

c. Airway protection: In the patient with altered mental status or a depressed gag reflex, insertion of an ETT before gastric lavage may protect against aspiration of gastric contents.

d. Method

    (1) Position patient on left side, with the head slightly lower than the body. Insert a large-bore orogastric tube (18 to 20 French [F] for children, 36 to 40F for adults).

    (2) Lavage with normal saline (NS), 15 mL/kg per cycle, to maximum of 200 mL/cycle in adults, until gastric contents are clear. This may require several liters. Save initial return for toxicologic examination.

4. Ipecac

a. Indications: Ipecac remains the drug of choice for home GI decontamination of selected ingestions within 30 minutes of onset (under the guidance of a health care provider or poison control center). It is rarely indicated for emergency department use.

b. Dosage (give with clear fluid):

    Ages 6 to 12 months: 10 mL

    1 to 12 years: 15 mL

    Over 12 years: 30 mL

Note: **Ipecac can cause drowsiness. Children who have taken ipecac should be laid prone or on their side when falling asleep to prevent aspiration after emesis.**

c. Contraindications: Ingestions with a potential for seizure and decreased or fluctuating level of consciousness (e.g., tricyclic antidepressant ingestions), caustic ingestions, hematemesis, prior vomiting, history of seizure, and age 6 months or less.

d. Relative contraindications: Severe cardiorespiratory disease, late-stage pregnancy, uncontrolled hypertension, and bleeding diathesis.

5. Whole-bowel irrigation

a. Indications: Administering polyethylene glycol solution via continuous NG infusion has been shown to be useful in certain ingestions when charcoal is not effective. Examples include ingestion of toxic iron or lithium, vials or whole packets of illicit substances (cocaine and heroin), or lead chips. Polyethylene glycol may also be useful in delayed therapy of enteric-coated or sustained-release preparations such as salicylates, calcium channel blockers, and β-blockers.

b. Contraindications: GI hemorrhage or obstruction, ileus, obtunded or comatose patient who is not intubated.

c. Method

    (1) Children: Use polyethylene glycol electrolyte lavage solution (GOLYTELY, Colyte) at a rate of 25 to 40 mL/kg/hr NG for 4 to 6 hours or until rectal effluent is clear.

    (2) Adults: Use the same solution as for children at a rate of 1 to 2 L/hr NG for 4 to 6 hours or until rectal effluent is clear.

B. ENHANCED ELIMINATION[3,4]

1. pH Alteration: Urinary alkalinization.

a. Indications: Elimination of weak acids such as salicylates, barbiturates, and methotrexate.

b. Method: Intravenous bolus of $NaHCO_3$ 1 to 2 mEq/kg is recommended, followed by continuous infusion of D_5W with $NaHCO_3$ 132 mEq/L (3 ampules of $NaHCO_3$ added to D_5W to make 1 liter, with each ampule containing 44 mEq $NaHCO_3$) at 1.5 to 2 times maintenance. Goal is urinary pH of 7 to 8. CAUTION: **Monitor for electrolyte disturbances, such as acute hypocalcemia.**

2. Hemodialysis: Useful for low-molecular-weight substances that have a low volume of distribution and low binding to plasma proteins, such as aspirin, theophylline, lithium, phenobarbital, and alcohols.

IV. TABLE OF SPECIFIC POISONINGS

Table 2-1 lists signs, symptoms, management, and treatment options for specific types of poisonings. Table 2-2 lists antidotes for specific poisonings.

2

POISONINGS

TABLE 2-1

SPECIFIC POISONINGS

Poisoning	Signs and Symptoms	Management and Treatment

Acetaminophen[5-8,36]	*Initial 24 hours after ingestion:* Nausea, vomiting, malaise. *24-36 hours after ingestion:* Improving symptoms, clinical evidence of hepatic dysfunction. Aspartate transaminase (AST) and international normalized ratio (INR) are the earliest and most sensitive lab tests of hepatotoxicity. Death can occur from fulminant hepatic failure.	1. A single dose of >150 mg/kg in an otherwise healthy child requires evaluation.
		2. Draw plasma level at least 4hr after ingestion and plot on nomogram (Fig. 2-1). For extended-release acetaminophen, obtain a second level at least 4hr after the initial level. Initiate NAC (see below) if either level is above the lower line on the nomogram.
		3. *N*-Acetylcysteine (NAC): This is most effective if administered within the first 8hr of ingestion, but should be administered within 24hr. If time of ingestion is greater than 24hr, NAC is indicated if hepatotoxicity is present. Dosing should be as follows:
		  a. Oral NAC regimen PO or NG (may be given as a slow bolus or continuous infusion): Give 20% NAC diluted 1:4 in a carbonated beverage as a loading dose of 140 mg/kg, then 70 mg/kg Q4hr for 17 doses.
		  b. Metoclopramide, droperidol, or ondansetron can be used as an antiemetic.
		4. Although charcoal adsorbs oral NAC, NAC and charcoal can be given together (when dosed at least 1 hr apart from each other) without any measurable difference in NAC's efficacy.
		5. In selected patients, a shortened course of NAC may be appropriate if:
		  a. Acetaminophen level is undetectable at 36hr
		    AND
		  b. Liver transaminases and INR are normal.
		If both criteria are fulfilled, NAC therapy may be discontinued.
		6. Intravenous NAC regimen is indicated for the following: oral NAC not tolerated despite adequate antiemetic therapy, GI bleeding or obstruction, neonatal acetaminophen toxicity from maternal overdose.

Alcohols[2,9]
Ethanol (often >50% in mouthwashes, colognes, and aftershave), isopropanol, methanol (windshield wiper fluid), ethylene glycol (antifreeze)

Blindness (methanol), inebriation, central nervous system (CNS) depression, seizures, coma, hypoglycemia, metabolic acidosis, renal failure (ethylene glycol)

NOTE: **Toxic effects are primarily the result of the metabolites of methanol and ethylene glycol.**

NOTE: **Blood volatile toxicology testing and specific levels are useful in confirming the diagnosis of alcohol poisoning.**

a. *Dosage:* Dilute 20% NAC solution to 3% solution with D_5W. Administer 140 mg/kg loading dose over 1hr using an in-line 0.2 micromillipore filter. Then administer maintenance dose of 70 mg/kg per dose over 1hr Q4hr for 12 doses.[6]

b. Check plasma acetaminophen level at 24hr. Small risk of anaphylaxis with IV NAC.

NOTE: **Oral preparation of NAC is not pyrogen free and should be used only as an IV preparation under the guidance of the hospital pharmacy.**

1. Measure anion gap (increase is due to metabolites, lactate, and ketones).

   Anion gap = $Na - (Cl + HCO_3)$

2. Measure osmolar gap (increased, though may be normal late in course of toxicity).

   Serum osmolarity = $2 [Na] + [Glucose (mg/dL)/18] + [BUN (mg/dL)/2.8]$

NOTE: **The osmolar gap is the difference between the calculated and measured osmolality. A gap >10 is suggestive of significant alcohol ingestion.**

3. Charcoal is generally not useful because it adsorbs alcohols poorly, and most alcohols are rapidly absorbed through the GI tract.

4. Ethanol: Support blood glucose as necessary with IV dextrose. There is a risk of hypoglycemia in significant ingestions.

5. Methanol, ethylene glycol:

   a. Fomepizole is an antidote for methanol and ethylene glycol poisoning.

      (1) Indications for use are for levels ≥20 mg/dL or high anion gap metabolic acidosis.

cont'd

TABLE 2-1

SPECIFIC POISONINGS—cont'd

Poisoning	Signs and Symptoms	Management and Treatment
Alcohols[2,9] (cont'd)		(2) Loading dose of 15 mg/kg followed by doses of 10 mg/kg Q12hr for 4 doses, then 15 mg/kg Q12hr until levels are below 20 mg/dL. A separate dosing schedule is recommended for patients requiring hemodialysis.
		b. Ethanol may be used when fomepizole is not available.
		6. Consider hemodialysis in severe cases (i.e., level >50 mg/dL, renal failure, blindness, and severe metabolic acidosis refractory to bicarbonate therapy).
Anticholinergics[9]	Dry mucous membranes,	1. Supportive care may be all that is necessary in mild cases.
Antihistamines, antiparkinsonian agents, scopolamine, belladonna alkaloids, plants (jimsonweed, deadly nightshade, selected mushrooms), ophthalmic mydriatics, diphenoxylate/atropine (e.g., Lomotil), phenothiazines, glycopyrrolate, antispasmodics, muscle relaxants, tricyclic antidepressants, and carbamazepine	swallowing difficulties, decreased GI motility, thirst, blurred vision, photophobia, mydriasis, skin flushing, tachycardia, fever, urinary retention, delirium, hallucinations, cardiovascular collapse. *"Mad as a hatter, red as a beet, blind as a bat, hot as a hare, dry as a bone."*	2. Give activated charcoal. 3. Benzodiazepines should be used to control agitation. Avoid phenytoin for seizures. 4. Physostigmine: a. May reverse symptoms in life-threatening emergencies secondary to pure anticholinergic poisoning unresponsive to standard therapy (dysrhythmias, hypertension, seizures, severe hallucinations). b. *Dosage:* Physostigmine 0.02 mg/kg per dose (up to 0.5 mg) IV every 5 min until a therapeutic effect is seen (maximum total dose 2 mg). **Note: Each dose should be given over 5 min.** c. Atropine should be available to reverse excess cholinergic side effects. Give 0.5 mg for every milligram of physostigmine given.

2

Barbiturates[1] Pentobarbital, phenobarbital, secobarbital, amobarbital	Ataxia, lethargy, headache, vertigo, coma, hypothermia, pulmonary edema, respiratory depression, hypotension, skin bullae.	1. Give activated charcoal. 2. Urinary alkalinization can increase phenobarbital excretion. 3. Consider hemodialysis or hemoperfusion in severe phenobarbital toxicity (levels >100 mg/L). 4. Electroencephalogram (EEG) may correlate with progression of coma.

Benzodiazepines[9]
Alprazolam, chlorazepate,
chlordiazepoxide,
clonazepam, diazepam,
flurazepam, lorazepam,
midazolam, oxazepam,
temazepam, trizolam
	Dizziness, ataxia, slurred speech,
	respiratory depression,
	hypotension, and coma.
		1. If airway and breathing are secure, there is rarely need for other intervention.
		2. Give activated charcoal.
		3. Flumazenil (should not be used routinely in setting of overdose).
		   a. May be used as a diagnostic tool in pure benzodiazepine toxicity. Use in 0.1-0.2 mg increments up to 1 mg. Re-sedation occurs within 20-120 min.
		   b. Contraindicated in patients with seizure disorders, chronic use of benzodiazepines, co-ingestion of substances that can cause seizures (includes tricyclic antidepressants [TCAs], theophylline, chloral hydrate, isoniazid, and carbamazepine).
		   c. May precipitate seizures that are difficult to control.
		4. May be present in urine for 3 days after single dose, up to 4-6 weeks for habitual users.

β-Blockers[10]
Atenolol, esmolol,
labetalol, metoprolol,
nadolol, propranolol,
timolol
	Bronchospasm (in those with
	preexisting bronchospastic
	disease), respiratory
	depression, bradydysrhythmias
	(such as atrioventricular [AV]
	block), hypotension,
	hypoglycemia, altered mental
	status, hallucinations, seizures,
	and coma.
		1. Give activated charcoal; consider whole-bowel irrigation for sustained-release preparations. Consider lavage in very serious intoxication.
		2. Give glucagon
		   Pediatric dosage: 0.05-0.1 mg/kg per bolus, followed by 0.1 mg/kg/hr infusion.
		   Adult dosage: 3-5 mg bolus, followed by 1-5 mg/hr infusion. Useful in reversing bradycardia and hypotension in β-blocker overdoses.
		3. Atropine, isoproterenol, and amrinone can be used if bradycardia or hypotension persists after glucagon administration.
		4. Consider pacing for severe bradycardia.
		5. *For cardiac arrest:* Massive doses of epinephrine (10 to 20 times standard dose) may be required.

cont'd

TABLE 2-1

SPECIFIC POISONINGS—cont'd

Poisoning	Signs and Symptoms	Management and Treatment
Calcium channel blockers[9] Amlodipine, bepridil, diltiazem, felodipine, isradipine, nicardipine, nifedipine, nimodipine, verapamil	Hypotension, bradycardia, altered mental status, seizures, hyperglycemia, atrioventricular conduction abnormalities (such as atrioventricular [AV] block, sinoatrial node abnormalities, idioventricular rhythms, or asystole).	1. Give activated charcoal. Consider whole-bowel irrigation for sustained-release preparations. 2. Use calcium chloride (20 mg/kg of 10% CaCl) or calcium gluconate (100 mg/kg of 10% calcium gluconate) for hypotension and bradydysrhythmias. 3. Give glucagon (see above), amrinone, isoproterenol, atropine, and dopamine for hypotension unresponsive to fluids and calcium. 4. Consider pacing for dysrhythmias.
Carbamazepine[9-11]	Ataxia, mydriasis, nystagmus, tachycardia, altered mental status, coma, seizures, nausea, vomiting, respiratory depression, hypotension or hypertension, dystonic posturing, and abnormal DTRs. Electrocardiogram (ECG) may show prolonged PR, QRS, or QT intervals, but malignant dysrhythmias are rare. Chronic toxicity may lead to AV block and syndrome of inappropriate antidiuretic hormone (SIADH).	1. Multiple doses of activated charcoal may be used for serious acute intoxications. 2. Seizures should be treated with benzodiazepines. NOTE: **Serum levels correlate poorly with toxicity.**

Carbon monoxide[9,11,12]
Fire, automobile exhaust, gasoline or propane engines operating in enclosed spaces, faulty furnaces or gas stoves, charcoal burners, paint remover with methylene chloride

Mild-to-moderate exposures can cause headache, dizziness, nausea, confusion, chest pain, dyspnea, gastroenteritis, and weakness. Severe exposures can cause syncope, seizures, coma, myocardial ischemia, dysrhythmias, pulmonary edema, skin bullae, and myoglobinuria.
NOTE: **Pulse oximetry may be misleadingly normal.**

1. Administer 100% oxygen.
2. Ensure adequate airway, prevent hypercapnia.
3. Obtain COHgb level; however, toxicity does not necessarily correlate with levels. Symptoms are usually seen with levels >20%.
4. In fires, consider the possibility of concomitant cyanide poisoning.
5. Chest radiograph should be obtained to rule out pneumonitis, atelectasis, and pulmonary edema.
6. Electrocardiogram (ECG) should be obtained to rule out cardiac dysrhythmias and myocardial ischemia.
7. Consider hyperbaric O_2 therapy if:
   a. There is evidence of myocardial ischemia or dysrhythmias.
   b. Patient has any serious neurologic or neuropsychiatric impairment.
   c. COHgb level is >40%.
   d. Patient is pregnant with a COHgb level >15% or shows evidence of fetal distress.
   e. Patient has persistent symptoms after 4hr of 100% O_2.
   If hyperbaric O_2 is unavailable, administer 100% O_2 until COHgb level decreases to <10%.

cont'd

2

POISONINGS

TABLE 2-1

SPECIFIC POISONINGS—cont'd

Poisoning	Signs and Symptoms	Management and Treatment
Caustic ingestions[9,13-15]	Stridor, hoarseness, dyspnea, aphonia, chest pain, abdominal pain, vomiting (often with blood or tissue), drooling, persistent salivation. Potential exists for airway swelling or esophageal perforation, even if there are no symptoms initially or no oropharyngeal burns.	1. Stabilize airway. Flexible fiberoptic intubation over an endoscope is preferable to a standard orotracheal intubation. Intubation may further traumatize damaged areas or perforate the pharynx; therefore blind nasotracheal intubation is contraindicated. Emergent cricothyrotomy may be necessary.
Strong acids and alkalis: hair relaxers, drain and oven cleaners, dishwater detergent crystals, rust removers, toilet bowl cleaners		2. Chest radiographic examination may demonstrate esophageal perforation or free intraperitoneal air.
		3. Maintain NPO status. Attempts to neutralize the caustic substance are ineffective and obscure and delay endoscopy. Ipecac or lavage is contraindicated.
		4. Obtain surgical consultation; proceed to endoscopy. Do not pass a nasogastric tube. Discontinue endoscopy immediately if esophageal burn is identified.
		5. Use of IV steroid therapy is controversial. For cases of airway compromise or stridor, it is probably indicated.
		Dosage: Methylprednisolone at 2 mg/kg/24hr divided Q6-8hr.
		6. Button or disk batteries:
		a. Ingestion can lead to esophageal and gastric burns.
		b. If initial radiographic examination shows battery lodged in esophagus, immediate endoscopic retrieval is indicated.
		c. If the battery is beyond the esophagus, the patient may be discharged, with follow-up radiographic studies required if battery has not passed in 4-7 days.
		d. For batteries >23 mm in diameter, a 48-hr radiographic study should be done to exclude retained foreign body, thus requiring endoscopic retrieval.

Digoxin[9]
Quinidine, amiodarone, and poor renal function can increase levels

Any new cardiac rhythm on ECG, especially induction of ectopic pacemakers and impaired conduction, atrial tachycardias with 2:1 block, premature ventricular contractions (PVCs), and junctional tachycardia. Anorexia, nausea and vomiting, headache, disorientation, somnolence, seizures, fatigue, weakness, blurry vision, and aberrations of color vision such as yellow halos around light.

1. Determine serum digoxin level. Therapeutic level is between 0.5 and 2 ng/mL. Toxic symptoms predict a serum level >2 ng/mL, but toxicity can develop in initially asymptomatic patients and can occur at therapeutic levels, especially in chronic users.
2. Determine electrolytes. Low potassium (K^+), magnesium (Mg^{2+}), or thyroxine (T4) will increase digoxin toxicity at a given level, as will high calcium (Ca^{2+}). Initial hyperkalemia results from release of intracellular K^+ and indicates serious acute toxicity.
3. Provide continuous ECG monitoring.
4. Give activated charcoal (even several hours after ingestion).
5. Correct electrolyte abnormalities:
   a. *Hypokalemia*: If any dysrhythmias are present, give potassium IV at 0.5-1 mEq/kg/dose as infusion of 0.5 mEq/kg/hr over 1-2 hr (max rate 1 mEq/kg/hr).
   b. *Hyperkalemia*: If [K^+] >5 mEq/L, then give insulin and dextrose, sodium bicarbonate, and Kayexalate. **Do not give calcium chloride or calcium gluconate because these can potentiate ventricular dysrhythmias.**
   c. *Hypomagnesemia*: May result in refractory hypokalemia if not treated. Give Mg^{2+} cautiously because high levels can cause AV block.
6. Digoxin-specific Fab:
   a. Indicated for ventricular dysrhythmias, supraventricular bradydysrhythmias unresponsive to atropine, hyperkalemia (K^+ >5 mEq/L), hypotension, second- and third-degree heart block, and ingestion of ≥10 mg of digoxin by adults or >4 mg of digoxin by children.

cont'd

2

POISONINGS

TABLE 2-1

SPECIFIC POISONINGS—cont'd

Poisoning	Signs and Symptoms	Management and Treatment
Digoxin[9] (cont'd)		b. *Dosage* (based on total body load of digoxin): Digoxin-immune Fab (Digibind) is available in 40-mg vial. Each vial will bind approximately 0.6 mg digoxin. Estimate total body load in milligrams using either of the following methods: (1) Use the known acutely given dose in milligrams for IV doses, as well as liquid-filled capsules. For PO tablets or elixir, multiply dose by 0.8 to correct for incomplete absorption. (2) Calculate total body load. Total body load (TBL) = serum digoxin concentration (ng/mL) × volume of distribution × weight of patient in kg ÷ 1000 (volume of distribution in this case is 5.6). Then, number of vials to be given equals the total body load (mg)/0.5 mg of digoxin neutralized per vial. Administer IV over 30 minutes. If cardiac arrest is imminent, give as bolus injection. **Note: If ingested dose is unknown, level is not available, and patient is symptomatic, then give 10 vials of Fab (i.e., 400 mg).** 7. Cardiac rhythm disturbances: a. *Bradydysrhythmias*: Atropine alone 0.01-0.02 mg/kg IV may reverse sinus bradycardia or AV block and may be used before digoxin Fab. Phenytoin improves AV conduction. If atropine, digoxin Fab, and phenytoin fail, may use external pacing first, followed by transvenous ventricular pacing if external pacing fails. Avoid propranolol, quinidine, procainamide, isoproterenol, or disopyramide if AV block is present.

Hydrocarbons[16-17]
Aliphatic: Gasoline, kerosene, mineral seal oil, lighter fluid, tar mineral oil, lubricating oils
Aromatic: Benzene, toluene, camphor, turpentine
Halogenated: Carbon tetrachloride, methylene chloride, trichloroethane, perchloroethylene

Tachypnea, dyspnea, tachycardia, cyanosis, grunting, cough, lethargy, seizures, coma, acute liver failure, dysrhythmias. **Note: Aliphatic hydrocarbons have the greatest risk for aspiration and pulmonary toxicity. Aromatic hydrocarbons have systemic toxicity.**

b. *Tachydysrhythmias:* Phenytoin and lidocaine are effective for ventricular dysrhythmias; propranolol is useful for both ventricular and supraventricular tachydysrhythmias. Cardioversion is indicated when pharmacotherapy fails in the hemodynamically unstable patient.
1. Decontamination
   a. Avoid emesis or lavage because of the risk of aspiration.
   b. Consider intubation with cuffed ETT followed by lavage if the hydrocarbon contains a potentially toxic substance (e.g., insecticide, heavy metal, camphor) and a toxic amount has been ingested.
   c. Avoid activated charcoal unless there is co-ingestion. It does not bind aliphatics and will increase the risk of aspiration.
2. Obtain chest radiograph and arterial blood gases (ABGs) on patients with pulmonary symptoms.
3. Observe patient for 6hr.
   a. If child is asymptomatic for 6hr and chest radiograph is normal, discharge home.
   b. If child is asymptomatic but chest radiograph is abnormal, consider admission for further observation. Discharge only if close follow-up can be ensured.
   c. If child becomes symptomatic in 6-hr period, admit.
4. Treat pneumonitis with oxygen and positive end-expiratory pressure (PEEP).
5. Routine administration of antibiotics and steroids is not warranted.

cont'd

2

POISONINGS

TABLE 2-1

SPECIFIC POISONINGS—cont'd

Poisoning	Signs and Symptoms	Management and Treatment
Iron[18-20,42]	*First stage:* GI toxicity (30 min to 6 hr after ingestion). Nausea, vomiting, diarrhea, abdominal pain, hematemesis, and melena. Rarely, this phase may progress to shock, seizures, and coma. *Second stage:* Latent period (6-24 hr after ingestion). Improvement and sometimes resolution of clinical symptoms. *Third stage:* Systemic toxicity (6-48 hr after ingestion). Hepatic injury or failure, hypoglycemia, metabolic acidosis, bleeding, shock, coma, convulsions, and death. *Fourth stage:* Late complications (4-8 wks after ingestion). Pyloric or antral stenosis.	1. Determine serum iron concentration 2-6 hr after ingestion (time of peak concentration varies with iron product ingested). A level >350 mcg/dL is frequently associated with systemic toxicity. **Note: Iron is rapidly cleared from plasma and distributed; thus serum levels obtained after peak do not accurately reflect degree of intoxication.** 2. Obtain abdominal radiograph because most iron tablets are radiopaque (except chewable vitamins and children's liquid). If present, consider lavage. 3. If ingestion of elemental iron <20 mg/kg, no treatment is needed. 4. Consider gastric emptying with ipecac for all ingestions of unknown amount or those 20-60 mg/kg. If the patient does not develop symptoms in the first 6 hr, no further treatment is needed. 5. Consider gastric lavage if dose ingested ≥60 mg/kg and/or presence of large amount of pills on radiograph. If iron tablets are present in the stomach despite lavage, begin whole-bowel irrigation, especially if abdominal radiograph reveals iron tablets distal to the pylorus. 6. Give deferoxamine IV at 15 mg/kg/hr via continuous infusion in all cases of serious poisoning (e.g., presence of significant clinical symptoms, positive abdominal radiograph with significant number of pills, or serum iron level >500 mcg/dL). Give continuous infusion until all symptoms and signs of toxicity have resolved and 24 hr after vinrose urine color disappears. 7. Supportive care is the most important therapy. Large IV fluid volumes may be needed in the first 24 hr to avoid hypovolemic shock and acidemia. Urine output should be maintained at >2 mL/kg/hr. 8. Correct metabolic acidosis with sodium bicarbonate.

Lead[21-25]

Environmental exposures:

1. Residence (primary, secondary, daycare, etc.) built before 1960, with lead-based paint.
2. Recent or ongoing renovation.
3. Nearby industry, such as battery plants, smelters.
4. Old furniture, vinyl mini-blinds, ceramics, leaded crystal, imported food cans, leaded toys, art supplies, cosmetics.
5. Presence of lead in water pipes, lead solder in connecting pipes, and brass or bronze plumbing fittings.
6. Use of lead-based insecticides and folk remedies such as azarcon, greta, surma.

Gastrointestinal: Anorexia, constipation, abdominal pain, colic, vomiting, failure to thrive, and diarrhea. Abdominal radiograph may show opacities in the GI tract.

Neurologic: Irritability, overactivity, lethargy, decreased play, increased sleep, ataxia, incoordination, headache, decreased nerve conduction velocity, encephalopathy, cranial nerve paralysis, papilledema, seizures, coma, death.

Hematologic: Microcytic anemia, basophilic stippling, increased free erythrocyte protoporphyrin (FEP).

Skeletal: Lead lines may be seen in the metaphyseal regions of long bones of leg and arm.

Note: **Most children with lead poisoning are asymptomatic. A blood test is the only way to determine the lead level.**

Blood lead level <9 mcg/dL (Class I): Rescreen annually, unless high risk.

Blood lead level 10-14 mcg/dL (Class IIA): Re-screen every 3-4 months, until two consecutive measurements are 10 or below then retest in 1 year. If there are a large number of children in the community in this range, community-wide prevention should be started.

Blood lead level 15-19 mcg/dL (Class IIB):
a. Obtain comprehensive environmental history.
b. Education on environment, cleaning, and nutrition should be started.
c. Remove child from the lead source.
d. Alert local health department.
e. Test for iron deficiency; if iron deficient, may begin iron (unless British Anti-Lewisite [BAL] is to be used).
f. Rescreen every 3-4 mo until two consecutive levels are ≤10 mcg/dL.
g. Consider abatement (see prevention below).

Blood lead level 20-44 mcg/dL (Class III):
a. As above.
b. These children require close follow-up, chelation may be considered in selected children.
c. Refer to lead poisoning specialist.

Blood lead level 45-69 mcg/dL (Class IV):
a. Begin both medical and environmental intervention.
b. Chelation treatment (either oral or IV/IM) should begin within 48 hrs with close follow-up (see below).

Blood lead level ≥70 mcg/dL (Class V): This is a MEDICAL EMERGENCY requiring immediate intervention and hospitalization for chelation (see below).

cont'd

TABLE 2-1

SPECIFIC POISONINGS—cont'd

Poisoning	Signs and Symptoms	Management and Treatment
Lead[21-25] (cont'd) 7. Other sources include maternal transmission such as breastfeeding and prenatal exposure via placenta. *Screening:* All children below the age of 6 yr should be screened at least once. Start screening at age 9-12 mo. However, children with high-risk factors, such as the above environmental exposures, should be screened at age 6 mo. Subsequent screens are determined by the blood lead level.		CHELATION 1. Chelation is a process to bind lead chemically in a form that is easily excreted. Most agents bind lead so it is soluble in water and excreted through the kidneys. Examples of agents: BAL, CaNa$_2$EDTA, succimer (DMSA). a. Before starting chelation administer two pediatric Fleet enemas to clear the GI tract of lead particles. b. Obtain baseline laboratory results: Venous lead level, complete blood count (CBC) with differential, chemistry panel (including electrolytes, blood urea nitrogen [BUN] and creatinine, hepatic function tests), reticulocyte count, urinalysis). 2. *Oral chelation:* This is used for children with blood lead levels between 45 and 69 mcg/dL. Chelation must occur in an environment free of lead, which may be the hospital. *Succimer (dimercaptosuccinic acid [DMSA])* a. *First 5 days:* 1050 mg/m^2/day or 30 mg/kg/day divided every 8 hr. b. *Next 14 days:* 700 mg/m^2/day or 20 mg/kg/day divided every 12 hr. c. Mix capsule contents in warm ginger ale and administer within 5 min. Give on empty stomach to improve GI absorption. d. Obtain weekly laboratory studies, including CBC with differential, chemistry panel, and lead level, to ensure response to treatment and monitor for possible drug side effects (decreased absolute neutrophil count and elevated liver function tests). 3. Parenteral chelation (blood lead level >45 mcg/dL). a. CaNa$_2$EDTA: (1) First begin multivitamin to replenish copper and zinc. (2) Start 1000 mg/m^2/day IM Q12hr for 5 days.

(3) 12 hr after the tenth injection, obtain CBC with differential, chemistry panel, venous lead level; if this lead level is still ≥45 mcg/dL, start the second 5-day therapy with CaNa$_2$EDTA after a 3-day break from chelation therapy.

(4) For pain control use EMLA (eutectic mixture of local anesthetics) cream and mix CaNa$_2$EDTA with 0.5% procaine.

NOTE: **It is important to use CaNa$_2$EDTA, not Na$_2$EDTA because the latter may cause tetany and life-threatening hypocalcemia.**

b. BAL: (recommended only for levels ≥70 mcg/dL). NOTE: **Toxic if given with iron.**

(1) Initial dose of 75 mg/m^2 is given as deep IM injection.

(2) Establish adequate urine output.

(3) 4 hr later start CaNa$_2$EDTA 1500 mg/m^2/day via continuous IV infusion for 48 hr. If there is risk of cerebral edema, dose may be given IM Q4 hr to decrease IV fluids.

(4) BAL is then continued simultaneously at 75 mg/m^2/dose IM Q4hr for 48 hr.

(5) Use of EMLA cream and 0.5% procaine is recommended for IM doses.

(6) After 48 hr obtain serum lead level to determine whether to continue chelation.

NOTE: **Side effects of BAL include fever, tachycardia, hypertension, salivation, tingling around the mouth, anaphylaxis (BAL is suspended in peanut oil, which may cause severe allergic reaction), and hemolysis (in patients with G6PD deficiency).**

4. Follow-up:

a. Repeat venous lead level and CBC 2 weeks after completion of chelation therapy. Venous lead level may rebound to 50%-75% of pretreatment value.

cont'd

POISONINGS **2**

TABLE 2-1
SPECIFIC POISONINGS—cont'd

Poisoning	Signs and Symptoms	Management and Treatment
Lead[21-25] (cont'd)		b. Repeat chelation with DMSA for levels ≥45 mcg/dL may be indicated.
		c. Neuropsychologic evaluation, speech evaluation, and monitoring of school progress.
		5. Prevention:
		a. *Nutrition:* Balanced diet, more frequent meals high in iron, vitamin C, and calcium and low in added fat.
		b. *Hygiene:* Wash hands regularly, avoid hand-to-mouth behavior.
		c. *House cleaning:* Damp-cleaning methods; use high-phosphate detergent such as powdered dishwasher detergent; can use special vacuum cleaner (HEPA-VAC) for picking up microscopic lead particles.
		d. *Abatement:* Must be performed by trained workers.
Methemoglobinemia[39] Exposures to sulfonamides, quinines, phenacetin, benzocaine, nitrates, nitrites, aniline dyes, naphthalene (mothballs) **Note: Also consider other etiologies (i.e., G6PD deficiency, acidosis from gastroenteritis)**	*Symptoms associated with % total hemoglobin:* <10%: No symptoms 10%-20%: Cyanosis 20%-30%: Anxiety, lightheadedness, headache, tachycardia 30%-50%: Dyspnea, increased tachycardia, dizziness, fatigue confusion 50%-70%: Severe lethargy, stupor, coma, seizures, arrhythmias, acidosis >70%: Death	1. *Rapid screening test:* Place drop of blood on filter paper; it should remain reddish-brown when waved in the air for 30-60 sec. 2. Measure level of methemoglobin. 3. Low arterial blood O_2 saturation by blood oximetry. Normal Po_2. Can have normal pulse oximetry. 4. Treatment: a. <30%: No treatment. b. 30%-70%: Methylene blue, 1-2 mg/kg of a 1% solution IV over 5 min. May repeat dose (1 mg/kg with max total dosage 7 mg/kg) if symptoms still present 1 hr later. c. If severely ill and no response to methylene blue, consider hyperbaric O_2 or exchange transfusion. **Note: Caution when using methylene blue in patients with G6PD deficiency; may induce paradoxical response (i.e., causing methemoglobinemia).**

Organophosphates[40]
Pesticides

Agitation, drowsiness, seizures, respiratory depression, DUMBELS (Diarrhea, Urination, Miosis, Bronchospasm, Emesis, Lacrimation, Salivation)

1. *Decontamination:* Remove affected clothing.
2. Measure plasma or red blood cell (RBC) pseudocholinesterase activity level (low in organophosphate poisoning).
3. Administer atropine
   Pediatric dosage: 0.05-0.1 mg/kg/dose IV.
   Adult dosage: 2-5 mg/dose IV.
   May repeat Q10-30 min to titrate to effect (reduces bronchorrhea and oral secretions).
4. *Antidote:* Pralidoxime; shortens duration.
   Pediatric dosage: 20-50 mg/kg/dose IM, IV, SQ.
   Adult dosage: 1-2 g/dose.
   May repeat in 1-2 hr if muscle weakness not relieved, then space doses to Q6-8 hr for 24-48 hr.

Opiates[26-28]
Codeine, fentanyl, heroin, hydromorphone, meperidine, methadone, morphine, oxycodone, proproxyphene

Depressed mental status, pinpoint pupils, respiratory depression, and hypotension

1. Administer naloxone 0.1 mg/kg/dose IV (max dose 2 mg) if there is respiratory or CNS depression. Repeat every 2 min as needed to improve respiratory and mental status. Higher doses may be required for ingestions of synthetic opioids (i.e., fentanyl).
2. Careful inpatient monitoring is required because of the short half-life of naloxone compared with most opiates. Indications for continuous naloxone infusion include the following:
   a. Repetitive bolus doses.
   b. Ingestion of large amount of opiate or long-acting opiate (e.g., methadone, or poorly antagonized opiates such as proproxyphene.

cont'd

2

POISONINGS

TABLE 2-1
SPECIFIC POISONINGS—cont'd

Poisoning	Signs and Symptoms	Management and Treatment

Opiates[26-28] (cont'd)		Suggested regimen is as follows:
		  a. Repeat the previously successful bolus as a loading dose.
		  b. Administer two thirds of loading dose as an hourly infusion dose.
		  c. Wean naloxone drip in 50% decrements as tolerated over 6-12 hr depending on the half-life of the opiate ingested. For methadone, may require infusion for up to 48 hours.
		Note: Naloxone can potentiate acute withdrawal (nausea, vomiting, hyperactive bowel sounds, yawning, piloerection, and pupillary dilatation) in patients with opiate addiction.
		3. Opiates may be present in urine for up to 2 days, for methadone up to 3 days.

Phenothiazine and butyrophenone[4,9]
Chlorpromazine,
fluphenazine,
haloperidol,
perphenazine,
prochlorperazine,
promethazine,
thioridazine,
trifluoperazine
	Symptoms (may be delayed 6-24 hr after ingestion):
	Depressed neurologic status, lethargy, coma, miosis, hypotension, dysrhythmias (including prolonged QTC intervals and occasionally QRS interval), extrapyramidal signs (oculogyric crisis, dysphagia, tremor, rigidity, torticollis, opisthotonus, trismus), neuroleptic malignant syndrome (fever, diaphoresis, rigidity, tachycardia, altered mental status), anticholinergic symptoms.
		1. Administer activated charcoal.
		2. Obtain ECG.
		3. Extrapyramidal symptoms:
		  a. Diphenhydramine:
		    Dosing for children: 1 mg/kg/dose (maximum 50 mg) slowly over 2-5 min.
		    Dosing for adults: 25-50 mg; give Q6hr for 48 hr. May be given IV, IM, or PO.
		  b. Intravenous benztropine:
		    Dosing for children:
		    >3 years: 0.02-0.05 mg/kg/dose (1-2 doses per day).
		    Children <3 years: Use only in severe life-threatening situations.
		    Adults: 1-2 mg IM or IV.
		4. Neuroleptic malignant syndrome:
		  a. Reduce hyperthermia with cooling blankets, external sponging, fanning, and gastric/colonic lavage. Antipyretics are not helpful.
		  b. Support respiratory and cardiovascular status; monitor neurologic and fluid status.

Phenytoin[29]

Ataxia, dysarthria, drowsiness, tremor, nystagmus, seizures, and hyperglycemic nonketotic coma. Intravenous preparations may cause bradycardia, dysrhythmia, and hypotension. (Above symptoms seen with serum levels >20 mg/L.)

   c. Neuromuscular paralysis with or without benzodiazepines for severe hyperthermia and muscle rigidity.

   d. Dantrolene and bromocriptine may be used in selected cases of severe toxicity.

1. *Supportive care:*

   a. Benzodiazepines or phenobarbital may be used for seizures.

   b. Insulin may be required for hyperglycemic nonketotic coma. Give fluid and monitor glucose.

2. *Activated charcoal:* Consider multiple-dose activated charcoal for selected cases to enhance elimination.

Salicylates[11,30]

Many preparations, (*children's:* 81-mg tablets; *adult:* 325-mg tablets), methyl salicylate (i.e., oil of wintergreen 5 mL = 22 ½ tablets of adult aspirin), Pepto Bismol (236 mg nonaspirin salicylate/15 mL)

Acute: Vomiting, hyperpnea, tinnitus, lethargy, hyperthermia, seizures, coma. *Chronic:* Confusion, dehydration, metabolic acidosis, cerebral edema, pulmonary edema.

1. Establish severity of ingestion. Acute toxicity can occur at doses of 150 mg/kg, whereas chronic overdose can produce toxicity at much lower doses.

2. Serum salicylate level

   a. Toxicity of salicylates correlates poorly with serum levels, and levels are less useful in chronic toxicity.

   b. Serial salicylate levels (Q2-4hr) are mandatory after ingestion to monitor for peak levels. In seriously ill patients, frequent determination of salicylate concentration is necessary to monitor efficacy of treatment and possible need for hemodialysis.

   c. Signs and symptoms of acute toxicity can occur at levels >30 mg/dL.

   d. 6-hr serum salicylate level of ≥100 mg/dL is considered potentially lethal and is an indication for hemodialysis. Be cautious of different laboratories reporting different units (10 mg/L = 1.0 mg/dL).

3. Consider multiple doses of activated charcoal if serum salicylate levels continue to increase after 6 hours. Consider whole-bowel irrigation in ingestions of enteric-coated preparations.

cont'd

POISONINGS

2

TABLE 2-1
SPECIFIC POISONINGS—cont'd

Poisoning	Signs and Symptoms	Management and Treatment
Salicylates[11,30] (cont'd)		4. Monitor serum electrolytes, calcium, arterial blood gases, glucose, urine pH and specific gravity, and coagulation studies as needed.
		5. Treat fluid and solute deficits; alkalinization is important in increasing the excretion of salicylate and decreasing the entry of salicylate into the CNS.
		a. Begin alkalinization by initial bolus of $NaHCO_3$ (1-2 mEq/kg). Then begin infusing D_5W with 132 mEq $NaHCO_3$/L (three ampules of 44 mEq $NaHCO_3$ each) and 20-40 mEq K^+/L at rates of 2-3L/m^2/24hr (i.e., 1.5 to 2 times maintenance fluids).
		b. Aim for a urine output of 2 mL/kg/hr.
		c. Adjust concentrations of electrolytes as needed to correct serum electrolyte abnormalities (especially hypokalemia, which inhibits salicylate excretion), and maintain a urinary pH >7.5.
		6. Hemodialysis may be required in the presence of metabolic acidosis or electrolyte abnormality unresponsive to appropriate therapy, renal or hepatic failure, persistent CNS impairment, pulmonary edema, progressive clinical deterioration despite adequate therapy, or salicylate level >100 mg/dL at 6 hr after ingestion.
Serotonin syndrome[38] SSRIs: sertraline, fluoxetine, paroxetine, fluvoxamine, clomipramine, venlafaxine, nefazodone Note: Most common precipitating events is combination of MAO inhibitor and SSRI	Classic triad of altered mental status, autonomic dysfunction, and neuromuscular abnormalities. Agitation, delirium, coma, mydriasis, diaphoresis, hyperthermia, tachycardia, fluctuating blood pressure, mutism, tremor, rigidity, myoclonus, seizures.	1. Discontinue drug, provide supportive care. 2. Usually resolves completely within 24-72 hr. 3. External cooling measures, sedatives, paralysis, mechanical ventilation for severe hyperthermia. 4. Consider cyproheptadine, methysergide, benzodiazepines (though none have been shown to be truly effective).

POISONINGS

2

Theophylline[9]

Vomiting, hematemesis, abdominal pain, bloody diarrhea, tachycardia, dysrhythmias, hypotension, cardiac arrest, seizures, agitation, coma, hallucinations, metabolic acidosis, hypokalemia, hyperglycemia, leukocytosis.

1. Obtain a theophylline level immediately and in 1-4 hr to determine the pattern of absorption. Peak absorption can be delayed as long as 13-17 hr after ingestion. Serial theophylline levels should be obtained to assess for rising levels, monitor efficacy of treatment, and determine need for hemodialysis.
   a. Levels >20 mcg/mL are associated with clinical symptoms of toxicity.
   b. Levels >40 mcg/mL or patients with neurotoxicity require admission and careful monitoring.
2. Obtain serum electrolyte, glucose, and blood gas levels.
3. Give initial dose of charcoal followed by a cathartic, regardless of the length of time after ingestion. For severe intoxication consider multiple-dose charcoal. If there is persistent vomiting, give metoclopramide or ondansetron, and administer charcoal by NG tube.
4. Continue use of cardiac monitor until level <20 mcg/mL. Treat dysrhythmias.
5. Monitor serum K^+, Mg^{2+}, PO_4^{3-}, Ca^{2+}, acid-base balance in moderate to severe intoxication.
6. Treat seizures aggressively with benzodiazepines and phenobarbital.
7. Hemodialysis is as effective as charcoal hemoperfusion, more readily available, and lower risk. Indications are as follows:
   a. Theophylline level ≥90 mg/mL at any time.
   b. Theophylline level ≥70 mg/mL 4 hr after ingestion of sustained-release preparation.
   c. Theophylline level ≥40 mcg/mL and seizures, dysrhythmias, and protracted vomiting unresponsive to antiemetics.
8. Exchange transfusion may be indicated in neonate with severe toxicity.

cont'd

TABLE 2-1
SPECIFIC POISONINGS—cont'd

Poisoning	Signs and Symptoms	Management and Treatment

Tricyclic antidepressants[31-34]
Amitriptyline, desipramine, doxepin, imipramine, nortriptyline
	Agitation, delirium, psychosis, seizures, lethargy, coma, conduction abnormalities, dysrhythmias, hypotension, anticholinergic symptoms.	1. Signs of toxicity usually appear within 4 hr of ingestion. Any ingestion should be observed for at least 6 hr.
		2. *ECG (acute overdose):* QRS duration >0.10 sec and R wave in lead aVR ≥3 mm are associated with increased risk of seizures and ventricular dysrhythmias. ECG must be monitored for at least 12-24 hr if these conduction abnormalities are present in the first 6 hr.
		3. Serum drug levels do not necessarily predict outcome and are not helpful in acute management.
		4. Start continuous ECG monitoring, even in the patient who is asymptomatic at presentation. If the patient remains asymptomatic, has normal bowel sounds, and has no ECG abnormalities in the 6-hr period after ingestion, then no further medical intervention is necessary.
		5. Treat seizures with benzodiazepines, then phenobarbital if seizures persist. Phenytoin is contraindicated because it may precipitate ventricular dysrhythmias.
		6. For cardiac conduction abnormalities, dysrhythmias, and hypotension:
		  a. Administer NaHCO₃ (1-2 mEq/kg) bolus until reversal of cardiovascular abnormalities or pH between 7.45-7.5 (multiple boluses may be required).
		  b. Start continuous infusion of D₅W with 132 mEq/L of NaHCO₃ at 1.5-2 times maintenance.
		  c. Manage hypotension initially with fluid boluses.
		  d. High-dose dopamine and norepinephrine may be used for hypotension unresponsive to fluids.
		7. Physostigmine, flumazenil, and Type Ia and Ic antidysrhythmics are contraindicated in patients with TCA ingestions.
		8. Admit patient if he or she exhibits any signs of major toxicity, such as change in mental status, conduction delays on ECG, dysrhythmias, seizures, or hypotension; place patient on cardiac monitor until symptom-free for 24 hr.

cont'd

DRUGS OF ABUSE

Amphetamines[35,37] Methamphetamine (Crank, speed; smoked form: ice); dextroamphetamine; methylenedioxy-methamphetamine (MDMA or Ecstasy); ephedrine (Ma Huang, Herbal Ecstasy) **NOTE: Insufflation of Ritalin is becoming popular**	Pupils dilated and reactive, increased blood pressure (BP), tachycardia, hyperthermia, cardiac dysrhythmias, dry mouth, diaphoresis, tremors, confused or hyperacute sensorium, paranoid ideation, impulsivity, hyperactivity, stereotypy, convulsions, exhaustion.	Supportive care (elimination half-life about 3 hr): 1. Administer activated charcoal if co-ingestion is suspected. 2. For agitation/seizures: Administer benzodiazepines. 3. For hyperthermia: Use external cooling measures, sedation, hydration. 4. For severe hypertension unresponsive to benzodiazepines: Consider phentolamine or IV sodium nitroprusside. 5. Monitor creatine phosphokinase (CPK) for rhabdomyolysis. Treatment for rhabdomyolysis includes IV hydration, urinary alkalinization. 6. Hyponatremia has been seen with use of Ecstasy and is thought to be due to SIADH or excessive free water intake. 7. May be present in urine for up to 48 hr.
Cocaine[35]	Excitement, restlessness, euphoria, garrulousness, increased motor activity, decreased sense of fatigue, increased tremors, convulsive movements, tachypnea, tachycardia, hypertension, fever, chills. Angina, myocardial infarction (MI) in acute cocaine exposure. Tachyarrhythmias, hyperexia, rhabdomyolysis with acute renal failure.	See above for management and treatment. 1. Obtain serial ECGs and cardiac isoenzymes/troponin levels to evaluate for signs of ischemia. 2. Cocaine metabolites can be detected in urine for up to 3 days after exposure, up to 2 weeks in a habitual user.

TABLE 2-1

SPECIFIC POISONINGS—cont'd

Poisoning	Signs and Symptoms	Management and Treatment
GHB/GBL[35,37] Gamma hydroxybutryate (GHB) and gamma butyrolactone (GBL); GBL is precursor to GHB (euphoriants and aphrodisiacs, also known as "date-rape" agent, *Liquid Ecstasy*)	Rapid onset of deep sleep. Can lead to coma and respiratory depression. Seizure activity, hypothermia, bradycardia. Coma lasts 1-2 hr.	1. Provide supportive measures. 2. Give atropine for severe bradycardia. 3. Blood pressure support is rarely necessary. 4. Not detected on routine urine toxicology screens.
Hallucinogens[35] PCP (phencyclidine)	Staggering gait, slurred speech, nystagmus, diaphoresis, catatonic muscular rigidity with blank stare, hypertension, tachycardia, seizures, coma. **Note: Typical high 4-6 hr, followed by extended "coming down."**	1. Diagnosis with urine: Half life is 18 hr. May be detected up to 1 week in acute user and 3 weeks in habitual user. 2. Provide GI decontamination with activated charcoal if ingested. 3. Treat seizures. For agitation consider benzodiazepines or haloperidol. 4. Watch for rhabdomyolysis. Avoid physical restraints if possible. 5. Never acidify urine to enhance excretion; may promote deposition of myoglobin in renal tubules and worsen metabolic acidosis.
LSD, psilocybin, mescaline	*Sympathomimetic:* Papillary dilation, hypertension, tachycardia, hyperreflexia, hyperpyrexia. Euphoria, alteration of time (passes slowly), mood lability, hallucination, psychosis, visual perceptive distortions.	1. Action lasts on average 6-12 hr. 2. Rarely associated with life-threatening events. 3. GI decontamination is unnecessary. 4. Place in quiet room, try to talk down. 5. Benzodiazepines or haloperidol for agitation or anxiety.

Inhalants[35,41] Hydrocarbons (benzene, glues), nitrous oxide (food product propellants [whipped cream]), nitrites, aliphatics (butane, propane), halides (paint additives, strippers, spot remover), ethers/ketones (solvents)	Euphoria; light-headedness; hyperactivity; ataxia; hallucinations; mental status changes, including coma with respiratory depression or aspiration. Can cause methemoglobinemia. *Halogenated hydrocarbons:* Cardiotoxicity and dysrhythmias, including ventricular fibrillation. *Sudden sniffing death:* Syndrome of simple asphyxiation from act of bagging.	1. Treat dysrhythmias; use of epinephrine relatively contraindicated because of worsening rhythm disturbances. 2. Obtain complete metabolic panel, including calcium, phosphate, magnesium, and amylase levels, liver function tests, CPK, and urinalysis. 3. Treat methemoglobinemia with methylene blue. 4. For respiratory symptoms, use caution with β-agonists. 5. With low-dose exposures, rapid recovery in 30 min to 2 hrs is typical.
Marijuana[35] Tetrahydrocannabinol (THC)	Euphoria, relaxation, impaired short-term memory, increased appetite, dry mouth, altered time perception, hallucinations, delusions, paranoia, tachycardia, hypertension, conjunctival injection.	1. Symptoms last 4-6 hr. 2. Drug screen may be positive for up to 2 weeks after single use. 3. May treat psychosis or delirium with benzodiazepines.

The author would like to thank Maryland Poison Control Center for providing information critical to the development of this chapter.

2

POISONINGS

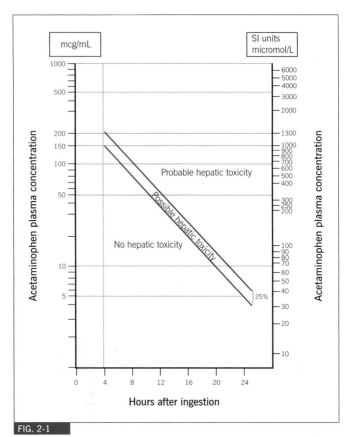

FIG. 2-1

Semilogarithmic plot of plasma acetaminophen levels versus time. *(From Jones AL. J Toxicol Clin Toxicol 1998; 36:277-285.)*

NOTE: This nomogram is valid for use after acute single ingestions of acetaminophen. The need for treatment cannot be extrapolated based on a level before 4 hours. In chronic overdose, toxicity can be seen with much lower plasma levels.

TABLE 2-2	
CHILDHOOD ANTIDOTES	
Drug	**Antidote**
Acetaminophen	*N*-Acetylcysteine
Anticholinergics	Physostigmine
Benzodiazepine	Flumazenil
β-blockers	Glucagon
Calcium channel blockers	Calcium chloride, calcium gluconate, glucagon
Carbon monoxide	Oxygen, hyperbaric oxygen
Coumadin	Vitamin K
Cyanide	Sodium nitrite/thiosulfate
Digitalis	Specific FAB antibody fragments
Ethylene glycol/Mehanol	Ethanol
Iron	Deferoxamine
Isoniazid	Pyridoxine
Lead	$CaNa_2EDTA$, penicillamine, BAL
Methemoglobinemia	Methylene blue
Opiates	Naloxone
Organophosphates	Atropine/pralidoxime
Phenothiazines	Diphenhydramine
Rattlesnake bite	Crotalid antivenom
Sulfonylureas	Octreotide

Modified from Weaver DR, Camfield P, Fraser A. Neurology 1988; 38:755 and Liebelt EL, Francis PD, Woolf AD. Ann Emerg Med 1995; 26:195-201.

REFERENCES

1. Ellenhorn MJ. Ellenhorn's medical toxicology, New York: William & Wilkins; 1997.
2. Tenenbein M. Recent advancements in pediatric toxicology. Pediatr Clin North Am 1999; 46:6.
3. Kulig K. Initial management of ingestions of toxic substances. N Engl J Med 1992; 326:1677.
4. Olson KR. Poisoning and drug overdose. Norwalk, Conn: Appleton & Lange; 1994.
5. Jones AL. Mechanism of action and value of *N*-acetylcysteine in the treatment of early and late acetaminophen poisoning: a critical review. J Toxicol Clin Toxicol 1998; 36:277-285.
6. Anker AL, Smilkstein MJ. Acetaminophen concepts and controversies. Emerg Med Clin North Am 1994; 12:335.
7. Smilkstein MJ et al. Acetaminophen overdose: a 48 hour intervenous, *N*-acetylcysteine treatment protocol. Ann Emerg Med 1991; 20:1058-1063.
8. Yip L, Dart RC, Hurlbut KM. Intravenous administration of oral *N*-acetylcysteine. Crit Care Med 1998; 26:40-43.
9. Goldfrank LR. Toxicologic emergencies. Norwalk, Conn: Appleton & Lange; 1998.
10. Weaver DF, Camfield P, Fraser A. Massive carbamazepine overdose: clinical and pharmacological observation in five episodes. Neurology 1988; 38:755.
11. Woolf AD. Poisoning in children and adolescents. Pediatr Rev 1993; 14:472.
12. Walker AR. Emergency department management of house fire burns and carbon monoxide poisoning in children. Curr Opin Pediatr 1996; 8:239-242.
13. Rothstein FC. Caustic injuries to the esophagus in children. Pediatr Clin North Am 1986; 33:665.
14. Moore WR. Caustic ingestion: pathophysiology, diagnosis, and treatment. Clin Pediatr 1986; 25:192.
15. Wason S. The emergency management of caustic ingestion. Emerg Med 1985; 2:175.
16. Tenenbein M. Pediatric toxicology: current controversies and recent advances. Curr Probl Pediatr 1986; 16:185.
17. Klein BL. Hydrocarbon poisonings. Pediatr Clin North Am 1986; 33:411.

18. Schauben JL et al. Iron poisoning: report of three cases and a review of therapeutic interventions. J Emerg Med 1990; 8:309.

19. Mills KC, Curry SC. Acute iron poisoning. Emerg Med Clin North Am 1994; 12:397.

20. Lovejoy FH, Nizet V, Priebe CJ. Common etiologies and new approaches to management of poisoning in pediatric practice. Curr Opin Pediatr 1993; 5:524-530.

21. Personal communication. Dr Cecilia T. Davoli, Lead poisoning prevention program, Kennedy Krieger Institute.

22. Schonfeld DJ, Needham D. Lead: a practical perspective. Contemp Pediatr 1994; 11:64-96.

23. Committee on Drugs. Treatment guidelines for lead exposure in children. Pediatrics 1995; 96: 155-160.

24. Centers for Disease Control and Prevention. Guidelines for lead poisoning prevention. Atlanta, GA: CDC; 1997.

25. Liebelt EL, Shannon MW. Oral chelators for childhood lead poisoning. Pediatr Ann 1994; 23: 616-626.

26. Moore R et al. Naloxone: under dosage after narcotic poisoning. Am J Dis Child 1980; 134:156.

27. Tenenbein M. Continuous naloxone infusion for opiate poisoning in infancy. J Pediatr 1984; 105:645.

28. Berlin CM. Advances in pediatric pharmacology and toxicology. Adv Pediatr 1993; 40:404-439.

29. Larsen LS et al. Adjunctive therapy of phenytoin overdose: a case report using plasmapheresis. Clin Toxicol 1986; 24:37.

30. Yip L, Dart RC, Gabow PA. Concepts and controversies in salicylate toxicity. Emerg Med Clin North Am 1994; 12:351.

31. Boehnert MT, Lovejoy FH. Value of the QRS duration versus the serum drug level in predicting seizures and ventricular arrhythmias after an acute overdose of tricyclic antidepressant. N Engl J Med 1985; 313:474.

32. Pimentel L, Trommer L. Cyclic antidepressant overdoses: a review. Emerg Med Clin North Am 1994; 12:533.

33. Shannon M, Liebelt EL. Toxicology reviews: targeted management strategies for cardiovascular toxicity from tricyclic antidepressant overdose—the pivotal role for alkalinization and sodium loading. Pediatr Emerg Care 1998; 14:293-298.

34. Liebelt EL, Francis PD, Woolf AD. ECG lead aVR versus QRS interval in predicting seizures and arrhythmias in acute tricyclic antidepressant toxicity. Ann Emerg Med 1995; 26:195-201.

35. Osterhondt KC, Shannon M, Henretig FM. Toxicologic emergencies. In Fleisher GR et al, editors. Textbook of pediatric emergency medicine, 4th ed. Williams & Wilkins, 2000.

36. Woo O et al. Shorter duration of oral *N*-acetylcysteine therapy for acute acetaminophen overdose. Ann Emerg Med 2000; 35:4 363-368.

37. Doyon S. The many faces of ecstasy. (submitted for publication) 2001.

38. Martin T. Serotonin syndrome. Ann Emer Med 1996; 28:520-525.

39. Wright R, Lewander W, Woolf A. Methemoglobinemia: etiology, pharmacology, and clinical management. Ann Emerg Med 1999; 34:5.

40. Eisenstein E, Amitai Y. Pediatrics in review 2000; 21:6.

41. Henretig F. Inhalant abuse in children and adolescents. Pediatr Ann 1996; 25:1.

42. McGuigan M. Acute iron poisoning. Pediatr Ann 1996; 25:1.

PROCEDURES

"See one, do one, teach one"

Matthew Grady, MD

I. GENERAL GUIDELINES

Before performing any procedure, it is crucial to obtain informed consent by explaining the procedure, the indications, any risks involved, and any alternatives. NOTE: **All invasive procedures involve pain and the risk of infection and bleeding.** Specific complications are listed by procedure. Sedation and analgesia should be planned in advance. In general, 1% lidocaine buffered with sodium bicarbonate (see Formulary) is adequate for local analgesia.

3

II. BLOOD SAMPLING AND VASCULAR ACCESS

A. HEELSTICK/FINGERSTICK

1. **Indications:** Blood sampling in infants for laboratory studies unaffected by hemolysis.
2. **Complications:** Infection, bleeding, osteomyelitis.
3. **Procedure**
   a. Warm heel or finger.
   b. Clean with alcohol.
      (1) Puncture heel using a lancet on the lateral part of the heel, avoiding the posterior area.
      (2) Puncture finger using a lancet on the palmar lateral surface of the finger near the tip.
   c. Wipe away the first drop of blood, then collect the sample using a capillary tube or container.
   d. Alternate between squeezing blood from the leg toward the heel (or from the hand toward the finger) and then releasing the pressure for several seconds.

B. INTRAVENOUS PLACEMENT AND ACCESS SITES

1. **Indications:** To obtain access to peripheral venous circulation to deliver fluid, medications, or blood products.
2. **Complications**
   a. Thrombosis.
   b. Infection.
3. **Procedure**
   a. Choose IV placement site and prepare with alcohol (Fig. 3-1).
   b. Apply tourniquet and then insert IV catheter, bevel up, at angle almost parallel to the skin, advancing until "flash" of blood is seen in the catheter hub. Advance the plastic catheter only, remove the needle, and secure the catheter.
   c. Attach T connector filled with saline to the catheter, flush with several mL of normal saline (NS) to ensure patency of the IV line.

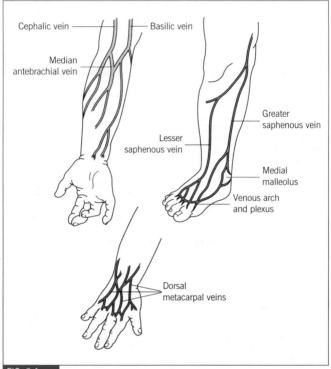

FIG. 3-1

Venous access sites. *(Courtesy Josie Pirro, RN, Johns Hopkins Children's Center.)*

C. EXTERNAL JUGULAR PUNCTURE[1]

1. **Indications:** Blood sampling in patients with inadequate peripheral vascular access or during resuscitation.
2. **Complications:** Infection, bleeding, pneumothorax.
3. **Procedure** (Fig. 3-2)
a. Restrain infant securely. Place infant with head turned away from side of blood sampling. Position with towel roll under shoulders or with head over side of bed to extend neck and accentuate the posterior margin of the sternocleidomastoid muscle on the side of the venipuncture.
b. Prepare area with povidone-iodine and alcohol in a sterile fashion.
c. The external jugular vein will distend if its most proximal segment is occluded or if the child cries. The vein runs from the angle of the mandible to the posterior border of the lower third of the sternocleidomastoid muscle.

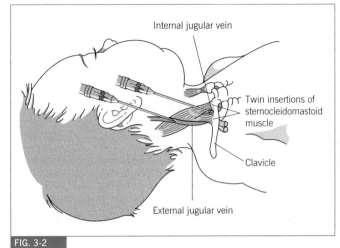

Internal jugular vein

Twin insertions of sternocleidomastoid muscle

Clavicle

External jugular vein

FIG. 3-2

Approach for external and internal jugular puncture. *(Courtesy Josie Pirro, RN, Johns Hopkins Children's Center.)*

3

PROCEDURES

d. With continuous negative suction on the syringe, insert the needle at about a 30-degree angle to the skin. Continue as with any peripheral venipuncture.

e. Apply a sterile dressing and pressure on the puncture site for 5 minutes.

D. FEMORAL ARTERY AND FEMORAL VEIN PUNCTURE[1,2]

1. **Indications:** Venous or arterial blood sampling in patients with inadequate vascular access or during resuscitation.

2. **Contraindications:** Femoral puncture is particularly hazardous in neonates and is not recommended in this age group. It is also discouraged in children because of the risk of trauma to the femoral head and joint capsule. Avoid femoral punctures in children who have thrombocytopenia or coagulation disorders, or those who are scheduled for cardiac catheterization.

3. **Complications:** Infection, bleeding, hematoma of femoral triangle, thrombosis of vessel, osteomyelitis, and septic arthritis of hip.

4. **Procedure** (Fig. 3-3)

a. Hold child securely in frog-leg position with the hips flexed and abducted.

b. Prepare area in sterile fashion.

c. Locate femoral pulse just distal to the inguinal crease (note that vein is medial to pulse). Insert needle 2 cm distal to the inguinal ligament and 0.5 to 0.75 cm into the groin. Aspirate while maneuvering the needle until blood is obtained.

d. Apply direct pressure for minimum of 5 minutes.

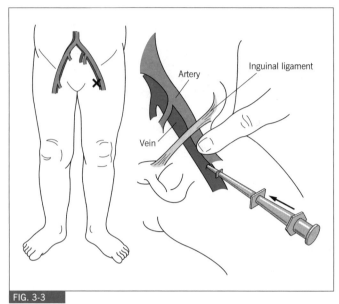

FIG. 3-3

Femoral puncture technique. *(Modified from Nichols DG et al. Golden hour: the handbook of advanced pediatric life support. St. Louis: Mosby; 1996.)*

E. RADIAL ARTERY PUNCTURE AND CATHETERIZATION[1,2]

1. **Indications:** Arterial blood sampling or for frequent blood gases and blood pressure monitoring in an intensive care setting.
2. **Complications:** Infection, bleeding, occlusion of artery by hematoma or thrombosis, ischemia if ulnar circulation is inadequate.
3. **Procedure**
a. Before procedure, test adequacy of ulnar blood flow with the Allen test. Clench the hand while simultaneously compressing ulnar and radial arteries. The hand will blanch. Release pressure from the ulnar artery and observe the flushing response. Procedure is safe to perform if entire hand flushes.
b. Locate the radial pulse. It is optional to infiltrate the area over the point of maximal impulse with lidocaine. Avoid infusion into the vessel by aspirating before infusing. Prepare the site in sterile fashion.
   (1) Puncture: Insert butterfly needle attached to a syringe at a 30- to 60-degree angle over the point of maximal impulse; blood should flow freely into the syringe in a pulsatile fashion; suction may be required for plastic tubes. Once the sample is obtained, apply firm, constant pressure for 5 minutes and then place a pressure dressing on the puncture site.

(2) Catheter placement: Secure the patient's hand to an arm board. Leave the fingers exposed to observe any color changes. Prepare the wrist with sterile technique and infiltrate over the point of maximal impulse with 1% lidocaine. Make a small skin puncture over the point of maximal impulse with a needle, then discard the needle. Insert an intravenous (IV) catheter with its needle through the puncture site at a 30-degree angle to the horizontal; pass the needle and catheter through the artery to transfix it, then withdraw the needle. Very slowly withdraw the catheter until free flow of blood is noted. Then advance the catheter and secure in place via sutures or tape. Apply an antibiotic ointment dressing. Infuse heparinized isotonic fluid (1 unit heparin/mL) at 1 mL/hr. A pressure transducer may be attached to monitor blood pressure.

NOTE: Do not infuse any medications, blood products, or hypotonic or hypertonic solutions through an arterial line.

F. POSTERIOR TIBIAL AND DORSALIS PEDIS ARTERY PUNCTURE[2]

1. **Indications:** Arterial blood sampling when radial artery puncture is unsuccessful or inaccessible.
2. **Complications:** Infection, bleeding, ischemia if inadequate circulation.
3. **Procedure** (see Radial Artery Puncture, p. 54, for technique)
a. Posterior tibial artery: Puncture the artery posterior to the medial malleolus while holding the foot in dorsiflexion.
b. Dorsalis pedis artery: Puncture the artery at the dorsal midfoot between the first and second toe while holding the foot in plantar flexion.

G. CENTRAL VENOUS CATHETER PLACEMENT[1,3]

1. **Indications:** To obtain emergency access to central venous circulation, to monitor central venous pressure, to deliver high-concentration parenteral nutrition or prolonged IV therapy, or to infuse blood products or large volumes of fluid.
2. **Complications:** Infection, bleeding, arterial or venous laceration, pneumothorax, hemothorax, thrombosis, catheter fragment in circulation, air embolism, and atrioventricular fistula.
3. **Access sites**
a. External jugular vein.
b. Subclavian vein.
c. Internal jugular vein.
d. Femoral vein.

NOTE: Femoral vein catheterization is contraindicated in severe abdominal trauma, and internal jugular catheterization is contraindicated in patients with elevated intracranial pressure (ICP).

4. **Procedure:** The Seldinger technique (Fig. 3-4)
a. Secure patient, prepare site, and drape in sterile fashion.
b. Insert needle, applying negative pressure to locate vessel.
c. When there is blood return, insert a guidewire through the needle into the vein to about one fourth to one third of the length of the wire.
d. Remove the needle, holding the guidewire firmly.

3

PROCEDURES

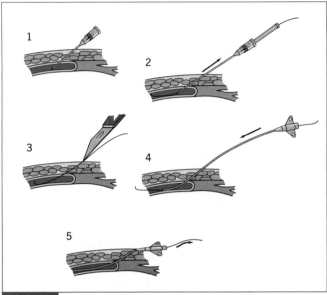

FIG. 3-4

The Seldinger technique for central venous catheter placement. *(Courtesy Josie Pirro, RN, Johns Hopkins Children's Center.)*

e. Slip a catheter that has been preflushed with sterile saline over the wire into the vein in a twisting motion. The entry site may be enlarged with a small skin incision or dilator. Pass the entire catheter over the wire until the hub is at the skin surface. Slowly remove the wire, secure the catheter by suture, and attach IV infusion.

f. Apply a sterile dressing over the site.

g. For neck vessels, obtain a chest radiograph to rule out pneumothorax.

5. **Approach**

a. External jugular (see Fig. 3-2): Place patient in 15- to 20-degree angle Trendelenburg position. Turn the head 45 degrees to the contralateral side. Enter the vein at the point where it crosses the sternocleidomastoid muscle.

b. Internal jugular (see Fig. 3-2): Place patient in 15- to 20-degree angle Trendelenburg position. Hyperextend the neck to tense the sternocleidomastoid muscle, and turn head away from the site of line placement. Palpate the sternal and clavicular heads of the muscle and enter at the apex of the triangle formed. Insert the needle at a 30-degree angle to the skin and aim toward the ipsilateral nipple. When blood flow is obtained, continue with Seldinger technique.

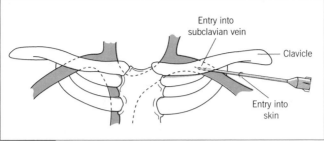

FIG. 3-5

Approach for catheterization of subclavian vein. *(Courtesy Josie Pirro, RN, Johns Hopkins Children's Center.)*

c. Subclavian vein (Fig. 3-5): Position the child in the Trendelenburg position with a towel roll under the thoracic spine to hyperextend the back. Aim the needle under the distal third of the clavicle toward the sternal notch. When blood flow is obtained, continue with Seldinger technique.

NOTE: **This is the least common site for central lines because of the increased risk of complications.**

d. Femoral vein (see Fig. 3-3): Hold the child securely with the hip flexed and abducted. Locate the femoral pulse just distal to the inguinal crease. Place the thumb of the nondominant hand on the femoral artery. Insert the needle medial to the thumb. The needle should enter the skin 2 to 3 cm distal to the inguinal ligament at a 30-degree angle to avoid entering the abdomen. When blood flow is obtained, continue with Seldinger technique.

H. INTRAOSSEOUS (IO) INFUSION[1,2]

1. **Indications:** Obtain emergency access in children <8 years old. This is very useful during circulatory collapse and/or cardiac arrest. The needle should be removed once adequate vascular access has been established.
2. **Complications:** Infection, bleeding, osteomyelitis, compartment syndrome, fat embolism, fracture, epiphyseal injury.
3. **Sites of entry (in order of preference)**
a. Anteromedial surface of the proximal tibia, 2 cm below and 1 to 2 cm medial to the tibial tuberosity on the flat part of the bone (Fig. 3-6).
b. Distal femur 3 cm above the lateral condyle in the midline.
c. Medial surface of the distal tibia 1 to 2 cm above the medial malleolus (may be a more effective site in older children).
4. **Procedure**
a. Prepare the patient for a sterile procedure.
b. If the child is conscious, anesthetize the puncture site down to the periosteum with 1% lidocaine (optional in emergency situations).

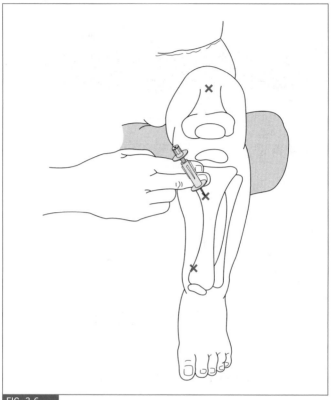

FIG. 3-6

Intraosseous insertion (anterior tibia). *(Courtesy Josie Pirro, RN, Johns Hopkins Children's Center.)*

c. Insert a 15-gauge IO needle perpendicular to the skin and advance to the periosteum. With a boring rotary motion, penetrate through the cortex until there is a decrease in resistance, indicating that you have reached the marrow. The needle should stand firmly without support. Secure the needle carefully.

d. Remove the stylet and attempt to aspirate marrow. (Note that it is not necessary to aspirate marrow.) Flush with 10 to 20 mL normal saline (NS). Observe for fluid extravasation. Marrow can be sent for determination of glucose levels, chemistries, blood type and crossmatch, but not for a complete blood count (CBC).

e. Attach standard IV tubing. Any crystalloid, blood product, or drug that may be infused into a peripheral vein may also be infused into the IO space, but an increased pressure (via pressure bag or push) is needed for infusion. There is a high risk of obstruction if continuous high-pressure fluids are not flushed through the IO needle.

I. UMBILICAL ARTERY (UA) AND VEIN (UV) CATHETERIZATION[1]

1. **Indications:** Vascular access (via UV), blood pressure (via UA), and blood gas (via UA) monitoring in critically ill neonates.

2. **Complications:** Infection; bleeding; hemorrhage; perforation of vessel; thrombosis with distal embolization; ischemia/infarction of lower extremities, bowel, or kidney; arrhythmia if the catheter is in the heart; air embolus.

3. **Caution:** UA catheterization should never be performed if omphalitis is present; it is contraindicated in the presence of possible necrotizing enterocolitis or intestinal hypoperfusion.

4. **Line placement**

a. Arterial line: Low line versus high line.

   (1) Low line: The tip of the catheter should lie just above the aortic bifurcation between L3 and L5. This avoids renal and mesenteric arteries near L1, perhaps decreasing the incidence of thrombosis or ischemia.

   (2) High line: The tip of the catheter should be above the diaphragm between T6 and T9. A high line may be recommended in infants weighing less than 750 g, in which a low line could easily slip out.

b. UV catheters should be placed in the inferior vena cava above the level of the ductus venosus and the hepatic veins and below the level of the right atrium.

c. Catheter length: Determine the length of catheter required using either a standardized graph or the regression formula. Add length for the height of the umbilical stump.

   (1) Standardized graph: Determine the shoulder-umbilical length by measuring the perpendicular line dropped from the tip of the shoulder to the level of the umbilicus. Use the graph in Fig. 3-7 to determine the arterial catheter length, and the one in Fig. 3-8 to determine venous catheter length.

   (2) Birth weight (BW) regression formula:
   Low line: UA catheter length (cm) = BW (kg) + 7.
   High line: UA catheter length (cm) = [3 × BW (kg)] + 9.
   UV catheter length (cm) = [0.5 × high line UA (cm)] + 1.

NOTE: Formula may not be appropriate for small-for-gestational-age (SGA) or large-for-gestational-age (LGA) infants.

5. **Procedure for UA line** (Fig. 3-9)

a. Determine the length of the catheter to be inserted for either high (T6 to T9) or low (L3 to L5) position.

b. Restrain the infant. Prepare and drape the umbilical cord and adjacent skin using sterile technique. Maintaining the infant's temperature is critical.

c. Flush the catheter with a sterile saline solution before insertion.

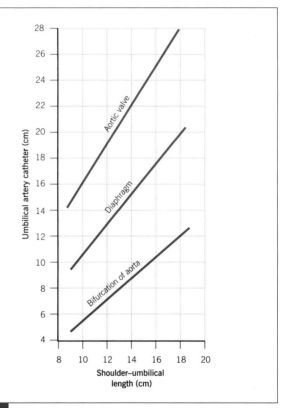

FIG. 3-7
Umbilical artery catheter length.

d. Place sterile umbilical tape around the base of the cord. Cut through the cord horizontally about 1.5 to 2.0 cm from the skin; tighten the umbilical tape to prevent bleeding.
e. Identify the one large, thin-walled umbilical vein and two smaller, thick-walled arteries. Use one tip of open, curved forceps to probe and dilate one artery gently; use both points of closed forceps and dilate artery by allowing forceps to open gently.
f. Grasp the catheter 1 cm from its tip with toothless forceps and insert the catheter into the lumen of the artery. Aim the tip toward the feet, and gently advance the catheter to the desired distance. Do not force. If resistance is encountered, try loosening umbilical tape; applying steady, gentle pressure; or manipulating the angle of the umbilical cord to skin.

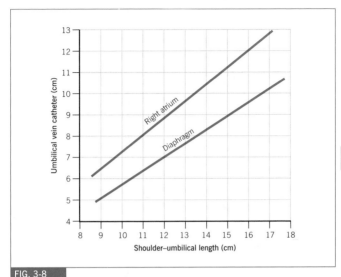

FIG. 3-8

Umbilical vein catheter length.

Often the catheter cannot be advanced because of creation of a "false luminal tract."

g. Confirm the position of the catheter tip radiologically. Secure the catheter with a suture through the cord, a marker tape, and a tape bridge. The catheter may be pulled back but not advanced once the sterile field is broken.

h. Observe for complications: Blanching or cyanosis of lower extremities, perforation, thrombosis, embolism, or infection. If any complications occur, the catheter should be removed.

NOTE: There are no definitive guidelines on feeding with a UA catheter in place. There is concern (up to 24 hours after removal) that the UA catheter or thrombus may interfere with intestinal perfusion. A risk/benefit assessment should be individualized. Use isotonic fluids, which contain 0.5 unit/mL of heparin. Never use hypoosmolar fluids in the UA.

6. Procedure for UV line (see Fig. 3-9)

a. Follow steps A-D for UA catheter placement. However, determine catheter length using Fig. 3-8.

b. Isolate the thin-walled umbilical vein, clear thrombi with forceps, and insert catheter, aiming the tip toward the right shoulder. Gently advance the catheter to the desired distance. Do not force. If resistance is encountered, try loosening the umbilical tape; applying steady, gentle pressure; or manipulating the angle of the umbilical cord to skin.

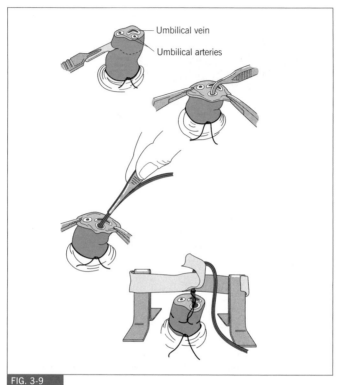

Umbilical vein
Umbilical arteries

FIG. 3-9

A four-step technique for placing and securing umbilical catheters. *(Courtesy Josie Pirro, RN, Johns Hopkins Children's Center.)*

c. Confirm position of the catheter tip radiologically. Secure catheter as described in step G for UA placement.

III. BODY FLUID SAMPLING

A. LUMBAR PUNCTURE[1,2]

1. **Indications:** Examination of spinal fluid for suspected infection or malignancy, instillation of intrathecal chemotherapy, or measurement of opening pressure.
2. **Complications:** Infection, bleeding, spinal fluid leak, hematoma, spinal headache, or acquired epidermal spinal cord tumor (caused by implantation of epidermal material into spinal canal if no stylet is used on skin entry).
3. **Cautions/contraindications**

a. Increased ICP: Before lumbar puncture (LP), perform funduscopic examination. The presence of papilledema, retinal hemorrhage, or clinical suspicion of increased ICP may be contraindications to the procedure. A sudden drop in intraspinal pressure by rapid release of cerebrospinal fluid (CSF) may cause fatal herniation. If LP is to be performed, proceed with extreme caution. Computed tomography (CT) may be indicated before LP if there is suspected intracranial bleeding, focal mass lesion, or increased ICP. A normal CT scan does not rule out increased ICP but usually excludes conditions that may put the patient at risk of herniation.

b. Bleeding diathesis: A platelet count >50,000/mm^3 is desirable before LP, and correction of any clotting factor deficiencies can minimize the risk of bleeding and subsequent cord or nerve root compression.

c. Overlying skin infection may result in inoculation of CSF with organisms.

d. LP should be deferred in an unstable patient, and appropriate therapy should be initiated, including antibiotics if indicated.

4. Procedure (Fig. 3-10)

a. Apply eutectic mixture of local anesthetics (EMLA) if sufficient time is available.

b. Position the child in either the sitting position or lateral recumbent position, with hips, knees, and neck flexed. Do not compromise a small infant's cardiorespiratory status by positioning.

c. Locate the desired intervertebral space (either L3-L4 or L4-L5) by drawing an imaginary line between the top of the iliac crests.

d. Prepare the skin in sterile fashion. Drape conservatively so it is possible to monitor the infant. Use a 20- to 22-gauge spinal needle with stylet (1½-inch for children younger than 12 years of age, 3½ inches for children 12 and over). A smaller-gauge needle will decrease the incidence of spinal headache and CSF leak.

e. The overlying skin and interspinous tissue can be anesthetized with 1% lidocaine.

f. Puncture the skin in the midline just caudad to the palpated spinous process, angling slightly cephalad toward the umbilicus. Advance several millimeters at a time and withdraw the stylet frequently to check for CSF flow. The needle may be advanced without the stylet once it is completely through the skin. In small infants, one may not feel a change in resistance or "pop" as the dura is penetrated.

g. If resistance is met initially (you hit bone), withdraw needle to the skin surface and redirect angle slightly.

h. Send CSF for appropriate studies (see Chapter 24, p. 557 for normal values). Send the first tube for culture and Gram stain, the second tube for measurement of glucose and protein levels, and the last tube for cell count and differential. If subarachnoid hemorrhage is suspected, send the first and fourth tubes for cell count and ask the laboratory to examine the CSF for xanthochromia.

i. Accurate measurement of CSF pressure can be made only with the

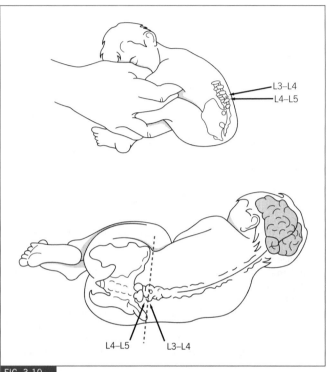

FIG. 3-10

Lumbar puncture. *(Courtesy Josie Pirro, RN, Johns Hopkins Children's Center.)*

patient lying quietly on his or her side in an unflexed position. Once free flow of spinal fluid is obtained, attach the manometer and measure CSF pressure.

B. BONE MARROW ASPIRATION[4]

1. **Indications:** Examination of bone marrow in a hematologic or oncologic workup.
2. **Complications:** Hematoma, osteomyelitis, or bone spur formation (if biopsy is performed).
3. **Procedure**
   a. Identify site for aspiration. For most children the posterior iliac crest is preferred, although the anterior iliac crest may be used. For some children younger than 3 months of age the tibia can be used.
   b. Position patient in the prone position with a pillow elevating the pelvis (for posterior iliac crest).

c. Prepare the site in sterile fashion and anesthetize the skin, soft tissue, and periosteum with 1% lidocaine.

d. Insert needle (16- or 18-gauge) with steady pressure in a boring motion. Needle should be directed perpendicular to the surface of the bone. Enter the ilium at the posterior superior iliac spine, which is a visible and palpable bony prominence superior and lateral to the intergluteal cleft. Needle will enter cortex and "pop" into the marrow space; the needle should be firmly anchored in bone.

e. Remove stylet, and aspirate marrow with a 20-mL or larger syringe. Apply pressure after procedure.

NOTE: In young infants and those with infiltrated leukemia, marrow aspiration may be impossible; bone marrow biopsy thus may be necessary.

C. CHEST TUBE PLACEMENT AND THORACENTESIS[1,3]

1. **Indications:** Evacuation of a pneumothorax, hemothorax, chylothorax, large pleural effusion, or empyema for diagnostic or therapeutic purposes.

2. **Complications:** Infection; bleeding; pneumothorax; hemothorax; pulmonary contusion or laceration; puncture of diaphragm, spleen or liver; or bronchopleural fistula.

3. **Procedure:** Needle decompression.

NOTE: For tension pneumothoraces it is imperative to attempt decompression quickly by sterilely inserting a large-bore needle (16 to 22 gauge, based on size) in the anterior second intercostal space in the midclavicular line.

a. Attach to a three-way stopcock and syringe, and aspirate air.

b. Use of a chest tube is still necessary.

4. **Procedure:** Chest tube insertion (see inside front cover for chest tube sizes; Fig. 3-11)

a. Position child supine or with affected side up.

b. Point of entry is the third to fifth intercostal space in the mid to anterior axillary line, usually at the level of the nipple (avoid breast tissue).

c. Prepare and drape in sterile fashion.

d. Patient may require sedation (see Formulary). Locally anesthetize skin, subcutaneous tissue, periosteum of rib, chest-wall muscles, and pleura with 1% lidocaine.

e. Make sterile incision one intercostal space below desired insertion point, and bluntly dissect with a hemostat through tissue layers until the superior portion of the rib is reached, avoiding the neurovascular bundle on the inferior portion of the rib.

f. Push the hemostat over the top of the rib, through the pleura, and into the pleural space. Enter the pleural space cautiously, and not deeper than 1 cm. Spread hemostat to open, place chest tube in clamp, and guide through entry site to desired distance.

g. For a pneumothorax, insert the tube anteriorly toward the apex. For a pleural effusion, direct the tube inferiorly and posteriorly.

3

PROCEDURES

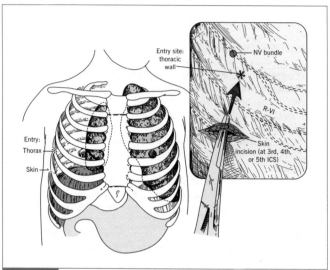

FIG. 3-11

Technique for insertion of chest tube. *ICS,* intercostal space; *NV,* neurovascular; *R-VI,* sixth rib. *(Modified from Fleisher G, Ludwig S. Pediatric emergency medicine, 3rd ed. Baltimore: Williams & Wilkins; 2000.)*

h. Secure the tube with purse-string sutures in which the suture is first tied at the skin, then wrapped around the tube once and tied at the tube.

i. Attach to a drainage system with −20 to −30 cm H_2O pressure.

j. Apply a sterile occlusive dressing.

k. Confirm position and function with chest radiograph.

5. Procedure: Thoracentesis (Fig. 3-12).

a. Confirm fluid in pleural space via clinical examination and radiographs or sonography.

b. If possible, place child in sitting position leaning over table; otherwise place supine.

c. Point of entry is usually in the seventh intercostal space and posterior axillary line.

d. Sterilely prepare and drape area.

e. Anesthetize skin, subcutaneous tissue, rib periosteum, chest wall, and pleura with 1% lidocaine.

f. Advance an 18- to 22-gauge IV catheter or large-bore needle attached to a syringe onto the rib and then "walk" over the superior aspect into the pleural space while providing steady negative pressure; often a

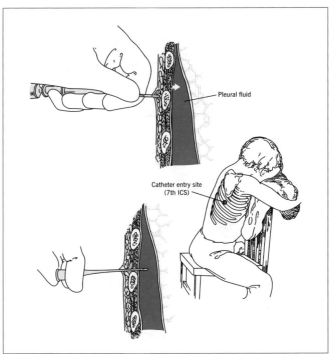

FIG. 3-12

Thoracentesis. *ICS,* Intercostal space. *(Modified from Fleisher G, Ludwig S. Pediatric emergency medicine, 3rd ed. Baltimore: Williams & Wilkins; 2000.)*

"popping" sensation is generated. Be careful not to advance too far into the pleural cavity. If an IV catheter is used, the soft catheter may be advanced into the pleural space aiming downward.

g. Attach syringe and stopcock device to remove fluid for diagnostic studies and symptomatic relief (see Chapter 24, p. 557 for evaluation of pleural fluid.)

h. After removing needle or catheter, place an occlusive dressing over the site and obtain a chest radiograph to rule out pneumothorax.

D. PERICARDIOCENTESIS[1,3]

1. **Indications:** To obtain pericardial fluid emergently for diagnostic or therapeutic purposes.

2. **Complications:** Bleeding, infection, puncture of cardiac chamber, cardiac dysrhythmia, hemopericardium/pneumopericardium, pneumothorax, or hemothorax.

3

PROCEDURES

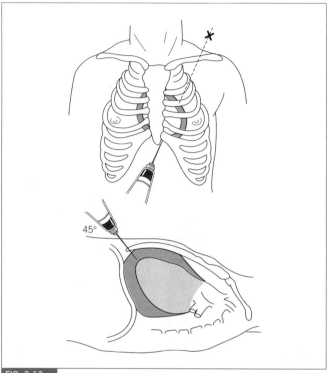

Pericardiocentesis. *(Modified from Nichols DG et al. Golden hour: the handbook of advanced pediatric life support. St. Louis: Mosby; 1996.)*

3. Procedure (Fig. 3-13)

a. Unless contraindicated, provide sedation and/or analgesia for the patient. Monitor electrocardiogram (ECG).

b. Place patient at a 30-degree angle (reverse Trendelenburg). Have patient secured.

c. Sterilely prepare and drape puncture site. A drape across the upper chest is unnecessary and may obscure important landmarks.

d. Anesthetize the puncture site with 1% lidocaine.

e. Insert an 18- or 20-gauge needle just to the left of the xiphoid process, 1 cm inferior to the bottom rib at about a 45-degree angle to the skin.

f. While gently aspirating, advance needle toward the patient's left shoulder until pericardial fluid is obtained.

g. Upon entering the pericardial space, clamp the needle at the skin edge to prevent further penetration. Attach a 30-mL syringe with a stopcock.

h. Gently and slowly remove the fluid. Rapid withdrawal of the pericardial fluid can result in shock or myocardial insufficiency.

i. Send fluid for appropriate laboratory studies (see Chapter 24).

E. PARACENTESIS[2]

1. **Indications:** Removal of intraperitoneal fluid for diagnostic or therapeutic purposes.

2. **Complications:** Bleeding, infection, puncture of viscera.

3. **Cautions**

a. Do not remove a large amount of fluid too rapidly because hypovolemia and hypotension may result from rapid fluid shifts.

b. Avoid scars from previous surgery; localized bowel adhesions increase the chances of entering a viscus in these areas.

c. The bladder should be empty to avoid perforation.

d. Never perform paracentesis through an area of cellulitis.

4. **Procedure**

a. Prepare and drape the abdomen as for a surgical procedure. Anesthetize the puncture site.

b. With the patient in semisupine, sitting, or lateral decubitus position, insert a 16- to 22-gauge IV catheter attached to a syringe in midline 2 cm below the umbilicus; in neonates, insert just lateral to the rectus muscle in the right or left lower quadrants, a few centimeters above the inguinal ligament.

c. Aiming cephalad, insert the needle at a 45-degree angle while one hand pulls the skin caudally until entering the peritoneal cavity. This creates a "Z" tract when the skin is released and the needle removed. Apply continuous negative pressure.

d. Once fluid appears in the syringe, remove introducer needle and leave catheter in place. Attach a stopcock and aspirate slowly until an adequate amount of fluid has been obtained for studies or symptomatic relief.

e. If, on entering the peritoneal cavity, air is aspirated, withdraw the needle immediately. Aspirated air indicates entrance into a hollow viscus. (In general, penetration of a hollow viscus during paracentesis does not lead to complications.) Repeat paracentesis with sterile equipment.

f. Send fluid for appropriate laboratory studies (see Chapter 24).

F. URINARY BLADDER CATHETERIZATION[2]

1. **Indications:** To obtain urine for urinalysis and culture sterilely and to monitor hydration status.

2. **Complications:** Hematuria, infection, trauma to urethra or bladder, intravesical knot of catheter (rarely occurs).

3. **Procedure**

a. Infant/child should not have voided within 1 hour of procedure.

NOTE: **Catheterization is contraindicated in pelvic fractures, known trauma to the urethra, or blood at the meatus.**

b. Prepare the urethral opening using sterile technique.

3

PROCEDURES

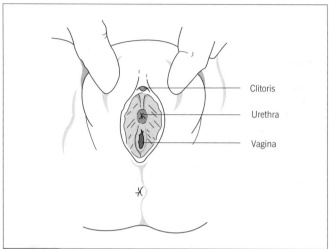

FIG. 3-14

Female urethra. *(Courtesy Josie Pirro, RN, Johns Hopkins Children's Center.)*

c. In boys, apply gentle traction to the penis to straighten the urethra.

d. Gently insert a lubricated catheter into the urethra. Slowly advance the catheter until resistance is met at the external sphincter. Continued pressure will overcome this resistance, and the catheter will enter the bladder. In girls, the urethral orifice may be difficult to visualize, but it is usually immediately anterior to the vaginal orifice (Fig. 3-14). Only a few centimeters of advancement is required to reach the bladder in girls. In boys, insert a few centimeters longer than the shaft of the penis.

e. Carefully remove the catheter once the specimen is obtained, and cleanse skin of iodine.

G. SUPRAPUBIC BLADDER ASPIRATION[1]

1. **Indications:** To obtain urine for urinalysis and culture sterilely in children less than 2 years of age (avoid in children with genitourinary tract anomalies).

2. **Complications:** Infection, hematuria (usually microscopic), intestinal perforation.

3. **Procedure**

a. Anterior rectal pressure in girls or gentle penile pressure in boys may be used to prevent urination during the procedure. Child should not have voided within 1 hour of procedure.

b. Restrain the infant in the supine, frog-leg position. Prepare suprapubic area in sterile fashion.

c. The site for puncture is 1 to 2 cm above the symphysis pubis in the midline. Use a syringe with a 22-gauge, 1-inch needle, and puncture

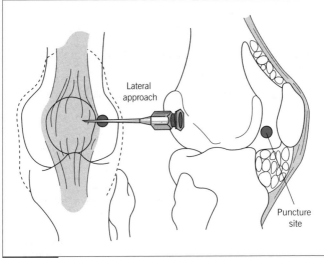

FIG. 3-15

Knee joint aspiration. *(Modified from Fleisher G, Ludwig S. Pediatric emergency medicine, 3rd ed. Baltimore: Williams & Wilkins; 2000.)*

at a 10- to 20-degree angle to the perpendicular, aiming slightly caudad.

d. Exert suction gently as the needle is advanced until urine enters syringe. The needle should not be advanced more than 1 inch. Aspirate the urine with gentle suction.

e. Cleanse skin of iodine.

H. KNEE JOINT ASPIRATION[1]

1. **Indications:** Removal of joint effusion causing severe pain or limitation of function and to obtain fluid for diagnosis of systemic illness (collagen vascular disease) or septic arthritis.

2. **Complications:** Bleeding, infection, damage to articular cartilage.

3. **Relative contraindications:** Bleeding diathesis, fracture (increased risk of infection).

4. **Procedure** (Fig. 3-15)

a. Secure the child with knee actively extended.

b. Prepare in sterile fashion.

c. Anesthetize the aspiration site with 1% lidocaine. Anesthetize the subcutaneous tissue down to the joint capsule.

d. Lateral approach: Site of entry is the lateral undersurface of the midpatella. Extend the knee as much as possible. Localize the undersurface of the patella. Insert an 18-gauge or larger-bore needle with a syringe. With continuous suction, advance needle at a 10- to 20-degree angle until fluid is obtained.

e. Aspiration of joint contents confirms an intraarticular placement.
f. Collect fluid for appropriate studies (see Chapter 24).
g. Place a dry, sterile dressing over aspiration site when finished.

I. TYMPANOCENTESIS[5]

1. **Indications:** Removal of middle ear fluid for diagnostic or therapeutic purposes.
2. **Complications:** Persistent perforation, tympanic membrane scar. Very rare: incostapedial joint dislocation, facial nerve injury, puncture of exposed jugular bulb.
3. **Procedure**
a. Prepare patient for the procedure. Consider use of an anxiolytic, such as midazolam (see Formulary). Restrain patient securely; a papoose board is recommended.
b. Remove all cerumen from canal (e.g., with No. 0 Buck cure). Gently swab ear canal with an alcohol-soaked applicator as a "wet mop" (e.g., 5-mm Farrell applicator tip wrapped with alcohol-soaked cotton).
c. Attach an 18- to 22-gauge, 2½ to 3-inch spinal needle, bevel upward, to the Luer-Lok adaptor of a disposable tympanocentesis aspirator. Alternatively, attach the needle to a 1-mL tuberculin syringe and bend needle 30 to 45 degrees (to allow for visualization during puncture).
d. Visualize the point of maximal bulge in the inferior portion (posteriorly or anteriorly) of the tympanic membrane through an otoscope fitted with an operating head (Fig. 3-16).

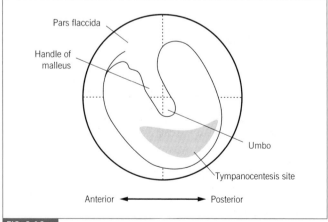

FIG. 3-16

Tympanocentesis in the left ear. *(Modified from Dieckmann R, Fiser D, Selbst S. Illustrated textbook of pediatric emergency and critical care procedures. St. Louis: Mosby; 1997.)*

e. Perforate the tympanic membrane and apply negative pressure to remove fluid in 1 to 2 seconds. Remove needle, avoiding contamination in the canal.

f. Send fluid for appropriate cultures and Gram's stain.

g. Place a small cotton pledget in the outer portion of the external auditory canal to absorb extra blood and discharge. Perforation usually heals in 3 to 5 days.

IV. IMMUNIZATION AND MEDICATION ADMINISTRATION[2]

A. SUBCUTANEOUS INJECTIONS

1. **Indications:** Immunizations and other medications.
2. **Complications:** Bleeding, infection, allergic reaction, lipohypertrophy/lipoatrophy after repeated injections.
3. **Procedure**
a. Locate injection site: Upper outer arm or outer aspect of upper thigh.
b. Clean skin with alcohol.
c. Insert 0.5-inch, 25- or 27-gauge needle into the subcutaneous layer at a 45-degree angle to the skin. Aspirate for blood, then inject medication.

B. INTRAMUSCULAR INJECTIONS

1. **Indications:** Immunizations and other medications.
2. **Complications:** Bleeding, infection, allergic reaction, nerve injury.
3. **Cautions**
a. Avoid intramuscular (IM) injections in a child with a bleeding disorder or thrombocytopenia.
b. Maximum volume to be injected is 0.5 mL in a small infant, 1 mL in an older infant, 2 mL in a school-age child, and 3 mL in an adolescent.
4. **Procedure**
a. Locate injection site: Anterolateral upper thigh (vastus lateralis muscle) in smaller child, or outer aspect of upper arm (deltoid) in older one. The dorsal gluteal region is less commonly used because of risk of nerve or vascular injury. To find the ventral gluteal site, form a triangle by placing your index finger on the anterior iliac spine and your middle finger on the most superior aspect of the iliac crest. The injection should occur in the middle of the triangle formed by the two fingers and the iliac crest.
b. Clean skin with alcohol.
c. Pinch muscle with free hand and insert 1-inch, 23- or 25-gauge needle until the hub is flush with the skin surface. For deltoid and ventral gluteal muscles, the needle should be perpendicular to the skin. For the anterolateral thigh, the needle should be 45 degrees to the long axis of the thigh. Aspirate for blood, then inject medication.

V. BASIC LACERATION REPAIR[1]

A. SUTURING

1. **Techniques** (Fig. 3-17)
a. Simple interrupted.
b. Horizontal mattress: Provides eversion of wound edges.

3

PROCEDURES

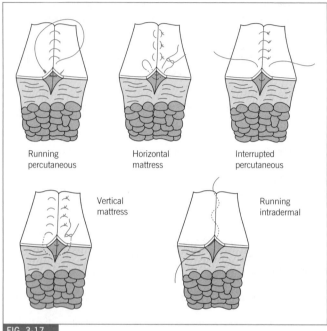

Running percutaneous

Horizontal mattress

Interrupted percutaneous

Vertical mattress

Running intradermal

FIG. 3-17

Basic skin-closure techniques. *(Courtesy Josie Pirro, RN, Johns Hopkins Children's Center.)*

c. Vertical mattress: For added strength in areas of thick skin or areas of skin movement; provides eversion of wound edges.

d. Running intradermal: For cosmetic closures.

2. Procedure

NOTE: Lacerations of the face, lips, hands, genitalia, mouth, or periorbital area may require consultation with a specialist. Ideally, lacerations at increased risk of infection (areas with poor blood supply, contaminated/ crush injury) should be sutured within 6 hours of injury. Clean wounds in cosmetically important areas may be closed up to 24 hours after injury in the absence of significant contamination or devitalization. In general, bite wounds should not be sutured except in areas of high cosmetic importance (face). The longer sutures are left in place, the greater the scarring and potential for infection. Sutures in cosmetically sensitive areas should be removed as soon as possible. Sutures in high-tension areas, such as extensor surfaces, should stay in longer (Table 3-1).

a. Prepare child for procedure with appropriate sedation, analgesia, and restraint.

	TABLE 3-1		

GUIDELINES FOR SUTURE MATERIAL, SIZE, AND REMOVAL

Body Region	Monofilament* (for Superficial Lacerations)	Absorbable[†] (for Deep Lacerations)	Duration (Days)
Scalp	5-0 or 4-0	4-0	5-7
Face	6-0	5-0	3-5
Eyelid	7-0 or 6-0	—	3-5
Eyebrow	6-0 or 5-0	5-0	3-5
Trunk	5-0 or 4-0	3-0	5-7
Extremities	5-0 or 4-0	4-0	7
Joint surface	4-0	—	10-14
Hand	5-0	5-0	7
Foot sole	4-0 or 3-0	4-0	7-10

*Examples of monofilament nonabsorbable sutures: nylon, polypropylene.
[†]Examples of absorbable sutures: polyglycolic acid and polyglactin 910 (Vicryl).

b. Anesthetize the wound with topical anesthetic or with lidocaine/bicarbonate by injecting the anesthetic into the subcutaneous tissues (see Formulary).

c. Forcefully irrigate the wound with copious amounts of sterile NS. Use at least 250 mL for smaller, superficial wounds and more for larger wounds. This is the most important step in preventing infection. Avoid high-pressure irrigation of deep puncture wounds.

d. Prepare and drape the patient for a sterile procedure.

e. Debride the wound when indicated. Probe for foreign bodies as indicated. Consider obtaining a radiograph if a radiopaque foreign body was involved in the injury.

f. Select suture type for percutaneous closure (see Table 3-1).

g. When suturing is complete, apply topical antibiotic and sterile dressing. If laceration is in proximity of a joint, splinting of the affected area to limit mobility often speeds healing and prevents wound separation.

h. Check wounds at 48 to 72 hours in cases in which wounds are of questionable viability, if wound was packed, or for patients prescribed prophylactic antibiotics. Change dressing at check.

i. For hand lacerations, close skin only; do not use subcutaneous stitches. Elevate and immobilize the hand.

j. Consider the child's need for tetanus prophylaxis (see Table 16-6).

VI. MUSCULOSKELETAL

A. BASIC SPLINTING[1]

1. **Indications:** To provide short-term stabilization of limb injuries.
2. **Complications:** Pressure sores, dermatitis, neurovascular impairment.
3. **Procedure**

a. Determine style of splint needed.

b. Measure and cut fiberglass or plaster to appropriate length. If using plaster, upper-extremity splints require 8 to 10 layers, and lower-extremity splints require 12 to 14 layers.

c. Pad extremity with cotton Webril, taking care to overlap each turn by 50%. In prepackaged fiberglass splints, additional padding is not generally required. Bony prominences may require additional padding. Place cotton between digits if they are in a splint.

d. Immerse plaster slabs into room-temperature water until bubbling stops. Smooth out wet plaster slab, avoiding any wrinkles.
WARNING: Plaster becomes hot after drying.

e. Position splint over extremity and wrap externally with gauze. When dry, an elastic wrap can be added.

f. Alternatively, wet one side of fiberglass until saturated. Roll or fold to remove excess water. Mold splint as indicated. **NOTE: Using warm water will decrease drying time. This may result in inadequate time to mold splint.** Turn edge of the splint back on itself to produce a smooth surface. Take care to cover the sharp edges of fiberglass. When dry, wrap with elastic bandage.

g. Use crutches or slings as indicated.

h. The need for orthopedic referral should be individually assessed.

B. LONG ARM POSTERIOR SPLINT (Fig. 3-18)
Indications: Immobilization of elbow and forearm injuries.

C. SUGAR TONG FOREARM SPLINT (Fig. 3-19)
Indications: For distal radius and wrist fractures, to immobilize the elbow and minimize pronation and supination.

D. ULNAR GUTTER SPLINT

1. **Indications:** Nonrotated fourth or fifth (boxer) metacarpal metaphyseal fracture with less than 20 degrees of angulation, uncomplicated fourth and fifth phalangeal fracture.

2. **Assess** for malrotation, displacement (especially Salter I type fracture), angulation, and joint stability before splinting.

3. **Procedure:** Elbow in neutral position, wrist in neutral position, metacarpophalangeal (MP) joint at 70 degrees, interphalangeal (IP) joint at 20 degrees. Apply splint in U shape from the tip of the fifth digit to 3 cm distal to the volar crease of the elbow. The splint should be wide enough to enclose the fourth and fifth digits.

E. THUMB SPICA SPLINT

1. **Indications:** Nonrotated, nonangulated, nonarticular fractures of the thumb metacarpal or phalanx, ulnar collateral ligament injury (gamekeeper/skier's thumb), scaphoid fracture or suspected scaphoid fracture (pain in anatomic snuff box).

2. **Procedure:** Wrist in slight dorsiflexion, thumb in some flexion and abduction, IP joint in slight flexion. Apply splint in U shape from tip of thumb to mid-forearm. Mold the splint along the long axis of the thumb so that thumb position is maintained. This will result in a spiral configuration along the forearm.

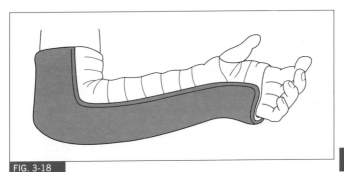

FIG. 3-18
Long arm posterior splint.

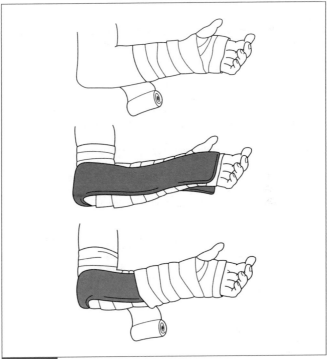

FIG. 3-19
Sugar tong forearm splint.

F. VOLAR SPLINT

1. **Indications:** Wrist immobilization.
2. **Procedure:** Wrist in slight dorsiflexion. Apply splint on palmar surface from the MP joint to 2 to 3 cm distal to the volar crease of the elbow. It is useful to curve the splint to allow the MP joint to rest at an 80- to 90-degree angle.

G. POSTERIOR ANKLE SPLINT

1. **Indications:** Immobilization of ankle sprains and fractures of the foot, ankle, and distal fibula.
2. **Procedure:** Measure leg for appropriate length of plaster. The splint should extend to base of toes and the upper portion of the calf. A sugar tong (stirrup) splint can be added to increase stability for ankle fractures.

H. RADIAL HEAD SUBLUXATION REDUCTION (NURSEMAID'S ELBOW)

1. **Presentation:** Commonly occurs in children ages 1 to 4 years with a history of inability to use an arm after it was pulled. The child presents with the affected arm held at the side in pronation, with elbow slightly flexed.
2. **Caution:** Rule out a fracture clinically before doing procedure. Consider radiograph if mechanism of injury or history is atypical.
3. **Procedure**

a. Support the elbow with one hand and place your thumb laterally over the radial head at the elbow. With your other hand, grasp the child's hand in a handshake position.

b. Quickly and deliberately supinate the forearm and flex the elbow. Alternatively, hyperpronation alone may be used. You may feel a click as reduction occurs.

c. Most children will begin to use the arm within 15 minutes, some immediately after reduction. If reduction occurs after a prolonged period of subluxation, it may take the child longer to recover use of the arm. In this case, the arm should be immobilized with a posterior splint.

d. If procedure is unsuccessful, consider obtaining a radiograph. Maneuver may be repeated if needed.

REFERENCES

1. Fleisher G, Ludwig S. Pediatric emergency medicine, 3rd ed. Baltimore: Williams & Wilkins; 2000.
2. Dieckmann R, Fiser D, Selbst S. Illustrated textbook of pediatric emergency and critical care procedures. St Louis: Mosby; 1997.
3. Nichols DG et al. Golden hour: the handbook of advanced pediatric life support. St Louis: Mosby; 1996.
4. Barone MA, Rowe PC. Pediatric procedures. In Oski's Pediatrics: principles and practice, 3rd ed. Baltimore: Lippincott Williams & Wilkins; 1999.
5. Hoberman A, Paradise JL, Wald ER. Tympanocentesis technique revisited. Pediatr Infect Dis J 1997; 16(2):S25-S26.

TRAUMA AND BURNS

Karyn Kassis, MD, MPH and Matthew Grady, MD

I. TRAUMA: OVERVIEW[1]

A. PRIMARY SURVEY

The primary survey includes assessment of the ABCs: **a**irway, **b**reathing, and **c**irculation. See Chapter 1 for a complete algorithm.

B. SECONDARY SURVEY

Procedures included in a secondary survey are listed in Table 4-1.

C. "AMPLE" HISTORY

Obtain an AMPLE history: **a**llergies, **m**edications, **p**ast illnesses, **l**ast meal, **e**vents preceding injury.

4

II. SPECIFIC TRAUMATIC INJURIES

A. CLOSED HEAD TRAUMA[2]

1. **Introduction:** (See Chapter 1 for treatment of severe closed head trauma [CHT]). Head injury can be caused by penetrating trauma, blunt force, rotational acceleration, or acceleration-deceleration injury. CHT may result in depressed or nondepressed skull fracture, epidural hematoma, subdural hematoma, cerebral contusion, brain edema, increased intracranial pressure (ICP), brain herniation, concussion (mild to moderated diffuse brain injury), and/or coma (diffuse axonal injury [DAI]). CHT not warranting intensive care or surgical management can be termed *minor CHT* and should be managed according to the following principles.

2. **Evaluation**

a. Initial assessment: Follow basic trauma principles, including assessment of ABCs and cervical spine immobilization.

b. Physical examination
   (1) Evaluate patient using Glasgow Coma Scale (GCS).
   (2) Obtain vital signs (look for Cushing's triad with hypertension, bradycardia, and abnormal respirations).
   (3) Perform secondary survey with careful neurologic evaluation (see Table 4-1).
   (4) If severe symptoms are present, or if CHT is not minor, follow procedures for emergency management of increased ICP and coma (see pp. 14-16).

c. Associated symptoms: Loss of consciousness (LOC), amnesia (before, during, or after the event), mental status change, behavior change, seizure activity, vomiting, headache, gait disturbance, visual change, altered level of consciousness, and altered level of activity since time of event.

d. Mechanism of injury
   (1) Linear forces are less likely to cause LOC; they more commonly lead to skull fractures, intracranial hematoma, or cerebral contusion.
   (2) Rotational forces commonly cause LOC and are occasionally associated with DAI.

TABLE 4-1

SECONDARY SURVEY

Remove all of patient's clothing, and perform a thorough head-to-toe examination, with special emphasis on the following. Remember to keep the child warm throughout the examination.

Organ System	Secondary Survey
Head	Scalp/skull injury.
	Raccoon eyes: Periorbital ecchymoses, which suggests orbital roof fracture.
	Battle's sign: Ecchymoses behind pinna, which suggests mastoid fracture.
	CSF leak from ears/nose, or hemotympanum suggests basilar skull fracture.
	Pupil size, symmetry, and reactivity: Unilateral dilation of one pupil suggests compression of cranial nerve III (CNIII) and possibly impending herniation; bilateral dilation of pupils is ominous and suggests bilateral CNIII compression or severe anoxia and ischemia.
	Corneal reflex.
	Funduscopic examination for papilledema as evidence of increased ICP.
	Hyphema.
Neck	Cervical spine tenderness, deformity, injury.
	Trachea midline.
	Subcutaneous emphysema.
Chest	Clavicle deformity, tenderness.
	Breath sounds, heart sounds.
	Chest wall symmetry, paradoxical movement, rib deformity/fracture.
	Petechiae over chest/head suggest traumatic asphyxia.
Abdomen	Serial examinations to evaluate tenderness, distention, ecchymosis.
	Shoulder pain suggests referred subdiaphragmatic process.
	Orogastric aspirates with blood or bile suggest intraabdominal injury.
	Splenic laceration suggested by left upper quadrant rib tenderness, flank pain, and/or flank ecchymoses.

cont'd

(3) If mechanism of injury is not consistent with sustained injuries, suspect abuse.

e. Medications and illicit drug use: Determining if a patient takes any medications or uses illicit drugs is helpful in determining the complete etiology of mental status changes.

3. Management

a. Initial management of minor CHT: Conduct according to basic trauma principles, with attention to ABCs, secondary survey, cervical spine immobilization, and basic radiologic evaluation of cervical spine. Apply basic wound management to any lacerations sustained to the scalp or face. (See also Chapter 3.)

b. Computed tomography (CT) scan of the head: A CT scan is warranted in the child with documented LOC. In the child with an unwitnessed event, unknown LOC, or no documented LOC, the decision to obtain a head

TABLE 4-1	
SECONDARY SURVEY—cont'd	
Organ System	Secondary Survey
Pelvis	Tenderness, symmetry, deformity, stability.
Genitourinary	Laceration, ecchymoses, hematoma, bleeding.
	Rectal tone, blood, displaced prostate.
	Blood at urinary meatus suggests urethral injury; do not catheterize.
Back	Log roll patient to evaluate spine for step-off along spinal column.
	Tenderness.
	Open or penetrating wound.
Extremities	*Neurovascular status:* Pulse, perfusion, pallor, paresthesias, paralysis, pain.
	Deformity, crepitus, pain.
	Motor/sensory examination.
	Compartment syndrome: Pain out of proportion to expected; distal pallor/pulselessness.
Neurologic	*Quick screen:* **AVPU** (**A**lert, **V**ocal stimulation response, **P**ainful stimulation response, **U**nresponsive).
	Glasgow Coma Scale (see Chapter 1)
Skin	Capillary refill, perfusion.
	Lacerations, abrasions.
	Contusion:
	Blue-purple: 0-5 days old.
	Green: 5-7 days old.
	Yellow: 7-10 days old.
	Brown: 10-14 days old.
	Resolution: 2-4 weeks old.

4

TRAUMA AND BURNS

CT scan must be based on the mechanism of injury, severity of known injuries, and persistence of complaints or deficits. Confusion and amnesia can occur without LOC and may not always warrant head CT when present without other concerns or complaints. Noncontrast CT is the preferred study in the emergency setting.

c. Observation: All children with significant CHT should be monitored for at least 4 to 6 hours to detect delayed signs or symptoms of intracranial injury. This commonly occurs with epidural bleeds, in which a symptom-free lucid period can precede variable degrees of acute-onset mental status change. The patient should also be observed for at least 48 hours after CHT. The decision of where (home versus hospital) to continue this observation period can be based on the degree of identified head injury or associated injuries, follow-up and reliability of the caretaker, and persistence of symptoms.

   d. Indications for hospitalization
      (1) Depressed or declining level of consciousness or prolonged unconsciousness.
      (2) Neurologic deficit.
      (3) Increasing headache or persistent vomiting.
      (4) Seizures.
      (5) Cerebrospinal fluid (CSF) otorrhea or rhinorrhea, hemotympanum, Battle's sign, or raccoon eyes.
      (6) Linear skull fracture crossing the groove of the middle meningeal artery, a venous sinus of the dura, or the foramen magnum.
      (7) Compound skull fracture or fracture into the frontal sinus.
      (8) Depressed skull fracture.
      (9) Bleeding disorder or patient receiving anticoagulation therapy.
     (10) Intoxication or illness obscuring neurologic state.
     (11) Suspected child abuse.
   e. If a child is stable for discharge, counsel parents on indications for reevaluation, including excessive sleepiness, more than two or three episodes of emesis, gait disturbance, severe headache not relieved with standard doses of acetaminophen or ibuprofen, drainage of blood or liquid from nose or ears, visual change, unequal pupil size, and/or seizure activity.

4. Sports-related closed head trauma[3]
   a. CHT occurring during sporting events frequently results in concussion, defined as alteration in cerebral function caused by trauma. See Box 4-1 for signs and symptoms of concussion.
   b. Guidelines for return to play: Patient needs to be symptom free both at rest and with exertion for at least 1 week to prevent second impact syndrome (fatality rate of 50%). Refer patient for sports medicine/neurology consultation for more than one concussion, amnesia for more than 24 hours, or prolonged loss of consciousness.

B. NECK INJURIES[2]
1. Introduction
   a. Infants and toddlers: At risk for subluxation of atlantooccipital joint (skull base-C1) or atlantoaxial joint (C1-C2).
   b. School-age children: Lower cervical spine involvement (C5-C6).
   c. Cervical spine injury is more likely to occur in children with an acceleration-deceleration injury such as a motor vehicle crash or fall. Assume cervical spine injury in the child with multiple injuries of any cause. Neurologic recovery after acute spinal cord injury is improved with prompt administration of methylprednisolone.

2. Evaluation
   a. Immobilize cervical spine, then perform careful history and physical examination.
   b. Radiographic studies: Obtain posteroanterior (PA) view, lateral view to include seventh cervical vertebra, and odontoid view. Additional flexion and extension views of the cervical spine should be obtained if there is point tenderness, symptoms on palpation, or any suspicion of abnormality on PA or lateral views. Flexion and extension views may be con-

BOX 4-1
CONCUSSION
EARLY SYMPTOMS
Amnesia
Headache
Nausea/emesis
Difficulty concentrating
Cognitive and/or memory dysfunction
Lightheadedness, dizziness, balance disturbance or vertigo
Blurred vision or photophobia
Tinnitus
LATE SYMPTOMS
Sleep irregularities
Fatigue
Depression
Lethargy
Personality or behavioral changes
Mental status changes
PHYSICAL EXAMINATION
Detailed neurologic examination
Funduscopy
Spinal tenderness
Facial or skull trauma
NEUROPSYCHOLOGICAL TESTING
Orientation
Memory/concentration
Mini-mental status
INDICATIONS FOR IMAGING
Seizure
Focal neurologic deficit
LOC greater than 5 min
LOC with severe headache

4

TRAUMA AND BURNS

traindicated if an unstable cervical spine injury is suspected. To read cervical spine films, the following ABCDs mnemonic is useful:

(1) **A**lignment: The anterior vertebral body line, posterior vertebral body line, facet line, and spinous process line should each form a straight line, with smooth contour and no step-offs.

(2) **B**ones: Assess each bone, looking for chips or fractures.

(3) **C**ount: You must see the C7 body in its entirety.

(4) **D**ens: Examine for chips or fractures.

(5) **D**isc spaces: Should see consistent distance between each vertebral body.

(6) **S**oft tissue: Assess for swelling, especially in the prevertebral area.

c. SCIWORA: **S**pinal **C**ord **I**njury **W**ith **O**ut **R**adiographic **A**bnormality; a functional cervical spine injury that cannot be excluded by abnormality on a radiograph; thought to be attributable to the increased mobility of a child's spine. Suspect in the setting of normal cervical spine images, when clinical signs or symptoms (e.g., point tenderness or focal neurologic symptoms) suggest cervical spine injury. If neurologic symptoms persist despite normal cervical spine and flexion/extension views, magnetic resonance imaging (MRI) is indicated to rule out swelling or intramedullary hemorrhage of the spinal cord.

d. Clinically clear the cervical spine: Patient must be awake; examiner must palpate posterior neck for localized tenderness. If there is no pain, assess active and passive range of motion. If there is any direct pain over bone, a cervical-spine collar should be maintained until further evaluation can definitively rule out injury.

C. BLUNT THORACIC TRAUMA[4]

1. **Internal injuries:** Often internal injuries present without external signs of trauma secondary to pliable rib cage and mediastinal mobility.

2. **Injury type (and frequency):** Pulmonary contusion/laceration (53%), pneumothorax/hemothorax (38%), rib/sternal fractures (36%), cardiac (5%), diaphragm (2%), major blood vessel (1%).

3. **Evaluation**

a. Careful history and physical examination.

b. Laboratory studies: Pulse oximetry, complete blood count (CBC); consider assessment of arterial blood gases (ABG) if patient is in severe distress, and type and crossmatch if patient is unstable.

c. Obtain a chest radiograph and chest CT with intravenous (IV) contrast if patient is stable.

4. **Treatment**

a. Tension pneumothorax: Presents as severe respiratory distress, distended neck veins, contralateral tracheal deviation, diminished breath sounds, and compromised systemic perfusion by obstruction of venous return. Perform needle decompression followed by chest tube placement directed to the lung apex (see pp. 65-67).

b. Open pneumothorax: An open pneumothorax, also known as a *sucking chest wound,* is rare but allows free flow of air between atmosphere and hemithorax. Cover defect with an occlusive dressing (i.e., petroleum jelly gauze), give positive pressure ventilation, and insert chest tube (see pp. 65-67).

c. Hemothorax: Provide fluid resuscitation followed by placement of a chest tube directed posteriorly and inferiorly.

D. BLUNT ABDOMINAL TRAUMA[4]

1. **Anatomic risk factors** in children include small, pliable rib cages; solid organs proportionally larger than those of adults, and underdeveloped abdominal muscles.

2. **Serious injuries** in children from blunt abdominal trauma (with frequency of injury) include splenic contusion/laceration (30%), liver contusion/laceration (28%), renal injury (28%), gastrointestinal (GI) tract/duodenal hematoma (14%), genitourinary (GU) tract injury (4%), pancreatic injury (3%), and disruption of major blood vessels (3%).

3. Evaluation

a. Careful history and physical examination.

b. Laboratory studies: Consider CBC, electrolytes, liver function tests (LFTs), amylase, lipase, urinalysis and microscopy; type and crossmatch if patient is unstable.

c. Consider abdominal CT scan with IV contrast (routine oral contrast is not indicated secondary to high false-negative rate for hollow viscus injury).

d. Consider focused abdominal ultrasound or diagnostic peritoneal lavage (DPL) when other co-existing injuries (i.e., neurologic or significant orthopedic) prevent CT scan. If DPL is used, the open method is preferred in small children, with warmed isotonic saline lavage (10 to 15 mL/kg).

4. If significant abdominal trauma is suspected or diagnosed, a pediatric surgeon should be consulted.

E. ORTHOPEDIC/LONG BONE TRAUMA[5]

1. **Fractures:** Some fracture patterns are unique to children (Fig. 4-1); growth-plate injuries are classified by the Salter-Harris classification

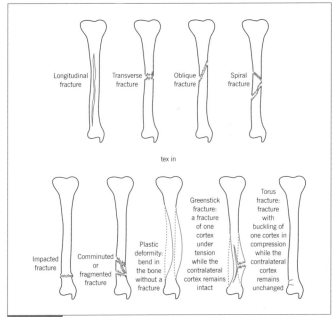

FIG. 4-1

Fracture patterns unique to children. *(Modified from Ogden JA. Skeletal injury in the child, 2nd ed. Philadelphia: WB Saunders; 1990.)*

TABLE 4-2				
SALTER-HARRIS CLASSIFICATION OF GROWTH-PLATE INJURY				
Class I	Class II	Class III	Class IV	Class V
Fracture along growth plate	Fracture along growth plate with metaphyseal extension	Fracture along growth plate with epiphyseal extension	Fracture across growth plate, including metaphysis and epiphysis	Crush injury to growth plate without obvious fracture

(Table 4-2). Ligaments are stronger than bones or growth plates in children; thus dislocations and sprains are relatively uncommon, whereas growth-plate disruption and bone avulsion are more common. For basic splinting techniques, see pp. 75-78.

2. **Compartment syndrome:**[6] Elevated muscle compartment venous pressure (enclosed by surrounding fascia) impairs blood flow and oxygenation, resulting in nerve and muscle damage.

a. Can be seen in open or closed fractures, crush injuries, burns, and necrotizing fasciitis; most common with tibial fractures but also occurs with displaced forearm and supracondylar humerus fractures. Chronic compartment syndrome is occasionally seen in athletes.

b. Severe, unremitting pain exacerbated by passive motion of the fingers or toes; swollen extremity that is tense to palpation.

c. 6 Ps: **P**ain (earliest symptom), **P**allor, **P**aresthesias, **P**aralysis, **P**oikilothermia, **P**ulselessness (late finding).

d. Studies: Reading of intracompartmental pressure (normal = 10 mm Hg; 20 to 30 mm Hg usually produces clinical symptoms).

e. Management: Emergent (within 6 hours of symptom onset) surgical fasciotomy (absolutely indicated if pressure ≥30 mm Hg).

III. ANIMAL BITES[2]

A. WOUND CONSIDERATIONS

1. **Wound location** suggests potential damage or infection of underlying structures, including tendon sheaths, bones, vessels, and nerves. Radiographs should be considered for deep bite wounds in which there is the possibility of foreign body, bone disruption, or fracture, especially when involving the scalp or hand. For bites in the periorbital area, ophthalmologic evaluation is suggested to rule out corneal abrasion,

lacrimal duct involvement, or other ocular damage. Bites of the hand are prone to infection because of the small, compact anatomy involved. Osteomyelitis is most common after hand bites. Bites to the nose must be evaluated for cartilage injury.

2. **Animal species**

a. Dog bites usually cause a crush injury, resulting in infection-prone devitalized tissue. Common organisms include *Staphylococcus aureus* and *Pasteurella multocida.*

b. Cat bite: Cats typically leave a deep puncture wound. Wound hygiene is difficult and there is increased risk of infection. *P. multocida* is the most common organism inoculated; infection may present in a fulminant manner, with rapid development of erythema, swelling, and pain in 12 to 24 hours. These infections respond slowly to drainage and appropriate antibiotics.

c. Human bite: In teens, a human bite commonly involves injury to the hand after fist-to-mouth contact. In younger children, a bite to the face or trunk is more common. Consider child abuse when human bites are involved. Consider risk of spread of systemic infection, such as human immunodeficiency virus (HIV), hepatitis B, and herpes simplex virus. Organisms most commonly isolated are *Streptococcus viridans* and *S. aureus*, and *Bacteroides* and *Peptostreptococcus* spp. More serious morbidity of human bites correlates with *S. aureus* and *Eikenella corrodens* infection.

d. Rodent bite: A rodent bite carries a low incidence of secondary infection; rat bite fever is rare but can present with fever, chills, headache, malaise, and rash 1 to 3 weeks after the bite. Causative agents, *Streptobacillus moniliformis* and *Spirillum minus*, are sensitive to IV penicillin.

e. Rabbit bites: *Francisella tularensis,* which causes tularemia (most frequently of the ulceroglandular type), is spread to humans via rabbit bites, contact with infected animals, or ingestion of infected animals.

B. MANAGEMENT

1. **Wound hygiene:** Copious irrigation of the wound is most important (a 19-gauge catheter and 35-mL syringe provide 8 lb/in^2 water pressure, using a minimum of 200 mL normal saline [NS]), in addition to debridement of all devitalized tissue, foreign bodies, and contaminants in the wound. Only 1% povidone-iodine should be used for cleansing because stronger antiseptics may damage the wound surface and delay healing. Peroxide should not be used because it prevents migration of white blood cells into the wound. Cultures of wounds are indicated if evidence of infection is present.

2. **Closure:** Wounds at high risk of infection include puncture wounds, minor hand or foot wounds, wounds with care delayed beyond 12 hours, cat or human bite wounds, and wounds in asplenic or immunosuppressed patients. In general, these wounds should not be sutured. Wounds that involve tendons, joints, deep fascial layers, or

4

TRAUMA AND BURNS

major vasculature should be evaluated by a plastic or hand surgeon and, if indicated, closed in the operating room.

a. Suturing: When indicated, closure should be done with a minimal number of simple, interrupted, nylon sutures and loose approximation of wound edges. Deep sutures should be avoided.

b. Head and neck: The head and neck can usually be safely sutured (with the exceptions noted above) after copious irrigation and wound debridement if within 6 to 8 hours of injury and with no signs of infection. Facial wounds often require primary closure for cosmetic reasons; infection risk is lower given the good vascular supply.

c. Extremities: In large hand wounds, the subcutaneous dead space should be closed with minimal absorbable sutures, with delayed cutaneous closure in 3 to 5 days if there is no evidence of infection.

3. **Antibiotics:** Prophylactic antibiotics are only indicated for wounds at risk for infection, as listed above. Antibiotics of choice include amoxicillin/clavulanic acid, or trimethoprim-sulfamethoxazole in combination with clindamycin for the penicillin-allergic patient. Initial doses should be given in the emergency department and continued for 3 to 5 days.

4. **Rabies and tetanus prophylaxis:** See Chapter 15.

5. **Disposition**

a. Outpatient care: Careful follow-up of all bite wounds, especially those requiring surgical closure, should be obtained within 24 to 48 hours. Extremity wounds, especially the hands, should be immobilized in position of function and kept elevated. Local care is of paramount importance; the wound should be kept clean and dry. Signs and symptoms of infection should be discussed.

b. Inpatient care: Consider hospitalization for observation and parenteral antibiotics for significant human bites, immunocompromised or asplenic hosts, established deep or severe infections, bites associated with systemic complaints, bites with significant functional or cosmetic morbidity, and/or unreliable follow-up or care by the parent/guardian. Hospitalization and IV antibiotics should be considered if a subsequent infection develops.

6. **The infected wound:** Drainage and debridement are required for wounds that subsequently become infected. Gram stain and aerobic/anaerobic cultures should be performed before start or change of antibiotics; in the case of cellulitis, aspirated cultures of leading edges may be useful. If deep tissue layers or structures are involved, exploration and debridement under general anesthesia may be indicated.

IV. BURNS[2,7]

A. EVALUATION OF PEDIATRIC BURNS (Tables 4-3 and 4-4)

NOTE: The extent and severity of burn injury may change over the first few days after injury; therefore, be cautious in discussing prognosis with the victim or victim's family.

TABLE 4-3	
THERMAL INJURY	
Type of Burn	**Description/Comment**
Flame	Most common type of burn; when clothing burns, the exposure to heat is prolonged, and the severity of the burn is worse.
Scald/contact	Mortality is similar to that in flame burns when total BSA involved is equivalent; see text for description of patterns of scald injury and burns suspicious of intentional injury.
Chemical	Tissue damaged by protein coagulation or liquefaction rather than hyperthermic activity.
Electrical	Injury is often extensive, involving skeletal muscle, and other tissues in addition to the skin damage. Extent of damage may not be initially apparent. The tissues that have the least resistance are the most heat sensitive. Bone has the greatest resistance, nerve tissue the least. Cardiac arrest may occur from passage of the current through the heart.
Inhalation	Present in 30% of victims of major flame burns and should be considered when there is evidence of fire in enclosed space, singed nares, facial burns, charred lips, carbonaceous secretions, posterior pharynx edema, hoarseness, cough, or wheezing. Inhalation injury increases mortality.
Cold injury/frostbite	Freezing results in direct tissue injury. Toes, fingers, ears, and nose are commonly involved. Initial treatment includes rewarming in tepid (105°-110° F) water for 20-40 min. Excision of tissue should not be done until complete demarcation of nonviable tissue has occurred.

TABLE 4-4	
BURN DEGREE	
Burn Depth/Degree	**Description/Comment**
First degree	Only epidermis involved; painful and erythematous.
Second degree	Epidermis and dermis involved, but dermal appendages spared. Superficial second-degree burns are blistered and painful. Any blistering qualifies as a second-degree burn. Deep second-degree burns may be white and painless, require grafting, and progress to full-thickness burns with wound infection.
Third degree	Full-thickness burns involving epidermis and all of the dermis, including dermal appendages; leathery and painless; require grafting.

B. BURN MAPPING

1. **Burn assessment chart:** Use chart (Fig. 4-2) to map areas of second- and third-degree burns.
2. **Calculate total body surface area (BSA) burned,** based only on percent of second- and third-degree burns.

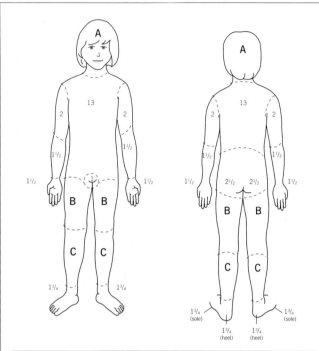

	<1yr	1yr	5yr	10yr	15yr	Adult
A half of head	$9^1/_2$	$8^1/_2$	$6^1/_2$	$5^1/_2$	$4^1/_2$	$3^1/_2$
B half of thigh	$2^3/_4$	$3^1/_4$	4	$4^1/_4$	$4^1/_2$	$4^3/_4$
C half of leg	$2^1/_2$	$2^1/_2$	$2^3/_4$	3	$3^1/_4$	$3^1/_2$

FIG. 4-2

Burn assessment chart. All numbers are percentages. *(From Barkin RM, Rosen P. Emergency pediatrics: a guide to ambulatory care, 4th ed. St Louis: Mosby; 1994.)*

C. EMERGENT MANAGEMENT OF PEDIATRIC BURNS

1. **Acute stabilization:** Special considerations of basic trauma principles.
a. Airway
   (1) Intubation: For pulmonary toilet or if there is evidence of inhalation. Neuromuscular blockade with succinylcholine for intubation is

appropriate for patients less than 48 hours postburn, but it is contraindicated after this time frame because of the risk of worsening hyperkalemia. (See also Chapter 1.)

(2) Inhalation injury: All patients with large burns and/or closed space burns should be assumed to have carbon monoxide (CO) poisoning until examination and evaluation of blood carboxyhemoglobin is undertaken (see Chapter 2). Humidified 100% O_2 should be administered during initial assessment. Delivery of 100% O_2 counteracts the effects of CO and speeds its clearance. Carboxyhemoglobin absorbs light at the same wavelength as oxyhemoglobin, so oxygen saturation, as determined by pulse oximetry, is not altered; a Pao_2 level must be obtained.

(3) Cyanide poisoning, via inhalation of combustible materials, can produce almond-scented breath and may cause profound positive anion gap metabolic acidosis (see Chapter 2).

b. Breathing

(1) Monitor pulmonary status with serial ABGs and chest radiographs as indicated.

(2) Increasing tachypnea may be seen in patients with pulmonary insufficiency caused by acute asphyxia and CO toxicity, upper airway obstruction secondary to edema, or overwhelming parenchymal damage.

c. Circulation/initial fluid resuscitation: Start IV fluid resuscitation of infants with burns greater than 10% of BSA, children with burns greater than 15% BSA, or children with evidence of smoke inhalation. Consider a bolus of 20 mL/kg lactated Ringer's (LR) or NS solutions. Further fluid resuscitation should maintain a urine output of 0.5 to 2 mL/kg/hr.

d. Secondary survey: Consider associated traumatic injuries. Electrical injury can produce deep tissue damage, intravascular thrombosis, cardiac and respiratory arrest, fractures secondary to muscle contraction, and cardiac arrhythmias. Look for exit site for electrical injury.

e. Laboratory evaluation: Consider CBC, type and crossmatch, carboxyhemoglobin, coagulation studies, chemistry panel, ABGs, and chest radiograph (may not show changes for 24 to 72 hours).

f. GI: Place nasogastric tube for decompression; patient should receive nothing by mouth (NPO); begin stress ulcer prophylaxis with H_2-receptor blockers and/or antacids.

g. Obtain bladder decompression and monitor urine output with Foley catheter.

h. Cardiac: Consider electrocardiogram (ECG).

i. Eye: Carefully examine patient for burns or abrasions to eyes, with referral to ophthalmology if suspected. Use topical ophthalmic antibiotics if abrasions are present.

j. Special considerations

(1) Tetanus immunoprophylaxis (see Chapter 15).

(2) Temperature management: Cooling decreases the severity of the

4

TRAUMA AND BURNS

burn if administered within 30 minutes of injury; it also helps to relieve pain. If burn is less than 10% of BSA, apply clean towels soaked in cold water to help prevent burn progression. If burns are more than 10% of BSA, apply clean, dry towels to burn to avoid hypothermia.

(3) Chemical burns: It is important to wash away or neutralize the chemical. Except in rare circumstances, the most efficacious first-aid treatment for chemical burns is lavaging with copious volumes of water for about 20 minutes.

(4) Analgesia: IV analgesia is often necessary to treat pain. Do not attribute combativeness or anxiety to pain until adequate perfusion, oxygenation, and ventilation are established. Consider narcotic therapy for pain management (see Formulary).

D. TRIAGE AND FURTHER MANAGEMENT OF PEDIATRIC BURNS

1. Outpatient management

a. Considerations: If burn is less than 10% of an infant's BSA, or less than 15% of a child's BSA and involves no full-thickness areas, patient may be treated as an outpatient.

b. Management

(1) Cleanse with warm saline or mild soap and water. Consider debridement with forceps or sterile gauze to pick up the edges and peel tissue off the base of the burn. Leave blisters intact.

(2) Apply topical antibacterial agent (Table 4-5).

(3) Daily follow-up is recommended.

(4) Have patient cleanse burn at home twice daily with mild soap followed by application of an antibacterial agent and sterile dressing, as above. Once epithelialization has begun, dressing may be changed once daily.

(5) Pain management: Oral narcotic or nonsteroidal antiinflammatory drugs (NSAIDs) may be taken (see Formulary).

2. Inpatient management

a. Considerations: Inpatient management should be considered for more extensive burns; electrical or chemical burns; burns of critical areas such as face, hands, feet, perineum, or joints; burns suspicious of abuse or unsafe home environment; and burns in a child with underlying chronic illness, evidence of smoke inhalation, cyanide poisoning, or CO poisoning. Consider transfer to a burn center if any of the following conditions occur: burns of at least 20% to 30% BSA; major burns to the hand, face, joints, or perineum; electrical burns; or burns associated with potentially life-threatening injuries.

b. Fluid therapy: Provide sufficient fluid to prevent shock and renal failure from excessive fluid losses and third spacing. Assess adequacy of perfusion using urine output, blood pressure, heart rate, peripheral circulation, and sensorium. Monitor electrolytes and blood gases for acidosis. Consider central venous access for burns greater than 25% BSA. Use the Parkland formula (below) as a guideline to estimate fluid

TABLE 4-5

TOPICAL ANTIBACTERIAL AGENTS

Agent	Action	Side Effects	Use
Silver sulfadiazine (Silvadene)	Broad antibacterial, painless, fair eschar penetration	Sulfonamide sensitivity, occasional leukopenia, contraindicated in pregnancy	Q12hr; cover with light dressings; leave face and chest open
Bacitracin ointment	Limited antibacterial action, poor eschar penetration, transparent, easy to apply	Rapid development of resistance; conjunctivitis develops if ointment comes into contact with eye	Q12hr, apply to small areas; acceptable with facial burns
Mafenide (Sulfamylon)	Excellent antibacterial for gram-positive and gram-negative bacteria, and *Clostridium;* rapid eschar penetration	Painful, sulfonamide sensitivity, carbonic anhydrase inhibition may lead to acidosis	Q12hr; cover with light dressings; leave face, chest, abdomen open
Aqueous silver nitrate solution	Universal antibacterial action, poor eschar penetration	Strong tissue staining, hypochloremic alkalosis	Q12hr, light gauze dressing
Iodophores (Efodine)	Universal antibacterial action, poor eschar penetration	Strong tissue staining, iodine absorption	Q12hr, light gauze dressing

need (note that this formula provides for replacement and losses, not maintenance fluids, so one must add maintenance fluid requirements).

(1) First 24 hours: Give 4 mL/kg of crystalloid per % BSA burned over the first 24 hours; give half of total dose over the first 8 hours calculated from the time of injury. Give the remaining half over the next 16 hours.

(2) Second 24 hours: Fluid requirements average 50% to 75% of the first day's requirements. Determine concentrations and rates by monitoring weight, serum electrolytes, urine output, nasogastric losses, etc.

(3) Consider adding colloid after 18 to 24 hours (albumin 1g/kg/day) to maintain serum albumin >2 g/dL.

(4) Withhold potassium generally for the first 48 hours because of a large release of potassium from damaged tissues. To manage electrolytes most effectively, monitor urine electrolytes twice weekly and replace urine losses accordingly. Urine output should be maintained at ≥0.5 mL/kg/hour.

3. **Prevention of burns:** Measures include child-proofing the home, installing smoke detectors, and turning hot water tap temperature down to 49° to 52° C (<120° F). It takes 2 minutes of immersion at 52° C to cause a full-thickness burn, compared with 5 seconds of immersion at 60° C.

V. CHILD ABUSE

A. INTRODUCTION

Involve the medical professional, social worker, and community agencies such as emergency medical service providers, police, social services, and prosecutors.

B. MANAGEMENT[2]

The medical professional should suspect, diagnose, treat, report, and document all cases of child abuse, neglect, or maltreatment.

1. **Suspect:** Be suspicious whenever there is inconsistent or inadequate history of injury, inappropriate parental response to the situation, delay in seeking medical attention, discrepancy between mechanism of injury and physical examination findings, evidence of neglect or failure to thrive, evidence of disturbed emotions or expressions in a child, prior history of suspicious events, or parental substance abuse.

2. **Diagnose:** Characteristic or concerning injuries.

a. Bruises: Shape, color, and dating of bruises are important (see Table 4-1); correlate with history. Be suspicious of bruises in protected areas (chest, abdomen, back, buttocks). Looped marks or railroad track marks may indicate injury from cords, belts, and ropes.

b. Bites: Shape, size, and location are important; correlate with history and dental anatomy of questioned perpetrator. Intercanine distances of more than 3 cm are suggestive of human bites; they generally crush more than lacerate.

c. Burns: Absence of splash marks and/or clearly demarcated edges are suggestive of nonaccidental injury. Stocking glove patterns, symmetrically burned buttocks and/or lower legs, spared inguinal creases, and symmetric involvement of palms or soles all suggest intentional injury.

d. Hemorrhage: Retinal hemorrhages are suggestive of abuse and always warrant evaluation for head trauma. Duodenal hematoma, causing eventual upper GI obstruction secondary to blunt trauma, is suspicious for intentional injury.

e. Skeletal injury: Correlate mechanism of injury with physical finding; rule out any underlying bony pathology.

   (1) Long bones: Classic fracture of abuse is the epiphyseal/metaphyseal chip fracture, seen as the "bucket handle" or "corner" fracture at the end of long bones, secondary to jerking or shaking of a child's limb.

Spiral fractures of the femur and humerus may be suspicious of abuse, especially if no history of rotational force is given as mechanism of injury. However, spiral fractures of the tibia in a toddler (i.e., "toddler's fracture") are commonly caused by minor accidental trauma.

(2) Ribs: Nonaccidental rib fractures are usually nondisplaced and often are posterior, near the attachment to the spine; they may not be readily visible on acute plain-film radiographs. Pleural thickening, pleural fluid, and contusion may suggest an undetected rib fracture. Fractures are secondary to direct blows or severe squeezing of the rib cage. Closed-chest compressions from cardiopulmonary resuscitation do not appear to cause rib fractures in children.

(3) Skull: Fractures suggestive of force greater than that sustained with minor household trauma are suspicious for abuse; these include fractures more than 3 mm wide, complex fractures, bilateral fractures, and nonparietal fractures.

f. Genital injury: Vaginal bleeding in the prepubertal female, or injury to external genitalia, especially the posterior region, are suspicious for abuse. The hymen should be examined for irregularity outside the realm of normal variation. Note: **A normal examination does not rule out abuse.** The anus should be evaluated for bruising, laceration, hemorrhoids, scars that extend beyond the anal verge, absence of anal wink, and evidence of infection, such as genital warts. Circumferential hematoma of the anal sphincter is associated with forced penetration. When recent (within 72 hours) sexual abuse is suspected, defer interview and detailed GU examination whenever possible until a multidisciplinary forensic team with expertise in the clinical and laboratory evaluation of sexual abuse can be involved. Avoid collection of laboratory specimens without input from this team. Note also that only cultures, not polymerase chain reaction (PCR), for gonorrhea and chlamydia are currently acceptable in this setting.

g. Shaken baby syndrome: Classically presents with retinal hemorrhages, long bone or rib fractures, and central nervous system (CNS) dysfunction, such as seizure, apnea, or lethargy secondary to intracranial injury. Shaken baby syndrome is usually found in children less than 6 months of age.

3. Useful studies

a. Skeletal surveys (see Chapter 23 for components) are suggested to evaluate suspicious bony trauma in any child; these studies are mandatory for children less than 2 years of age.

b. A bone scan may be indicated to identify early or difficult-to-detect fractures.

c. CT scan of the head is unreliable for detection of skull fractures but useful in detecting intracranial pathology secondary to trauma.

d. MRI may identify lesions not detected by CT scan; for example, posterior fossa injury and diffuse axonal injury. MRI also provides more useful information about the dating of injuries identified.

4

TRAUMA AND BURNS

e. Ophthalmologic evaluation for retinal hemorrhages is useful in suspected shaken baby syndrome.

4. **Treat:** Refer to basic principles of trauma management. Special attention should be paid to "stabilizing" the existing and immediate environment of the child (utilizing available social and protective services) so as to protect the child from incurring further injury during the work-up.

5. **Report:** All health care providers are required by law to report suspected maltreatment of a child to the local police and/or welfare agency. Suspicion, supported by objective evidence, is criterion for reporting and should first be discussed with not only the rest of the involved medical team but also the family. The professional who makes such reports is immune from any civil or criminal liability.

6. **Document:** Write legibly, carefully documenting the following: reported and suspected history and mechanisms of injury; any history given by the victim in his or her own words (use quotation marks); information provided by other providers or services; and physical examination findings, including drawings of injuries and details of dimensions, color, shape, and texture. Always consider early utilization of police crime laboratory photography to document injuries.

REFERENCES

1. American College of Surgeons. Advanced trauma life support for doctors, 6th ed. Chicago: American College of Surgeons; 1997.
2. Fleisher GR, Ludwig S, editors. Textbook of pediatric emergency medicine, 4th ed. Philadelphia: Lippincott, Williams & Wilkens; 2000.
3. Proctor M, Cantu R. Head and neck injuries in young athletes. Clin Sports Med 2000; 19(4): 693-714.
4. Sachez J, Paidas C: Childhood trauma: now and in the new millennium. Surg Clin North Am 1999; 79(6):1503-1535.
5. Ogden JA. Skeletal injury in the child, 2nd ed. Philadelphia: WB Saunders; 1990.
6. Mabee JR, Bostwick TL. Pathophysiology and mechanisms of compartment syndrome. Orthopaed Rev 1993; 22(2):175-181.
7. Barkin RM, Rosen P. Emergency pediatrics: a guide to ambulatory care, 4th ed. St Louis: Mosby; 1994.

PART II

Diagnostic and Therapeutic Information

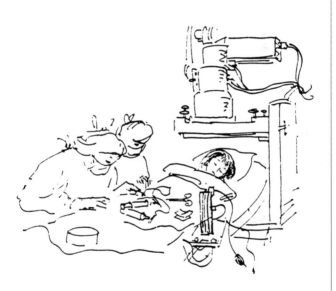

ADOLESCENT MEDICINE

Dominique Foulkes, MD and Karyn Kassis, MD, MPH

I. ADOLESCENT HEALTH MAINTENANCE[1,2] (Table 5-1)

A. MEDICAL HISTORY

Medical history includes any information regarding immunizations, chronic illness, chronic medications (including hormonal contraception), recent dental care, hospitalizations, or surgeries.

B. FAMILY HISTORY

Family history includes any information regarding psychiatric disorders, suicide, alcoholism/substance abuse, or chronic medical conditions. Assess familial risk factors (e.g., for cholesterol screening).

C. REVIEW OF SYSTEMS

1. **Dietary habits:** Typical foods consumed, types and frequency of meals skipped, vomiting, use of laxatives or other weight-loss methods, dietary sources of calcium.
2. **Recent weight gain or loss, body image.**

D. PSYCHOSOCIAL/MEDICOSOCIAL HISTORY (HEADSS)

1. **H(ome):** Household composition; family dynamics and relationships with adolescent; living/sleeping arrangements; guns in the home.
2. **E(ducation):** School attendance/absences; ever failed a grade(s); grades as compared to previous years; attitude toward school; favorite, most difficult, best subjects; special educational needs; goals for the future, including vocational/technical school, college, career.
3. **A(ctivities):** Physical activity, exercise, hobbies, sports participation, job, weapon carrying, and fighting.
4. **D(rugs):** Cigarettes/smokeless tobacco: age at first use, packs per day; alcohol and/or other drugs: use at school or parties, use by friends, type of substance (i.e., beer, wine coolers), frequency, and quantity used. If yes, administer CAGE questionnaire: Have you ever felt the need to **C**ut down; have others **A**nnoyed you by commenting on your use; have you ever felt **G**uilty about your use; have you ever needed an **E**yeopener (alcohol first thing in morning)? Any affirmative answer on CAGE indicates high risk of alcoholism/dependence and requires further assessment.
5. **S(exuality):** Sexual feelings toward opposite or same sex; sexual intercourse: age at first intercourse, number of lifetime and current partners, age of partners, recent change in partners; contraception/sexually transmitted disease (STD) prevention; history of STDs, prior pregnancies, abortions/ever fathered a child; history of nonconsensual intimate physical contact/sex.
6. **S(uicide)/depression:** Feelings about self, both positive and negative; history of depression or other mental health problems, prior suicidal thoughts, prior suicide attempts; sleep problems: difficulty getting to sleep, early waking.

TABLE 5-1

ADOLESCENT ANNUAL HEALTH MAINTENANCE VISITS

Age (years)	11	12	13	14	15	16	17	18	19	20	21
HISTORY	•	•	•	•	•	•	•	•	•	•	•
MEASUREMENTS											
Height and weight	•	•	•	•	•	•	•	•	•	•	•
Blood pressure	•	•	•	•	•	•	•	•	•	•	•
SENSORY SCREEN											
Vision	S	O	S	S	O	S	S	O	S	S	S
Hearing	S	O	S	S	O	S	S	O	S	S	S
BEHAVIOR ASSESSMENT											
HEADSS and CAGE	•	•	•	•	•	•	•	•	•	•	•
PHYSICAL EXAMINATION	•	•	•	•	•	•	•	•	•	•	•
GENERAL PROCEDURES											
Immunization[a]	Td	Td	—	—	—	—	—	—	—	—	—
Hematocrit or hemoglobin	*	*	*	*	*	*	*	*	*	*	*
Urinalysis	#	#	#	#	#	#	#	#	#	#	#

AT RISK PROCEDURES

Tuberculin test (PPD)	◆	◆	◆	◆	◆	◆	◆	◆
Cholesterol screening	◆	◆	◆	◆	◆	◆	◆	◆
STD screening (includes HIV and syphilis)	◆	◆	◆	◆	◆	◆	◆	◆
Pelvic examination	◆	◆	◆	◆	◆	◆	◆	◆

ANTICIPATORY GUIDANCE

Injury prevention	•	•	•	•	•	•	•	•
Violence prevention	•	•	•	•	•	•	•	•
Nutrition counseling	•	•	•	•	•	•	•	•
Sexuality (abstinence/contraception)	•	•	•	•	•	•	•	•
Substance abuse prevention	•	•	•	•	•	•	•	•

Modified from AAP Practice Guidelines. Pediatrics 2000; 105(3):645 with additions from Joffe A. Adolescent medicine. In Oski FA et al. Principles and practice of pediatrics. Philadelphia: JB Lippincott; 1999.

•, To be performed; ◆, to be performed for patients at risk; S, subjective, by history; O, objective, by standard testing; *, all menstruating females should be screened at least once, consider annual screen if symptoms or history of anemia; #, all sexually active adolescents should be screened annually; —, update or complete immunizations.

[a] Td booster should be given at age 11 or 12.

E. PHYSICAL EXAMINATION (MOST PERTINENT ASPECTS)

1. **Skin:** Acne (type and distribution of lesions), piercings, tattoos.
2. **Thyroid.**
3. **Spine:** Scoliosis (see Section V, p. 109).
4. **Breasts:** Tanner stage (Fig. 5-1), masses.
5. **External genitalia.**
   a. Pubic hair distribution: Tanner stage (Figs. 5-2 and 5-3).
   b. Testicular examination: Tanner stage (Table 5-2), masses (hydrocele, varicocele, hernia).
6. **Pelvic examination:** For any age female who is sexually active and/or has a gynecologic complaint; suggest to all females ages 18 to 21 that a screening Papanicolaou (PAP) smear be obtained.

F. LABORATORY TESTS

1. **Purified protein derivative (PPD):** If patient is high risk for tuberculosis, see Chapter 16 for screening recommendations.

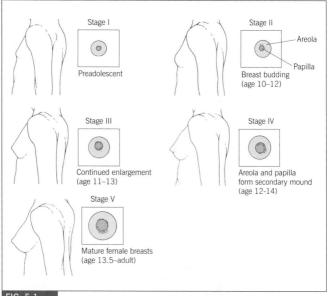

FIG. 5-1

Tanner stages of breast development in females. *(Modified from Johnson TR, Moore WM, Jefferies JE. Children are different: development physiology, 2nd ed. Columbus, Ohio: Ross Laboratories, Division of Abbott Laboratories; 1978. Age range [one standard deviation around mean] from Oski FA et al. Principles and practice of pediatrics. Philadelphia: JB Lippincott; 1999 and Marshall WA, Tanner JM. Variations in pattern of pubertal changes in girls. Arch Dis Child 1969; 44:291.)*

2. **Hemoglobin/hematocrit:** Levels should be obtained once during puberty for males, and at least once after menarche for females.
3. **Sexually active adolescents:** Serologic tests for syphilis and human immunodeficiency virus (HIV) should be obtained annually.
a. Males: First-part voided urinalysis/leukocyte esterase screen with positive results confirmed by detection tests for gonorrhea and chlamydia (i.e., cultures, ligase/polymerase chain reaction [PCR]).
b. Females: Detection tests for gonorrhea and chlamydia (i.e., cultures, LCR/PCR), wet preparation, potassium hydroxide (KOH), cervical Gram's stain, PAP smear, mid-vaginal pH.

G. IMMUNIZATIONS

See Chapter 15 for dosing, route, formulation, and schedules.
1. **Tetanus and diphtheria (Td):** Booster at age 11 to 12 years.
2. **Measles:** Two doses of live attenuated vaccine are required after the first birthday. Use measles, mumps, rubella (MMR) vaccine if not previously

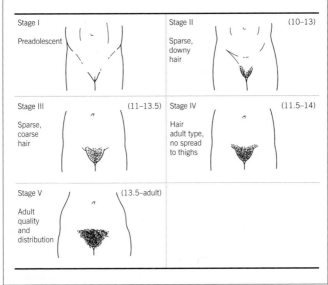

Stage I			Stage II		(10–13)
Preadolescent			Sparse, downy hair		
Stage III		(11–13.5)	Stage IV		(11.5–14)
Sparse, coarse hair			Hair adult type, no spread to thighs		
Stage V		(13.5–adult)			
Adult quality and distribution					

FIG. 5-2

Tanner stages of pubic hair development in females. *(Modified from Neinstein LS. Adolescent health care: a practical guide, 2nd ed. Baltimore: Urban & Schwarzenberg; 1991, with age range [one standard deviation around mean] from Oski FA et al. Principles and practice of pediatrics. Philadelphia: JB Lippincott; 1999 and Marshall WA, Tanner JM. Variations in pattern of pubertal changes in girls. Arch Dis Child 1969; 44:291.)*

ADOLESCENT MEDICINE

5

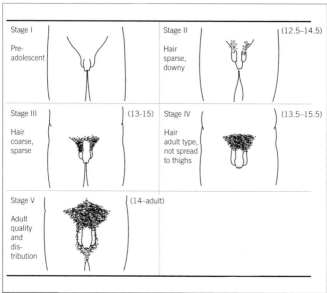

FIG. 5-3

Pubic hair development in males. Tanner stages 1-5 with age range. *(Modified from Neinstein LS. Adolescent health care: a practical guide, 2nd ed. Baltimore: Urban & Schwarzenberg; 1991. Age range from Marshall WA, Tanner JM: Arch Dis Child 1970; 45:13.)*

TABLE 5-2

GENITAL DEVELOPMENT (MALE)

Stage	Comment (One standard deviation around mean age)
I	*Preadolescent:* Testes, scrotum, and penis about same size and proportion as in early childhood
II	Enlargement of scrotum and testes; skin of scrotum reddens and changes in texture; little or no enlargement of penis (10.5-12.5)
III	Enlargement of penis, first mainly in length; further growth of testes and scrotum (11.5-14)
IV	Increased size of penis with growth in breadth and development of glans; further enlargement of testes and scrotum and increased darkening of scrotal skin (13.5-15)
V	Genitalia adult in size and shape (14-adult)

From Oski FA et al. Principles and practice of pediatrics. Philadelphia: JB Lippincott; 1999, as modified by Marshall WA, Tanner JM. Arch Dis Child 1969; 44:291 and Marshall WA, Tanner JM. Arch Dis Child 1970; 45:13.

immunized for mumps or rubella. Assess pregnancy status, and do not administer rubella vaccine to any woman anticipating pregnancy within 90 days.

3. **Hepatitis B vaccine (HBV):** Recommended for all adolescents if not previously vaccinated. Recent data indicate that a two-dose HBV vaccination regimen (Recombivax NB 10 mcg/1.0 mL given at 0 and 4 to 6 months) may be as effective as the standard three-dose regimen.[3]

4. **Varicella vaccine:** Two doses at least 1 month apart are recommended for adolescents over 13 years of age with no history of disease.

H. ANTICIPATORY GUIDANCE

See Table 5-1.

5

II. PUBERTAL EVENTS AND TANNER STAGE DIAGRAMS

The temporal interrelationship of the biologic and psychosocial events of adolescence are illustrated in Figs. 5-1 to 5-4 and Table 5-2. Age limits for the events and stages are approximations and may differ from those used by other authors.

III. CONTRACEPTIVE INFORMATION

A. METHODS OF CONTRACEPTION (Table 5-3)

B. ORAL CONTRACEPTIVE PILL (OCP) INFORMATION

1. **OCP contraindications** (for all OCPs containing estrogen).[4]

a. *Refrain from providing* (World Health Organization [WHO] category 4): Patients with a history of thrombophlebitis/thromboembolic disease, stroke, ischemic (coronary) heart disease, complicated structural heart disease, breast cancer, estrogen-dependent neoplasia, liver disease (including liver cancer, benign hepatic adenoma, active viral hepatitis, severe cirrhosis), diabetes with complications, headaches with focal neurologic symptoms, major surgery with prolonged immobilization, any surgery on the legs, hypertension with pressures 160+/100+ mmHg.

b. *Exercise caution* (WHO category 3): Undiagnosed abnormal vaginal/ uterine bleeding, use of drugs that affect liver enzymes, gallbladder disease.

c. *Advantages generally outweigh disadvantages* (WHO category 2): Headaches without focal neurologic symptoms, diabetes without complications, major surgery without prolonged immobilization, sickle cell disease, moderate hypertension (140-159/100-109 mmHg), undiagnosed breast mass, mental retardation, drug or alcohol abuse, severe psychiatric disorders.

2. **Instructions for use.**

a. Sunday start is the most common method.

b. Start with a low-dose estrogen pill (≤30 to 35 mcg).

c. 21 days hormone pills, 7 days inactive pills.

d. Advise patient about need for back-up methods during first month of use and need for STD prevention.

ADOLESCENT MEDICINE

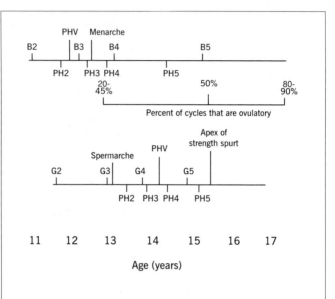

FIG. 5-4

Pubertal events and Tanner stages. *B,* Breast (stage); *G,* genital (stage); *PH,* pubic hair (stage); *PHV,* peak height velocity. *(Modified from Joffe A. Adolescent medicine. In Oski FA et al. Principles and practice of pediatrics. Philadelphia: JB Lippincott; 1999.)*

e. Another method of contraception should be used if more than two consecutive pills are missed in any menstrual cycle.

f. A pelvic examination is recommended at baseline or during first 3 to 6 months of use, then annually.

g. Two to three follow-up visits per year are recommended to monitor patient compliance, blood pressure, and side effects.

3. **Complications** (ACHES).

a. **A**bdominal pain (pelvic vein/mesenteric vein thrombosis, pancreatitis).

b. **C**hest pain (pulmonary embolism).

c. **H**eadaches (thrombotic/hemorrhagic stroke, retinal vein thrombosis).

d. **E**ye symptoms (thrombotic/hemorrhagic stroke, retinal vein thrombosis).

e. **S**evere leg pain (thrombophlebitis of the lower extremity).

TABLE 5-3

METHODS OF CONTRACEPTION

Method	Failure Rate in Typical User (%)	Benefits	Risk/Disadvantages
HORMONAL			
Combined oral contraceptives*	3.0 (may be increased among adolescents)	Intercourse independent; decreased risk of dysmenorrhea, benign breast disorders, rheumatoid arthritis, iron deficiency anemia, ovarian and uterine cancers, ovarian cysts, acne, ectopic pregnancy	Thromboembolic phenomena, cerebrovascular accident, hypertension, worsening of migraines, nausea, weight gain, breakthrough bleeding, amenorrhea, depression
Injectable contraceptives (Depo-Provera)	0.3	Intercourse independent, long-acting (3 mo), can be used when breast-feeding, no estrogen, decreased risk of endometrial/ovarian cancer, no drug interactions	Injection every 3 mo, delayed return to fertility, menstrual irregularity/amenorrhea, weight gain, reversible osteopenia, mood changes
(Lunelle)†	0.1–1.0	Benefits same as with oral combined hormonal contraceptives, long-acting (1 mo)	Same as with OCPs, monthly injections
NONHORMONAL			
Condom	12.0	No major risks, low cost, nonprescription, male involvement, protects against STD and cervical cancer	Decreased sensation, use with each act of coitus; polyurethane condoms are now available for those with latex allergy
Diaphragm with contraceptive cream or jelly	18.0	Some protection against many STDs	Allergy (rare), toxic shock syndrome (rare), increased incidence of urinary tract infection, vaginal ulceration, requires motivation
Spermicide	21.0	Nonprescription, no major medical risks, some STD protection	Allergy (rare), use related to coitus

Modified from Wilson MD. Adolescent pregnancy and contraception. In Oski FA et al. Principles and practice of pediatrics. Philadelphia: JB Lippincott; 1994.

*See pp. 105–106 for further information on oral contraceptive pills.

†Lunelle for Healthcare Professionals. Pharmacia and Upjohn Inc; 2001.

Note: Progestin-only pills and Norplant are generally not recommended for use in adolescents. Hormonal methods of birth control do not afford protection against STDs. Intrauterine device and natural family planning are generally not recommended for adolescents.

ADOLESCENT MEDICINE 5

TABLE 5-4			
EMERGENCY CONTRACEPTIVE PILL			
Trade Name	Ethinyl Estradiol Per Dose (mg)	Levonorgestrel Per Dose (mg)	Pills Per Dose
Ovral	0.1	0.5	2 white
Lo-Ovral	0.12	0.6	4 white
Nordette	0.12	0.6	4 light-orange
Levlen	0.12	0.6	4 light-orange
Triphasil	0.12	0.5	4 yellow
Trilevlen	0.12	0.5	4 yellow
Alesse	0.1	0.5	5 pink
Plan B*	0	0.75	1 white
Preven*	0.1	0.5	2 blue

Modified from Brill SR, Rosenfeld WD. Med Clin North Am, Adolesc Med 2000; 84:12.
*Manufactured solely for the purpose of emergency contraception

C. EMERGENCY CONTRACEPTIVE PILL (ECP) (Table 5-4)

1. Instructions for use.[4]

a. To reduce the chance of nausea, recommend patient take diphenhydramine 1 hour before the first dose of ECPs.

b. A pregnancy test should be administered to check for preexisting pregnancy before the patient takes an ECP.

c. The first ECP dose should be taken as soon as possible, within 72 hours after unprotected sex. There is a linear relationship between efficacy and the time from intercourse to treatment.[5]

d. The second ECP dose should be taken 12 hours after the first dose; the patient should not take any extra pills.

e. The patient should use only one type of pill.

f. Recommend the use of condoms, spermicides, or a diaphragm during sex after taking ECPs until the next menstrual period; ensure proper use of regular birth control for the future.

g. Perform pregnancy test if there is no menstrual period within 3 weeks of ECP treatment.

IV. VAGINAL INFECTIONS, GENITAL ULCERS, AND WARTS

See Chapter 16 for discussion of infection with *Chlamydia* sp., gonorrhea, pelvic inflammatory disease (PID), HIV, and further discussion of syphilis. See Part IV, Formulary, for additional information and comments regarding specific medications. After diagnosis of an STD, encourage the patient to refrain from intercourse until full therapy is complete, the partner is treated, and all visible lesions are resolved.

A. DIAGNOSTIC FEATURES AND MANAGEMENT OF VAGINAL INFECTION (Table 5-5)

B. DIAGNOSTIC FEATURES AND MANAGEMENT OF GENITAL ULCERS AND WARTS (Table 5-6)

V. SCOLIOSIS[6]

Refer to Fig. 5-5 for routine screening for scoliosis. Many curves that are detected on screening are nonprogressive and/or too slight to be significant.

A. ASSESSMENT

1. **Radiographic determination of the Cobb angle** (Fig. 5-6): If clinical suspicion exists of significant scoliosis, use erect thoracoabdominal spinal view.
2. **Bone scan +/− magnetic resonance imaging (MRI):** If there is pain that is worse at night, progressive, well localized, or otherwise suspicious, obtain bone scan or MRI.
3. **MRI:** If patient is less than 10 years old, or "opposite" curves are present (left-sided thoracic, right-sided lumbar), obtain an MRI.

B. TREATMENT

Treatment plan is determined according to the Cobb angle and skeletal maturity, which is assessed by grading the ossification of the iliac crest.

1. **Skeletally immature.**
   a. <10 Degrees: Obtain a single follow-up radiograph in 4 to 6 months to ensure there has been no significant progression of the scoliosis.
   b. 10 to 20 Degrees: Obtain follow-up radiographs every 4 to 6 months.
   c. 20 to 40 Degrees: Bracing is required.
   d. >40 Degrees: Surgical correction is necessary.
2. **Skeletally mature.**
   a. <40 Degrees: No further evaluation or intervention is indicated.
   b. >40 Degrees: Surgical correction is required.
3. **Orthopedic referral** is indicated if the patient is skeletally immature with a curve >20 degrees, skeletally mature with a curve >40 degrees, and/or in the presence of suspicious pain or neurologic symptoms.

VI. RECOMMENDED COMPONENTS OF THE PREPARTICIPATION PHYSICAL EVALUATION

A. MEDICAL HISTORY

The medical history should include information regarding illnesses or injuries since the last examination or preparticipation physical examination (PPE); chronic conditions and medications; hospitalizations or surgeries; medications used by athletes (including those they may be taking to enhance performance); use of any special equipment or protective devices during sports participation; allergies, particularly those associated with anaphylaxis or respiratory compromise and those provoked by exercise; immunization status, including hepatitis B, MMR, tetanus, and varicella.

B. REVIEW OF SYSTEMS/PHYSICAL EXAMINATION ITEMS[7]

Examination items are in italics.

1. **Height and weight.**
2. **Vision:** Visual problems, corrective lenses; *visual acuity*.
3. **Cardiac:** History of congenital heart disease; symptoms of syncope, dizziness, or chest pain during exercise; history of high blood pressure or

TABLE 5-5
DIAGNOSTIC FEATURES AND MANAGEMENT OF VAGINAL INFECTIONS

	Normal Vaginal Examination	Yeast Vaginitis	Trichomoniasis	Bacterial Vaginosis
Etiology	Uninfected; *Lactobacillus* predominant	*Candida albicans* and other yeasts	*Trichomonas vaginalis*	Associated with *Gardnerella vaginalis*, various anaerobic bacteria, and mycoplasma
Typical symptoms	None	Vulvar itching and/or irritation, increased discharge	Malodorous purulent discharge, vulvar itching	Malodorous, slightly increased discharge
DISCHARGE				
Amount	Variable; usually scant	Scant to moderate	Profuse	Moderate
Color*	Clear or white	White	Yellow-green	Usually white or gray
Consistency	Nonhomogeneous, floccular	Clumped; adherent plaques	Homogeneous	Homogeneous, low viscosity; smoothly coating vaginal walls
Inflammation of vulvar or vaginal epithelium	No	Yes	Yes	No
pH of vaginal fluid†	Usually <4.5	Usually <4.5	Usually >5.0	Usually >4.5
Amine ("fishy") odor with 10% KOH	None	None	May be present	Present

	Normal	Candidiasis	Trichomoniasis	Bacterial vaginosis
Microscopy[‡]	Normal epithelial cells; Lactobacillus predominate	Leukocytes, epithelial cells, yeast, mycelia, or pseudomycelia in 40%-80% of cases	Leukocytes; motile trichomonads seen in 50%-70% of symptomatic patients, less often in the absence of symptoms	Clue cells; few leukocytes; Lactobacillus outnumbered by profuse mixed flora, nearly always including G. vaginalis plus anaerobic species, on Gram's stain
Usual treatment	None	Single dose of oral fluconazole, or miconazole or clotrimazole vaginal suppository	Metronidazole, single dose or 7-day course	Oral or topical metronidazole or oral clindamycin
Note: Refer to Formulary for dosing information				
Usual management of sex partners	None	None; topical treatment if candidal dermatitis of penis is present	Treatment recommended	Examine for STD; routine treatment not recommended

From Holmes KK et al. Sexually transmitted diseases. New York: McGraw-Hill; 1990 and Centers for Disease Control and Prevention. MMWR 1998; 47(RR-1):1-118.

*Color of discharge is determined by examining vaginal discharge against the white background of a swab.

†pH determination is not useful if blood is present.

‡To detect fungal elements, vaginal fluid is digested with 10% KOH before microscopic examination; to examine for other features, fluid is mixed (1:1) with physiologic saline.

Note: Gram's stain is also excellent for detecting yeasts and pseudomycelia and for distinguishing normal flora from the mixed flora seen in bacterial vaginosis, but it is less sensitive than the saline preparation for detection of T. vaginalis.

ADOLESCENT MEDICINE **5**

TABLE 5-6

DIAGNOSTIC FEATURES AND MANAGEMENT OF GENITAL ULCERS AND WARTS

Infection	Clinical Presentation	Presumptive Diagnosis	Definitive Diagnosis	Treatment/Management of Sex Partners
Genital herpes	Grouped vesicles, painful shallow ulcers; tender inguinal adenopathy	Tzanck smear looking for multinucleated giant cells	Viral culture	No known cure. Prompt initiation of therapy shortens duration of first episode. For severe recurrent disease, initiate therapy at start of prodrome or within 1 day of onset of lesions. See formulary for dosing of acyclovir, famciclovir, or valacyclovir. Transmission can occur during asymptomatic periods.
Primary syphilis	Indurated, well defined, usually single painless ulcer or "chancre"; nontender inguinal adenopathy	Nontreponemal serologic test: VDRL, RPR, or STS	Treponemal serologic test: FTA-ABS or MHA-TP; darkfield microscopy or direct fluorescent antibody tests of lesion exudates or tissue	Parenteral penicillin G is preferred treatment; preparation(s), dosage, and length of treatment depend on stage and clinical manifestations (see Chapter 16). All sexual contacts of persons with acquired syphilis should be evaluated. Contacts within the previous 3 months may be falsely seronegative; presumptive treatment recommended.
HPV infection (genital warts)	Single or multiple soft, fleshy, papillary or sessile, painless growth around the anus, vulvovaginal area, penis, urethra, or perineum; no inguinal adenopathy	Typical clinical presentation	Papanicolaou smear revealing typical cytologic changes	Treatment does not eradicate infection. *Goal:* Removal of exophytic warts. Exclude cervical dysplasia before treatment. Patient-administered therapies include podofilox and imiquimod cream. Clinician-applied therapies include podophyllin 10%–25% in compound tincture of benzoin, bichloroacetic or trichloroacetic acid, and surgical removal. Podofilox, imiquimod, and podophyllin are contraindicated in pregnancy. Period of communicability is unknown.

NOTE: Chancroid, lymphogranuloma venereum (LGV), and granuloma inguinale should be considered in the differential diagnosis of genital ulcers if the clinical presentation is atypical and testing for herpes and syphilis are negative.

Modified from Centers for Disease Control and Prevention. MMWR 1998; 47(RR-1):1-118 and Adger H. Sexually transmitted diseases. In Oski FA et al: Principles and practice of pediatrics, Philadelphia: Lippincott, Williams & Wilkins; 1999.

FTA-ABS, Fluorescent treponemal antibody absorbed; *HPV,* human papilloma virus; *MHA-TP,* microhemagglutination assay for antibody to *T. pallidum; RPR,* rapid plasma reagin; *STS,* serologic test for syphilis; *VDRL,* Venereal Disease Research Laboratory.

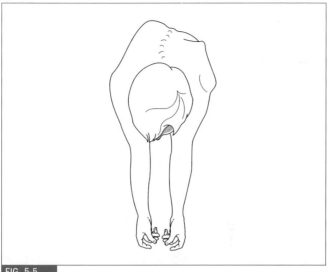

FIG. 5-5

Forward bending test. This emphasizes any asymmetry of the paraspinous muscles and rib cage.

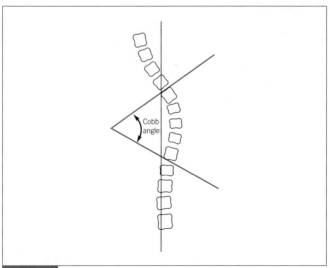

FIG. 5-6

Cobb angle. This is measured using the superior and inferior endplates of the most tilted vertebrae at the end of each curve.

5

ADOLESCENT MEDICINE

heart murmurs; family history of heart disease; previous history of disqualification or limited participation in sports because of a cardiac problem; *blood pressure, heart rate and rhythm, pulses (including radial/femoral lag), auscultation for heart sounds, murmurs.*

4. **Respiratory:** Asthma, coughing, wheezing, or dyspnea during exercise.
5. **Genitourinary:** Age at menarche, last menstrual period, regularity of menstrual periods, number of periods in the last year, longest interval between periods, dysmenorrhea; *palpation of the abdomen, palpation of the testicles, examination of the inguinal canals.*
6. **Orthopedic:** Previous injuries that have limited sports participation; injuries that have been associated with pain, swelling, or the need for medical intervention; *screening orthopedic examination* (Fig. 5-7).
7. **Neurology:** History of a significant head injury or concussion; numbness or tingling in the extremities; severe headaches; seizure disorder.
8. **Psychosocial:** Weight control and body image; stresses at home or in school; use or abuse of drugs and alcohol; *attention to signs of eating disorders, including oral ulcerations, eroded tooth enamel, edema, lanugo hair, calluses/ulcerations on knuckles.*

VII. SPORTS INJURIES[s]

A. SHOULDER[8] (Fig. 5-8)

1. **Clavicular fracture:** Obtain chest radiograph to rule out pneumothorax; treat with sling for 3 weeks followed by restriction from sports for 3 weeks. Consider figure-8 bandage for optimal alignment, but this is usually unnecessary to achieve adequate healing.
2. **Separation:** Laxity of the acromioclavicular joint; usually occurs secondary to a fall and directly landing on the shoulder or an outstretched hand. Examination may reveal a positive crossover test (pain when patient reaches across chest to touch contralateral shoulder) and localized pain, crepitus, and/or swelling; conservative management with a sling is adequate in lower-grade (most) injuries.
3. **Dislocation:** Displacement of the humeral head from the glenoid socket, usually anteriorly. Patient often holds injured arm in abduction and external rotation (if posterior dislocation, arm is usually held across the chest). There is usually obvious asymmetry and deformity, with limited range of motion. Neurovascular status may be compromised (usually axillary nerve; impaired sensation over lateral aspect of shoulder). With first-time dislocation, anteroposterior, lateral, and axillary/scapular radiographs are necessary to rule out fracture. Immediate reduction is indicated to minimize neurovascular injury; referral to an orthopedist or sports medicine physician is indicated for further evaluation.
4. **Subluxation:** Repetitive partial dislocation, indicating unidirectional or multidirectional instability. May involve anterior (apprehension with abduction and external rotation), posterior (excessive movement with posteromedial force on elbow while shoulder/elbow are flexed at 90 degrees), and/or inferior (sulcus sign [dimple over deltoid with humeral

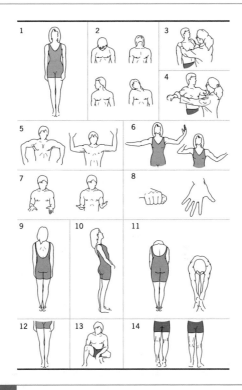

FIG. 5-7

Screening orthopedic examination. The general musculoskeletal screening examination consists of the following: (1) Inspection, athlete standing, facing examiner (symmetry of trunk, upper extremities); (2) forward flexion, extension, rotation, lateral flexion of neck (range of motion, cervical spine); (3) resisted shoulder shrug (strength, trapezius); (4) resisted shoulder abduction (strength, deltoid); (5) internal and external rotation of shoulder (range of motion, glenohumeral joint); (6) extension and flexion of elbow (range of motion, elbow); (7) pronation and supination of elbow (range of motion, elbow and wrist); (8) clenching of fist, then spreading of fingers (range of motion, hand and fingers); (9) inspection, athlete facing away from examiner (symmetry of trunk, upper extremities); (10) back extension, knees straight (spondylolysis/spondylolisthesis); (11) back flexion with knees straight, facing toward and away from examiner (range of motion, thoracic and lumbosacral spine; spine curvature; hamstring flexibility); (12) inspection of lower extremities, contraction of quadriceps muscles (alignment symmetry); (13) "duck walk" four steps (motion of hips, knees, and ankles; strength; balance); (14) standing on toes, then on heels (symmetry, calf; strength; balance). *(Modified from American Academy of Family Physicians. Preparticipation physical examination, 2nd ed. Kansas City, MO: American Academy of Family Physicians; 1997.)*

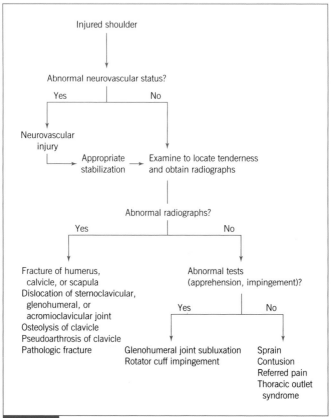

FIG. 5-8

Approach to the patient with an injured shoulder. *(From Fleisher GR, Ludwig S, editors. Textbook of pediatric emergency medicine, 4th ed. Philadelphia: Lippincott, Williams & Wilkins; 2000.)*

distraction]) instability. Physical therapy is indicated (strengthening only, not flexibility); some instability may require surgical correction.

5. **"Little League Shoulder:"**[9] Stress fracture through the proximal humeral physis; patient is usually 10 to 14 years old, with insidious onset of shoulder pain with motion. Examination may reveal generalized weakness and limited active range of motion in abduction and external and internal rotation. Radiographs can show widening of the proximal humeral physis with fragmentation and sclerosis.

6. **Impingement syndrome:**[10] Anterior shoulder pain is present only when the shoulder is abducted to 90 degrees. Supraspinatus tendinitis is secondary to chronic anterior glenohumeral instability. Tenderness is apparent over the greater tuberosity; there is pain with forward shoulder flexion/adduction (impingement test). Treat with rest, nonsteroidal anti-inflammatory drugs (NSAIDs), physical therapy, and ice after activity.

B. KNEE

Must also evaluate for hip pathology (Fig. 5-9).

1. **Instability.**

a. Anterior cruciate ligament: Likely history of falling on a hyperextended leg, or twisting a knee while the foot is planted. There is usually a large effusion, with or without blood, within the initial few hours after injury and limited or exaggerated range of motion. Administer the Lachman test (usually helpful only in the acute setting before compensation by hamstrings; with patient supine and knee flexed 20 to 30 degrees, evaluate excursion and endpoint when displacing the tibia anteriorly with one hand on the tibia and the other on the distal femur) and pivot shift (more helpful with older injuries; patient is supine with the knee extended and in slight valgus, and the foot/tibia internally rotated; a positive test equals pain with progressive knee flexion).

b. Posterior cruciate ligament (less common): Posterior drawer test (one hand on the femur, the other on the tibia; laxity when pushing the tibia posteriorly), step-off, posterior/tibial sag sign (backward subluxation of the tibia on the femur with patient supine and muscles relaxed, knee flexed 90 degrees, and hip flexed 45 degrees).

c. Medial/lateral collateral ligaments: There is usually a history of direct contact at the lateral knee; patient has pain and tenderness with palpation, and varus/valgus stress to the knee at 0 and 30 degrees.

d. Medial/lateral menisci: There is usually a history of twisting motion. May have effusion, tenderness to palpation at joint line with knee flexed 90 degrees, positive McMurray test (with knee fully flexed, rotate externally/internally; apply varus stress to the knee by pushing/pulling ankle medially while stabilizing the femur and then the knee and extend to 90 degrees; repeat using valgus stress to the knee by pushing/pulling ankle laterally, then extend 90 degrees; pain and a palpable click or grinding indicate a positive test). If there is limited extension, refer patient to an orthopedist for likely "bucket-handle" tear.

e. Management for instability: Rest, crutches, ice, NSAIDs, and immobilization; referral to an orthopedist is indicated if there is severe injury, persistent pain, or instability.

2. **Osgood-Schlatter apophysitis:** Knee pain and tenderness over tibial tuberosities (greater than 50% bilateral) with occasional avulsion; most common with open tibial physes (usually between 6 and 16 years); radiographs, which are necessary only if clinical presentation is unclear, are usually normal with soft tissue swelling but may reveal an avulsion

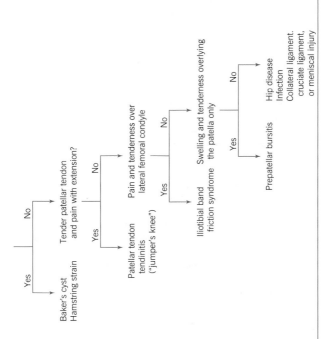

FIG. 5-9

Approach to the patient with a subacute knee injury. *(From Fleisher GR, Ludwig S, editors. Textbook of pediatric emergency medicine, 4th ed. Philadelphia: Lippincott, Williams & Wilkins; 2000.)*

ADOLESCENT MEDICINE **5**

or occult pathology; conservative management with NSAIDs and relative rest is sufficient.

3. **Osteochondritis dissecans (OCD):** Partial or complete separation of hyaline cartilage from supporting bone, most common in the distal femur/medial femoral condyle. Most cases occur in teenage years. Symptoms include increasing pain with activity and a positive Wilson test (flex knee 90 degrees and rotate tibia internally; anterior knee pain just before full extension, relieved by external rotation of tibia). Radiographs (including notch or tunnel view for femoral condyles) may show sclerosis or fragmentation. Nonoperative treatment with a non-weight-bearing cylinder cast is often successful with open physes, otherwise fragment removal and/or fixation may be necessary.

4. **Patellar instability:** Dislocation of patella out of the trochlear groove, usually from direct contact or pivoting maneuver. Accompanied by pain, swelling, and occasionally crepitus, which is often recurrent with disruption of the medial retinaculum. Patient is usually apprehensive before attempted patellar distraction; there is pain over the medial adductor tubercle. Radiographs should include a "sunrise" view; management includes symptomatic treatment and rehabilitation with flexibility and strength training; surgery is recommended if persistent hypermobility exists.

5. **Patellofemoral dysfunction:** Includes malalignment, lateral patellar compression syndrome (LPCS), and chondromalacia. There is a gradual onset of pain, and a possible history of overuse or distant trauma; pain is usually caused by squatting maneuvers, going up and down stairs, and prolonged knee flexion ("theater sign"); examination may reveal muscle tightness or crepitus. Radiographs may be helpful and may show patellar variants. Management should focus on physical therapy with strengthening and flexibility exercises.

C. **FOOT/ANKLE**

1. **Sprains.**

a. Sprains are classified as grade I (stretching, minor ligamentous injury), grade II (partial tear of anterior talofibular [ATF] ligament), and grade III (complete ligamentous disruption with inability to bear weight).

b. Examination includes anterior drawer test (integrity of ATF ligament) and talar tilt (inversion stress to heel and ankle, integrity of calcaneofibular ligament); palpation must include first and fifth metatarsophalangeal (MTP) joints and metatarsal heads, navicular and peroneal tubercles, head and dome of talus, bilateral malleoli, calcaneus, sinus tarsi (anterior to lateral malleolus), ligaments (anterior/posterior talofibular, calcaneofibular, deltoid), tendons, and proximal tibia/fibula.

c. Look for hidden injuries, including high sprain, disruption of syndesmosis (squeeze distal fibular shaft toward tibia, palpate interosseus membrane), Maisonneuve fracture with diastasis of mortise and fibular fracture, and subtalar sprain.

d. Radiographs (anteroposterior [AP], lateral, and oblique) are recommended if there is pain near the malleoli, inability to bear weight, and point tenderness at the posterior edge or tip of either malleolus. Tenderness over the navicular, cuboid, and base of the fifth metatarsal should prompt additional views of the foot.[11]

e. Conservative management with RICE (rest, ice for 24 to 48 hours, compression with elastic wrap and stirrup or posterior ankle splint, and elevation) and avoidance of weight bearing by using crutches for at least 48 to 72 hours is recommended. Also important is early stress-controlled rehabilitation (maintain proprioception, strength). There is infrequent indication for application of a weight-bearing cast with grade III injuries. Persistent pain may indicate anterolateral soft tissue impingement or occult fracture. Repetitive injury may result from peroneal weakness or loss of subtalar motion.

2. **Severe (calcaneal) apophysitis:** Inflammation of the open calcaneal growth plate. Heel pain with direct pressure, medial-lateral compression. Conservative management with ice, NSAIDs, heel cup, orthotics, and Achilles tendon stretching is warranted. Evaluate older adolescents for stress fracture.

3. **Islen apophysitis:** Traction apophysitis, overuse osteochondritis, and inflammation of fifth metatarsal tuberosity. Conservative management (ice, NSAIDs, arch support, foot taping) is warranted; healing can be complicated by nonunion and/or intermittent pain.

4. **Accessory navicular:** Normal variant (5% to 10% incidence); can cause medial ankle pain, usually chronic and insidious, that worsens with activity. Evaluation can include tenderness on palpation of ossicle and visualization of ossicle on radiographs. Conservative management is initially indicated, using orthotics and NSAIDs; a walking cast can be applied if there is an acute fracture, or surgery is necessary if treatment fails.

5. **Fractures:** Indications for radiographic examination include point tenderness and inability to bear weight; management includes non-weight-bearing immobilization; refer patient to an orthopedist for casting and definitive management.

D. CLOSED HEAD TRAUMA

See Chapter 4 for treatment of concussions and return-to-play guidelines.

5

ADOLESCENT MEDICINE

REFERENCES

1. Joffe A. Adolescent medicine. In Oski FA et al. Principles and practice of pediatrics. Philadelphia: JB Lippincott; 1999.
2. AAP Practice Guidelines. Recommendations for preventive pediatric health care. Pediatrics 2000; 105(3):645.
3. Cassidy WM et al. A randomized trial of alternative two- and three-dose hepatitis B vaccine regimens in adolescents. Pediatrics 2001; 10(11):626-631.
4. Hatcher RA et al: Contraceptive technology, 17th rev. ed. New York: Ardent Media, Inc; 1998: 420-424.

5. Brill SR, Rosenfeld WD. Contraception. Med Clin North Am, Adolesc Med 2000; 84:12.
6. Kautz SM, Skaggs DL. Getting an angle on spinal deformities. Contemp Pediatr 1998; 15: 112-289.
7. Andrews J. Making the most of the sports physical. Contemp Pediatr 1997; 14:182-205.
8. Glockner SM. Shoulder pain: a diagnostic dilemma. Am Fam Physician 1995; 51(7): 1677-1687, 1690-1692.
9. Gomez JE. Injuries unique to young athletes. Paper presented at the 22nd Annual Sports Medicine Symposium, The University of Wisconsin-Madison, May 7, 1999.
10. Oski FA et al. Principles and practice of pediatrics. Philadelphia: JB Lippincott; 1999.
11. Morrisy RT, Weinstein SC. Lovell and Winter's pediatric orthopedics. Philadelphia: Lippincott-Raven Publishers; 1996.

CARDIOLOGY

Brett H. Siegfried, MD and Tara O. Henderson, MD

6

I. WEBSITES

www.americanheart.org (Open the Heart and Stroke Encyclopedia)
www.cincinnatichildrens.org/heartcenter/encyclopedia/

II. THE CARDIAC CYCLE (Fig. 6-1)

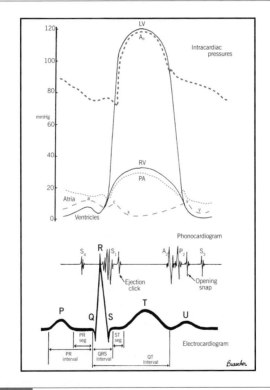

FIG. 6-1

The cardiac cycle.

III. PHYSICAL EXAMINATION

A. PRESSURE

1. **Pulse pressure** = Systolic pressure − Diastolic pressure.

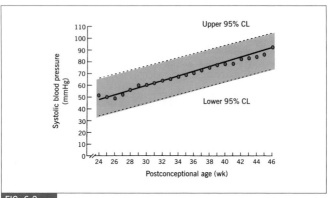

FIG. 6-2

Linear regression of mean systolic blood pressure on postconceptional age (gestational age in weeks + weeks after delivery). *(From Zubrow AB et al. J Perinatol 1995; 15:470.)*

a. If pulse pressure is wide (>40 mmHg), consider thyrotoxicosis, arteriovenous (AV) fistula, patent ductus arteriosus (PDA), or aortic insufficiency.

b. If pulse pressure is narrow (<25 mmHg), consider pericarditis, pericardial effusion, pericardial tamponade, aortic stenosis (AS), or significant tachycardia.

2. **Mean arterial pressure (MAP)** = Diastolic pressure + (Pulse pressure/3). In preterm infants and newborns, generally a normal MAP = gestational age in weeks + 5.

3. **Blood pressure**

a. Four limb blood pressures can be used to assess for coarctation of the aorta; pressure must be measured in both the right and left arm because of the possibility of an aberrant subclavian artery.

b. Pulsus paradoxus is an exaggeration of the normal drop in systolic blood pressure (SBP) seen with inspiration. Determine the SBP at the end of exhalation and then during inhalation; if the difference in SBP is greater than 10 mmHg, consider pericardial effusion, tamponade, pericarditis, severe asthma, or restrictive cardiomyopathies.

c. See Figs. 6-2 to 6-6[1,2] and Tables 6-1 and 6-2 for blood pressure norms.

B. HEART SOUNDS

1. **S1 is best heard at the apex or left lower sternal border (LLSB).** Wide splitting is unusual in children and may suggest Ebstein's anomaly or right bundle-branch block (RBBB).

2. **S2, heard best at the left upper sternal border (LUSB), has a normal physiologic split that increases with inspiration.** If the S2 split is wide and fixed, consider volume overload from an atrial septal defect (ASD)

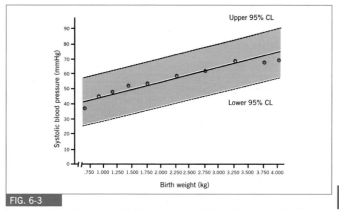

FIG. 6-3

Linear regression of mean systolic blood pressure on birth weight on day 1 of life.
(From Zubrow AB et al. J Perinatol 1995; 15:470.)

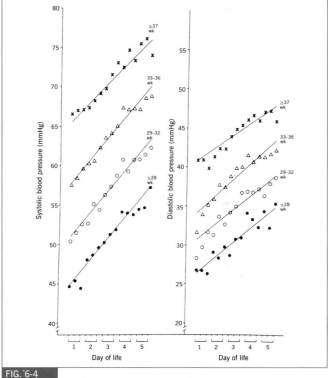

FIG. 6-4

Systolic and diastolic blood pressure in the first 5 days of life. *(From Zubrow AB et al. J Perinatol 1995; 15:470.)*

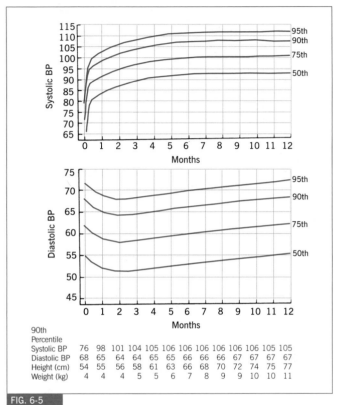

FIG. 6-5

Age-specific percentile of blood pressure (BP) measurements in girls from birth to 12 months of age; Korotkoff phase IV (K4) used for diastolic BP. *(From Horan MJ et al. Pediatrics 1987; 79(1):1-25.)*

90th Percentile												
Systolic BP	76	98	101	104	105	106	106	106	106	106	106	105	105
Diastolic BP	68	65	64	64	65	65	66	66	66	67	67	67	67
Height (cm)	54	55	56	58	61	63	66	68	70	72	74	75	77
Weight (kg)	4	4	4	5	5	6	7	8	9	9	10	10	11

or partial anomalous pulmonary venous return (PAPVR), valve abnormalities as in pulmonary stenosis (PS), electrical delay from RBBB, early aortic closure from mitral regurgitation (MR), or normal variation. Conditions that delay aortic valve closure or accelerate pulmonic valve closure will narrow S2. Examples are pulmonary hypertension, AS, left bundle branch block (LBBB), and normal variant (Box 6-1, p. 132).[3]

3. **S3, heard best at the apex or LLSB, can be commonly heard in healthy children and adults but may also be seen in patients with dilated ventricles (large ventricular septal defect [VSD] or congestive heart failure [CHF]).**

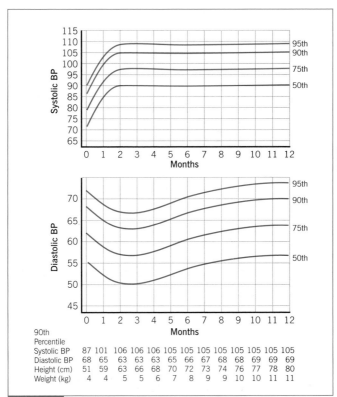

FIG. 6-6

Age-specific percentiles of blood pressure (BP) measurements in boys from birth to 12 months of age; Korotkoff phase IV (K4) used for diastolic BP. *(From Horan MJ et al. Pediatrics 1987; 79(1):1-25.)*

4. S4, heard at the apex, is always considered pathologic and suggests decreased ventricular compliance.

C. SYSTOLIC AND DIASTOLIC SOUNDS

1. **An ejection click sounds like splitting of the S1 but is most audible at the apex rather than at the LLSB.** The ejection click is associated with stenosis of the semilunar valves and large great arteries (e.g., systemic hypertension; pulmonary hypertension; idiopathic dilation of the pulmonary artery [PA]; tetralogy of Fallot [TOF], in which the aorta is dilated; and persistent truncus arteriosus).

Text continued on p. 132

TABLE 6-1

BLOOD PRESSURE LEVELS FOR THE 90TH AND 95TH PERCENTILES OF BLOOD PRESSURE FOR GIRLS AGED 1-17 YEARS BY PERCENTILES OF HEIGHT

Age (yr)	Height* → BP† ↓	Systolic BP (mmHg) by Percentile of Height							Diastolic BP (DBP) (mmHg) by Percentile of Height						
		5%	10%	25%	50%	75%	90%	95%	5%	10%	25%	50%	75%	90%	95%
1	90th	97	98	99	100	102	103	104	53	53	53	54	55	56	56
	95th	101	102	103	104	105	107	107	57	57	57	58	59	60	60
2	90th	99	99	100	102	103	104	105	57	57	58	58	59	60	61
	95th	102	103	104	105	107	108	109	61	61	62	62	63	64	65
3	90th	100	100	102	103	104	105	106	61	61	61	62	63	63	64
	95th	104	104	105	107	108	109	110	65	65	65	66	67	67	68
4	90th	101	102	103	104	106	107	108	63	63	64	65	65	66	67
	95th	105	106	107	108	109	111	111	67	67	68	69	69	70	71
5	90th	103	103	104	106	107	108	109	65	66	66	67	68	68	69
	95th	107	107	108	110	111	112	113	69	70	70	71	72	72	73
6	90th	104	105	106	107	109	110	111	67	67	68	69	69	70	71
	95th	108	109	110	111	112	114	114	71	71	72	73	73	74	75
7	90th	106	107	108	109	110	112	112	69	69	69	70	71	72	72
	95th	110	110	112	113	114	115	116	73	73	73	74	75	76	76
8	90th	108	109	110	111	112	113	114	70	70	71	71	72	73	74
	95th	112	112	113	115	116	117	118	74	74	75	75	76	77	78

Age	BP %ile	SBP							DBP						
9	90th	110	110	112	113	114	115	116	71	72	72	73	74	74	75
	95th	114	114	115	117	118	119	120	75	76	76	77	78	78	79
10	90th	112	112	114	115	116	117	118	73	73	73	74	75	75	76
	95th	116	116	117	119	120	121	122	77	77	77	78	79	79	80
11	90th	114	114	116	117	118	119	120	74	74	74	75	76	76	77
	95th	118	118	119	121	122	123	124	78	78	78	79	80	80	81
12	90th	116	116	118	119	120	121	122	75	75	75	76	77	77	78
	95th	120	120	121	123	124	125	126	79	79	79	80	81	81	82
13	90th	118	118	119	121	122	123	124	76	76	76	77	78	78	78
	95th	121	122	123	125	126	127	128	80	80	80	81	82	82	82
14	90th	119	120	121	122	124	125	126	77	77	77	78	79	79	80
	95th	123	124	125	126	128	129	130	81	81	81	82	83	83	84
15	90th	121	121	122	124	125	126	127	78	78	78	79	80	80	81
	95th	124	125	126	128	129	130	131	82	82	82	83	84	84	85
16	90th	122	122	123	125	126	127	128	79	79	79	80	81	81	82
	95th	125	126	127	129	130	131	132	83	83	83	84	85	85	86
17	90th	122	123	124	125	126	128	128	79	79	79	80	81	81	82
	95th	126	126	127	129	130	131	132	83	83	83	84	85	85	86

*Height percentile determined by standard growth curves.

†Blood pressure percentile determined by a single measurement.

6

CARDIOLOGY

TABLE 6-2

BLOOD PRESSURE LEVELS FOR THE 90TH AND 95TH PERCENTILES OF BLOOD PRESSURE FOR *BOYS* AGED 1-17 YEARS BY PERCENTILES OF HEIGHT

Age (yr)	Height* → BP† ↓	Systolic BP (mmHg) by Percentile of Height							Diastolic BP (DBP) (mmHg) by Percentile of Height						
		5%	10%	25%	50%	75%	90%	95%	5%	10%	25%	50%	75%	90%	95%
1	90th	94	95	97	98	100	102	102	50	51	52	53	54	54	55
	95th	98	99	101	102	104	106	106	55	55	56	57	58	59	59
2	90th	98	99	100	102	104	105	106	55	55	56	57	58	59	59
	95th	101	102	104	106	108	109	110	59	59	60	61	62	63	63
3	90th	100	101	103	105	107	108	109	59	59	60	61	62	63	63
	95th	104	105	107	109	111	112	113	63	63	64	65	66	67	67
4	90th	102	103	105	107	109	110	111	62	62	63	64	65	66	66
	95th	106	107	109	111	113	114	115	66	67	67	68	69	70	71
5	90th	104	105	106	108	110	112	112	65	65	66	67	68	69	69
	95th	108	109	110	112	114	115	116	69	70	70	71	72	73	74
6	90th	105	106	108	110	111	113	114	67	68	69	70	70	71	72
	95th	109	110	112	114	115	117	117	72	72	73	74	75	76	76
7	90th	106	107	109	111	113	114	115	69	70	71	72	72	73	74
	95th	110	111	113	115	116	118	119	74	74	75	76	77	78	78
8	90th	107	108	110	112	114	115	116	71	71	72	73	74	75	75
	95th	111	112	114	116	118	119	120	75	76	76	77	78	79	80

9	90th	109	110	112	113	115	117	117	72	73	73	74	75	76	77
	95th	113	114	116	117	119	121	121	76	77	77	79	80	80	81
10	90th	110	112	113	115	117	118	119	73	74	74	75	76	77	78
	95th	114	115	117	119	121	122	123	77	78	78	79	80	81	82
11	90th	112	113	115	117	119	120	121	74	74	75	76	77	78	78
	95th	116	117	119	121	123	124	125	78	79	79	80	81	82	83
12	90th	115	116	118	120	121	123	123	75	75	76	77	78	78	79
	95th	119	120	121	123	125	126	127	79	79	80	81	82	83	83
13	90th	117	118	120	122	124	125	126	75	76	76	77	78	79	80
	95th	121	122	124	126	128	129	130	79	80	81	82	83	83	84
14	90th	120	121	123	125	126	128	128	76	76	77	78	79	80	80
	95th	124	125	127	128	130	132	132	80	81	81	82	83	84	85
15	90th	123	124	125	127	129	131	131	77	77	78	79	80	81	81
	95th	127	128	129	131	133	134	135	81	82	83	83	84	85	86
16	90th	125	126	128	130	132	133	134	79	79	80	81	82	82	83
	95th	129	130	132	134	136	137	138	83	83	84	85	86	87	87
17	90th	128	129	131	133	134	136	136	81	81	82	83	84	85	85
	95th	132	133	135	136	138	140	140	85	85	86	87	88	89	89

*Height percentile determined by standard growth curves.
†Blood pressure percentile determined by a single measurement.

6

CARDIOLOGY

BOX 6-1	
SUMMARY OF ABNORMAL S2	
ABNORMAL SPLITTING	
Widely Split and Fixed S2	
Volume overload (e.g., ASD, PAPVR)	
Abnormal pulmonary valve (e.g., PS)	
Electrical delay (e.g., RBBB)	
Early aortic closure (e.g., MR)	
Occasional normal child	
Narrowly Split S2	
Pulmonary hypertension	
AS	
LBBB	
Occasional normal child	
Single S2	
Pulmonary hypertension	
One semilunar valve (e.g., pulmonary atresia, aortic atresia, truncus arteriosus)	
P2 not audible (e.g., TGA, TOF, severe PS)	
Severe AS	
Occasional normal child	
Paradoxically Split S2	
Severe AS	
LBBB, Wolff-Parkinson-White syndrome (type B)	
ABNORMAL INTENSITY OF P2	
Increased P2 (e.g., pulmonary hypertension)	
Decreased P2 (e.g., severe PS, TOF, TS)	

From Park MK. Pediatric cardiology for practitioners, 3rd ed. St. Louis: Mosby; 1996. *PAPVR*, Partial anomalous pulmonary venous return; *MR*, mitral regurgitation; *LBBB*, left bundle-branch block; *TS*, tricuspid stenosis; *ASD*, atrial septal defect; *PS*, pulmonary stenosis; *RBBB*, right bundle-branch block; *AS*, aortic stenosis; *TGA*, transposition of the great arteries; *TOF*, tetralogy of Fallot.

2. A midsystolic click with or without a late systolic murmur is heard near the apex in mitral valve prolapse (MVP).
3. Diastolic opening snap is audible at the apex or LLSB in mitral stenosis.

D. **MURMURS**[4]

1. **Benign heart murmurs are caused by a disturbance of the laminar flow of blood,** frequently produced as the diameter of the blood's pathway decreases and the velocity increases. Over 80% of children have innocent murmurs sometime during childhood, most commonly beginning around age 3 or 4. All innocent murmurs are accentuated in high-output states, especially with fever and anemia, and are associated with normal electrocardiogram (ECG) and radiographic findings. However, note that an ECG and chest radiograph are not routinely useful

TABLE 6-3
COMMON INNOCENT HEART MURMURS

Type (Timing)	Description of Murmur	Age Group
Classic vibratory murmur (Still's murmur; systolic)	Maximal at MLSB or between LLSB and apex Grade 2-3/6 in intensity Low-frequency vibratory, twanging string, groaning, squeaking, or musical	3-6 yr; occasionally in infancy
Pulmonary ejection murmur (systolic)	Maximal at ULSB Early to midsystolic Grade 1-3/6 in intensity Blowing in quality	8-14 yr
Pulmonary flow murmur of newborn (systolic)	Maximal at ULSB Transmits well to left and right chest, axillae, and back Grade 1-2/6 in intensity	Premature and full-term newborns Usually disappears by 3-6 mo of age
Venous hum (continuous)	Maximal at right (or left) supraclavicular and infraclavicular areas Grade 1-3/6 in intensity Inaudible in supine position Intensity changes with rotation of head and disappears with compression of jugular vein	3-6 yr
Carotid bruit (systolic)	Right supraclavicular area over carotids Grade 2-3/6 in intensity Occasional thrill over carotid	Any age

From Park MK. Pediatric cardiology for practitioners, 3rd ed. St. Louis: Mosby, 1996.
LLSB, Lower left sternal border; *MLSB,* middle left sternal border; *ULSB,* upper left sternal border.

6

CARDIOLOGY

or cost-effective screening tools for distinguishing benign from pathologic murmurs. Clinical characteristics of these murmurs are summarized in Table 6-3.[3] When one or more of the following are present, the murmur is likely to be pathologic and require cardiac consultation:
- Symptoms
- Cyanosis
- Systolic murmur that is loud (grade 3/6 or with a thrill) and long in duration
- Diastolic murmur
- Abnormal heart sounds
- Abnormally strong or weak pulses
2. **Systolic murmurs** (Fig. 6-7)
3. **Diastolic murmurs** (see Fig. 6-7)

IV. ELECTROCARDIOGRAPHY
A. BASIC ELECTROCARDIOGRAPHY PRINCIPLES
1. **Lead placement** (Fig. 6-8): For pediatric ECGs, V3R is typically recorded instead of V3 (i.e., V1, V2, V3R, V4, V5, V6).

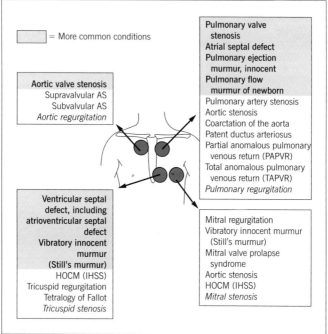

FIG. 6-7

The location at which various murmurs may be heard. Diastolic murmurs are in italics. *AS,* Aortic stenosis; *HOCM,* hypertrophic obstructive cardiomyopathy; *IHSS,* idiopathic hypertrophic subaortic stenosis. *(From Park MK. Pediatric cardiology for practitioners, 3rd ed. St. Louis: Mosby; 1996.)*

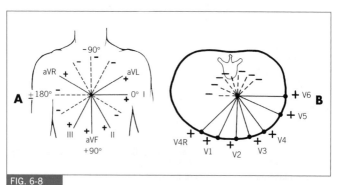

FIG. 6-8

A, Hexaxial reference system. **B,** Horizontal reference system. *(Modified from Park MK, Guntheroth WG. How to read pediatric ECGs, 3rd ed. St. Louis: Mosby; 1992.)*

2. **ECG complexes** (see Fig. 6-1)
a. P wave: Represents atrial depolarization.
b. QRS complex: Represents ventricular depolarization.
c. T wave: Represents ventricular repolarization.
d. U wave: May follow T wave, representing late phases of ventricular repolarization.
3. **Systematic approach for evaluating ECGs:** (See Table 6-4 for normal ECG parameters.)[3,5]
a. Rate
   (1) Standardization: Paper speed is 25 mm/sec. One small square = 1 mm = 0.04 sec. One large square = 5 mm = 0.2 sec. Amplitude standard: 10 mm = 1 millivolt.
   (2) Calculation: Heart rate (beats per minute) = 60 divided by the average R-R interval in seconds, or 1500 divided by the R-R interval in millimeters.
b. Rhythm
   (1) Sinus rhythm: Every QRS complex is preceded by a P wave, normal PR interval (the PR interval may be prolonged, as in first-degree atrioventricular [AV] block), and normal P wave axis (upright P in lead I and aVF).
   (2) There is normal respiratory variation of the R-R interval without morphologic changes of the P wave or QRS complex.
c. Axis: Determine quadrant and compare with age-matched normal values (Fig. 6-9; see Table 6-4).
d. Intervals: (PR, QRS, QT_c). See Table 6-4 for normal PR and QRS intervals. The QT_c is calculated as:

$$QT_c = QT\ (sec)/\sqrt{\text{R-R(sec)}}$$

The R-R interval should extend from the R wave in the QRS complex in which you are measuring QT to the preceding R wave. Normal values for QT_c:
   (1) 0.440 sec is 97th percentile for infants 3 to 4 days old[6]
   (2) ≤0.45 sec in infants <6 months old
   (3) ≤0.44 sec in children
   (4) ≤0.44 sec in adults
e. P-wave size and shape: Normal P wave should be <0.10 sec in children, <0.08 sec in infants, with amplitude <30 mV (3 mm in height, with normal standardization).
f. R-wave progression: There is generally a normal increase in R-wave size and decrease in S-wave size from leads V1 to V6 (with dominant S waves in right precordial leads and dominant R waves in left precordial leads), representing dominance of left ventricular forces. However, newborns and infants have a normal dominance of the right ventricle.
g. Q waves: Normal Q waves are usually <0.04 second (1 mm) in duration and less than 25% of the total QRS amplitude. Q waves are <5mm

6

CARDIOLOGY

TABLE 6-4
NORMAL PEDIATRIC ECG PARAMETERS

Age	Heart Rate (bpm)	QRS Axis*	PR Interval (sec)*	QRS Duration (sec)†	Lead V$_1$			Lead V$_6$		
					R Wave Amplitude (mm)†	S Wave Amplitude (mm)†	R/S Ratio	R Wave Amplitude (mm)†	S Wave Amplitude (mm)†	R/S Ratio
0-7 days	95-160 (125)	+30 to 180 110	0.08-0.12 (0.10)	0.05 (0.07)	13.3 (25.5)	7.7 (18.8)	2.5	4.8 (11.8)	3.2 (9.6)	2.2
1-3 wk	105-180 (145)	+30 to 180 110	0.08-0.12 (0.10)	0.05 (0.07)	10.6 (20.8)	4.2 (10.8)	2.9	7.6 (16.4)	3.4 (9.8)	3.3
1-6 mo	110-180 (145)	+10 to +125 (+70)	0.08-0.13 (0.11)	0.05 (0.07)	9.7 (19)	5.4 (15)	2.3	12.4 (22)	2.8 (8.3)	5.6
6-12 mo	110-170 (135)	+10 to +125 (+60)	0.10-0.14 (0.12)	0.05 (0.07)	9.4 (20.3)	6.4 (18.1)	1.6	12.6 (22.7)	2.1 (7.2)	7.6
1-3 yr	90-150 (120)	+10 to +125 (+60)	0.10-0.14 (0.12)	0.06 (0.07)	8.5 (18)	9 (21)	1.2	14 (23.3)	1.7 (6)	10
4-5 yr	65-135 (110)	0 to +110 (+60)	0.11-0.15 (0.13)	0.07 (0.08)	7.6 (16)	11 (22.5)	0.8	15.6 (25)	1.4 (4.7)	11.2
6-8 yr	60-130 (100)	-15 to +110 (+60)	0.12-0.16 (0.14)	0.07 (0.08)	6 (13)	12 (24.5)	0.6	16.3 (26)	1.1 (3.9)	13
9-11 yr	60-110 (85)	-15 to +110 (+60)	0.12-0.17 (0.14)	0.07 (0.09)	5.4 (12.1)	11.9 (25.4)	0.5	16.3 (25.4)	1.0 (3.9)	14.3
12-16 yr	60-110 (85)	-15 to +110 (+60)	0.12-0.17 (0.15)	0.07 (0.10)	4.1 (9.9)	10.8 (21.2)	0.5	14.3 (23)	0.8 (3.7)	14.7
>16 yr	60-100 (80)	-15 to +110 (+60)	0.12-0.20 (0.15)	0.08 (0.10)	3 (9)	10 (20)	0.3	10 (20)	0.8 (3.7)	12

New data compiled from Park MK. Pediatric cardiology for practitioners, 3rd ed. St Louis: Mosby; 1996 and Davignon A et al. Pediatr Cardiol 1979; 1:123-131.
*Normal range and (mean).
†Mean and (98th percentile).

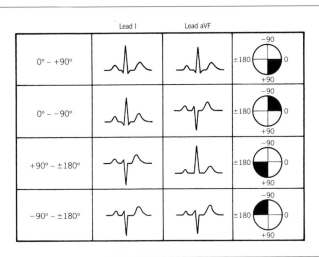

FIG. 6-9

Locating quadrants of mean QRS axis from leads 1 and aVF. *(From Park MK, Guntheroth WG. How to read pediatric ECGs, 3rd ed. St. Louis: Mosby; 1992.)*

6

CARDIOLOGY

TABLE 6-5

NORMAL T-WAVE AXIS

Age	V1, V2	AVF	I, V5, V6
Birth-1 day	±	+	±
1-4 days	±	+	+
4 days to adolescent	−	+	+
Adolescent to adult	+	+	+

+, T wave positive; −, T wave negative; ±, T wave normally either positive or negative.

deep in left precordial leads and aVF and ≤8 mm deep in lead III for children <3 years of age.

h. ST-segment and T-wave evaluation: ST-segment elevation or depression >1 mm in limb leads and >2 mm in precordial leads is consistent with myocardial injury. Tall, peaked T waves may be seen in hyperkalemia. Flat or low T waves may be seen in hypokalemia, hypothyroidism, normal newborn, and in myocardial and pericardial ischemia and inflammation (Table 6-5 and Fig. 6-10).

i. Hypertrophy.

(1) Atrial: See Fig. 6-11

(2) Ventricular: Diagnosed by QRS axis, voltage, and R/S ratio (see Table 6-4).

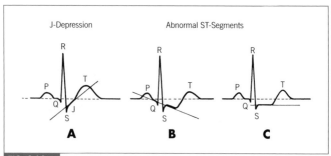

FIG. 6-10

Nonpathologic (nonischemic) and pathologic (ischemic) ST and T changes. **A,** Characteristic nonischemic ST segment alteration called *J depression;* note that the ST slope is upward. **B** and **C,** Ischemic or pathologic ST segment alterations. **B,** Downward slope of the ST segment. **C,** Horizontal segment is sustained. *(From Park MK, Guntheroth WG. How to read pediatric ECGs, 3rd ed. St. Louis: Mosby; 1992.)*

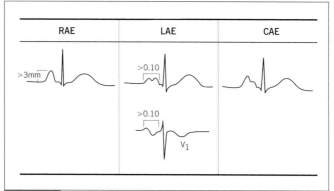

FIG. 6-11

Criteria for atrial enlargement. *CAE,* combined atrial enlargement; *LAE,* left atrial enlargement; *RAE,* right atrial enlargement. *(From Park MK. Pediatric cardiology for practitioners, 3rd ed. St. Louis: Mosby; 1996.)*

(a) Right ventricular hypertrophy (RVH) criteria (at least one of the following):
  (i) Increased right and anterior QRS voltage (with normal QRS duration):
    • R in lead V1 >98th percentile for age.
    • S in lead V6 >98th percentile for age.
  (ii) Upright T wave in lead V1 after 3 days of age to adolescence.
  (iii) Supplemental criteria include presence of q wave in V1 (qR or qRs pattern), right axis deviation (RAD) for patient's age, and right ventricle (RV) strain (associated with inverted T wave in V1 with tall R wave).
(b) Left ventricular hypertrophy (LVH) criteria:
  (i) Increased QRS voltage in left leads (with normal QRS duration):
    • R in lead V6 (and I, aVL, V5) >98th percentile for age.
    • S in lead V1 >98th percentile for age.
  (ii) Supplemental criteria include left axis deviation (LAD) for patient's age, volume overload (associated with Q wave >5 mm and tall T waves in V5 or V6), and left ventricle (LV) strain (associated with inverted T wave in leads V6, I, or aVF).

B. ECG ABNORMALITIES
1. **Nonventricular arrhythmias** (Table 6-6)[7]
2. **Ventricular arrhythmias** (Table 6-7): Abnormal rhythm resulting from ectopic focus in ventricles. Characterized by wide QRS complex, T wave in opposite direction to QRS, random relation of QRS to P wave (i.e., AV dissociation); see Fig. 6-13.
3. **Nonventricular conduction disturbances** (Table 6-8, Fig. 6-14)[8]
4. **Ventricular conduction disturbance** (Table 6-9): Abnormal transmission of electrical impulse through ventricles leading to prolongation of QRS complex (≥0.08 second for infants, ≥0.10 second for adults)

C. MYOCARDIAL INFARCTION IN CHILDREN
1. **Etiology:** Myocardial infarction (MI) in children is rare but could occur in children with anomalous origin of the left coronary artery, Kawasaki disease, congenital heart disease (presurgical and postsurgical), and dilated cardiomyopathy. It is rarely seen in children with hypertension, lupus, myocarditis, cocaine ingestion, and use of adrenergic drugs (e.g., β-agonists used for asthma).
2. **Frequent ECG findings in children with acute MI**[9]
a. New-onset wide Q waves (>0.035 sec), with or without Q-wave notching, seen within first few hours (and persistent over several years).
b. ST segment elevation (>2 mm), seen within first few hours.
c. Diphasic T waves, seen within first few days (becoming sharply inverted, then normalizing over time).

Text continued on p. 145

6

CARDIOLOGY

TABLE 6-6

NONVENTRICULAR ARRHYTHMIAS

Name/Description	Cause	Treatment
SINUS		
Tachycardia		
Normal sinus rhythm with HR >95th percentile for age (usually less than 230 beats/min)	Hypovolemia, shock, anemia, sepsis, fever, anxiety, CHF, PE, myocardial disease, drugs (e.g., β-agonists, aminophylline, atropine)	Address underlying cause
Bradycardia		
Normal sinus rhythm with HR <5th percentile for age	Normal (especially in athletic individuals), increased ICP, hypoxia, hyperkalemia, hypercalcemia, vagal stimulation, hypothyroidism, hypothermia, drugs (e.g., digoxin, β-blockers), long QT syndrome	Address underlying cause; if symptomatic, **refer to inside back cover for bradycardia algorithm**
SUPRAVENTRICULAR		
Abnormal rhythm resulting from ectopic focus in atria or AV node, or from accessory conduction pathways. Characterized by varying P-wave shape and abnormal P-wave axis. QRS morphology usually normal. See Fig. 6-12.[7]		
Premature Atrial Contraction		
Narrow QRS. Ectopic focus in atria or in AV node. Abnormal P wave and normal QRS	Digitalis toxicity, medications (e.g., caffeine, theophylline, sympathomimetics)	Treat digitalis toxicity, otherwise no treatment needed
Atrial Flutter		
Atrial rate between 250 and 350 beats/min, yielding characteristic sawtooth or flutter pattern (no discrete P waves) with variable ventricular response rate and normal QRS complex	Dilated atria, previous intraatrial surgery, valvular or ischemic heart disease, digitalis toxicity	Digoxin ± β-blockers, synchronized cardioversion or overdrive pacing; treat underlying cause (consult cardiologist)

6

TABLE 6-6		
NONVENTRICULAR ARRHYTHMIAS—cont'd		
Name/Description	Cause	Treatment
SUPRAVENTRICULAR—cont'd		
Atrial Fibrillation		
Ectopic atrial foci with atrial rate between 350 and 600 beats/min, yielding characteristic fibrillatory pattern (no discrete P waves) and irregularly irregular ventricular response rate of about 110-150 beats/min with normal QRS complex	See above	See Atrial Flutter (p. 140), may need anticoagulation pretreatment
SVT		
Sudden run of three or more premature supraventricular beats at >230 beats/min, with narrow QRS complex and abnormal P wave. Either sustained (>30 sec) or unsustained.	Most commonly idiopathic but may be seen in congenital heart disease (e.g., Ebstein's anomaly, transposition)	Vagal maneuvers, adenosine; if unstable, need immediate synchronized cardioversion (0.5 j/kg up to 1 j/kg). Consult cardiologist. **See "Tachycardia with Poor Perfusion" and "Tachycardia with Adequate Perfusion" algorithms in back of handbook.**
I. AV Reentrant: Presence of accessory bypass pathway, in conjunction with AV node, establishes cyclic pattern of signal reentry, independent of SA node. Most common cause of nonsinus tachycardia in children (see "Wolff-Parkinson-White syndrome").		
II. AV nodal/junctional: Cyclical reentrant pattern resulting from dual AV node pathways. Simultaneous depolarization of atria and ventricles yields invisible P wave or retrograde P wave		
III. Ectopic atrial: Rapid firing of ectopic focus in atrium.		
Nodal Escape/Junctional Rhythm		
Abnormal rhythm driven by AV node impulse, giving normal QRS complex and invisible P wave (buried in preceding QRS or T wave) or retrograde P wave (negative in lead II, positive in aVR)		

AV, Atrioventricular; *CHF,* congestive heart failure; *HR,* heart rate; *ICP,* intracranial pressure; *PE,* pulmonary embolism; *SA,* sinoatrial; *SVT,* supraventricular tachycardia.

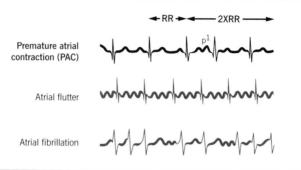

FIG. 6-12

Supraventricular arrhythmias. p^1, Premature atrial contraction. *(From Garson A Jr. The electrocardiogram in infants and children: a systematic approach. Philadelphia: Lea & Febiger; 1983.)*

TABLE 6-7

VENTRICULAR ARRHYTHMIAS

Name/Description	Cause	Treatment
PVC		
Ectopic ventricular focus causing early depolarization. Abnormally wide QRS complex appears prematurely, usually with full compensatory pause. May be unifocal or multifocal. **Bigeminy** is alternating normal and abnormal QRS complexes; **trigeminy** is two normal QRS complexes followed by an abnormal QRS complex. A **couplet** is two consecutive PVCs.	Myocarditis, myocardial injury, cardiomyopathy, long QT syndrome, congenital and acquired heart disease, drugs (e.g., digitalis, catecholamines, theophylline, caffeine, anesthetics), MVP, anxiety, hypokalemia, hypoxia, hypomagnesemia	More worrisome if associated with underlying heart disease, if worse with activity, if symptomatic, or if they are multiform (especially couplets). Address underlying cause, rule out structural heart disease.
VENTRICULAR TACHYCARDIA		
Series of three or more PVCs at rapid rate (120-250 beats/min), with wide QRS complex and dissociated, retrograde, or no P wave.	See above (70% have abnormal cardiac anatomy)	**See "Tachycardia with Poor Perfusion" and "Tachycardia with Adequate Perfusion" algorithms in back of handbook.**
VENTRICULAR FIBRILLATION		
Depolarization of ventricles in uncoordinated, asynchronous pattern, yielding abnormal QRS complexes of varying size and morphology with irregular, rapid rate. Rare in children.	Myocarditis, MI, postoperative state, digitalis or quinidine toxicity, catecholamines, severe hypoxia, electrolyte disturbances	**Requires immediate defibrillation. See algorithm for "Asystole and Pulseless Arrest" inside back cover.**

MI, Myocardial infarction; MVP, mitral valve prolapse; PVC, premature ventricular contraction.

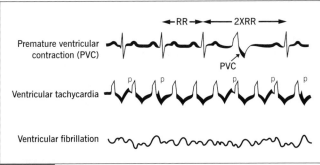

FIG. 6-13

Ventricular arrhythmias. *P,* P wave.

TABLE 6-8

Name/Description*	Cause	Treatment
NONVENTRICULAR CONDUCTION DISTURBANCES		
FIRST-DEGREE HEART BLOCK		
Abnormal but asymptomatic delay in conduction through AV node, yielding prolongation of PR interval	Acute rheumatic fever, tick-borne (i.e., Lyme) disease, connective tissue disease, congenital heart disease, cardiomyopathy, digitalis toxicity, postoperative state and normal children	None necessary except address the underlying cause
SECOND-DEGREE HEART BLOCK: MOBITZ TYPE I (WENCKEBACH)		
Progressive lengthening of PR interval until a QRS is not conducted and ventricular contraction does not occur. Does not usually progress to complete heart block.	Myocarditis, cardiomyopathy, congenital heart disease, postoperative state, MI, toxicity (digitalis, β-blocker), normal children	Address underlying cause
SECOND-DEGREE HEART BLOCK: MOBITZ TYPE II		
Paroxysmal skipped ventricular conduction without lengthening of the PR interval. Block is at the level of the bundle of His and may progress to complete heart block.	Same as for Mobitz Type I (not found in normal children)	Address underlying cause, may need pacemaker
THIRD-DEGREE (COMPLETE) HEART BLOCK		
Complete dissociation of atrial and ventricular conduction. P wave and PR interval regular; RR interval regular and much slower (driven by junctional or ectopic ventricular pacemaker with intrinsic rate of 30-50 beats/min). Width of QRS will be narrow with junctional pacemaker, wide with ventricular pacemaker.	Congenital, maternal lupus or other connective tissue disease, structural heart disease, or acquired (acute rheumatic fever, myocarditis, Lyme carditis, postoperative, cardiomyopathy, MI, drug overdose)	If bradycardic, consider pacing and **see "Bradycardia" algorithm on inside back cover.**

AV, Atrioventricular; *MI,* myocardial infarction.
*Higher AV block: Conduction of atrial impulse at regular intervals, yielding 2:1 block (two atrial impulses for each ventricular response), 3:1 block, etc.

TABLE 6-9 °

VENTRICULAR CONDUCTION DISTURBANCES

Name/Description	Criteria	Causes/Treatment
RIGHT BUNDLE BRANCH BLOCK (RBBB)		
Delayed right bundle conduction prolongs RV depolarization time, leading to wide QRS	1. RAD 2. Long QRS with terminal slurred R′ (M-shaped RSR′ or RR′) in V1, V2, aVR 3. Wide and slurred S wave in leads I and V6	ASD, surgery with right ventriculostomy, Ebstein's anomaly, coarctation in infants <6 mo, endocardial cushion defect, and partial anomalous pulmonary venous return; occasionally occurs in normal children
LEFT BUNDLE BRANCH BLOCK (LBBB)		
Delayed left bundle conduction prolongs septal and LV depolarization time, leading to wide QRS with loss of usual septal signal; there is still a predominance of left ventricle forces. Rare in children.	1. Wide negative QS complex in lead V1 with loss of septal R wave 2. Entirely positive wide R or RR′ complex in lead V6 with loss of septal Q wave	Hypertension, ischemic or valvular heart disease, cardiomyopathy
WOLFF-PARKINSON-WHITE (WPW)		
Atrial impulse transmitted via anomalous conduction pathway to ventricles, bypassing AV node and normal ventricular conduction system. Leads to premature and prolonged depolarization of ventricles. Bypass pathway is a predisposing condition for SVT.	1. Shortened PR interval 2. Delta wave 3. Wide QRS	Acute management of SVT if necessary as previously described; consider ablation of accessory pathway if recurrent SVT

ASD, Atrial septal defect; *AV,* atrioventricular; *LV,* left ventricle; *RAD,* right axis deviation; *RV,* right ventricle; *SVT,* supraventricular tachycardia.

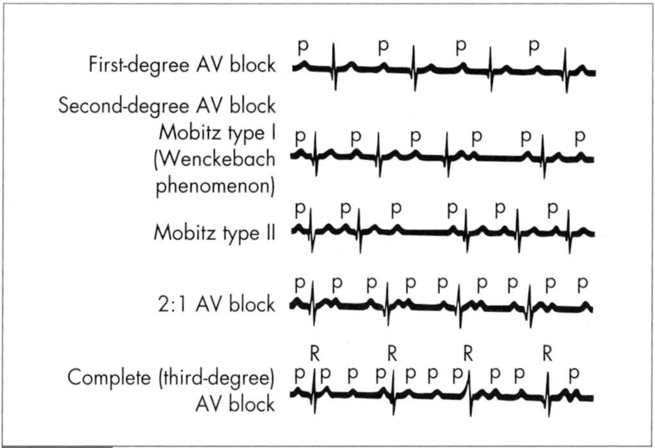

FIG. 6-14

Conduction blocks. *P,* P wave; *R,* QRS complex. *(From Park MK, Guntheroth WG. How to read pediatric ECGs, 3rd ed. St. Louis: Mosby; 1992.)*

d. Prolonged QT_c interval (>0.44 sec) with accompanying abnormal Q waves.
e. Deep, wide Q waves in leads I, aVL, or V6, without Q waves in II, III, aVF, suggestive of anomalous origin of the left coronary artery.

3. **Other criteria:**
a. An elevated creatine phosphokinase (CK)/MB fraction, although this is not specific for detection of acute MI in children.
b. Cardiac troponin I is likely to be a more sensitive indicator of early myocardial damage in children. It becomes elevated within hours of cardiac injury, persists for 4 to 7 days, and is specific for cardiac injury.[10]

D. **ECG FINDINGS SECONDARY TO ELECTROLYTE DISTURBANCES, MEDICATIONS, AND SYSTEMIC ILLNESSES**

1. **Digitalis**
a. Digitalis effect: Associated with shortened QT_c interval, ST depression ("scooped" or "sagging"), mildly prolonged PR interval, and flattened T wave.
b. Digitalis toxicity: Primarily arrhythmias (bradycardia, supraventricular tachycardia [SVT], ectopic atrial tachycardia, ventricular tachycardia, AV block).

2. **Other conditions:** Table 6-10.[7,11]

TABLE 6-10

SYSTEMIC EFFECTS ON ELECTROCARDIOGRAM

	Short QT	Long QT-U	Prolonged QRS	ST-T Changes	Sinus Tachycardia	Sinus Bradycardia	AV Block	Ventricular Tachycardia	Miscellaneous
CHEMISTRY									
Hyperkalemia			X	X			X	X	Low voltage Ps; peaked Ts
Hypokalemia	X	X	X	X					
Hypercalcemia	X					X	X		
Hypocalcemia		X			X			X	
Hypermagnesemia							X		
Hypomagnesemia		X							
DRUGS									
Digitalis	X			X		T	X	T	
Phenothiazines		T						T	
Phenytoin	X								
Propranolol	X					X	T		
Quinidine		X	X			T	T	T	
Tricyclics		T	T	T	T		T		

					T	
Verapamil				X		
Imipramine				X	T	Atrial flutter
MISCELLANEOUS						
CNS injury			X	X	T	
Freidreich's ataxia		X	X			Atrial flutter
Duchenne's muscular dystrophy		X	X			Atrial flutter
Myotonic dystrophy	X	X	X	X		
Collagen vascular disease		X	X	X	X	
Hypothyroidism			X	X		Low voltage
Hyperthyroidism	X	X	X			
Other diseases	Romano-Ward	Lyme disease	X	Holt-Oram, maternal lupus		

From Garson A Jr. The electrocardiogram in infants and children: a systematic approach. Philadelphia: Lea & Febiger; 1983 and Walsh EP. In Fyler DC, Nadas A, editors. Pediatric cardiology. Philadelphia: Hanley & Belfus; 1992.

CNS, Central nervous system; *T,* present only with drug toxicity; *X,* present.

V. IMAGING

A. CHEST RADIOGRAPH

1. Evaluate the heart

a. Size: The cardiac shadow should be less than 50% of the thoracic width, which is the maximal width between inner margins of the ribs, as measured on a posteroanterior (PA) radiograph during inspiration.

b. Shape: The shape of the heart can aid in the diagnosis of chamber/vessel enlargement and some congenital heart disease (CHD) (Fig. 6-15).

c. Situs (levocardia, mesocardia, dextrocardia).

2. Evaluate the lung fields

a. Decreased pulmonary blood flow is seen in pulmonary or tricuspid stenosis/atresia, TOF, pulmonary hypertension ("peripheral pruning").

b. Increased pulmonary blood flow can be seen as increased pulmonary vascular markings (PVMs) with redistribution from bases to apices of lungs and extension to lateral lung fields, as with large ASD, VSD, or PDA, transposition of the great arteries (TGA), and total anomalous pulmonary venous return (TAPVR).

c. Venous congestion, or congestive heart failure (CHF) causes increased PVMs centrally, interstitial and alveolar pulmonary edema (air bronchograms), septal lines, and pleural effusions, as with obstructed TAPVR and mitral valve stenosis/regurgitation.

3. Evaluate the airway: The trachea usually bends slightly to the right above the carina in normal patients with a left-sided aortic arch. A

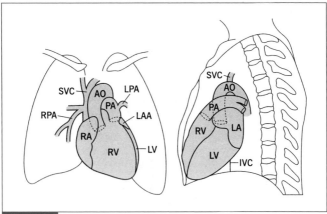

FIG. 6-15

Radiologic contours of the heart. *AO,* Aorta; *IVC,* inferior vena cava; *LA,* left atrium; *LAA,* left atrial appendage; *LPA,* left pulmonary artery; *LV,* left ventricle; *PA,* pulmonary artery; *RA,* right atrium; *RPA,* right pulmonary artery; *RV,* right ventricle; *SVC,* superior vena cava.

perfectly straight or left-bending trachea suggests a right aortic arch, which may be associated with other defects (TOF, truncus arteriosus, vascular rings, chromosome 22 microdeletion).

4. **Skeletal anomalies**

a. Rib notching (e.g., from collateral vessels in patients >5 years of age with coarctation of the aorta).

b. Sternal abnormalities (e.g., Holt-Oram syndrome; pectus excavatum in Marfan, Ehlers-Danlos, and Noonan syndromes).

c. Vertebral anomalies (e.g., VATER/VACTERL syndrome: **V**ertebral anomalies, **A**nal atresia, **T**racheo**E**sophageal fistula, **R**adial and **R**enal, **C**ardiac, and **L**imb anomalies).

NOTE: See Tables 6-12 and 6-13 for typical findings on a chest radiograph in CHD. Please see Chapter 23 for more information on the chest radiograph.

B. ECHOCARDIOGRAPHY

1. **Approach**

a. Transthoracic echocardiography (TTE) does not require general anesthesia, is simpler to perform than transesophageal echocardiography (TEE), but does have limitations in some patients (e.g., uncooperative, obese) or in patients with suspected valvular endocarditis.

b. TEE uses an ultrasound transducer on the end of a modified endoscope to view the heart from the esophagus and stomach, allowing for better imaging of the aorta, atria, and obese or intraoperative patients. TEE is also useful for visualizing valvular anatomy, including valvular vegetations.

2. **Shortening fraction:** Very reliable index of left ventricle (LV) function. Normal values range from approximately 30% to 45%, depending on age.[12]

VI. CONGENITAL HEART DISEASE

See Table 6-11 for common genetic syndromes associated with cardiac lesions.

TABLE 6-11
COMMON GENETIC SYNDROMES ASSOCIATED WITH CARDIAC DEFECTS

Syndrome	Dominant Cardiac Defect
CHARGE	Ventricular, atrioventricular, and ASDs
DiGeorge	Aortic arch anomalies, tetralogy of Fallot
Down	Atrioventricular septal defects, VSD
Marfan	Aortic root dissection, mitral valve prolapse
Noonan	Pulmonic stenosis, ASD
Turner	Coarctation of the aorta, bicuspid aortic valve
Williams	Supravalvular aortic stenosis

From Pelech AN: Pediatr Clin North Am 1999; 46(2):167-168.

ASD, Atrial septal defect; *CHARGE,* a syndrome of associated defects, including coloboma of the eye, heart anomaly, choanal atresia, retardation, and genital and ear anomalies; *VSD,* ventricular septal defect.

A. ACYANOTIC LESIONS (Table 6-12)
B. CYANOTIC LESIONS (Table 6-13)

An oxygen challenge test is used to evaluate the etiology of cyanosis in neonates. Obtain baseline arterial blood gas (ABG) with saturation at $FiO_2 = 0.21$, then place infant in an oxygen hood at $FiO_2 = 1$ for a minimum of 10 minutes, and repeat ABG. Pulse oximetry will not be useful for following the change in oxygenation once the saturations reach 100% (approximately $Pao_2 > 90$) (Table 6-14).[13-16] See Table 6-15 for acute management of hypercyanotic spells in Tetralogy of Fallot.

C. SURGICAL PROCEDURES

1. **Atrial septostomy:** Atrial septostomy creates an intraatrial opening to allow for mixing or shunting between atria (i.e., for TGA, tricuspid atresia, mitral atresia).

2. **Palliative systemic-to-pulmonary artery shunts** use systemic arterial flow to increase pulmonary blood flow in cardiac lesions with impaired pulmonary perfusion (e.g., TOF, hypoplastic right heart, tricuspid atresia, PS) (Fig. 6-16). Types of shunt include the following:
   a. Blalock-Taussig shunt
   b. Waterston-Cooley shunt
   c. Potts shunt

3. **Palliative cava-to-pulmonary artery shunts** use systemic venous flow to increase pulmonary blood flow (usually performed in older children who have lower pulmonary vascular resistance) as an intermediate step to a Fontan procedure (see Fig. 6-16). This is called a *unidirectional* or *bidirectional* Glenn shunt.

4. **Repair of TGA**
   a. Atrial inversion (Mustard or Senning)
   b. Arterial switch (of Jatene)

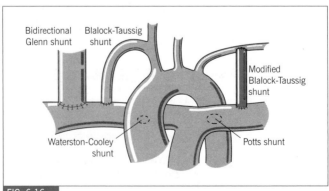

Bidirectional Glenn shunt

Blalock-Taussig shunt

Modified Blalock-Taussig shunt

Waterston-Cooley shunt

Potts shunt

FIG. 6-16

Schematic diagram of cardiac shunts.

5. **Fontan:** Anastomosis of the superior vena cava (SVC) to the right pulmonary artery (RPA) (Glenn shunt), together with anastomosis of the RA and/or inferior vena cava (IVC) to pulmonary arteries via conduits; separates systemic and pulmonary circulations in patients with functionally single ventricles (tricuspid atresia, hypoplastic left heart syndrome).

6. **Norwood:** Used for hypoplastic left heart syndrome.

a. Stage 1: Anastomosis of the proximal main pulmonary artery (MPA) to the aorta, with aortic arch reconstruction and transection and patch closure of the distal MPA; a modified right Blalock-Taussig shunt (subclavian artery to RPA) to provide pulmonary blood flow. ASD created to allow for adequate left to right flow.

b. Stage 2: Bidirectional Glenn shunt to reduce volume overload of single right ventricle and modified Fontan procedure to correct cyanosis.

7. **Ross:** Pulmonary root autograft for aortic stenosis; autologous pulmonary valve replaces aortic valve, and aortic or pulmonary allograft replaces pulmonary valve.

D. **EXERCISE RECOMMENDATIONS FOR CONGENITAL HEART DISEASE** (Table 6-16)[17]

VII. ACQUIRED HEART DISEASE

A. **ENDOCARDITIS**

1. **Common causative organisms:** About 70% of causes of endocarditis are streptococcal species (*Streptococcus viridans*, enterococci); 20% are staphylococcal species (*Staphylococcus aureus, Staphylococcus epidermidis*); 10% are other organisms (*Haemophilus influenzae*, Gram-negative bacteria, fungi).

2. **Clinical findings:** New heart murmur, fever, splenomegaly, petechiae, Osler's nodes (tender nodules at fingertips), Janeway's lesions (painless hemorrhagic areas on palms or soles), splinter hemorrhages, and Roth's spots (retinal hemorrhages).

B. **BACTERIAL ENDOCARDITIS PROPHYLAXIS**

See Tables 6-17 to 6-19 and Boxes 6-2 and 6-3.[16]

C. **MYOCARDIAL DISEASE**

1. **Dilated cardiomyopathy** is the end result of myocardial damage, leading to atrial and ventricular dilation with decreased contractile function of the ventricles.

a. Etiology: Infectious, toxic (alcohol, doxorubicin), metabolic (hypothyroidism, muscular dystrophy), immunologic, collagen vascular disease.

b. Symptoms: Fatigue, weakness, shortness of breath.

c. Examination: Look for signs of CHF, including tachycardia, tachypnea, rales, cold extremities, jugular venous distention, hepatomegaly, peripheral edema, S3 gallop, and displacement of point of maximal impulse (PMI) to the left and inferiorly.

Text continued on p. 161

CARDIOLOGY

6

TABLE 6-12

ACYANOTIC CONGENITAL HEART DISEASE

Lesion Type	Examination Findings	ECG Findings	Chest Radiograph Findings
Ventricular septal defect (VSD) 20%–25% of CHD	2-5/6 holosystolic murmur loudest at the LLSB A systolic thrill may be felt at the LLSB ± apical diastolic rumble with large shunt S2 may be narrow and P2 may be increased with large VSD and pulmonary hypertension	*Small VSD:* Normal *Medium VSD:* LVH ± LAE *Large VSD:* BVH ± LAE, pure RVH	May show cardiomegaly and increased PVMs dependent on the amount of left to right shunting
Atrial septal defect (ASD)	Wide, fixed split S2 with a grade 2-3/6 SEM at the LUSB May have mid-diastolic rumble at LLSB	*Small ASD:* Normal *Hemodynamically significant ASD:* RAD and mild RVH or RBBB with an RSR' in V1	May show cardiomegaly with increased PVMs if hemodynamically significant lesion
Patent ductus arteriosus (PDA) 5%-10% of CHD in term infants; 40%-60% in preterm infants weighing <1500 g	1-4/6 continuous "machinery" murmur loudest at the LUSB	*Small-moderate PDA:* Normal or LVH *Large PDA:* BVH	May have cardiomegaly and increased PVMs depending on size of shunt (see p. 390 for treatment)
Atrioventricular septal defects 30%–60% occur in Down syndrome	Hyperactive precordium with systolic thrill at LLSB and loud S2. There may be a grade 3-4/6 holosystolic regurgitant murmur along LLSB. May hear systolic rumble of MR at apex. May hear middiastolic rumble at LLSB or at apex. Gallop rhythm may be present.	Superior QRS axis RVH and LVH may be present	Cardiomegaly with increased PVMs

Pulmonary stenosis (PS)	Ejection click at LUSB with valvular PS. Click intensity will vary with respiration, decreasing with inspiration and increasing with expiration. S2 may split widely with P2 diminished in intensity. SEM (2-5/6) ± thrill at LUSB with radiation to the back and sides.	*Mild PS:* Normal *Moderate PS:* RAD and RVH *Severe PS:* RAE and RVH with strain	Normal heart size with normal to decreased PVMs
Aortic stenosis (AS)	Systolic thrill at RUSB, suprasternal notch, or over carotids. Ejection click, which does not vary with respiration, if valvular AS. Harsh SEM (2-4/6) at second RICS or third LICS with radiation to neck and apex. May have early diastolic decrescendo murmur as a result of AR. Narrow pulse pressure if severe stenosis.	*Mild AS:* Normal *Moderate-severe AS:* LVH ±strain	Usually normal
Coarctation of the aorta 8%-10% of CHD with male/female ratio of 2:1. May present as (1) infant in CHF; (2) child with HTN; (3) child with murmur	2-3/6 SEM at LUSB with radiation to the left interscapular area. Bicuspid valve is often associated and thus may have systolic ejection click at the apex and RUSB. BP in lower extremities will be lower than in upper extremities. Pulse oximetry discrepancy of >5% between upper and lower extremities is also suggestive of coarctation.	*In infancy:* RVH or RBBB *In older children:* LVH	Marked cardiomegaly and pulmonary venous congestion. Rib notching from collateral circulation not seen in infants because collaterals not yet established; usually seen after 5 years of age.

AR, Aortic regurgitation; *BP,* blood pressure; *BVH,* biventricular hypertrophy; *CHD,* congenital heart disease; *CHF,* congestive heart failure; *HTN,* hypertension; *LAE,* left atrial enlargement; *LICS,* left intercostal space; *LSB,* left lower sternal border; *LUSB,* left upper sternal border; *LVH,* left ventricular hypertrophy; *MR,* mitral regurgitation; *PVM,* pulmonary vascular markings; *RAD,* right axis deviation; *RAE,* right atrial enlargement; *RICS,* right intercostal space; *RBBB,* right bundle branch block; *RUSB,* right upper sternal border; *RVH,* right ventricular hypertrophy; *SEM,* systolic ejection murmur.

6

CARDIOLOGY

TABLE 6-13
CYANOTIC CONGENITAL HEART DISEASE

Lesion	Examination Findings	ECG Findings	Chest Radiograph Findings
Tetralogy of Fallot: 1. Large VSD 2. RVOT obstruction 3. RVH 4. Overriding aorta The degree of RVOT obstruction will determine whether there is clinical cyanosis. If there is only mild PS, there will be a left to right shunt and the child will be acyanotic. Increased obstruction leads to increased right to left shunting across the VSD and cyanosis.	Loud systolic ejection murmur at middle and upper LSB and a loud, single S2. May also have a thrill at the middle and lower LSB. *Tet spells:* Occur in young infants. As RVOT obstruction increases or systemic resistance decreases, right to left shunting across the VSD occurs. May present with tachypnea, increasing cyanosis, and decreasing murmur. See Table 6-15 for treatment.	RAD and RVH	Boot-shaped heart with normal heart size ± decreased PVMs
Transposition of the Great Arteries	Nonspecific findings. Extreme cyanosis. S2 will be single and loud. May have murmur from associated VSD or PS, but if not present, there may not be a murmur	Because RV acts as systemic ventricle, patient will have RAD and RVH. Upright T wave in V1 after 3 days old may be only abnormality.	Classic finding is "egg on a string" with cardiomegaly. Increased PVMs may also be present.
Tricuspid atresia Absent tricuspid valve and hypoplastic RV and PA. Must have ASD, PDA, or VSD for survival.	Single S2. A grade 2-3/6 systolic regurgitation murmur at the LLSB is present if there is a VSD. Occasionally, there is a PDA murmur.	Superior QRS axis. RAE or CAE, and LVH	Normal or slightly enlarged heart size. May have boot-shaped heart.

Total anomalous pulmonary venous return Pulmonary veins drain into RA or other location besides LA. Must have ASD or PFO for survival: 1. *Supracardiac* (most common): Common pulmonary vein into SVC. 2. *Cardiac:* Pulmonary vein into coronary sinus or RA. 3. *Subdiaphragmatic:* Common pulmonary vein into IVC, portal vein, ductus venosus or hepatic vein. 4. *Mixed type*	Hyperactive RV impulse, quadruple rhythm, S2 fixed and widely split, 2-3/6 SEM at LUSB and middiastolic rumble at LLSB.	RAD, RVH (RSR' in V1). May see RAE.	Cardiomegaly and increased PVMs. Classic is the "snowman in a snowstorm" finding, but this is rarely seen until after 4 months of age.

Other

Cyanotic CHDs that occur at a frequency of <1% each include pulmonary atresia, Ebstein's anomaly, truncus arteriosus, single ventricle, and double outlet right ventricle.

ASD, Atrial septal defect; *CAE,* common atrial enlargement; *IVC,* inferior vena cava; *LA,* left atrium; *LLSB,* left lower sternal border; *LSB,* left sternal border; *LUSB,* left upper sternal border; *LVH,* left ventricular hypertrophy; *PA,* pulmonary artery; *PDA,* patent ductus arteriosus; *PFO,* patent foramen ovale; *PVM,* pulmonary vascular markings; *PS,* pulmonary stenosis; *RA,* right atrium; *RAD,* right axis deviation; *RAE,* right atrial enlargement; *RV,* right ventricle; *RVH,* right ventricular hypertrophy; *RVOT,* right ventricular outflow tract; *SEM,* systolic ejection murmur; *SVC,* superior vena cava; *VSD,* ventral septal defect.

TABLE 6-14

INTERPRETATION OF OXYGEN CHALLENGE TEST

	$Fio_2 = 0.21$ Pao_2 (% Saturation)		$Fio_2 = 1.00$ Pao_2 (% Saturation)	$Paco_2$
Normal	70 (95)		>200 (100)	35
Pulmonary disease	50 (85)		>150 (100)	50
Neurologic disease	50 (85)		>150 (100)	50
Methemoglobinemia	70 (85)		>200 (85)	35
Cardiac disease				
Separate circulation*	<40 (<75)		<50 (<85)	35
Restricted PBF†	<40 (<75)		<50 (<85)	35
Complete mixing without restricted PBF‡	50 (85)		<150 (<100)	35
Persistent pulmonary hypertension	Preductal	Postductal		
PFO (no R to L shunt)	70 (95)	<40 (<75)	Variable	35-50
PFO (with R to L shunt)	<40 (<75)	<40 (<75)	Variable	35-50

From Lees MH. J Pediatr 1970; 77:484; Kitterman JA. Pediatr Rev 1982; 4:13; and Jones RW et al. Arch Dis Child 1976; 51:667.

PBF, Pulmonary blood flow; *PFO,* patent foramen ovale.

*D-Transposition of the great arteries (D-TGA) with intact ventricular septum.

†Tricuspid atresia with pulmonary stenosis or atresia; pulmonary atresia or critical pulmonary stenosis with intact ventricular septum; or tetralogy of Fallot.

‡Truncus, total anomalous pulmonary venous return, single ventricle, hypoplastic left heart, D-TGA with ventricular septal defect, tricuspid atresia without pulmonary stenosis or atresia.

TABLE 6-15

TREATMENT OPTIONS FOR "TET SPELLS"

Treatment	Rationale
Oxygen	Reduces hypoxemia (limited value)
Calm child, encourage knee-chest position	Decreases venous return and increases systemic resistance
Propranolol	Negative inotropic effect on infundibular myocardium; may block drop in systemic vascular resistance (0.15-0.25 mg/kg slow IV push)
Morphine	Decreases venous return, depresses respiratory center, relaxes infundibulum (morphine sulfate 0.1-0.2 mg/kg SC or IM). Do not try to establish IV access initially. Use the SC route.
Phenylephrine	Increases systemic vascular resistance (0.02 mg/kg IV)
Methoxamine	Increases systemic vascular resistance
Sodium bicarbonate	Reduces metabolic acidosis (1 mEq/kg IV)
Correct anemia	Increases delivery of oxygen to tissues
Correct pathologic tachyarrhythmias	May abort hypoxic spell
Infuse glucose	Avoids hypoglycemia from increased utilization and depletion of glycogen stores

IM, Intramuscular; *IV,* intravenous; *SC,* subcutaneous.

TABLE 6-16

EXERCISE RECOMMENDATIONS FOR CONGENITAL HEART DISEASE

SPORTS ALLOWED FOR SOME SPECIFIC CARDIAC LESIONS

Diagnosis	Sports Allowed
Small ASD or VSD	All
Mild aortic stenosis	All
MVP (without other risk factors)	All
Moderate aortic stenosis	IA, IB, IIA
Mild LV dysfunction	IA, IB, IC
Moderate LV dysfunction	IA only
Hypertrophic cardiomyopathy	None (or IA only)
Severe aortic stenosis	None
Long QT syndrome	None

	Low Dynamic (A)	Moderate Dynamic (B)	High Dynamic (C)
I. Low static	Billiards	Baseball	Badminton
	Bowling	Softball	Cross-country skiing
	Cricket	Table tennis	Field hockey*
	Curling	Tennis (doubles)	Orienteering
	Golf	Volleyball	Race walking
	Riflery		Racquetball
			Running (long distance)
			Soccer*
			Squash
			Tennis (singles)
II. Moderate static	Archery	Fencing	Basketball*
	Auto racing*,†	Field events (jumping)	Ice hockey*
	Diving*,†	Figure skating*	Cross-country skiing (skating technique)
	Equestrian*,†	Football (American)*	Football (Australian)*
	Motorcycling*,†	Rodeoing*,†	Lacrosse*
		Rugby*	Running (middle distance)
		Running (sprint)	Swimming
		Surfing*,†	Team handball
		Synchronized swimming†	
III. High static	Bobsledding*,†	Body building*,†	Boxing*
	Field events (throwing)	Downhill skiing*,†	Canoeing/kayaking
	Gymnastics*,†	Wrestling*	Cycling*,†
	Karate/judo*		Decathlon
	Luge*,†		Rowing
	Sailing		Speed skating
	Rock climbing*,†		
	Waterskiing*,†		
	Weight lifting*,†		
	Windsurfing*,†		

From 26th Bethesda Conference, 1994 and Washington RL et al. Medical conditions affecting sports participation. Pediatrics 2001; 107(5):1205-1209.

*Danger of bodily collision.

†Increased risk if syncope occurs.

6

CARDIOLOGY

TABLE 6-17

PROCEDURES AND ENDOCARDITIS PROPHYLAXIS

	Prophylaxis Recommended	Prophylaxis Not Recommended
Respiratory tract	Tonsillectomy, adenoidectomy, or both Surgical operations that involve respiratory mucosa Bronchoscopy with a rigid bronchoscope	Endotracheal intubation Bronchoscopy with a flexible bronchoscope, with or without biopsy* Tympanostomy tube insertion
Gastrointestinal tract†	Sclerotherapy for esophageal varices Esophageal stricture dilation Endoscopic retrograde cholangiography with biliary obstruction Biliary tract surgery Surgical operations that involve intestinal mucosa	Transesophageal echocardiography* Endoscopy with or without gastrointestinal biopsy*
Genitourinary tract	Prostatic surgery Cystoscopy Urethral dilation	Vaginal hysterectomy* Vaginal delivery* Cesarean section In uninfected tissue: Urethral catheterization Uterine dilation and curettage Therapeutic abortion Sterilization procedures Insertion or removal of intrauterine devices
Other		Cardiac catheterization, including balloon angioplasty Implanted cardiac pacemakers, implanted defibrillators, and coronary stents Incision or biopsy of surgically scrubbed skin Circumcision

From American Academy of Pediatrics. 2000 Red book: report of the Committee on Infectious Diseases, 25th ed. Elk Grove Village, Ill: the Academy; 2000.

*Prophylaxis is optional for high-risk patients.

†Prophylaxis is recommended for high-risk patients; optional for medium-risk patients.

TABLE 6-18

PROPHYLACTIC REGIMENS FOR DENTAL, ORAL, RESPIRATORY TRACT, OR ESOPHAGEAL PROCEDURES

Situation	Agent	Regimen*
Standard general prophylaxis	Amoxicillin	Adults: 2 g; children: 50 mg/kg orally 1 h before procedure
Unable to take oral medications	Ampicillin	Adults: 2 g intramuscularly (IM) or intravenously (IV); children: 50 mg/kg IM or IV within 30 min before procedure
Allergic to penicillin	Clindamycin	Adults: 600 mg; children: 20 mg/kg orally 1 h before procedure
	OR	
	Cephalexin† or cefadroxil†	Adults: 2 g; children: 50 mg/kg orally 1 h before procedure
	OR	
	Azithromycin or clarithromycin	Adults: 500 mg; children: 15 mg/kg orally 1 h before procedure
Allergic to penicillin and unable to take oral medications	Clindamycin	Adults: 600 mg; children: 20 mg/kg IV within 30 min before procedure
	OR	
	Cefazolin†	Adults: 1 g; children: 25 mg/kg IM or IV within 30 min before procedure

From American Academy of Pediatrics. 2000 Red book: report of the Committee on Infectious Diseases, 25th ed. Elk Grove Village, Ill: the Academy; 2000.

*Total children's dose should not exceed adult dose.

†Cephalosporins should not be used for persons with immediate-type hypersensitivity reaction to penicillins.

CARDIOLOGY

6

TABLE 6-19

PROPHYLACTIC REGIMENS FOR GENITOURINARY AND GASTROINTESTINAL TRACT (EXCLUDING ESOPHAGEAL) PROCEDURE

Situation	Agents*	Regiment†
High-risk patients	Ampicillin PLUS Gentamicin	Adults: Ampicillin 2 g intramuscularly (IM) or intravenously (IV) plus gentamicin 1.5 mg/kg (not to exceed 120 mg) within 30 min of starting the procedure; 6 h later, ampicillin 1 g IM or IV or amoxicillin 1 g orally Children: Ampicillin 50 mg/kg IM or IV (not to exceed 2 g) plus gentamicin 1.5 mg/kg within 30 min of starting the procedure; 6 h later, ampicillin 25 mg/kg IM or IV or amoxicillin 25 mg/kg orally
High-risk patients allergic to ampicillin or amoxicillin	Vancomycin PLUS Gentamicin	Adults: Vancomycin 1 g IV over 1-2 h plus gentamicin 1.5 mg/kg IV or IM (not to exceed 120 mg); complete injection/infusion within 30 min of starting the procedure Children: Vancomycin 20 mg/kg IV over 1-2 h plus gentamicin 1.5 mg/kg IV or IM; complete injection or infusion within 30 min of starting the procedure
Moderate-risk patients	Amoxicillin OR Ampicillin	Adults: Amoxicillin 2 g orally 1 h before procedure, or ampicillin 2 g IM or IV within 30 min of starting the procedure Children: Amoxicillin 50 mg/kg orally 1 h before procedure, or ampicillin 50 mg/kg IM or IV within 30 min of starting the procedure
Moderate-risk patients allergic to ampicillin or amoxicillin	Vancomycin	Adults: Vancomycin 1 g IV over 1-2 h; complete infusion within 30 min of starting the procedure Children: Vancomycin 20 mg/kg IV over 1-2 h; complete infusion within 30 min of starting the procedure

From American Academy of Pediatrics. 2000 Red book: report of the Committee on Infectious Diseases, 25th ed. Elk Grove Village, Ill: the Academy; 2000.
*Total children's dose should not exceed adult dose.
†No second dose of vancomycin or gentamicin is recommended.

BOX 6-2

CARDIAC CONDITIONS ASSOCIATED WITH ENDOCARDITIS

PROPHYLAXIS RECOMMENDED

High Risk

Prosthetic cardiac valves, including bioprosthetic and homograft valves

Previous bacterial endocarditis

Complex cyanotic congenital heart disease (e.g., single ventricle states, transposition of the great arteries, tetralogy of Fallot)

Surgically constructed systemic pulmonary shunts or conduits

Moderate Risk

Most other congenital cardiac malformations (other than those in the high-risk and negligible-risk categories)

Acquired valvular dysfunction (e.g., rheumatic heart disease)

Hypertrophic cardiomyopathy

Mitral valve prolapse with valvular regurgitation and/or thickened leaflets†

PROPHYLAXIS NOT RECOMMENDED

Negligible Risk*

Isolated secundum atrial septal defect

Surgical repair of atrial septal defect, ventricular septal defect, or patent ductus arteriosus (without residua and beyond 6 mo of age)

Previous coronary artery bypass graft surgery

Mitral valve prolapse without valvular regurgitation†

Physiologic, functional, or innocent heart murmurs†

Previous Kawasaki disease without valvular dysfunction

Previous rheumatic fever without valvular dysfunction

Cardiac pacemakers (intravascular and epicardial) and implanted defibrillators

From American Academy of Pediatrics. 2000 Red book: report of the Committee on Infectious Diseases, 25th ed. Elk Grove Village, Ill: the Academy; 2000.

*No greater risk than the general population.

†For further information, see Dajani AS et al. JAMA 1997; 277:1794-1801.

---

d. Chest radiograph: Generalized cardiomegaly, pulmonary congestion.

e. ECG: Sinus tachycardia, left ventricular hypertrophy (LVH), possible atrial enlargement, arrhythmias, conduction disturbances, ST segment/T wave changes.

f. Echocardiography: Enlarged ventricles (increased end-diastolic and end-systolic dimensions) with little or no wall thickening; decreased shortening fraction.

g. Treatment: Management of CHF (digoxin, diuretics, vasodilation, rest). Consider anticoagulants to decrease risk of thrombus formation.

2. **Hypertrophic cardiomyopathy** is an abnormality of myocardial cells leading to significant ventricular hypertrophy, particularly of the LV, with small to normal ventricular dimensions. Contractile function is increased, but filling is impaired secondary to stiff ventricles. The most common type is asymmetric septal hypertrophy, also called *idiopathic*

BOX 6-3
DENTAL PROCEDURES AND ENDOCARDITIS PROPHYLAXIS
PROPHYLAXIS RECOMMENDED*
Dental extractions
Periodontal procedures, including surgery, scaling and root planing, probing, and routine maintenance
Dental implant placement and reimplantation of avulsed teeth
Endodontic (root canal) instrumentation or surgery only beyond the apex
Subgingival placement of antibiotic fibers or strips
Initial placement of orthodontic bands but not brackets
Intraligamentary local anesthetic injections
Prophylactic cleaning of teeth or implants during which bleeding is anticipated
PROPHYLAXIS NOT RECOMMENDED
Restorative dentistry† (operative and prosthodontic) with or without retraction cord‡
Local anesthetic injections (nonintraligamentary)
Intracanal endodontic treatment; postplacement and buildup
Placement of rubber dams
Postoperative suture removal
Placement of removable prosthodontic or orthodontic appliances
Taking of oral impressions
Fluoride treatments
Taking of oral radiographs
Orthodontic appliance adjustment
Shedding of primary teeth

From American Academy of Pediatrics. 2000 Red book: report of the Committee on Infectious Diseases, 25th ed. Elk Grove Village, Ill: the Academy; 2000.
*Prophylaxis is recommended for patients with high- and moderate-risk cardiac conditions.
†This includes restoration of decayed teeth (filling cavities) and replacement of missing teeth.
‡Clinical judgment may indicate antibiotic use in selected circumstances that may create significant bleeding.

hypertrophic subaortic stenosis (IHSS), with varying degrees of obstruction. There is a 4% to 6% incidence of sudden death in children and adolescents.

a. Etiology: Genetic (autosomal dominant, 60% of cases) or sporadic (40% of cases).
b. Symptoms: Easy fatigability, anginal pain, shortness of breath, occasional palpitations.
c. Examination: Usually found in adolescents or young adults, signs include left ventricular heave, sharp upstroke of arterial pulse, murmur of mitral regurgitation.
d. Chest radiograph shows a globular-shaped heart with LV enlargement.
e. ECG indicates LVH, prominent Q waves (septal hypertrophy), ST segment/T wave changes, arrhythmias.
f. Echocardiography shows extent and location of hypertrophy, obstruction, increased contractility.

g. Treatment includes moderate restriction of physical activity, administration of negative inotropes (β-blocker, calcium channel blocker) to help improve filling, and subacute bacterial endocarditis (SBE) prophylaxis.

3. **Restrictive cardiomyopathy:** Myocardial/endocardial disease (usually infiltrative or fibrotic) resulting in stiff ventricular walls, with restriction of diastolic filling but normal contractile function. Results in atrial enlargement. Very rare in children.

4. **Myocarditis:** Inflammation of myocardial tissue.

a. Etiology: Viral (coxsackievirus, echovirus, poliomyelitis, mumps, rubella, cytomegalovirus [CMV], human immunodeficiency virus [HIV], arbovirus, adenovirus, influenza); bacterial, rickettsial, fungal, or parasitic infection; immune-mediated disease (Kawasaki disease, acute rheumatic fever); collagen vascular disease; toxin-induced condition.

b. Symptoms: Nonspecific and inconsistent, depending on severity of disease. Variably see anorexia, lethargy, emesis, lightheadedness, cold extremities, shortness of breath.

c. Examination: Look for signs of CHF (tachycardia, tachypnea, jugular venous distention, rales, gallop, hepatomegaly); occasionally, a soft, systolic murmur or arrhythmias may be noted.

d. Chest radiograph: Shows variable cardiomegaly and pulmonary edema.

e. ECG: Indicates low QRS voltages throughout (<5 mm), ST segment/T wave changes (e.g., decreased T-wave amplitude), prolongation of QT interval, arrhythmias (especially premature contractions, first- or second-degree AV block).

f. Echocardiography: Indicates enlargement of heart chambers, impaired LV function.

g. Treatment: Bed rest, diuretics, inotropes (dopamine, dobutamine), digoxin, gamma globulin (2 g/kg over 24 hours), afterload reducer (e.g., angiotensin-converting enzyme [ACE] inhibitor), possibly steroids. Further clinical study is needed to evaluate the efficacy of pleconaril in enteroviral myocarditis. May require heart transplantation.

D. PERICARDIAL DISEASE

1. **Pericarditis:** Inflammation of visceral and parietal layers of pericardium.

a. Etiology: Viral/idiopathic (especially echovirus, coxsackievirus B), tuberculous, bacterial, uremic, neoplastic, collagen vascular, post-MI or postpericardiotomy, radiation-induced, drug-induced (e.g., procainamide, hydralazine).

b. Symptoms: Chest pain (retrosternal or precordial, radiating to back or shoulder, pleuritic in nature, alleviated by leaning forward, aggravated by supine position), dyspnea.

c. Examination: Pericardial friction rub, fever, tachypnea.

d. ECG: Diffuse ST segment elevation in almost all leads (representing inflammation of adjacent myocardium); PR segment depression.

e. Treatment: Often self-limited. Treat underlying condition and provide symptomatic treatment with rest, analgesia, and antiinflammatory drugs.

2. **Pericardial effusion:** Accumulation of excess fluid in pericardial sac.
   a. Etiology: Associated with acute pericarditis (exudative fluid) or serous effusion resulting from increased capillary hydrostatic pressure (e.g., CHF), decreased plasma oncotic pressure (e.g., hypoproteinemia), and increased capillary permeability (transudative fluid).
   b. Symptoms: Can present with no symptoms, dull ache in left chest, or symptoms of cardiac tamponade, discussed below.
   c. Examination: Muffled distant heart sounds, dullness to percussion of posterior left chest (secondary to atelectasis from large pericardial sac), hemodynamic signs of cardiac compression (see next section).
   d. Chest radiograph: Globular, symmetric cardiomegaly.
   e. ECG: Decreased voltage of QRS complexes, electrical alternans (variation of QRS axis with each beat secondary to swinging of heart within pericardial fluid).
   f. Echocardiography: Fluid within pericardial cavity visualized by M-mode and two-dimensional (2-D) echocardiography.
   g. Treatment: Address underlying condition. Observe if asymptomatic; use pericardiocentesis if there is sudden increase in volume or hemodynamic compromise.

3. **Cardiac tamponade:** Accumulation of pericardial fluid under high pressure, causing compression of cardiac chambers, limiting filling, and decreasing stroke volume and cardiac output.
   a. Etiology: As above for pericardial effusion. Most commonly associated with neoplasm, uremia, viral infection, and acute hemorrhage.
   b. Symptoms: Dyspnea, fatigue, cold extremities.
   c. Examination: Jugular venous distention, hepatomegaly, peripheral edema, tachypnea, rales (from increased systemic and pulmonary venous pressure), hypotension, tachycardia, pulsus paradoxus (decrease in systolic BP by >10 mmHg with each inspiration), decreased capillary refill (from decreased stroke volume and cardiac output), quiet precordium, and muffled heart sounds.
   d. ECG: Sinus tachycardia, decreased voltage, electrical alternans.
   e. Echocardiography: Right ventricle (RV) collapse in early diastole, right atrial/left atrial (RA/LA) collapse in end-diastole and early systole.
   f. Treatment: Pericardiocentesis with temporary catheter left in place if necessary (see p. 67), pericardial window or stripping if it is a recurrent condition.

E. KAWASAKI DISEASE

Kawasaki disease is the leading cause of acquired heart disease in children in developed countries. It is seen almost exclusively in children under 8 years of age. Patients present with acute febrile vasculitis, which may lead to long-term cardiac complications from vasculitis of coronary arteries. The numbers of cases peaks in winter and spring.

1. **Etiology:** Unknown. Thought to be immune-regulated, in response to infectious agents and/or environmental toxins.

2. **Diagnosis:** Based on clinical criteria. These include high fever lasting 5 days or more, plus at least four of the following five criteria:
a. Bilateral bulbar conjunctival injection without exudate.
b. Erythematous mouth and pharynx, strawberry tongue, and/or red, cracked lips.
c. Polymorphous exanthem (may be morbilliform, maculopapular, or scarlatiniform).
d. Swelling of hands and feet, with erythema of palms and soles.
e. Cervical lymphadenopathy (>1.5 cm in diameter), usually single and unilateral.

NOTE: **Atypical Kawasaki disease, more often seen in infants, consists of fever with fewer than four of the above criteria, but findings of coronary artery abnormalities.**

3. **Other clinical findings:** Often associated with extreme irritability, abdominal pain, diarrhea, vomiting. Also seen are anterior uveitis (80%), arthritis/arthralgias (35%), aseptic meningitis (25%), pericardial effusion or arrhythmias (20%), gallbladder hydrops (<10%), carditis (<5%), and perineal rash with desquamation.

4. **Laboratory findings:** Leukocytosis with left shift, neutrophils with vacuoles or toxic granules, elevated C-reactive protein (CRP) or erythrocyte sedimentation rate (ESR) (seen acutely), thrombocytosis (after first week, peaking at 2 weeks), normocytic/normochromic anemia, sterile pyuria (70%), increased LFTs (40%).

5. **Subacute phase (11 to 25 days after onset of illness):** Resolution of fever, rash, and lymphadenopathy. Often, desquamation of fingertips or toes and thrombocytosis occur.

6. **Cardiovascular complications:** If untreated, 15% to 25% develop coronary artery aneurysms and dilation in this phase (peak prevalence occurs about 2 to 4 weeks after onset of disease; rarely appears after 6 weeks) and are at risk for coronary thrombosis acutely and coronary stenosis chronically. Carditis; aortic, mitral, and tricuspid regurgitation; pericardial effusion; CHF; MI; LV dysfunction; and ECG changes may also occur.

7. **Convalescent phase:** ESR, CRP, and platelet count return to normal. Those with coronary artery abnormalities are at increased risk for MI, arrhythmias, and sudden death.

8. **Management**[17] (Table 6-20)
a. Intravenous gamma globulin (IVIG) has been shown to reduce incidence of coronary artery dilation to <3% and decrease duration of fever if given in the first 10 days of illness. Current recommended regimen is a single dose of IVIG, 2 g/kg over 10 to 12 hours.
b. Aspirin is recommended for both its antiinflammatory and its antiplatelet effects. Some recommend initial high-dose aspirin (80 to 100 mg/kg/day divided in four doses) until fever resolves. Then continue with 3 to 5 mg/kg/day Q24hr for 6 to 8 weeks or until platelet count and ESR are normal (if there are no coronary artery abnormalities), or indefinitely if

TABLE 6-20

GUIDELINES FOR TREATMENT AND FOLLOW-UP OF CHILDREN WITH KAWASAKI DISEASE

Risk Level	Pharmacologic Therapy	Physical Activity	Follow-up and Diagnostic Testing	Invasive Testing
I (no coronary artery changes at any stage of illness)	None beyond initial 6-8 weeks	No restrictions beyond initial 6-8 weeks	None beyond first year unless cardiac disease suspected	None recommended
II (transient coronary artery ectasia that disappears during acute illness)	None beyond initial 6-8 weeks	No restrictions beyond initial 6-8 weeks	None beyond first year unless cardiac disease suspected; physician may see patient at 3- to 5-year intervals	None recommended
III (small to medium solitary coronary artery aneurysm)	3-5 mg/kg aspirin per day, at least until abnormalities resolve	For patients in first decade of life, no restriction beyond initial 6-8 weeks; for patients in second decade, physical activity guided by stress testing every other year; competitive contact athletics with endurance training discouraged	Annual follow-up with echocardiogram ± electrocardiogram in first decade of life	Angiography, if stress testing or echocardiography suggests stenosis

IV (one or more giant coronary artery aneurysms or multiple small to medium aneurysms, without obstruction)	Long-term aspirin (3-5 mg/kg/day) ± warfarin	For patients in first decade of life, no restriction beyond initial 6-8 weeks; for patients in second decade, annual stress testing guides recommendations; strenuous athletics are strongly discouraged; if stress test rules out ischemia, noncontact recreational sports allowed	Annual follow-up with echocardiogram ± electrocardiogram ± chest x-ray ± additional electrocardiogram at 6-mo intervals; for patients in first decade of life, pharmacologic stress testing should be considered	Angiography, if stress testing or echocardiography suggests stenosis; elective catheterization may be done in certain circumstances
V (coronary artery obstruction)	Long-term aspirin (3-5 mg/kg/day) ± warfarin; use of calcium channel blockers should be considered to reduce myocardial oxygen consumption	Contact sports, isometrics, and weight training should be avoided; other physical activity recommendations guided by outcome of stress testing or myocardial perfusion scan	Echocardiogram and electrocardiogram at 6-mo intervals and annual Holter and stress testing	Angiography recommended for some patients to aid in selecting therapeutic options; repeat angiography with new-onset or worsening ischemia

coronary artery abnormalities persist. Others recommend starting with low-dose aspirin (3 to 5 mg/kg/day) and continuing as above.

c. Dipyridamole, 4 mg/kg divided in three doses, is sometimes used as alternative to aspirin.

d. Follow-up: Serial echocardiography is recommended to assess coronary arteries and LV function (at time of diagnosis, at 6 to 8 weeks, and at 6 to 12 months). More frequent intervals and long-term follow-up are recommended if abnormalities are seen on echocardiography (see Table 6-20).

REFERENCES

1. Zubrow AB et al. Determinants of blood pressure in infants admitted to neonatal intensive care units: a prospective multicenter study—Philadelphia Neonatal Blood Pressure Study Group. J Perinatol 1995; 15:470.

2. Horan MJ et al. Report of the second task force on blood pressure control in children. Pediatrics 1987; 79(1):1-25.

3. Park MK. Pediatric cardiology for practitioners, 3rd ed. St Louis: Mosby; 1996.

4. Sapin SO. Recognizing normal heart murmurs: a logic-based mnemonic. Pediatrics 1997; 99(4): 616-619.

5. Davignon A et al. Normal ECG standards for infants and children. Pediatr Cardiol 1979; 1: 123-131.

6. Schwartz PJ et al. Prolongation of the QT interval and the sudden infant death syndrome. N Engl J Med 1998; 338:1709-1714.

7. Garson A Jr. The electrocardiogram in infants and children: a systematic approach. Philadelphia: Lea & Febiger; 1983.

8. Park MK, Guntheroth WG. How to read pediatric ECGs, 3rd ed. St Louis: Mosby; 1992.

9. Towbin JA, Bricker JT, Garson A Jr. Electrocardiographic criteria for diagnosis of acute myocardial infarction in childhood. Am J Cardiol 1992; 69:1545.

10. Hirsch R et al. Cardiac troponin I in pediatrics: normal values and potential use in assessment of cardiac injury. J Pediatr 1997; 130:872-877.

11. Walsh EP. In Fyler DC, Nadas A, editors. Pediatric cardiology. Philadelphia: Hanley & Belfus; 1992.

12. Colon SD et al. Developmental modulation of myocardial mechanics: age- and growth-related alterations in afterload and contractility. J Am Coll Cardiol 1992; 19:619.

13. Lees MH. Cyanosis of the newborn infant: recognition and clinical evaluation. J Pediatr 1970; 77:484.

14. Kitterman JA. Cyanosis in the newborn infant. Pediatr Rev 1982; 4:13-24.

15. Jones RW et al. Arterial oxygen tension and response to oxygen breathing in differential diagnosis of heart disease in infancy. Arch Dis Child 1976; 51:667.

16. American Academy of Pediatrics. 2000 Red book: report of the Committee on Infectious Diseases, 25th ed. Elk Grove Village, IL: The Academy; 2000.

17. Dajani AS et al. Guidelines for the long-term management of patients with Kawasaki disease: report from the Committee on Rheumatic Fever, Endocarditis, and Kawasaki Disease, Council on Cardiovascular Disease in the Young, American Heart Association. Circulation 1994; 89:916.

DERMATOLOGY

Monique Soileau-Burke, MD

I. WEBSITES

www.med.jhu.edu/peds/dermatlas

Please refer to Figs. 7-1 to 7-5 for pattern and distribution of rashes, and algorithms for evaluation of common skin disorders. Also, see color plates 1-16 (after p. 176) for pictures of common dermatologic findings.

II. HEMANGIOMAS

Hemangiomas are the most common soft tissue tumors of infancy and occur in 5% to 10% of 1-year-olds. Hemangiomas have a phase of rapid proliferation followed by spontaneous involution.

A. PATHOGENESIS

During the proliferative phase, densely packed endothelial cells form small capillaries. Subsequent vessels develop from existing vasculature.

B. CLINICAL MANIFESTATIONS

1. Appearance
a. Newborns demonstrate pale macules with threadlike telangiectasias.
b. The most recognizable form is a bright red, slightly elevated, noncompressible plaque. Frequently, both superficial and deep components are present, with deep components appearing bluish in color.
c. Size can range from a few millimeters to several centimeters.
2. **Incidence:** Hemangiomas have an increased incidence in premature infants and are three times more likely in girls than boys.
3. **Natural history:** Approximately 20% of hemangiomas are present at birth, with the remainder developing within the first 4 weeks of life. The most rapid growth phase occurs between 2 to 4 months, with regression beginning at 6 to 12 months.
4. **Diagnosis:** Although the majority of hemangiomas are diagnosed clinically, imaging techniques (e.g., ultrasound, computed tomography [CT], magnetic resonance imaging [MRI]) can be used to differentiate hemangiomas from vascular malformations or neoplastic processes.

C. COMPLICATIONS

1. **Ulceration is the most common complication** and may result in severe pain, infection, hemorrhage, or scarring.
a. Ulceration results from necrosis of superficial component.
b. Hemorrhage, although alarming in appearance, is usually minimal and can be controlled by direct pressure.
c. Superinfection may lead to cellulitis, osteomyelitis, or septicemia.
2. **Kasabach-Merritt phenomenon**
a. Kasabach-Merritt phenomenon, a complication of rapidly enlarging, usually deep lesions, is characterized by anemia, thrombocytopenia, and coagulopathy.
b. These lesions are differentiated from benign hemangiomas by their deep

7

169

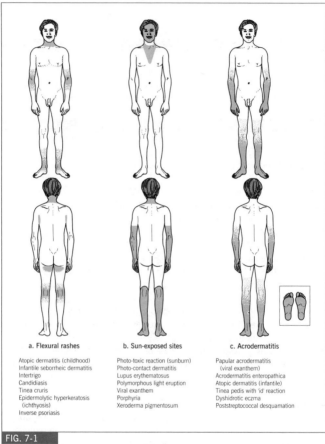

a. Flexural rashes	b. Sun-exposed sites	c. Acrodermatitis
Atopic dermatitis (childhood)	Photo-toxic reaction (sunburn)	Papular acrodermatitis
Infantile seborrheic dermatitis	Photo-contact dermatitis	(viral exanthem)
Intertrigo	Lupus erythematosus	Acrodermatitis enteropathica
Candidiasis	Polymorphous light eruption	Atopic dermatitis (infantile)
Tinea cruris	Viral exanthem	Tinea pedis with 'id' reaction
Epidermolytic hyperkeratosis	Porphyria	Dyshidrotic eczma
(ichthyosis)	Xeroderma pigmentosum	Poststreptococcal desquamation
Inverse psoriasis		

FIG. 7-1

Pattern diagnosis. *(From Cohen BA. Pediatric dermatology, 2nd ed. London: Mosby; 1999.)*

    red-blue appearance, marked firmness, and a different histologic appearance.

c. These lesions require aggressive medical management.

3. Regionally important lesions

a. Periorbital lesions: Hemangiomas in the periorbital region may cause amblyopia from obstruction of the visual axis or astigmatism from insidious compression of the globe or extension into the retrobulbar

7

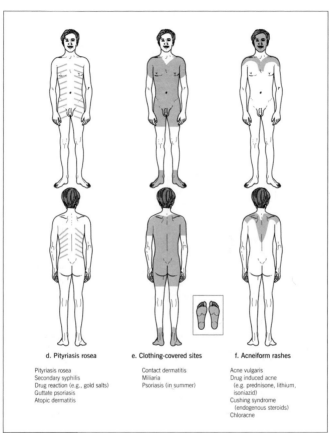

d. Pityriasis rosea

Pityriasis rosea
Secondary syphilis
Drug reaction (e.g., gold salts)
Guttate psoriasis
Atopic dermatitis

e. Clothing-covered sites

Contact dermatitis
Miliaria
Psoriasis (in summer)

f. Acneiform rashes

Acne vulgaris
Drug induced acne
  (e.g. prednisone, lithium,
  isoniazid)
Cushing syndrome
  (endogenous steroids)
Chloracne

FIG. 7-1—cont'd

Pattern diagnosis. *(From Cohen BA. Pediatric dermatology, 2nd ed. London: Mosby; 1999.)*

space. They require careful observation and evaluation by an ophthalmologist.

b. External auditory canal lesions may result in otitis or conductive hearing loss.

c. Multiple cutaneous hemangiomas and large facial hemangiomas are associated with visceral hemangiomas and may warrant abdominal ultrasound to look for organ involvement (i.e., liver hemangiomas).

Text continued on p. 180

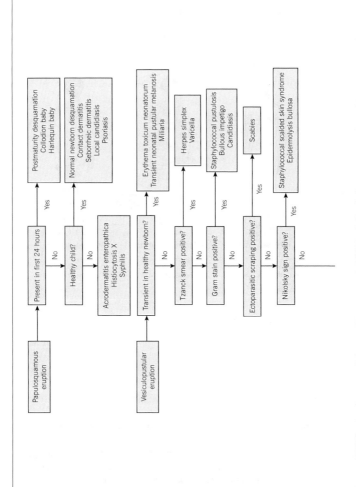

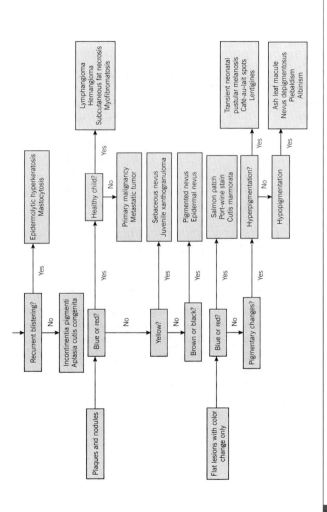

7

DERMATOLOGY

FIG. 7-2

Evaluation of neonatal rashes. *(From Cohen BA. Pediatric dermatology, 2nd ed. London: Mosby; 1999.)*

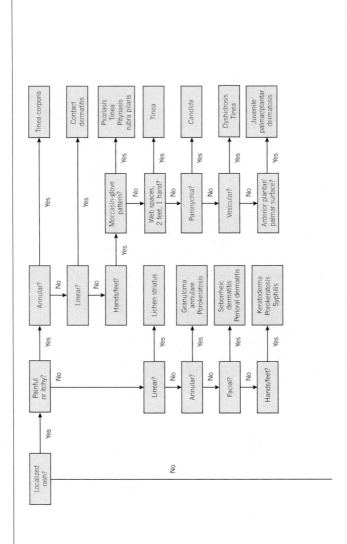

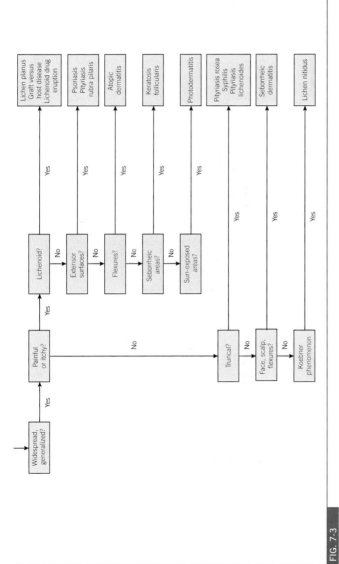

FIG. 7-3

Evaluation of papulosquamous rashes. *(From Cohen BA.*
Pediatric dermatology, 2nd ed. London: Mosby; 1999.)

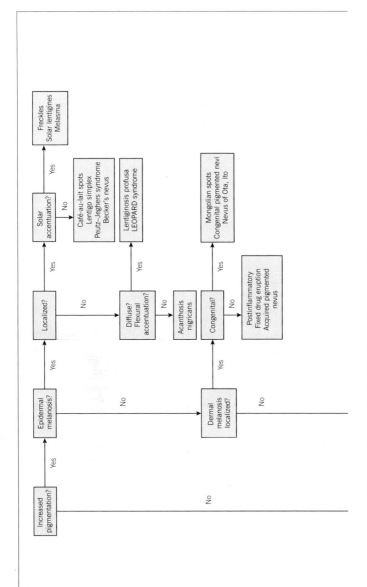

INFANT RASHES

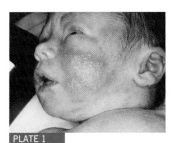

PLATE 1

Erythema toxicum. *(From Cohen B: www.med.jhu.edu/peds/dermatlas, 2001.)*

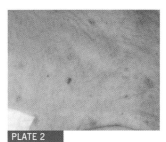

PLATE 2

Neonatal pustular melanosis. *(From Cohen B: Atlas of pediatric dermatology. St. Louis: Mosby; 1993.)*

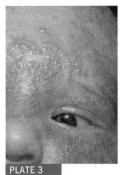

PLATE 3

Neonatal acne. *(From Cohen B: Atlas of pediatric dermatology. St. Louis: Mosby; 1993.)*

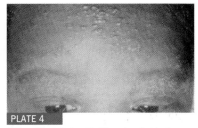

PLATE 4

Milia. *(From Cohen B: Atlas of pediatric dermatology. St. Louis: Mosby; 1993.)*

HAIR DISORDERS

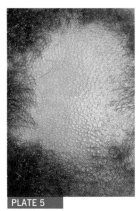

PLATE 5

Alopecia areata. *(From Cohen B: Atlas of pediatric dermatology. St. Louis: Mosby; 1993.)*

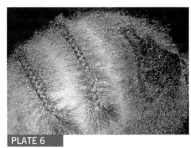

PLATE 6

Traction alopecia. *(From Cohen B: Atlas of pediatric dermatology. St. Louis: Mosby; 1993.)*

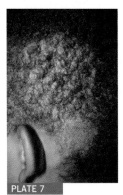

PLATE 7

"Black dot" tinea capitis. *(From Cohen B: www.med. jhu.edu/peds/dermatlas, 2001.)*

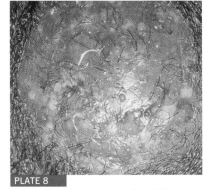

PLATE 8

Kerion. *(From Cohen B: Atlas of pediatric dermatology. St. Louis: Mosby; 1993.)*

INFLAMMATORY RASHES

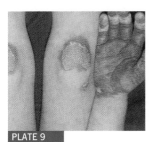

PLATE 9

Psoriasis. *(From Cohen B: Atlas of pediatric dermatology. St. Louis: Mosby; 1993.)*

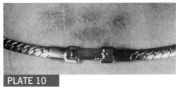

PLATE 10

Allergic contact dermatitis. *(From Cohen B: Atlas of pediatric dermatology. St. Louis: Mosby; 1993.)*

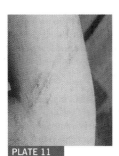

PLATE 11

Poison ivy (*Rhus* dermatitis). *(From Cohen B: Atlas of pediatric dermatology. St. Louis: Mosby; 1993.)*

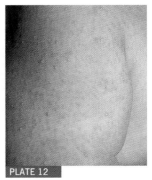

PLATE 12

Keratosis pilaris. *(From Cohen B: Atlas of pediatric dermatology. St. Louis: Mosby; 1993.)*

ECZEMATOUS RASHES

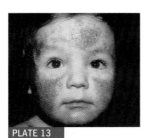

PLATE 13
Infantile eczema. *(From Cohen B: Atlas of pediatric dermatology. St. Louis: Mosby; 1993.)*

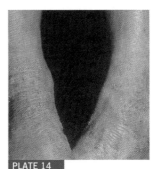

PLATE 14
Childhood eczema. *(From Cohen B: Atlas of pediatric dermatology. St. Louis: Mosby; 1993.)*

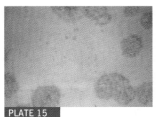

PLATE 15
Nummular eczema. *(From Cohen B: Atlas of pediatric dermatology. St. Louis: Mosby; 1993.)*

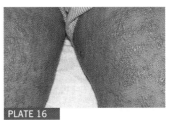

PLATE 16
Follicular eczema. *(From Cohen B: Atlas of pediatric dermatology. St. Louis: Mosby; 1993.)*

FUNGAL RASHES

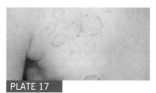

PLATE 17

Tinea corporis. *(From Cohen B: Atlas of pediatric dermatology. St. Louis: Mosby; 1993.)*

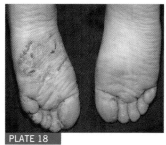

PLATE 18

Tinea pedis. *(From Cohen B: www.med. jhu.edu/peds/dermatlas, 2001.)*

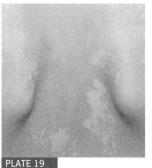

PLATE 19

Tinea versicolor. *(From Cohen B: Atlas of pediatric dermatology. St. Louis: Mosby; 1993.)*

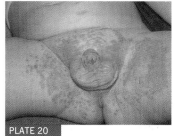

PLATE 20

Diaper candidiasis. *(From Cohen B: Atlas of pediatric dermatology. St. Louis: Mosby; 1993.)*

INFECTIOUS RASHES

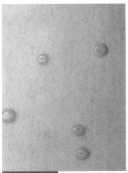

PLATE 21

Molluscum contagiosum. *(From Cohen B: Atlas of pediatric dermatology. St. Louis: Mosby; 1993.)*

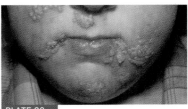

PLATE 22

Herpetic gingivostomatitis. *(From Cohen B: Atlas of pediatric dermatology. St. Louis: Mosby; 1993.)*

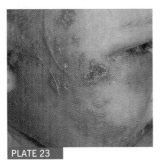

PLATE 23

Herpes zoster. *(From Cohen B: Atlas of pediatric dermatology. St. Louis: Mosby; 1993.)*

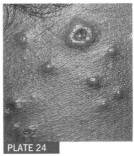

PLATE 24

Varicella. *(From Cohen B: Atlas of pediatric dermatology. St. Louis: Mosby; 1993.)*

EXANTHEMS

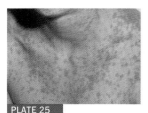

PLATE 25

Measles. *(From Cohen B: Atlas of pediatric dermatology. St. Louis: Mosby; 1993.)*

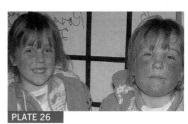

PLATE 26

Fifth disease. *(From Cohen B: Atlas of pediatric dermatology. St. Louis: Mosby; 1993.)*

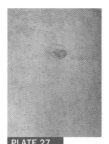

PLATE 27

Roseola. *(From Cohen B: Atlas of pediatric dermatology. St. Louis: Mosby; 1993.)*

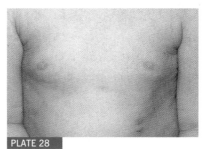

PLATE 28

Scarlet fever. *(From Cohen B: Atlas of pediatric dermatology. St. Louis: Mosby; 1993.)*

MISCELLANEOUS

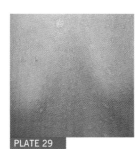

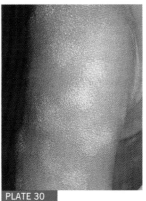

PLATE 29
Pityriasis rosea. *(From Cohen B: Atlas of pediatric dermatology. St. Louis: Mosby; 1993.)*

PLATE 30
Pityriasis alba. *(From Cohen B: Atlas of pediatric dermatology. St. Louis: Mosby; 1993.)*

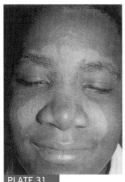

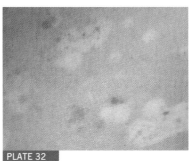

PLATE 31
Seborrhea dermatitis. *(From Cohen B: Atlas of pediatric dermatology. St. Louis: Mosby; 1993.)*

PLATE 32
Postinflammatory hypopigmentation. *(From Cohen B: Atlas of pediatric dermatology. St. Louis: Mosby; 1993.)*

7

DERMATOLOGY

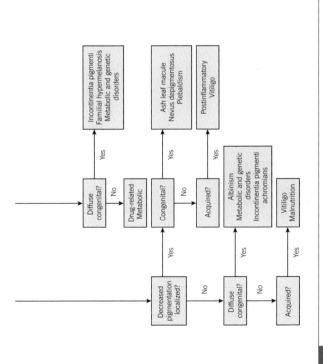

FIG. 7-4

Evaluation of disorders of pigmentation. *(From Cohen BA. Pediatric dermatology, 2nd ed. London: Mosby; 1999.)*

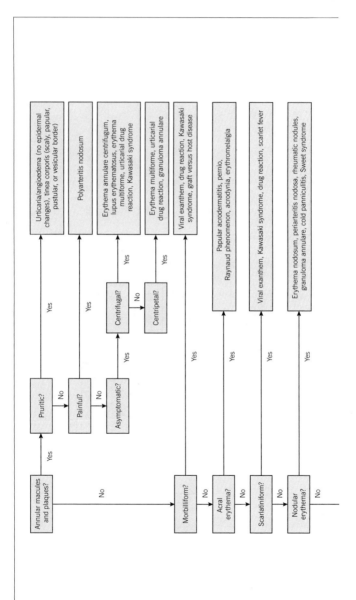

7

DERMATOLOGY

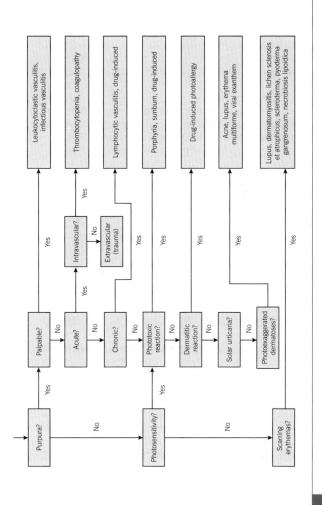

FIG. 7-5
Evaluation of reactive erythema. (From Cohen BA. Pediatric dermatology, 2nd ed. London: Mosby; 1999.)

Visceral hemangiomas are often characterized by high-flow patterns and may result in high-output cardiac failure and anemia. Large facial hemangiomas are also associated with posterior fossa vascular malformations and may require neuroimaging for evaluation.

d. Airway hemangiomas are often located in the subglottic region and may cause hoarseness and stridor. Infants with cutaneous lesions in a beard distribution (chin, lips, mandibular region, and neck) are at greatest risk for airway involvement.

e. Lumbosacral hemangiomas that span the midline are associated with spinal malformations and anomalies of the anorectal and urogenital regions.

D. MANAGEMENT

1. **Because the majority of hemangiomas require no intervention, the decision to treat should be based on location and depth of the lesion, age of the patient, and likelihood of complication.** Photo documentation is used to follow the growth/regression process.

2. **Systemic corticosteroids are the mainstay of therapy for lesions that require intervention to prevent subsequent complication** (i.e., periorbital or subglottic lesions). Usually, doses of 2 to 3 mg/kg/day of prednisone/prednisolone are used. One third of lesions demonstrate dramatic shrinkage, one third demonstrate stabilization of growth, and one third show no response.

3. **Laser ablation**

4. **Interferon**

5. **Embolization** can be used to treat cutaneous hemangiomas that have not responded to medical therapy.

6. **Surgical excision**[1]

III. WARTS

A. PATHOGENESIS

Warts are caused by more than 60 types of the human papillomavirus (HPV). The virus enters the skin through breaks in the epithelium, and then causes hyperplasia of the squamous epithelium.

B. MORPHOLOGY

1. **Common warts:** The lesions of common warts are skin-colored, rough, minimally scaly papules and nodules found on the exposed surfaces of the hands, face, arms, and legs. Lesions can be solitary or multiple, a few millimeters to several centimeters, and may form large plaques or a confluent, linear pattern secondary to autoinoculation.

2. **Flat warts** occur over the hands, arms, and face, and are usually less than 2 mm wide. They often present in clusters.

3. **Plantar warts** are found on the soles of the feet as sometimes painful but often asymptomatic, inward-growing, hyperkeratotic plaques and papules. Trauma on weight-bearing surfaces results in small black dots ("seeds" from thrombosed vessels on the surface of the wart).

4. **Anogenital warts**: See Chapter 5.

TABLE 7-1		
WART THERAPY		
Treatment	**Advantages**	**Disadvantages**
Keratolytics (lactic acid, salicylic acid, tretinoin)	Available without prescription, home therapy, low cost, low risk, little pain	Slow response, irritation
DESTRUCTIVE AGENTS		
Cryotherapy	Quick office procedure, relatively low cost	Pain, scarring, recurrence
Caustics (topical acids)	Home or office therapy, relatively low cost	Irritation, recurrence, systemic toxicity (podophyllin)
Cantharidin (vesicant)	Occasionally effective	High risk of recurrence, prominent pigmentary changes
Electrocautery and laser	Usually effective	Pain, scarring, recurrence, requires anesthesia, moderate cost

From Cohen BA. Contemp Pediatr 1997; 2:128-149.

C. TREATMENT (Table 7-1)

1. **Spontaneous resolution** occurs in over 75% of warts in otherwise healthy individuals within 3 years.
2. **Keratolytics** (i.e., topical salicylates) work by removing excess scale within and around warts and by triggering an inflammatory reaction. This is particularly effective in combination with adhesive tape occlusion; however, a response may take 4 to 6 months.
3. **Destructive techniques** depend on destruction of wart and surrounding normal skin.
a. Cryotherapy results in necrosis and blister formation. Treatment may produce scarring and warts may recur.
b. Caustic agents can be applied after warts have been shaved but require application for several weeks or months.
c. Cantharidin is a topical vesicant that causes the formation of intra-epidermal blisters. Recurrence risk is high and blister formation can be difficult to control.
d. Electrocautery and CO_2 laser ablation require local or general anesthesia. These can be particularly useful for treating large lesions on the trunk and extremities and discrete plantar warts. Both can leave scars, and recurrence is well documented. Open wounds and prolonged healing pose significant problems in weight bearing.
e. Intradermal bleomycin has also been used.
f. Destructive options for therapy are often not good choices in the treatment of young children.
4. **Immunotherapy**
a. Immunotherapy involves contact sensitization with a potent allergen

initially, followed by the application of a low concentration of the allergen in cream form to the wart site.

b. Cimetidine can be used in doses of 30 to 40 mg/kg/day divided into two doses for 2 months; however, it may be no better than placebo.[2]

IV. MOLLUSCUM CONTAGIOSUM

A. MORPHOLOGY

Molluscum contagiosum consists of dome-shaped, often umbilicated, translucent to white papules that range from 1 mm to 1 cm, with a tiny keratotic core at the center. They often are surrounded by scaling and erythema that resemble eczema. They may appear inflamed and secondarily infected when undergoing spontaneous involution.

B. TREATMENT

Lesions are benign and self-limited.

1. **Use a small curette** with gentle pressure to debride the lesion. This treatment is the least likely to cause scarring.
2. **Liquid nitrogen** may be an option in older children.
3. **Topical preparations** of salicylic-lactic acid combinations, cantharidin, and retinoic acid may also be used.[3]

V. ATOPIC DERMATITIS

A. PATHOPHYSIOLOGY

Atopic dermatitis involves a genetic predisposition and elevated IgE levels, which suggests an abnormal response to triggering agents, resulting in the release of histamine, prostaglandins, and cytokines. Inflammation causes itching and subsequent scratching, which produces the clinical lesions of eczema.

B. EPIDEMIOLOGY

1. **Atopic dermatitis affects 5% to 7% of children,** with the peak prevalence between 6 months and 8 to 10 years of age.
2. **Approximately 95% of children with atopic dermatitis will have asthma or allergic rhinitis.**

C. CLINICAL PRESENTATIONS (Box 7-1)

Acute changes include erythema, vesicles, crusting, and secondary infection. Chronic changes include lichenification, scaling, and postinflammatory hypopigmentation or hyperpigmentation.

1. **Infantile form:** Extensor surfaces are more affected than flexors. Truncal, facial, and scalp involvement are common, with sparing of the diaper area.
2. **Early to middle childhood:** Flexural surfaces are more severely involved.
3. **Late childhood and adolescence:** Lesions tend to be restricted to skin creases and hand dermatitis.

D. TREATMENT

1. **Chronic disease:** Bland lubricants, including petroleum jelly, Aquaphor, Eucerin, and vegetable shortening, are the mainstays of therapy. Lubricants should be used two to three times per day and immediately

BOX 7-1
IDENTIFYING CHARACTERISTICS OF ATOPIC DERMATITIS
Major Criteria (Seen in All Patients)
Pruritus
Typical morphology and distribution of lesions
Facial and extensor involvement in infants
Flexural lichenification in older children and adults
Tendency toward chronic or chronically relapsing dermatitis
Common Findings (At Least 2)
Personal or family history of atopic disease (asthma, allergic rhinitis, atopic dermatitis)
Immediate skin test reactivity
White dermatographism and/or delayed blanch to cholinergic agents
Anterior subcapsular cataracts
Associated Findings (At Least 4)
Xerosis/ichthyosis/hyperlinear palms and soles
Pityriasis alba
Keratosis pilaris
Facial pallor/infraorbital darkening
Dennie-Morgan infraorbital fold
Elevated serum IgE
Tendency toward nonspecific hand dermatitis
Tendency toward repeated cutaneous infections

From Cohen BA. Contemp Pediatr 1992; 7:64-81.

7

DERMATOLOGY

after bathing or swimming. Bathing time should be short (no more than 5 minutes), and the skin should be patted dry, not rubbed, before application of lubricant.

2. **Topical steroids** (Table 7-2)

a. Low and medium-potency steroid creams should be used once or twice per day in the most severely affected areas for eczema flares and for generally no more than 7 days. Severe flares may require a longer duration of therapy followed by a taper to lower-potency steroids. Even with low-potency steroids, special care is required in areas in which the skin is thin, such as the diaper area, groin, armpits, under the breasts, around the neck, and on the face. High-potency topical steroids should generally be used in consultation with a dermatologist.

b. Topical steroids can be applied at the same time as lubricants and can be mixed with lubricants when weaning from the topical steroid.

3. **Systemic steroids should generally be avoided.** They may be used for short periods of uncontrolled eczema flares or for severe disease requiring hospitalization.

4. **Antihistamines** may be used when hives cause scratching, thus exacerbating underlying eczema. Sedating antihistamines

TABLE 7-2

TOPICAL AND SYSTEMIC ANTIBIOTICS USED TO TREAT ACNE

Antibiotic	Characteristics
TOPICAL	
Erythromycin	*P. acnes* very sensitive; least lipophilic
Clindamycin	*P. acnes* very sensitive; more lipophilic than erythromycin, but less than benzoyl peroxide
Benzoyl peroxide plus erythromycin	*P. acnes* very sensitive; most lipophilic topical agent; less irritating than benzoyl peroxide alone
Benzoyl peroxide plus clindamycin	Similar to above
Azelaic acid	*P. acnes* sensitive; minimal lipophilia; can reduce abnormal desquamation
Metronidazole	*P. acnes* not sensitive; has antiinflammatory properties
Benzoyl peroxide plus glycolic acid	Glycolic acid may enhance penetration and reduce abnormal desquamation
SYSTEMIC	
Tetracycline	*P. acnes* sensitive; inexpensive; usually needs to be taken two to four times a day; compliance can be a problem because of need to take on an empty stomach
Erythromycin	*P. acnes* very sensitive; resistance emerging; gastrointestinal upset common; inexpensive
Doxycycline	Lipophilic; *P. acnes* very sensitive; resistance not yet seen; photosensitivity can occur; more expensive than tetracycline and erythromycin
Minocycline	Lipophilic; *P. acnes* very sensitive; resistance not yet seen; no photosensitivity; abnormal pigmentation in oral mucosa and skin; vertigo-like symptoms; most expensive
Trimethoprim-sulfamethoxazole	Lipophilic; *P. acnes* very sensitive; severe erythema multiforme and toxic epidermal necrolysis limit use
Clindamycin	*P. acnes* very sensitive; somewhat lipophilic; pseudomembranous colitis limits use

From Leyden JJ. N Engl J Med 1997; 16:1156-1162.

(i.e., diphenhydramine, hydroxyzine) are more effective for pruritus. Cetirizine is the most effective of the nonsedating antihistamines.

5. **Protective clothing** should be worn.
6. **Topical tacrolimus** is a newer agent that may be efficacious for severe, treatment-resistant atopic dermatitis (see Formulary for dosage information).

E. **COMPLICATIONS**
1. **For weeping or blistering lesions** with no evidence of infection, cold water compresses three or four times per day, or tepid baths followed by bland lubricant application may be used.
2. **Bacterial infection,** usually staphylococcal and sometimes streptococcal, must be recognized quickly. Localized infections can be treated with topical antibiotics, whereas more serious infections require systemic antibiotics.[4]

3. **Eczema herpeticum** must be treated systemically with acyclovir.

VI. ACNE VULGARIS

A. PATHOPHYSIOLOGY

Acne is the result of the obstruction of sebaceous follicles, located primarily on the face and trunk, by excessive amounts of sebum and desquamated epithelial cells. The resident anaerobic organism, *Propionibacterium acnes,* proliferates and produces chemotactic and inflammatory mediators that lead to inflammation.

1. Noninflammatory open comedones, or "blackheads."
2. Noninflammatory closed comedones, or "whiteheads."
3. Inflammatory papules, pustules, nodules, or cysts.

B. TREATMENT (see Table 7-2)

1. **Gentle, nonabrasive cleaning is best.** Vigorous scrubbing, abrasive cleaners, and mechanical devices can promote the development of inflammatory lesions.
2. **Dietary factors play no role in sebum production.**
3. **Comedonal acne:** The treatment goal for noninflammatory acne is first prevention and second to minimize the formation of new comedones and colonization with *P. acnes.* This type of acne is most common in the preadolescent and early adolescent years.
   a. Topical tretinoin or Adapalene and benzoyl peroxide (either or both) are the treatments of choice. Salicylic acid and topical antibiotics may also be used.
   b. Topical cream or gel should be applied sparingly once daily, starting with a low concentration and increasing concentration if local irritation does not occur. It may take several weeks for desired clinical results to become apparent.
   c. Continue therapy until it is clear that new lesions are not developing.
4. **Mild inflammatory acne:** Scattered small papules or pustules develop, with a minimum of comedones. Proliferation of *P. acnes* occurs at this stage. This often occurs in the early teens and in adult women in their 20s.
   a. Most patients improve after a 2- to 4-week course of topical antibiotics applied twice daily, topical benzoyl peroxide, or a combination of the two.
   b. Treatment should be continued until no new lesions develop and then should be slowly tapered.
5. **Inflammatory acne** is a generalized eruption of papules and pustules on the face and trunk. A few patients have a more destructive type of inflammation associated with large, deep inflammatory nodules.
   a. A topical retinoid plus a topical and/or systemic antibiotic should be used, depending on the severity of the lesions, for 4 to 6 weeks.
   b. Systemic antibiotics may be used with a topical antibiotic. In general, the dose of the antibiotic should not be reduced for 2 to 4 months.

7

DERMATOLOGY

c. Patients with nodular, cystic lesions may not respond to systemic antibiotics and may require systemic isotretinoin. This should be used in consultation with a dermatologist and requires two forms of effective and reliable contraception in women because of its teratogenic effects.

d. Women with persistent acne unresponsive to antibiotics and topical tretinoin may respond to therapy with oral contraceptives after appropriate gynecologic and endocrine evaluation, especially for polycystic ovarian syndrome and other androgen excess conditions.[5]

VII. COMMON CAUSES OF HAIR LOSS IN CHILDREN
A. TINEA CAPITIS
1. Epidemiology

a. *Trichophyton tonsurans* accounts for greater than 90% of tinea capitis in North America. It is an anthropophilic organism with no known natural reservoir. The fungus persists for long periods on fomites, such as hairbrushes, combs, furniture, stuffed toys, and clothing.

b. The majority of patients are between 1 and 10 years of age, but infection may occur at any age.

c. The incidence is highest in African-American children and second highest in Hispanic youths. This predisposition in African-American children is not completely understood, but it may be the result of the character of the hair follicle, tight braiding, or the use of pomades.

2. Clinical presentation

a. Classic tinea capitis presents as one or more round to oval patches of partial to complete alopecia, with varying degrees of erythema. Scale is present, and the border is slightly raised and more erythematous than the central area.

b. A kerion is an inflammatory presentation of tinea capitis. It presents as a boggy, tender, edematous plaque or cluster of nodules with erythema. It is usually solitary and is frequently accompanied by cervical or occipital adenopathy and papular morbilliform eruption classified as an "id" reaction.

c. The seborrheic dermatitis–like pattern may produce minimal or no alopecia and show diffuse scaling over the scalp, with pruritus.

d. Follicular pustules with crusting and scaling scattered over the scalp is a pattern seen predominantly in African-American children with tight braiding and constant pomade use. It often resembles bacterial folliculitis, but bacterial culture is negative.

3. Diagnosis:
The presumptive clinical diagnosis of tinea capitis may be confirmed by either direct microscopic examination or culture of scale (may be collected with a toothbrush on a culture plate or on a moistened culturette swab).

4. Treatment

a. Successful treatment requires oral therapy; griseofulvin is the agent of choice. It is best taken with fatty food to promote absorption (see Formulary for dosage information). Standard references suggest 4 to

6 weeks of therapy, although 8 to 12 weeks may be required for eradication. Patients should be reevaluated monthly, and repeat culture may be obtained 2 weeks after therapy is discontinued to document cure. Patients will often develop an eczema-like rash associated with the fungal infection, known as an "id" reaction. This is not a drug reaction, and griseofulvin therapy should be continued.

b. Kerions should be treated with prednisone or prednisolone if no contraindication exists (0.5 mg/kg/day for 7 to 10 days) in addition to standard griseofulvin therapy.

c. The use of sporicidal shampoos in addition to oral therapy promotes rapid elimination of spores, thus decreasing the contagion risk to family members and schoolmates. The use of selenium sulfide 2.5% shampoo twice weekly is recommended.[6] Ketoconazole 1% and 2% shampoo is also available for this purpose.

B. ALOPECIA AREATA

Alopecia areata is a common condition characterized by the sudden onset of asymptomatic, noninflammatory, round, bald patches located on any hair-bearing part of the body, most commonly the scalp.

1. **Alopecia areata is best differentiated by the absence of hair follicles in the bald spot.** There is also a lack of scaly erythema, pustules, and crusts.

2. **Although the course is irregular and unpredictable, most patients develop good regrowth of hair within 1 or 2 years.**

3. **Treatments include topical corticosteroids, topical minoxidil, tar preparations, anthralin, topical sensitizers, and ultraviolet light therapy.**[7] Systemic steroids should generally not be used because they do not alter prognosis. In adolescents and adults, hair loss often resolves over months to years, but in younger children the prognosis is more guarded.

C. TELOGEN EFFLUVIUM

Telogen effluvium is a form of alopecia characterized by diffuse hair loss that is usually not clinically obvious to anyone but the patient and parent.

1. **Growing hair follicles respond to physiologic and pathologic stress** (e.g., high fever, severe influenza, infection, surgery, drugs, pregnancy, hypothyroidism) by regressing to the resting, or telogen, state.

2. **Telogen effluvium usually occurs 3 to 5 months after the stressor and is self-limited.**

D. TRACTION ALOPECIA

Traction alopecia is often a result of hairstyles that apply tension for long periods of time.

1. **Traction alopecia is characterized by noninflammatory linear areas of hair loss** at the margins of the hairline, part line, or scattered regions, depending on hair styling procedures used.

2. **Treatment is avoidance of styling products or styles resulting in traction.**

7

DERMATOLOGY

E. HAIR PULLING

Hair pulling is a benign, self-limited activity common in young children.

F. TRICHOTILLOMANIA

Trichotillomania is a type of alopecia caused by the compulsion to pull out one's own hair, resulting in irregular areas of incomplete hair loss, mainly on the scalp, but the eyebrows and eyelashes may also be involved.

1. **The clinical appearance** is characterized by areas of hair loss within which are short, broken hair shafts of varying lengths.
2. **Most cases spontaneously resolve,** but in severe cases a psychiatric evaluation may be warranted.

REFERENCES

1. Drolet BA, Esterly NB, Frieden IJ. Hemangiomas and children. Primary Care 1999; 3:173-181.
2. Cohen BA. Warts and children: can they be separated? Contemp Pediatr 1997; 2:128-149.
3. Gellia SE. Warts and molluscum contagiosum in children. Pediatr Ann 1987; 1:69-76.
4. Cohen BA. Atopic dermatitis: breaking the itch-scratch cycle. Contemp Pediatr 1992; 7:64-81.
5. Leyden JJ. Therapy for acne vulgaris. N Engl J Med 1997; 16:1156-1162.
6. Smith ML. Tinea capitis. Pediatr Ann 1996; 25:101-105.
7. Cohen BA. Pediatric dermatology, 2nd ed. London: Mosby; 1999.

DEVELOPMENT AND BEHAVIOR

Lori Chaffin Jordan, MD

I. INTRODUCTION

8

Developmental disabilities are a group of interrelated, nonprogressive, neurologic disorders occurring in childhood. This chapter focuses on screening and assessment of neurodevelopment to identify possible developmental disability.

A. DEVELOPMENT

Development can be divided into five major streams or skill areas: visual-motor and language (the cognitive streams), motor, social, and adaptive. Each stream has a spectrum of normal and abnormal presentation. Abnormal assessment in one stream increases the risk of deficit in another stream and should alert the examiner to consider a careful assessment of all streams. A developmental diagnosis is a functional description and classification that does not specify an etiology or medical diagnosis.

1. **Motor stream:** Evaluating motor stream includes assessment of both fine and gross motor skills. A full neurologic examination should be performed, which includes examination of tone, strength, coordination, deep tendon reflexes (DTRs), primitive reflexes, and postural reactions.
2. **Cognitive streams:** Evaluating cognitive streams includes assessment of language skills (expressive and receptive) and of problem-solving/visual-motor skills.
3. **Social and adaptive streams:** Evaluating social and adaptive streams includes assessment of social skills, activities of daily living, affect, temperament, and interpersonal communication/interaction.

II. DEFINITIONS[1]

A. DEVELOPMENTAL QUOTIENT

The developmental quotient (DQ) can be calculated for any given stream as follows:

$$DQ = (Developmental\ age/Chronological\ age) \times 100$$

1. **The DQ reflects the child's percent of normal development for age present at the time of testing.** Two separate developmental assessments over time are more predictive than a single assessment.
2. **Language remains the best predictor of future intellectual endowment,** but an isolated mild expressive language delay often has a good

189

prognosis in the absence of other deficits. Language development can be divided into two categories—receptive and expressive—each assigned a separate DQ.

B. DELAY

Delay is defined as performance significantly below average (DQ <70) in a given area of skill. Delay may occur in a single stream or several streams.

C. DEVIANCY

Deviancy is defined as atypical development within a single stream, such as developmental milestones occurring out of sequence. Deviancy does not necessarily imply abnormality, but should alert one to the possibility that problems may exist. EXAMPLE: An infant who crawls before sitting, or an infant with early development of hand preference.

D. DISSOCIATION

Dissociation is defined as a substantial difference in the rate of development between two streams. EXAMPLE: Cognitive-motor difference in some children with mental retardation or cerebral palsy.

III. DISORDERS

A. COGNITIVE DISORDERS

1. **Mental retardation (MR):** MR is characterized by significantly below-average intellectual functioning (IQ <70 to 75) existing concurrently with related limitation in two or more of the following adaptive skill areas: communication, self-care, home living, social skills, community use, self-direction, health and safety, functional academics, leisure, and work (Table 8-1). MR manifests itself before age 18. Formal psychometric testing is needed to make the diagnosis of MR. Patients should be referred to a developmental pediatrician or psychologist for such testing if the DQ for any given stream is <70, or if there is significant learning difficulty.

2. **Communication disorders:** A group of disorders that can be subdivided into expressive language disorders, mixed receptive-expressive language disorders, phonologic disorders, and stuttering. Developmental language disorders can be characterized by deficits of comprehension, production, or use of language. Differential diagnosis includes hearing loss, specific language disability, expressive language disorder, mixed expressive and receptive language disorder, selective mutism, and autism (or another pervasive developmental disorder).

3. **Learning disabilities (LD):** LDs are a heterogeneous group of disorders that manifest as significant difficulties in one or more of the following seven areas (as defined by the federal government): basic reading skills, reading comprehension, oral expression, listening comprehension, written expression, mathematical calculation, and mathematical reasoning. Specific learning disabilities are diagnosed when the individual's achievement on standardized tests in a given area is substantially below that expected for age, schooling, and level of intelligence.[2]

TABLE 8-1
MENTAL RETARDATION

Level	IQ	Academic Potential	Daily Living	Work	Expected Mental Age as an Adult (yr)	Intensity of Support
Borderline	70-80	Educable to about the 6th grade	Fully independent	Employable; may need training to be competitive	—	Intermittent
Mild	50-69	Reading and writing to 4th-5th grade or less	Relatively independent with some training	Employable, often need training	9-11	Intermittent
Moderate	35-49	Limited reading to 1st or 2nd grade	Dress without help, use toilet, prepare food	Likely to need sheltered employment	5-8	Limited
Severe	20-34	Very unlikely to read or write	Can be toilet trained, dress with help, may be able to sign name	Sheltered employment	3-5	Extensive
Profound	<20	None	Occasionally can be toilet trained, dress with help, often nonverbal	Very limited	below 3	Pervasive

From American Association on Mental Retardation. Mental retardation: definition, classification and systems of supports, 9th ed. Washington, DC: AAMR; 1992.

DEVELOPMENT AND BEHAVIOR 8

TABLE 8-2

CLINICAL CLASSIFICATION OF CEREBRAL PALSY

Type	Pattern of Involvement
I. SPASTIC (increased tone, clasped knife, clonus, further classified by distribution)	
Hemiplegia	Ipsilateral arm and leg; arm worse than leg
Diplegia	Legs primarily effected
Quadriplegia	All four extremities impaired; legs worse than arms
Double hemiplegia	All four extremities; arms notably worse than legs
Monoplegia	One extremity, usually upper; probably reflects a mild hemiplegia
Triplegia	One upper extremity and both lower; probably represents a hemiplegia plus a diplegia or incomplete quadriplegia
II. EXTRAPYRAMIDAL (lead pipe or candle wax rigidity, variable tone, +/− clonus)	
Choreoathetosis, rigidity, dystonia	Complex movement/tone disorders reflecting basal ganglia pathology
Ataxia, tremor	Movement and tone disorders reflecting cerebellar origin
Hypotonia	Usually related to diffuse, often severe, cerebral and/or cerebellar cortical damage

From Capute AJ, Accardo PJ, editors. Cerebral palsy: developmental disabilities in infancy and childhood, 2nd ed. Baltimore: Paul H. Brookes; 1996.

B. MOTOR DISORDERS[3]
Cerebral palsy (CP) is a disorder of movement and posture resulting from a permanent, nonprogressive lesion of the immature brain. Manifestations, however, may change with brain growth and development. A child with significant motor impairment can be identified at any age. The diagnosis of CP should be made before age 12 months; however, the mean age of diagnosis is 13 months. CP is classified in terms of physiologic and topographic characteristics (Table 8-2).

C. BEHAVIORAL DISORDERS
1. **Age-specific behavioral issues:** Table 8-3.
2. **Attention deficit/hyperactivity disorder (ADHD):** ADHD is a neurobehavioral disorder characterized by inattention, impulsivity, and hyperactivity, all behaviors that are more frequent and severe than typically observed in individuals of the same developmental age. Symptoms must persist for more than 6 months, occur before 7 years of age, and be evident in two or more settings.
   a. Prevalence: Approximately 3% to 5% of school-age children are affected. The hyperactive-impulsive type of ADHD is more common in males.
   b. Diagnosis: Use the criteria provided in the American Psychiatric Association's *Diagnostic and statistical manual of mental disorders,* 4th ed (DSM-IV).[4] Subcategories listed in DSM-IV include inattentive type, hyperactive-impulsive type, and combined type.
   c. Evaluation: The diagnosis is clinical and is based primarily on parent and child interviews. Input from the school on learning, classroom behaviors, and attention needs to be integrated. Rating scales (e.g., Conners' Parent and Teacher Rating Scales [Fig. 8-1] and ADHD Rating

Scale IV) are used to measure the severity of symptoms at baseline and to monitor progress with treatment.

d. Management: A multimodal approach with possible components is listed below. Note that none of the psychosocial treatments have been shown to be very effective without medication. The presence of comorbid psychiatric disorders, coexisting academic and cognitive deficits, patient strengths, and level of family functioning and support need to be considered in the creation of an effective treatment plan.

(1) Pharmacotherapy: In most cases, psychostimulants (methylphenidate, dextroamphetamine, amphetamine [Adderall], and long-acting methylphenidate) are the first line of pharmacologic agents. With significant side effects and poor response to two or more adequate stimulant trials, consider a consultation with a specialist for the possible use of other agents, such as clonidine, bupropion, and magnesium pemoline (see the Formulary for dosage information).

(2) Psychosocial treatments: Options include behavior modification, parent training, classroom modifications (seating in the front row, smaller student-teacher ratios), social skills training, and support organizations for the family (e.g., Children and Adults with Attention Deficit Hyperactivity Disorder [CHADD]).

3. **Autism:** The essential features of autism are impaired social interaction and communication and a restricted group of activities and interests, with stereotyped behaviors, rituals, or mannerisms. Onset of abnormal functioning occurs before age 3. Of note, 75% of autistic children function in the mentally retarded range. See DSM-IV for full diagnostic criteria.

4. **Pervasive developmental disorders** include autism, Rett's disorder, childhood disintegrative disorder, Asperger's disorder, and pervasive developmental disorder, not otherwise specified. See DSM-IV for diagnostic criteria.

IV. DEVELOPMENTAL SCREENING AND EVALUATION

A. **DEVELOPMENTAL MILESTONES** (Table 8-4)

B. **DENVER DEVELOPMENT ASSESSMENT (DENVER II)** (see foldout)

1. **The Denver II is a tool for screening of the apparently normal child between the ages of 0 and 6 years;** its use is suggested at every well-child visit. This screen will allow the practitioner to identify those children who may have developmental delay. These children should be further evaluated for the purpose of definitive diagnosis. The test screens the child in four areas: personal-social, fine motor, gross motor, and language.

2. **Age calculation:** For children born before 38 weeks gestation, age should be corrected for prematurity, up to 2 years of age.

3. **Scoring:** Note that items that can be passed by report of caregiver are denoted with a letter R. Each item that intersects or is just adjacent to the age line should be scored. Items should be scored as

TABLE 8-3

AGE-APPROPRIATE BEHAVIORAL ISSUES IN INFANCY AND EARLY CHILDHOOD

Age	Behavioral Issue	Symptoms	Guidance
1-3 months	Colic	Paroxysms of fussiness/crying, 3+ hours per day, 3+ days per week, may pull knees up to chest, pass flatus	Crying usually peaks at 6 weeks and resolves by 3-4 months. Prevent overstimulation; swaddle infant; use white noise, swing, or car rides to soothe. Avoid medication and formula changes. Encourage breaks for the primary caregiver.
3-4 months	Trained night feeding	Night awakening	Comfort quietly, avoid reinforcing behavior (i.e., avoid night feeds). Do not play at night. Introducing cereal or solid food does not reduce awakening. Develop a consistent bedtime routine. Place baby in bed while drowsy and not fully asleep.
9 months	Stranger anxiety/ separation anxiety	Distress when separated from parent or approached by a stranger	Use a transitional object, such as a special toy or blanket; use routine or ritual to separate from parent; may continue until 24 months but can reduce intensity.
	Developmental night waking	Separation anxiety at night	Keep lights off. Avoid picking child up or feeding. May reassure verbally at regular intervals or place a transitional object in crib.
12 months	Aggression	Biting, hitting, kicking in frustration	Say "No" with negative facial cues. Begin time out (1 min/yr of age). No eye contact or interaction, place in a nonstimulating location. May restrain child gently until cooperation is achieved.
	Need for limit setting	Exploration of environment, danger of injury	Avoid punishing exploration or poor judgment. Emphasize child-proofing and distraction.
18 months	Temper tantrums	Occur with frustration, attention-seeking rage, negativity/refusal	Try to determine cause and react appropriately (i.e., help child who is frustrated, ignore attention-seeking behavior). Make sure child is in a safe location.

24 months	Toilet training	*Child needs to demonstrate readiness:* shows interest, neurologic maturity (i.e., recognizes urge to urinate or defecate), ability to walk to bathroom and undress self, desire to please/imitate parents, increasing periods of daytime dryness.	Age range for toilet training is usually 2 to 4 yr. Give guidance early; may introduce potty seat but avoid pressure or punishment for accidents. Wait until the child is ready. Expect some periods of regression, especially with stressors.
24-36 months	New sibling	Regression, aggressive behavior	Allow for special time with parent, 10-20 min daily of one-on-one time exclusively devoted to the older sibling(s). Child chooses activity with parent. No interruptions. May not be taken away as punishment.
36 months	Nightmare	Awakens crying, may or may not complain of bad dream	Reassure child, explain that they had a bad dream. Leave bedroom door open, use a nightlight, demonstrate there are no monsters under the bed. Discuss dream the following day. Avoid scary movies or television shows.
	Night terrors	Agitation, screaming 1-2 hr after going to bed. Child may have eyes open but not respond to parent. May occur at same time each night.	May be familial, not volitional. *Prevention:* For several nights, awaken child 15 min before terrors occur. Avoid over-tiredness. *Acute:* Be calm, speak in soft, soothing, repetitive tones, help child return to sleep. Protect child against injury.

From Dixon SD, Stein MT. Encounters with children: pediatric behavior and development. St. Louis: Mosby; 2000; Schmitt BD. Instructions for pediatric patients, 2nd ed. Philadelphia: WB Saunders; 1999; and Howard BJ. Audio Digest Pediatrics 2000; 46(2).

DEVELOPMENT AND BEHAVIOR

8

Conners' Parent Rating Scale – Revised (S)
by C. Keith Conners, Ph.D.

Child's Name: _____ Age: _____ School Grade: _____ Gender: M F

Birthdate: ___/___/___
Month Day Year

Parent's Name: _____

Today's Date: ___/___/___
Month Day Year

Instructions: Below are a number of common problems that children have. Please rate each item according to your child's behavior in the last month. For each item, ask yourself, "How much of a problem has this been in the last month?", and circle the best answer for each one. If none, not at all, seldom, or very infrequently, you would circle 0. If very much true, or it occurs very often or frequently, you would circle 3. You would circle 1 or 2 for ratings in between. Please respond to each item.

	NOT TRUE AT ALL (Never, Seldom)	JUST A LITTLE TRUE (Occasionally)	PRETTY MUCH TRUE (Often, Quite a Bit)	VERY MUCH TRUE (Very Often, Very Frequent)
1. Inattentive, easily distracted	0	1	2	3
2. Angry and resentful	0	1	2	3
3. Difficulty doing or completing homework	0	1	2	3
4. Is always "on the go" or acts as if driven by a motor	0	1	2	3
5. Short attention span	0	1	2	3
6. Argues with adults	0	1	2	3
7. Fidgets with hands or feet or squirms in seat	0	1	2	3
8. Fails to complete assignments	0	1	2	3
9. Hard to control in malls or while grocery shopping	0	1	2	3

10. Messy or disorganized at home or school	0	1	2	3
11. Loses temper	0	1	2	3
12. Needs close supervision to get through assignments	0	1	2	3
13. Only attends if it is something he/she is very interested in	0	1	2	3
14. Runs about or climbs excessively in situations where it is inappropriate	0	1	2	3
15. Distractibility or attention span a problem	0	1	2	3
16. Irritable	0	1	2	3
17. Avoids, expresses reluctance about, or has difficulties engaging in tasks that require sustained mental effort (such as schoolwork or homework)...	0	1	2	3
18. Restless in the "squirmy" sense	0	1	2	3
19. Gets distracted when given instructions to do something	0	1	2	3
20. Actively defies or refuses to comply with adults' requests.	0	1	2	3
21. Has trouble concentrating in class	0	1	2	3
22. Has difficulty waiting in lines or awaiting turn in games or groups situations.	0	1	2	3
23. Leaves seat in classroom or in other situations in which remaining seated is expected.	0	1	2	3
24. Deliberately does things to annoy other people	0	1	2	3
25. Does not follow through on instructions and fails to finish schoolwork, chores or duties in the workplace (not due to oppositional behavior or failure to understand instructions)	0	1	2	3
26. Has difficulty playing or engaging in leisure activities quietly.........	0	1	2	3
27. Easily frustrated in efforts.	0	1	2	3

FIG. 8-1

The Conners' Parent Rating Scale.

DEVELOPMENT AND BEHAVIOR

8

TABLE 8-4		
DEVELOPMENTAL MILESTONES		
Age	**Gross Motor**	**Visual-Motor/Problem Solving**
1 mo	Raises head from prone position	*Birth:* Visually fixes *1 mo:* Has tight grasp, follows to midline
2 mo	Holds head in midline, lifts chest off table	No longer clenches fists tightly, follows object past midline
3 mo	Supports on forearms in prone position, holds head up steadily	Holds hands open at rest, follows in circular fashion, responds to visual threat
4 mo	Rolls over, supports on wrists, and shifts weight	Reaches with arms in unison, brings hands to midline
6 mo	Sits unsupported, puts feet in mouth in supine position	Unilateral reach, uses raking grasp, transfers objects
9 mo	Pivots when sitting, crawls well, pulls to stand, cruises	Uses immature pincer grasp, probes with forefinger, holds bottle, throws objects
12 mo	Walks alone	Uses mature pincer grasp, can make a crayon mark, releases voluntarily
15 mo	Creeps up stairs, walks backwards independently	Scribbles in imitation, builds tower of two blocks in imitation
18 mo	Runs, throws objects from standing without falling	Scribbles spontaneously, builds tower of 3 blocks, turns 2-3 pages at a time
24 mo	Walks up and down steps without help	Imitates stroke with pencil, builds tower of 7 blocks, turns pages one at a time, removes shoes, pants, etc.
3 yr	Can alternate feet when going up steps, pedals tricycle	Copies a circle, undresses completely, dresses partially, dries hands if reminded, unbuttons
4 yr	Hops, skips, alternates feet going down steps	Copies a square, buttons clothing, dresses self completely, catches ball
5 yr	Skips alternating feet, jumps over low obstacles	Copies triangle, ties shoes, spreads with knife

From Capute AJ, Biehl RF. Pediatr Clin North Am 1973; 20:3; Capute AJ, Accardo PJ. Clin Pediatr 1978; 17:847; and Capute AJ et al. Am J Dis Child 1986; 140:694. Rounded norms from Capute AJ et al. Dev Med Child Neurol 1986; 28:762.

pass, fail, no opportunity, or refused to cooperate. Assess each item as follows:

a. Advanced: Child passes item that falls completely to the right of age line.
b. Normal: Child passes, fails, or refuses item on which the age line falls between the 25th and 75th percentile.
c. Caution: Child fails or refuses item on which the age line falls between the 75th and 90th percentile.
d. Delayed: Child fails or refuses item that falls completely to the left of age line.

Language	Social/Adaptive
Alerts to sound	Regards face
Smiles socially (after being stroked or talked to)	Recognizes parent
Coos (produces long vowel sounds in musical fashion)	Reaches for familiar people or objects, anticipates feeding
Laughs, orients to voice	Enjoys looking around
Babbles, ah-goo, razz, lateral orientation to bell	Recognizes that someone is a stranger
Says "mama, dada" indiscriminately, gestures, waves bye-bye, understands "no"	Starts exploring environment, plays gesture games (e.g., pat-a-cake)
Uses two words other than mama/dada or proper nouns, jargoning (runs several unintelligible words together with tone or inflection), one-step command with gesture	Imitates actions, comes when called, cooperates with dressing
Uses two words, follows one-step command without gesture	*15-18 mo:* Uses spoon and cup
Mature jargoning (includes intelligible words), 7-10 word vocabulary, knows 5 body parts	Copies parent in tasks (sweeping, dusting), plays in company of other children
Uses pronouns (I, you, me) inappropriately, follows two-step commands, has a 50-word vocabulary, uses two-word sentences	Parallel play
Uses minimum of 250 words, 3-word sentences, uses plurals, knows all pronouns, repeats two digits	Group play, shares toys, takes turns, plays well with others, knows full name, age, gender
Knows colors, says song or poem from memory, asks questions	Tells "tall tales," plays cooperatively with a group of children
Prints first name, asks what a word means	Plays competitive games, abides by rules, likes to help in household tasks

8

DEVELOPMENT AND BEHAVIOR

3. **Assessment:** A child fails a Denver screen if he or she has two or more delays noted. Re-evaluate the child in 3 months if there is one delay and/or two or more cautions. A child passes the screen with no delays and a maximum of one caution. Additionally, some children may be termed *untestable* if there are a significant number of refusal or no opportunity test items. Indications for referral are a failed test or a classification of untestable on two consecutive screenings.

C. CAT/CLAMS (CAPUTE SCALES) (Table 8-5)

1. **The Capute Scales** are an assessment tool that gives quantitative developmental quotients for visual-motor/problem-solving and language abilities. The CLAMS (Clinical Linguistic and Auditory Milestone Scale) was developed for the assessment of language milestones from birth to 36 months of age. The CAT (Clinical Adaptive Test) consists of problem-solving items for ages from birth to 36 months, adapted from standardized infant psychological tests.

2. **Scoring:** Scoring is done by calculating the basal age as the highest age group in which a child accomplishes all of the test tasks correctly. The age equivalent is then determined by adding the decimal number (recorded in parentheses) next to each correctly scored item passed at age groups beyond the basal age to the basal age itself. Each of these age equivalents (language and visual motor) is then divided by the child's chronologic age and multiplied by 100 to determine a developmental quotient. Again, a DQ <70 constitutes delay and warrants referral.

D. EVALUATION OF VISUAL-MOTOR AND PROBLEM-SOLVING SKILLS

For these tests, it is important to observe how they are done and to evaluate the final product.

1. **Goodenough-Harris Draw-a-Person Test**

a. Procedure: Give the child a pencil and a sheet of blank paper. Instruct the child to "draw a person; draw the best person you can." Supply encouragement if needed (e.g., "draw a whole person"); however, do not suggest specific supplementation or changes.

b. Scoring: Ask the child to describe or explain the drawing to you. Give the child one point for each detail present using the guide in Box 8-1 (maximum score: 51) and compare to norms for age in Table 8-6.

2. **Gesell figures** (Fig. 8-2): When using Gesell figures, the examiner is not supposed to demonstrate the drawing of the figures for the patient.

3. **Gesell block skills:** The structures in Fig. 8-3 should be demonstrated for the child. Fig. 8-3 includes the developmental age at which each structure can usually be accomplished.

V. EVALUATION OF A CHILD SUSPECTED TO HAVE DEVELOPMENTAL DELAY

A. HISTORY TO ELICIT RISK OF DELAY/DEVELOPMENTAL MILESTONES

1. Obtain patient history, to include complications of pregnancy, birth, neonatal period, past medical history, and family history.

2. Obtain history of developmental milestones to assess rate of acquisition of skills in the past.

3. Obtain history of education in school-age children.

B. EXAMINATION

1. Examination consists of a general physical, a careful search for

TABLE 8-5

CLAMS/CAT*

Age (mo)	CLAMS	Yes	No	CAT	Yes	No
1	1. Alerts to sound (0.5)†	—	—	1. Visually fixates momentarily upon red ring (0.5)	—	—
	2. Soothes when picked up (0.5)	—	—	2. Chin off table in prone position (0.5)	—	—
2	1. Social smile (1.0)†	—	—	1. Visually follows ring horizontally and vertically (0.5)	—	—
				2. Chest off table prone (0.5)	—	—
3	1. Cooing (1.0)	—	—	1. Visually follows ring in circle (0.3)	—	—
				2. Supports on forearms in prone position (0.3)	—	—
				3. Visual threat (0.3)	—	—
4	1. Orients to voice (0.5)†	—	—	1. Unfisted (0.3)	—	—
	2. Laughs aloud (0.5)	—	—	2. Manipulates fingers (0.3)	—	—
				3. Supports on wrists in prone position (0.3)	—	—
5	1. Orients toward bell laterally (0.3)†	—	—	1. Pulls down rings (0.3)	—	—
	2. Ah-goo (0.3)	—	—	2. Transfers (0.3)	—	—
	3. Razzing (0.3)	—	—	3. Regards pellet (0.3)	—	—
6	1. Babbling (1.0)	—	—	1. Obtains cube (0.3)	—	—
				2. Lifts cup (0.3)	—	—
				3. Radial rake (0.3)	—	—
7	1. Orients toward bell (1.0)† (upwardly/indirectly 90°)	—	—	1. Attempts pellet (0.3)	—	—
				2. Pulls out peg (0.3)	—	—
				3. Inspects ring (0.3)	—	—
8	1. Says "dada" inappropriately (0.5)	—	—	1. Pulls on ring by string (0.3)	—	—
	2. Says "mama" inappropriately (0.5)	—	—	2. Secures pellet (0.3)	—	—
				3. Inspects bell (0.3)	—	—
9	1. Orients toward bell (upward directly 180°) (0.5)†	—	—	1. Three-finger scissor grasp (0.3)	—	—
	2. Gesture language (0.5)	—	—	2. Rings bell (0.3)	—	—
				3. Over the edge for toy (0.3)	—	—

*See p. 200 for instructions.
†Indicates CLAMS item that must be demonstrated for examiner to receive credit.

cont'd

TABLE 8-5						
CLAMS/CAT*—cont'd						
Age (mo)	CLAMS	Yes	No	CAT	Yes	No
10	1. Understands "no" (0.3)	—	—	1. Combine cube-cup (0.3)	—	—
	2. Uses "dada" appropriately (0.3)	—	—	2. Uncovers bell (0.3)	—	—
	3. Uses "mama" appropriately (0.3)	—	—	3. Fingers pegboard (0.3)	—	—
11	1. One word (other than "mama" and "dada") (1.0)	—	—	1. Mature overhand pincer movement (0.5)	—	—
				2. Solves cube under cup (0.5)	—	—
12	1. One-step command with gesture (0.5)	—	—	1. Release one cube in cup (0.5)	—	—
	2. Two-word vocabulary (0.5)	—	—	2. Makes crayon mark (0.5)	—	—
14	1. Three-word vocabulary (1.0)	—	—	1. Solves glass frustration (0.6)	—	—
	2. Immature jargoning (1.0)	—	—	2. Out-in with peg (0.6)	—	—
				3. Solves pellet-bottle with demonstration (0.6)	—	—
16	1. Four- to six-word vocabulary (1.0)	—	—	1. Solves pellet-bottle spontaneously (0.6)	—	—
	2. One-step command without gesture (1.0)	—	—	2. Round block on form board (0.6)	—	—
				3. Scribbles in imitation (0.6)	—	—
18	1. Mature jargoning (0.5)	—	—	1. 10 cubes in cup (0.5)	—	—
	2. 7-10 word vocabulary (0.5)	—	—	2. Solves round hole in form board reversed (0.5)	—	—
	3. Points to one picture (0.5)†	—	—	3. Spontaneous scribbling with crayon (0.5)	—	—
	4. Knows body parts (0.5)	—	—	4. Pegboard completed spontaneously (0.5)	—	—

dysmorphisms, and a neurodevelopmental evaluation (neurologic examination and assessment of primitive and postural reflexes.)

2. **Primitive/postural reflexes:** Primitive reflexes are present at birth and disappear by 6 to 9 months. Postural reactions appear after suppression of the primitive reflexes and precede voluntary motor function. A reflex/reaction profile can be helpful in identifying infants at risk for cerebral palsy or other motor impairment when used in conjunction with a neurologic examination. An infant with an asymmetric neurologic exami-

TABLE 8-5 .
CLAMS/CAT*—cont'd

Age (mo)	CLAMS	Yes	No	CAT	Yes	No
21	1. 20-word vocabulary (1.0)	—	—	1. Obtains object with stick (1.0)	—	—
	2. Two-word phrases (1.0)	—	—	2. Solves square in form board (1.0)	—	—
	3. Points to two pictures (1.0)[†]	—	—	3. Tower of three cubes (1.0)	—	—
24	1. 50-word vocabulary (1.0)	—	—	1. Attempts to fold paper (0.7)	—	—
	2. Two-step command (1.0)	—	—	2. Horizontal four-cube train (0.7)	—	—
	3. Two-word sentences (1.0)	—	—	3. Imitates stroke with pencil (0.7)	—	—
				4. Completes form board (0.7)	—	—
30	1. Uses pronouns appropriately (1.5)	—	—	1. Horizontal-vertical stroke with pencil (1.5)	—	—
	2. Concept of one (1.5)[†]	—	—	2. Form board reversed (1.5)	—	—
	3. Points to 7 pictures (1.5)[†]	—	—	3. Folds paper with definite crease (1.5)	—	—
	4. Two digits forward (1.5)[†]	—	—	4. Train with chimney (1.5)	—	—
36	1. 250-word vocabulary (1.5)	—	—	1. Three-cube bridge (1.5)	—	—
	2. Three-word sentence (1.5)	—	—	2. Draws circle (1.5)	—	—
	3. Three digits forward (1.5)[†]	—	—	3. Names one color (1.5)	—	—
	4. Follows two preposi- tional commands (1.5)[†]	—	—	4. Draws a person with head plus one other part of body (1.5)	—	—

nation or persistent or exaggerated primitive reflexes is at high risk for developmental disability (Tables 8-7 and 8-8).

C. DEVELOPMENTAL SCREENING

1. **Appropriate screening tests vary with age** (Table 8-9). Significant delays on screening merit referral for formal testing.

2. **In assessing for delay, an individual DQ can be calculated for any given developmental stream;** if the quotient is <70%, a diagnosis of delay can be made and warrants further evaluation and/or referral. For example, a 13-month-old child who does not yet walk alone but is able

Text continued on p. 211

8

DEVELOPMENT AND BEHAVIOR

BOX 8-1
GOODENOUGH-HARRIS SCORING

General:
- ☐ Head Present
- ☐ Legs present
- ☐ Arms present

Trunk:
- ☐ Present
- ☐ Length greater than breadth
- ☐ Shoulders

Arms/legs:
- ☐ Attached to trunk
- ☐ At correct point

Neck:
- ☐ Present
- ☐ Outline of neck continuous with head, trunk, or both

Face:
- ☐ Eyes
- ☐ Nose
- ☐ Mouth
- ☐ Nose and mouth in two dimensions
- ☐ Nostrils

Hair:
- ☐ Present
- ☐ On more than circumference; nontransparent

Clothing:
- ☐ Present
- ☐ Two articles; nontransparent
- ☐ Entire drawing (sleeves and trousers) nontransparent
- ☐ Four articles
- ☐ Costume complete

Fingers:
- ☐ Present
- ☐ Correct number
- ☐ Two dimensions; length, breadth
- ☐ Thumb opposition
- ☐ Hand distinct from fingers and arm

Joints:
- ☐ Elbow, shoulder, or both
- ☐ Knee, hip, or both

Proportion:
- ☐ *Head:* 10% to 50% of trunk area
- ☐ *Arms:* Approximately same length as trunk
- ☐ *Legs:* 1-2 times trunk length; width less than trunk width
- ☐ *Feet:* To leg length
- ☐ Arms and legs in two dimensions
- ☐ Heel

Motor coordination:
- ☐ Lines firm and well connected
- ☐ Firmly drawn with correct joining
- ☐ Head outline
- ☐ Trunk outline
- ☐ Outline of arms and legs
- ☐ Features

Ears:
- ☐ Present
- ☐ Correct position and proportion

Eye detail:
- ☐ Brow or lashes
- ☐ Pupil
- ☐ Proportion
- ☐ Glance directed front in profile drawing

Chin:
- ☐ Present; forehead
- ☐ Projection

Profile:
- ☐ Not more than one error
- ☐ Correct

TABLE 8-6										
GOODENOUGH AGE NORMS										
Age (yr)	3	4	5	6	7	8	9	10	11	12	13
Points	2	6	10	14	18	22	26	30	34	38	42

From Taylor E. Psychological appraisal of children with cerebral defects. Boston: Harvard University; 1961.

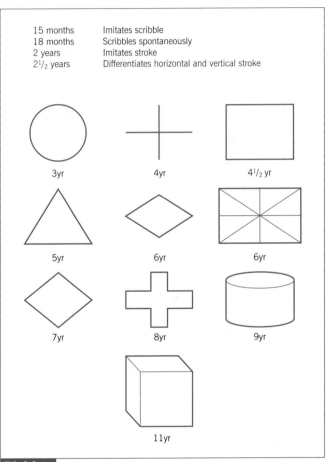

15 months	Imitates scribble
18 months	Scribbles spontaneously
2 years	Imitates stroke
2½ years	Differentiates horizontal and vertical stroke

3yr 4yr 4½ yr

5yr 6yr 6yr

7yr 8yr 9yr

11yr

FIG. 8-2

Gesell figures. *(From Illingsworth RS. The development of the infant and young child, normal and abnormal, 5th ed. Baltimore: Williams & Wilkins; 1972 and Cattel P. The measurement of intelligence of infants and young children. New York: The Psychological Corporation; 1960.)*

DEVELOPMENT AND BEHAVIOR

8

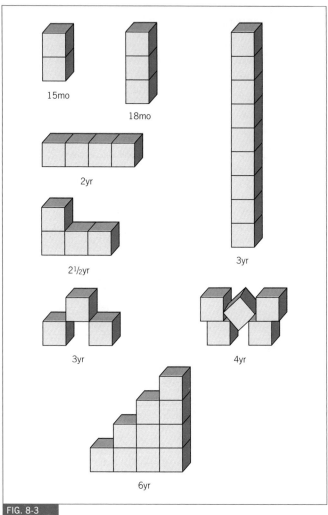

FIG. 8-3

Block skills. *(From Capute AJ, Accardo PJ. The pediatrician and the developmentally disabled child: a clinical textbook on mental retardation. Baltimore: University Press; 1979.)*

TABLE 8-7

POSTURAL REACTIONS

Postural Reaction	Age of Appearance	Description	Importance
Head righting	6 wk-3 mo	Lifts chin from tabletop in prone position	Necessary for adequate head control and sitting
Landau response	2-3 mo	Extension of head, then trunk and legs when held prone	Early measure of developing trunk control
Derotational righting	4-5 mo	Following passive or active head turning, the body rotates to follow the direction of the head	Prerequisite to independent rolling
Anterior propping	4-5 mo	Arm extension anteriorly in supported sitting	Necessary for tripod sitting
Parachute	5-6 mo	Arm extension when falling	Facial protection when falling
Lateral propping	6-7 mo	Arm extension laterally in protective response	Allows independent sitting
Posterior propping	8-10 mo	Arm extension posteriorly	Allows pivoting in sitting

Modified from Milani-Comparetti A, Gidoni EA. Dev Med Child Neurol 1967; 9:631; Capute AJ. Pediatr Ann 1986; 15:217; Capute AJ et al. Dev Med Child Neurol 1984; 26:375; and Palmer FB, Capute AJ. Developmental disabilities. In Oski FA, editor. Principles and practice of pediatrics. Philadelphia: JB Lippincott; 1994.

DEVELOPMENT AND BEHAVIOR

8

TABLE 8-8
PRIMITIVE REFLEXES

Primitive Reflexes	Elicitation	Response	Timing
Moro reflex (MR, "embrace" response) of fingers, wrists, and elbows	*Supine:* Sudden neck extension; allow head to fall back about 3 cm	Extension, adduction, and then abduction of UEs, with semiflexion	Present at birth; disappears by 3-6 mo
Galant reflex (GR)	*Prone suspension:* Stroking paravertebral area from thoracic to sacral region	Produces truncal incurvature with concavity toward stimulated side	Present at birth; disappears by 2-6 mo
Asymmetric tonic neck reflex (ATNR, "fencer" response)	*Supine:* Rotate head laterally about 45-90 degrees	Relative extension of limbs on chin side and flexion on occiput side	Present at birth; disappears by 4-9 mo
Symmetric tonic neck reflex (STNR, "cat" reflex)	*Sitting:* Head extension/flexion	Extension of UEs and flexion of LEs/flexion of UEs and LE extension	Appears at 5 mo; not present in most normal children; disappears by 8-9 mo
Tonic labyrinthine supine (TLS)	*Supine:* Extension of the neck (alters relation of the labyrinths)	Tonic extension of trunk and LEs, shoulder retraction and adduction, usually with elbow flexion	Present at birth; disappears by 6-9 mo
Tonic labyrinthine prone (TLP)	*Prone:* Flexion of the neck	Active flexion of trunk with protraction of shoulders	Present at birth; disappears by 6-9 mo
Positive support reflex (PSR)	Vertical suspension; bouncing hallucal areas on firm surface	*Neonatal:* Momentary LE extension followed by flexion	Present at birth; disappears by 2-4 mo
		Mature: Extension of LEs and support of body weight	Appears by 6 mo

DIRECTIONS FOR ADMINISTRATION

1. Try to get child to smile by smiling, talking or waving. Do not touch him/her.
2. Child must stare at hand several seconds.
3. Parent may help guide toothbrush and put toothpaste on brush.
4. Child does not have to be able to tie shoes or button/zip in the back.
5. Move yarn slowly in an arc from one side to the other, about 8" above child's face.
6. Pass if child grasps rattle when it is touched to the backs or tips of fingers.
7. Pass if child tries to see where yarn went. Yarn should be dropped quickly from sight from tester's hand without arm movement.
8. Child must transfer cube from hand to hand without help of body, mouth, or table.
9. Pass if child picks up raisin with any part of thumb and finger.
10. Line can vary only 30 degrees or less from tester's line. /
11. Make a fist with thumb pointing upward and wiggle only the thumb. Pass if child imitates and does not move any fingers other than the thumb.

12. Pass any enclosed form. Fail continuous round motions.

13. Which line is longer? (Not bigger.) Turn paper upside down and repeat. (pass 3 of 3 or 5 of 6)

14. Pass any lines crossing near midpoint.

15. Have child copy first. If failed, demonstrate.

When giving items 12, 14, and 15, do not name the forms. Do not demonstrate 12 and 14.

16. When scoring, each pair (2 arms, 2 legs, etc.) counts as one part.
17. Place one cube in cup and shake gently near child's ear, but out of sight. Repeat for other ear.
18. Point to picture and have child name it. (No credit is given for sounds only.)
    If less than 4 pictures are named correctly, have child point to picture as each is named by tester.

  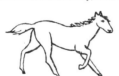

19. Using doll, tell child: Show me the nose, eyes, ears, mouth, hands, feet, tummy, hair. Pass 6 of 8.
20. Using pictures, ask child: Which one flies?... says meow?... talks?... barks?... gallops? Pass 2 of 5, 4 of 5.
21. Ask child: What do you do when you are cold?... tired?... hungry? Pass 2 of 3, 3 of 3.
22. Ask child: What do you do with a cup? What is a chair used for? What is a pencil used for?
    Action words must be included in answers.
23. Pass if child correctly places and says how many blocks are on paper. (1, 5).
24. Tell child: Put block **on** table; **under** table; **in front of** me, **behind** me. Pass 4 of 4.
    (Do not help child by pointing, moving head or eyes.)
25. Ask child: What is a ball?... lake?... desk?... house?... banana?... curtain?... fence?... ceiling? Pass if defined in terms of use, shape, what it is made of, or general category (such as banana is fruit, not just yellow). Pass 5 of 8, 7 of 8.
26. Ask child: If a horse is big, a mouse is __? If fire is hot, ice is __? If the sun shines during the day, the moon shines during the __? Pass 2 of 3.
27. Child may use wall or rail only, not person. May not crawl.
28. Child must throw ball overhand 3 feet to within arm's reach of tester.
29. Child must perform standing broad jump over width of test sheet (8 1/2 inches).
30. Tell child to walk forward, ⊂⊃⊂⊃⊂⊃⊂⊃➤ heel within 1 inch of toe. Tester may demonstrate.
    Child must walk 4 consecutive steps.
31. In the second year, half of normal children are non-compliant.

OBSERVATIONS:

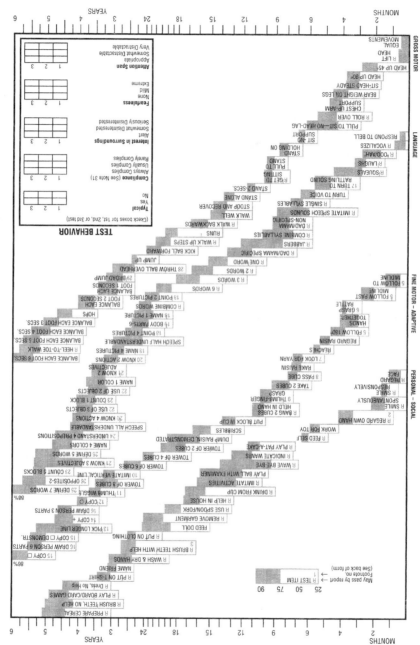

The Denver Development Assessment (Denver II). (From Frankenberg WE, Dodds JB. The Denver Development Assessment (Denver II). Denver: University of Colorado Medical School; 1990.)

Stepping reflex (SR, walking reflex)	Vertical suspension; hallucal stimulation	Stepping gait	Disappears by 2-3 mo
Crossed extension reflex (CER)	Prone; hallucal stimulation of an LE in full extension	Initial flexion, adduction, then extension of contralateral limb	Present at birth; disappears by 9 mo
Plantar grasp	Stimulation of hallucal areas	Plantar flexion grasp	Present at birth; disappears by 9 mo
Palmar grasp	Stimulation of palm	Palmar grasp	Present at birth; disappears by 9 mo
Lower extremity placing (LEP)	Vertical suspension; rubbing tibia or dorsum of foot against edge of tabletop	Initial flexion, then extension, then placing of LE on tabletop	Appears at 1 day
Upper extremity placing (UEP)	Rubbing lateral surface of forearm along edge of tabletop from elbow to wrist to dorsal hand	Flexion, extension, then placing of hand on tabletop	Appears at 3 mo
Downward thrust (DT)	Vertical suspension; thrust LEs downward	Full extension of LEs	Appears at 3 mo

UE, Upper extremity; *LE*, lower extremity.

DEVELOPMENT AND BEHAVIOR 8

TABLE 8-9

APPROPRIATE SCREENING IN EACH DEVELOPMENTAL STREAM BY AGE*

Age	Cognitive		Motor	Behavior
	Visual Motor	Language		
Infants and toddlers	CAT, Denver II	CLAMS, Denver II	Milestones, Denver II, neurologic examination, primitive reflexes	Temperament, social skills, activity level, Denver II
Preschool age	Draw-a-person, Gesell figures, block skills, Denver II	Articulation, comprehension (example: following commands), expression (example: estimate of vocabulary), Denver II	Milestones, neurologic examination, Denver II	Child behavior checklist, ADHD checklist, Denver II
School age	Draw-a-person, Gesell figures, handwriting	Reading, decoding comprehension, listening, written language	Coordination, neurologic examination, soft neurologic signs	Child behavior checklist, ADHD checklist

*If significant delays are noted, referral to a developmental pediatrician or psychologist is indicated.

to walk when led with two hands held (i.e., a 10-month level of motor development) has a DQ of $10/13 = 77\%$ and is not considered delayed.

REFERENCES

1. Capute AJ, Shapiro BK, Palmer FB. Spectrum of developmental disabilities: continuum of motor dysfunction. Orthoped Clin North Am 1981; 12:15-21.
2. Shapiro BK, Gallico RP. Learning disabilities. Pediatr Clin North Am 1993; 40:491-505.
3. Capute AJ, Accardo PJ, editors. Cerebral palsy: developmental disabilities in infancy and childhood, 2nd ed, vol 2. Baltimore: Paul H Brookes; 1996.
4. American Psychiatric Association. Diagnostic and statistical manual of mental disorders, 4th ed. Washington, DC: The Association; 1994.

8

DEVELOPMENT AND BEHAVIOR

ENDOCRINOLOGY

Irene Moff, MD and Renu Peterson, MD

I. WEBSITES

www.diabetes.org (American Diabetes Association)
www.jdrf.org (Juvenile Diabetes Research Foundation International)

II. DIABETES

A. DIABETIC KETOACIDOSIS

Diabetic ketoacidosis (DKA) is defined by hyperglycemia, ketonemia, ketonuria, and metabolic acidosis (pH <7.30, bicarbonate <15 mEq/L).

1. **Assessment**
a. History: In a known diabetic child, determine the usual insulin regimen, last dose, history of infection, or inciting event. In a suspected diabetic child, determine if there is a history of polydipsia, polyuria, polyphagia, weight loss, vomiting, or abdominal pain.
b. Examination: Assess for dehydration, Kussmaul's respiration, fruity breath, change in mental status, and current weight.
c. Laboratory tests: See Fig. 9-1 for a management algorithm. In addition, consider assessing the HgbA1c level in a known diabetic as an index of chronic hyperglycemia (normal values are 4.5% to 6.1%); in a new-onset diabetic, consider islet cell antibodies, insulin antibodies, thyroid antibodies, and thyroid function tests.
2. **Management: Because the fluid and electrolyte requirements of patients in DKA may vary greatly, the following guidelines should be taken as a starting point for therapy that must be individualized based on the dynamics of the patient. Cerebral edema is the most important complication of DKA; overaggressive hydration and overly rapid correction of hyperglycemia should be avoided because it may play a role in its development.** Remember that pH is a good indicator of insulin deficiency, and if acidosis is not resolving, the patient may need more insulin, whereas the degree of hyperglycemia is often a reflection of hydration status. See Figs. 9-1 and 9-2 for details.

B. DIAGNOSTIC CRITERIA

Under the American Diabetes Association's guidelines,[1] one of three criteria must be met to make the diagnosis of diabetes mellitus:

- Symptoms of diabetes (polyuria, polydipsia, and weight loss) and a random blood glucose ≥200 mg/dL.
- Fasting blood glucose (no caloric intake for at least 8 hours) ≥126 mg/dL.
- Oral glucose tolerance test (OGTT) with a 2-hour post-load blood glucose of ≥200 mg/dL.

1. **Pretest preparation:** A calorically adequate diet is required for 3 days before the test, with 50% of total calories taken as carbohydrate.
2. **Delay test 2 weeks after illness.** Discontinue all hyperglycemic and

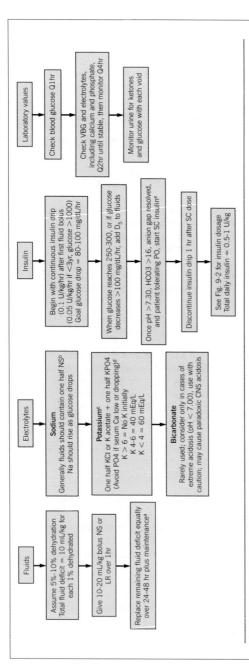

FIG. 9-1

Management of diabetic ketoacidosis. *CNS,* Central nervous system; *LR,* lactated Ringer's solution; *NS,* normal saline; *SC,* subcutaneous; *VBG,* venous blood gases. *(Modified from Hafeez W, Vuguin P. Contemp Pediatr 2000; 17(6):72-83.)*

Fluids

Assume 5%-10% dehydration
Total fluid deficit = 10 mL/kg for each 1% dehydrated

Give 10-20 mL/kg bolus or LR over 1 hr

Replace remaining fluid deficit equally over 24-48 hr plus maintenance[e]

Electrolytes

Sodium[b]
Generally fluids should contain one half NS[b]
Na should rise as glucose drops

Potassium[c]
One half KCl or K acetate + one half KPO4
(Avoid PO4 if serum Ca low or dropping)[d]
K > 6 = No K initially
K 4-6 = 40 mEq/L
K < 4 = 60 mEq/L

Bicarbonate
Rarely used; consider only in cases of extreme acidosis (pH < 7.00), use with caution; may cause paradoxic CNS acidosis

Insulin

Begin with continuous insulin drip (0.1 U/kg/hr) after first fluid bolus (0.05 U/kg/hr if <3yr, glucose >1000)
Goal glucose drop = 80-100 mg/dL/hr

When glucose reaches 250-300, or if glucose decreases >100 mg/dL/hr, add D5 to fluids

Once pH >7.30, HCO3 >16, anion gap resolved, and patient tolerating PO, start SC insulin[e]

Discontinue insulin drip 1 hr after SC dose

See Fig. 9-2 for insulin dosage
Total daily insulin = 0.5-1 U/kg

Laboratory values

Check blood glucose Q1hr

Check VBG and electrolytes, including calcium and phosphate, Q2hr until stable, then monitor Q4hr

Monitor urine for ketones and glucose with each void

[a]If urine output is high, include in maintenance until osmotic diuresis slows; therefore maintenance = urine output + insensible losses (one third of standard maintenance calculations).
[b]Some DKA protocols recommend using NS rather than half NS during part of the replacement period in an effort to further decrease risk of cerebral edema.
[c]Patients with DKA are total body K+ depleted and are at risk for severe hypokalemia during DKA therapy. However, serum K+ levels may be normal or elevated as a result of the shift of K+ to the extracellular compartment in the setting of acidosis.
[d]Phosphate is depleted in DKA and will drop further with insulin therapy. Consider replacing half of K as KPO4 for first 8hr, then all as KCl. Excessive phosphate may induce hypocalcemic tetany.
[e]Some protocols recommend also waiting for urine ketones to decrease or clear before starting SC insulin.

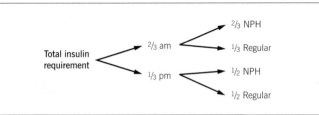

FIG. 9-2

Conversion to daily insulin dosage. *NPH,* Neutral protamine Hagedorn.

hypoglycemic agents (e.g., salicylates, diuretics, oral contraceptives, phenytoin).

3. **Give 1.75 g/kg (maximum of 100 g) of glucose orally after a 12-hour fast,** allowing up to 5 minutes for ingestion. Mix glucose with water and lemon juice as a 20% dilution. Quiet activity is permissible during the OGTT. Draw blood samples at 0, 30, 60, 120, 180, and 240 minutes after ingestion.

4. **Interpretation:** 2-hour blood glucose <140 mg/dL = normal; 140 to 199 mg/dL = impaired glucose tolerance; ≥200 mg/dL = diabetes mellitus.

C. **TYPE II DIABETES MELLITUS**

1. **There is an increasing prevalence of type II diabetes mellitus among children, especially among African-Americans, Hispanics, and Native Americans;** this increase is related to an increased prevalence of childhood obesity.

2. **An abnormality in glucose levels is caused by insulin resistance and an insulin secretory defect.**

3. **It can present in ketoacidosis** (chronic high glucose impairs beta cell function and increases peripheral insulin resistance).

4. **Consider screening by measuring fasting blood glucose levels among children who are overweight (body mass index [BMI] >85th percentile for age and gender) and have two of the following risk factors:** family history of type II diabetes in a first or second-degree relative; race/ethnicity of African-American, Native American, Hispanic, or Asian/Pacific Islander; signs associated with insulin resistance (acanthosis nigricans, hypertension, dyslipidemia, polycystic ovarian disease). Screening, if done, should begin at age 10 or onset of puberty (whichever occurs first) and repeated every 2 years.[2]

5. **Primary treatment is with diet and exercise,** although pharmacologic agents are often necessary for those who fail conservative management and/or are symptomatic at presentation. No validated treatment protocols currently exist in children. Metformin has been used for patients with serum glucose levels <350 mg/dL without ketones (see Chapter 26). Metformin is not approved by the Federal Drug Administration (FDA) for use in adolescents; use with caution and avoid

in patients with renal or hepatic impairment.[3] For patients with severe hyperglycemia and/or DKA on presentation, insulin and metformin may be initiated, with eventual discontinuation of the insulin. There has been no reported experience in adolescents with the newer insulin-sensitizing drugs (i.e., rosiglitazone and pioglitazone) or with sulfonylureas.

III. THYROID AND PARATHYROID FUNCTION

A. THYROID TESTS[5-7]

1. **Interpretation of thyroid function tests:** Table 9-1.
2. **Thyroid scan:** Used to assess thyroid clearance and to study structure and function of the thyroid. Localizes ectopic thyroid tissue and hyperfunctioning and nonfunctioning thyroid nodules.
3. **Technetium uptake:** Measures uptake of technetium by thyroid gland, levels are increased in hyperthyroidism and decreased in thyroxine-binding globulin (TBG) deficiency and in hypothyroidism (except dyshormonogenesis, when it may be increased).

B. HYPOTHYROIDISM

1. **Symptoms:** Clinical signs and symptoms of congenital hypothyroidism are rarely present at birth. They usually develop within the first few days to 2 weeks of life and are almost always present by 6 weeks. These may include lethargy, constipation, hoarse cry, large fontanelles, hypotonia, hypothermia, and jaundice. Acquired hypothyroidism can occur as early as the first 2 years of life, with deceleration of growth as the first manifestation.
2. **Diagnosis:** Initial laboratory evaluation includes measurement of T_4 and thyroid-stimulating hormone (TSH) levels. Also consider antithyroglobulin and antimicrosomal antibodies to evaluate for Hashimoto's thyroiditis.
3. **Treatment:** Begin with L-thyroxine (see Chapter 26). Monitor T_4 and TSH at the end of the first and second weeks to make sure replacement is not excessive. Thereafter, levels should be monitored at 1- to 3-month intervals during the first year, and more frequently if the dose is adjusted. After 2 years, monitoring levels every 6 to 12 months should be adequate because the need to change the dose is less frequent.

C. HYPERTHYROIDISM

1. **Thyroid storm** is a form of hyperthyroidism that is acute in onset and manifested by hyperthermia, tachycardia, and restlessness. Untreated, this may progress to delirium, coma, and death.
a. **Management:** Treat with propylthiouracil (PTU) or methimazole, which inhibit formation of thyroid hormone. Propranolol is used to suppress signs and symptoms of thyrotoxicosis. Potassium iodide, in a variety of preparations, may also be used for acute hyperthyroid management (see Chapter 26 for dosage information).
b. **Neonatal thyrotoxicosis** is seen almost exclusively in infants born to mothers with Graves' disease and it is caused by transplacental passage of maternal thyroid-stimulating immunoglobulin. Onset can range from

TABLE 9-1

THYROID FUNCTION TESTS: INTERPRETATION

	TSH	T_4	Free T_4
Primary hyperthyroidism	L	H	High N to H
Primary hypothyroidism	H	L	L
Hypothalamic/pituitary hypothyroidism	L, N, H*	L	L
TBG deficiency	N	L	N
Euthyroid sick syndrome	L, N, H*	L	L to low N
TSH adenoma or pituitary resistance	N to H	H	H
Compensated hypothyroidism†	H	N	N

H, High; *L,* low; *N,* normal; T_4, thyroxine; *TSH,* thyroid stimulating hormone.
*Can be normal, slightly low, or slightly high.
†Treatment may not be necessary

immediate to delayed for weeks, with duration of up to 6 months. Clinical signs and symptoms include microcephaly, frontal bossing, intrauterine growth retardation (IUGR), tachycardia, hypertension, irritability, failure to thrive, exophthalmos, goiter, flushing, vomiting/diarrhea, jaundice, thrombocytopenia, and cardiac failure/arrhythmias. Treat as described for hyperthyroidism. In addition, digoxin may be needed for cardiac failure.

2. **The most common cause of hyperthyroidism in children is Graves' disease.** Other rare causes include subacute thyroiditis, pituitary resistance to thyroid hormone, factitious hyperthyroidism (intake of exogenous hormone), and TSH-secreting pituitary tumor. Initial laboratory evaluation includes evaluation of TSH, T_4, and T_3 levels. Further tests include assessment of TSH receptor stimulating antibody, antithyroglobulin and antimicrosomal antibodies, free T_4, and free T_3.

D. HYPERPARATHYROIDISM

1. **Definition:** Primary hyperparathyroidism causes hypercalcemia from increased bone and renal resorption and increased intestinal absorption of calcium via increased activated vitamin D. Primary hyperparathyroidism is uncommon in childhood. It is associated with multiple endocrine neoplasia syndromes. Secondary hyperparathyroidism may develop in renal failure secondary to hyperphosphatemia. Symptoms of hypercalcemia include vomiting, constipation, abdominal pain, weakness, paresthesias, malaise, and bone pain.

2. **Laboratory abnormalities:** Table 9-2.

3. **Management:** Hydration is the mainstay of treatment by enhancing calciuria. Furosemide may be used with caution because hypercalcemia can be exacerbated if hydration is not adequate. Hydrocortisone, 1 mg/kg every 6 hours, reduces intestinal absorption of calcium. Calcitonin opposes bone resorption but only transiently. In severe hypercalcemia, bisphosphates may be considered.

TABLE 9-2

LABORATORY ABNORMALITIES IN ENDOCRINE DISEASE

Disorder	Laboratory Findings
Diabetes insipidus	Low urine specific gravity (<1.005)
	Low urine osmolarity (50-200)
	Low vasopressin (<0.5 pg/mL)
SIADH	Low serum Na^+ and chloride with normal HCO_3^-
	Hypouricemia
	Inappropriately concentrated urine
Hypoparathyroidism	Low serum calcium
	High serum phosphorus
	Normal or low alkaline phosphatase
	Low 1,25-hydroxy-vitamin D_3
	Low PTH (may be normal or elevated in pseudohypoparathyroidism)
Hyperparathyroidism	High serum calcium
	Low serum phosphorus
	Normal or high alkaline phosphatase
	High PTH
Congenital adrenal hyperplasia (classic 21-hydroxylase deficiency)	Low serum Na^+ and chloride
	High serum potassium
	High renin
	Low cortisol
	Elevated androgens and cortisol precursors
	Hypoglycemia

E. HYPOPARATHYROIDISM

1. **Definition:** True hypoparathyroidism results from a decrease in parathyroid hormone (PTH). Patients may also have PTH resistance (pseudohypoparathyroidism), in which PTH is normal or elevated. Clinical manifestations range from asymptomatic or mild muscle cramps to hypocalcemic tetany and convulsions.
2. **Laboratory abnormalities:** See Table 9-2.
3. **Management:** Therapy is calcium supplementation for documented hypocalcemia and vitamin D supplementation with calcitriol (see Chapter 26). Monitor serum calcium and phosphorous carefully during therapy.

IV. ADRENAL AND PITUITARY FUNCTION[8]

A. ADRENAL INSUFFICIENCY

1. **Etiology:** Most common causes are congenital adrenal hyperplasia (CAH) and long-term glucocorticoid treatment. Other causes include Addison's disease and hypothalamic or pituitary disease secondary to tumors, surgery, radiation therapy, or congenital defects.
2. **Acute adrenal crisis**
a. Assessment: Characterized by hypoglycemia, hyponatremia, hyperkalemia, hypotension, metabolic acidosis, and shock. The more

subtle signs of adrenal insufficiency include poor appetite, emesis, dehydration, and failure to gain weight.

b. Diagnosis: Obtain serum electrolytes and glucose to guide therapy. Serum cortisol and aldosterone are decreased and adrenocorticotropic hormone (ACTH) and renin are elevated. In infants with CAH, 17-hydroxyprogesterone (17-OHP) is increased. These studies are useful to obtain before steroid administration to confirm the diagnosis, but treatment should not be delayed.

c. Management: Requires rapid volume expansion to support blood pressure, sufficient dextrose to maintain blood glucose, close monitoring of electrolytes, and corticosteroid administration. Give 50 mg/m^2 of hydrocortisone in an intravenous (IV) bolus (rapid estimate: infants = 25 mg; children = 50 to 100 mg), followed by 50 mg/m^2/24 hours as a continuous drip (preferable) or divided every 3 to 4 hours. Hydrocortisone and cortisone are the only glucocorticoids that provide the necessary mineralocorticoid effects.

3. Congenital adrenal hyperplasia[9,10]

a. Definition: Group of autosomal-recessive disorders characterized by a defect in one of the enzymes required in the synthesis of cortisol from cholesterol. Cortisol deficiency results in oversecretion of ACTH and hyperplasia of the adrenal cortex. The enzymatic defect results in impaired synthesis of adrenal steroids beyond the enzymatic block, and overproduction of the precursors before the block.

b. Etiology: 21-Hydroxylase deficiency accounts for 90% of cases. See Fig. 9-3 for enzyme deficiencies that can cause CAH.

c. Diagnosis (see Table 9-2 for laboratory abnormalities)

(1) Classic or salt-losing form (complete enzyme deficiency): Adrenal insufficiency occurs under basal conditions and manifests as adrenal crisis in the neonatal period. Adrenal crisis in untreated patients occurs at 1 to 2 weeks of life, with signs and symptoms of adrenal insufficiency rarely occurring before 3 to 4 days of life. CAH is the most common cause of ambiguous genitalia in females. Diagnosis is based on elevated 17-OHP levels. Levels of testosterone in girls and androstenedione in boys and girls are also elevated.

(2) Nonclassic or simple virilizing form (partial enzyme deficiency): Adrenal insufficiency tends to occur only under stress and manifests as androgen excess after infancy (precocious pubarche, irregular menses, hirsutism, acne). Morning 17-OHP levels may be elevated, but diagnosis is based on the ACTH stimulation test (see p. 223). A significant rise in the 17-OHP level 60 minutes after ACTH injection is diagnostic. Cortisol response will be decreased.

4. Daily management of adrenal insufficiency

a. Glucocorticoid maintenance: Physiologic glucocorticoid production is approximately 9 to 12 mg/m^2/day. For congenital adrenal hyperplasia, 12.5 mg/m^2/day of hydrocortisone via IV or intramuscular (IM) route or 25 mg/m^2/day orally (PO) is recommended for daily mainte-

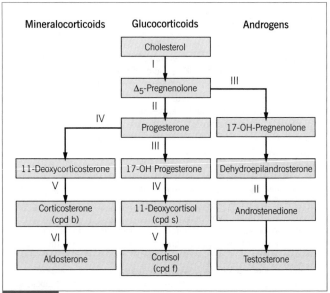

FIG. 9-3

Steroid hormone pathway and the enzymatic deficiencies in congenital adrenal hyperplasia. Enzyme deficiency: I, cholesterol (20, 22) desmolase; II, 3-B-hydroxysteroid dehydrogenase; III, 17-hydroxylase; IV, 21-hydroxylase; V, 11-hydroxylase; VI, 18-"oxidation" defect; Cpd, compound. *(From Bacon GE et al. A practical approach to pediatric endocrinology, 3rd ed. Chicago: Year Book Medical Publishers; 1990.)*

nance to allow for suppression of the ACTH axis. For pure adrenal insufficiency, daily dosing of 9 to 12 mg/m^2 of hydrocortisone PO is often sufficient and helps decrease the toxic effects seen at higher doses.

b. Mineralocorticoid maintenance: For salt-losing forms of adrenal insufficiency, 0.05 to 0.3 mg/day of fludrocortisone acetate PO once daily is recommended. Note that IV hydrocortisone at 50 mg/m^2/day will also supply a maintenance amount of mineralocorticoid activity for patients who cannot take the oral form. Always monitor blood pressure and electrolytes when supplementing mineralocorticoids.

c. Stress dose glucocorticoids: Increase the dose of glucocorticoids in patients with fever or other illness. The stress dose is 25 to 50 mg/m^2/day of hydrocortisone IV/IM (as a continuous drip or divided every 3 to 6 hours) or 75 mg/m^2/day PO. For surgery or severe illness, treatment with doses of 50 to 100 mg/m^2/day IV may be indicated.

B. **SYNDROME OF INAPPROPRIATE ANTIDIURETIC HORMONE SECRETION**[11]

1. **Definition:** The hallmark of syndrome of inappropriate antidiuretic hormone (SIADH) is hyponatremia (Na^+ <135) with inappropriately concentrated urine in the setting of euvolemia or hypervolemia. It is associated with many conditions, including central nervous system (CNS) trauma and CNS infection (see Table 9-2 for laboratory abnormalities).

2. **Management:** Hyponatremia should be corrected slowly with fluid restriction. A reasonable goal is a 10% increase in Na^+ per 24 hours. In the setting of coma or seizures, more rapid Na^+ correction should be undertaken by treating with hypertonic saline (see Chapter 10 for details). Definitive therapy is to identify and treat the underlying cause.

C. **DIABETES INSIPIDUS**[11]

1. **Definition:** The hallmark of diabetes insipidus (DI) is an impaired ability to concentrate urine (specific gravity is usually <1.005). Central DI is caused by vasopressin deficiency and is associated with CNS injury, including trauma and tumors. Nephrogenic DI is caused by renal tubular resistance to vasopressin and can be genetic or acquired. The water-deprivation test (see p. 228) is diagnostic for DI, and the vasopressin test (see p. 228) is used to differentiate between central and nephrogenic DI (see Table 9-2 for laboratory abnormalities).

2. **Management:** DDAVP (desmopressin acetate) in nasal spray, IV, PO, or subcutaneous (SC) preparation is used for management of central DI. Titrate the DDAVP dosage to urine output, aiming for at least one period of diuresis per day that is sufficient to stimulate thirst. Electrolytes must be monitored closely. Provision of free water and a diet that is low in salt is the cornerstone of therapy in nephrogenic DI. Definitive therapy is to identify and treat the underlying cause.

V. GROWTH AND SEXUAL DEVELOPMENT[12-17]

A. **GROWTH**

1. **Target height** range is calculated as mid-parental stature ± 2 SD (1 SD = 2 inches).

a. Mid-parental stature for boys is (paternal height + maternal height + 5 inches)/2.

b. Mid-parental stature for girls is (paternal height + maternal height − 5 inches)/2.

2. **Short stature**[12,13]

a. Differential diagnosis: It is important to differentiate constitutional growth delay (CGD) and familial short stature (FSS) from pathologic causes of short stature. CGD is characterized by slow growth rate during the first 2 to 3 years of life followed by a low-normal growth velocity. Family history of short stature and delayed puberty is often present. A short child with a normal linear growth velocity and a short target height is

9

ENDOCRINOLOGY

suggestive of FSS. Deceleration of linear growth in a well-nourished child is typical of growth hormone deficiency, hypothyroidism, or glucocorticoid excess. Initial decline in weight followed by decreased height velocity is suggestive of malnutrition or systemic illness. Dysmorphic features may indicate a chromosomal abnormality (Trisomy 21 or Turner's syndrome) or other specific syndrome. Disproportionate features or skeletal abnormalities are consistent with skeletal dysplasias or metabolic bone disease.

b. Initial evaluation: Begin with a thorough history, physical examination, and evaluation of growth curves. Initial screening tests include complete blood count (CBC), liver function tests (LFTs), electrolytes, erythrocyte sedimentation rate (ESR), and urinalysis (including pH and specific gravity). Also consider thyroid function tests, serum IGF-1 and IGFBP-3, antiendomysial and antigliadin antibodies for celiac disease, bone age, and karyotype. Bone age is delayed in CGD but consistent with chronologic age in FSS. Consider a skeletal survey in a patient with disproportionate features.

B. SEXUAL DEVELOPMENT[14-17]

1. Delayed puberty is defined as no signs of pubertal development by 13 years in girls and 14 years in boys, or an arrest in pubertal maturation. There are two major categories:

a. Hypergonadotropic hypogonadism (high luteinizing hormone [LH] and follicle-stimulating hormone [FSH]) is secondary to primary gonadal failure. Common causes are chemotherapy, radiation therapy, and autoimmune glandular failure. Other causes include androgen insensitivity, Turner's syndrome, and Klinefelter's syndrome. Karyotype should be obtained for initial evaluation.

b. Hypogonadotropic hypogonadism (low or normal LH and FSH) is secondary to constitutional delay or a central gonadotropin deficiency. Kallman's syndrome is the most common cause of isolated gonadotropin deficiency. Other causes include CNS tumors, hypopituitarism, Prader-Willi syndrome, and chronic disease.

2. Precocious puberty is traditionally defined as any sign of secondary sexual maturation before 8 years in girls and 9 years in boys. More recent data suggest early puberty may not warrant extensive evaluation or intervention if it occurs after 6 years in African-American girls or after 7 years in Caucasian girls.

a. *Central, true, isosexual,* or *complete precocious puberty (CPP)* refers to gonadotropin-releasing hormone (GnRH)–dependent puberty and involves activation of the hypothalamic-pituitary-gonadal axis. Most common causes are CNS lesions (congenital anomalies, tumors, trauma, infections) and idiopathic. Pathologic etiologies are more commonly seen in boys.

b. *Peripheral* or *pseudoprecocious puberty* refers to GnRH-independent puberty and involves adrenal, gonadal, ectopic, or exogenous sources of hormone production. Most common causes are CAH, adrenal tumors,

McCune-Albright syndrome, gonadal tumors, human chorionic gonadotropin (hCG)–producing tumors, and exogenous sex hormones. Hypothyroidism can also cause GnRH-independent precocity.

c. Initial evaluation: Begin with a complete history, physical examination, and evaluation of growth curves. Penile length is disproportionately greater than testicular size in pseudoprecocious puberty, and testicular volume is disproportionately greater than penile size in normal puberty and in CPP. Growth rate in precocious puberty is usually more rapid than along a single height percentile. Patients with suspected precocious puberty should have a bone age study to confirm the diagnosis. Bone age is generally more than 2 years in advance of chronologic age in long-standing precocious puberty because of the action of sex hormones. Further studies should include basal and/or GnRH-stimulated LH levels (see p. 231), estradiol measurement in girls, testosterone levels in boys, 17-OHP levels, dehydroepiandrosterone (DHEA) levels, and urinary 17-ketosteroids (see p. 231). A magnetic resonance imaging (MRI) scan of the brain to identify CNS lesions should be obtained in any patient suspected of having CPP.

3. **Ambiguous genitalia**

a. Clinical findings in a neonate that indicate possible ambiguous genitalia include anogenital ratio >0.5 (distance between anus and posterior fourchette divided by distance between anus and base of clitoris), phallus length <2.2 cm (mean newborn length – 2 SD), clitoromegaly (length >1 cm), nonpalpable gonads in an apparent male, and hypospadias associated with separation of scrotal sacs or undescended testis.

b. Etiology: The most common cause of ambiguous genitalia is CAH. Other causes include testicular regression syndrome, androgen insensitivity, testosterone biosynthesis disorders, and chromosomal abnormalities.

c. Diagnosis is based on karyotype, measurement of gonadotropins (LH, FSH), adrenal steroids (cortisol, 17-OHP, and ACTH stimulation test), testosterone precursors (DHEA, androstenedione), testosterone, dihydrotestosterone (DHT), and hCG stimulation test (see p. 232).

VI. NORMAL VALUES (Tables 9-3 to 9-22)

Normal values may differ among laboratories because of variation in technique and in type of radioimmunoassay used. Unless otherwise noted, the values below are reference ranges from the Johns Hopkins Hospital Laboratories or from SmithKline Beecham clinical laboratories in Baltimore, Maryland.

VII. TESTS AND PROCEDURES

1. **ACTH stimulation test**

a. The ACTH stimulation test measures the ability of the adrenal gland to produce cortisol in response to ACTH. It is most useful in diagnosis of adrenal insufficiency.

9

ENDOCRINOLOGY

TABLE 9-3
GONADOTROPINS

Age	FSH (mIU/mL)	LH (mIU/mL)
Prepubertal children	0.0-2.8	0.0-1.6
Men	1.4-14.4	1-10.2
Women, follicular phase	3.7-12.9	0.9-14

Normal infants have a transient rise in FSH (follicle-stimulating hormone) and LH (luteinizing hormone) to pubertal levels or higher within the first 3 mo, which then declines to prepubertal values by the end of the first year.

TABLE 9-4
TESTOSTERONE

Age	Testosterone, Serum Total (ng/dL)	Testosterone, Unbound (pg/mL)
Prepubertal children	10-20	0.15-0.6
Men	275-875	52-280
Women	23-75	1.1-6.3
Pregnancy	35-195	

TABLE 9-5
DIHYDROTESTOSTERONE (DHT)

Age	Males (ng/dL)	Females (ng/dL)
Cord blood	<2-8	<2-5
1-6 mo	12-85	<5
Prepubertal	<5	<5
Tanner stage II-III	3-33	5-19
Tanner stage IV-V	22-75	3-30

TABLE 9-6
ESTRADIOL

Age	pg/mL
Prepubertal children	<25
Men	6-44
Women	
Luteal phase	26-165
Follicular phase	None detected-266
Midcycle	118-355
Adult women on OCPS	None detected-102

Normal infants have an elevated estradiol at birth, which decreases to prepubertal values during the first week of life. Estradiol levels increase again between 1 and 2 mo of age and return to prepubertal values by 6-12 mo of age.

TABLE 9-7

ANDROSTENEDIONE, SERUM

Age	Male (ng/dL)	Female (ng/dL)
Preterm infants		
26-28 wk to day 4 of life	92-892	92-892
31-35 wk to day 4 of life	80-446	80-446
Full-term infants		
1-7 day	20-290	20-290
1-12 mo	6-68	6-68
Prepubertal children	8-50	8-50
Tanner II	31-65	42-100
Tanner III	50-100	80-190
Tanner IV	48-140	77-225
Tanner V	65-210	80-240
Adults	78-205	85-275

TABLE 9-8

DEHYDROEPIANDROSTERONE (DHEA)

Age	HEA (ng/D/mL)	DHEA Sulfate (mcg/dL)
Newborn infants	—	1.7-3.6
Prepubertal children	0-100	0.1-0.6
Men	195-915	1.4-7.9 (to age 30)
Women	215-855	0.7-4.5 (to age 30)

TABLE 9-9

17-HYDROXYPROGESTERONE, SERUM

Age	Baseline (ng/dL)	60 min after ACTH Stimulation (ng/dL)
Premature infants (31-35 wks)	≤360	N/A
Term infants, 1st wk of life	≤63	N/A
1-5 days	80-420	N/A
<1 yr	11-170	85-465
1-5 yr	4-115	50-350
6-12 yr	7-69	75-220
Male, Tanner Stages II-III	12-130	69-310
Female, Tanner Stages II-III	18-220	80-420
Male, Tanner Stages IV-V	51-190	105-230
Female, Tanner Stages IV-V	36-200	80-225
Adult Male	50-250	42-250
Adult Female, Premenopausal		
Follicular phase	20-100	42-250
Midcycle peak	100-250	
Luteal phase	100-500	

8 AM level is most accurate given diurnal variation. Levels are normally increased in newborns for the first few days of life. Be aware that infant serum contains substances that may cross-react in the assay for 17-hydroxyprogesterone and artificially elevate the level, unless they are separated by chromatography. Before interpreting results on infants, be sure that the laboratory has prepared HS samples appropriately.

9

ENDOCRINOLOGY

TABLE 9-10

CORTISOL, SERUM WITH ACTH STIMULATION TEST

Condition	mcg/dL
Any gender/any age/pre-ACTH, 8 AM	5.7-16.6
1 hr post-ACTH	16-36

TABLE 9-11

CORTISOL, URINE

Age	mcg/g Creatinine	mcg/24hr
Prepubertal children	7-25	3-9
Men	7-45	11-84
Women	9-32	10-34

TABLE 9-12

17-KETOSTEROIDS, URINE

Age	mg/24hr
<1 mo	<2.0
1 mo-5 yr	<0.5
6-8 yr	1.0-2.0
Men	9-22
Women	5-15

TABLE 9-13

17-HYDROXYCORTICOSTEROIDS, URINE

Children (body weight variable)	3 ± 1 mg/m^2/24 hr
Men	3-9 mg/24 hr
Women	2-8 mg/24 hr

TABLE 9-14

CATECHOLAMINES, URINE

Compound	Amount/24hr Urine Collection
Dopamine	100-440 mcg
Epinephrine	<15 mcg
Norepinephrine	15-86 mcg
Metanephrines	<0.4 mg
Normetanephrines	<0.9 mg
Homovanillic acid (HVA)	0-10 mg
Vanillyl mandelic acid (VMA)	2-10 mg

Catecholamines are elevated in a variety of tumors including neuroblastoma, ganglioneuroma, ganglioblastoma, and pheochromocytoma.

TABLE 9-15

CATECHOLAMINES, SERUM

Compound	Supine (mcg)	Sitting (mcg)
Dopamine	<87	<87
Epinephrine	<50	<60
Norepinephrine	110-410	120-680

TABLE 9-16

INSULIN-LIKE GROWTH FACTOR 1 (IGF-1)

Age	Males (units)	Females (units)
2 mo-6 yr	17-248	17-248
6-9 yr	88-474	88-474
9-12 yr	110-565	117-771
12-16 yr	202-957	261-1096
16-26 yr	182-780	182-780
>26 yr	123-463	123-463

A clearly normal IGF-1 level argues against GH deficiency, although in young children there is considerable overlap between normals and those with GH deficiency.

TABLE 9-17

INSULIN-LIKE GROWTH FACTOR-BINDING PROTEIN (IGF-BP3)

Age (years)	Males (mg/L)	Females (mg/L)
0-2	0.94-1.76	0.66-2.51
2-4	1.12-2.33	0.84-3.77
4-6	1.16-3.13	1.32-3.60
6-8	1.32-3.38	1.21-4.66
8-10	1.35-3.94	1.58-3.99
10-12	1.53-5.02	1.93-6.46
12-14	1.73-5.11	1.78-6.08
14-16	1.90-6.40	2.02-5.44
16-18	1.70-6.04	1.88-5.29
18-20	1.52-6.01	1.63-6.02
20-22	1.79-5.41	1.82-5.35
Adult (continues to vary with age)	1.15-5.18	1.19-5.69

Levels below the 5th percentile suggest a GH deficiency. This test may have greater discrimination than the IGF-1 test in younger patients.

9

ENDOCRINOLOGY

b. Method: Give 250 mcg ACTH IV/IM and measure cortisol at 0, 30, and 60 minutes.

c. Interpretation: With a normal pituitary-adrenal axis, there is a rise in serum cortisol after ACTH administration (see Table 9-10 for values). With ACTH deficiency or prolonged adrenal suppression, there is no rise in cortisol after a single ACTH dose. A decreased rise in cortisol is indicative of CAH. A lack of response after 3 consecutive days of ACTH stimulation is pathognomonic of Addison's disease.

TABLE 9-18
VITAMIN D

Compound	Value
25-Hydroxy-vitamin D	ng/mL
Newborns	8-21
Children	17-54
Adults	10-55
1,25-Dihydroxy-vitamin D	pg/mL
Newborns	8-72
Children	15-90
Adults	24-64

Note that 1,25-dihydroxy-vitamin D is the physiologically active form; however, 25-hydroxyvitamin D is the value to monitor for vitamin D deficiency, since this approximates body stores of vitamin D.

2. **Water deprivation test**

a. The water deprivation test determines ability to concentrate urine and is useful in the diagnosis of DI. It requires careful supervision because dehydration and hypernatremia may occur.

b. Method: Begin the test after a 24-hour period of adequate hydration and stable weight. Obtain a baseline weight after bladder emptying. Restrict fluids for 7 hours. Measure body weight and urinary specific gravity and volume hourly. Check serum Na^+ and urine and serum osmolality every 2 hours. Hematocrit and blood urea nitrogen (BUN) levels may also be obtained at these times but are not critical. Monitor carefully to ensure that fluids are not ingested during the test. Terminate the test if weight loss approaches 5%.

c. Interpretation

   (1) Normal individuals and those with psychogenic DI who are water deprived will concentrate their urine to 500 to 1400 mOsm/L, and plasma osmolality will be 288 to 291 mOsm/L. Urinary specific gravity rises to at least 1.010, urinary:plasma osmolality ratio is >2, urine volume decreases significantly, and there should be no appreciable weight loss.

   (2) In patients with central or nephrogenic DI, specific gravity remains <1.005. Urine osmolality remains <150 mOsm/L, with no significant reduction of urine volume. A weight loss of up to 5% usually occurs. At the end of the test, a serum osmolality >290 mOsm/L, Na+ >150 mEq/L, and a rise of BUN and hematocrit provide evidence that the patient did not receive water.

3. **Vasopressin test**

a. A vasopressin test is used for differentiation between central (ADH-deficient) and nephrogenic DI.

b. Method: Vasopressin is given SC, preferably at the end of the water deprivation test. Urine output, urine specific gravity, and water intake are monitored.

c. Interpretation: Patients with central DI concentrate their urine (>1.010)

TABLE 9-19

ROUTINE STUDIES (THYROID)

Test	Age	Normal	Comments
T_4 RIA (mcg/dL)	Cord	6.6-17.5	Measures total T_4 by radioimmunoassay
	1-3 dy	11.0-21.5	
	1-4 wk	8.2-16.6	
	1-12 mo	7.2-15.6	
	1-5 yr	7.3-15.0	
	6-10 yr	6.4-13.3	
	11-15 yr	5.6-11.7	
	16-20 yr	4.2-11.8	
	21-50 yr	4.3-12.5	
Free T_4 (ng/dL)	1-10 dy	0.6-2.0	Metabolically active form; the normal range for free T_4 is very assay dependent
	>10 dy	0.7-1.7	
T_3 RIA (ng/dL)	Cord	14-86	Measures T_3 by RIA
	1-3 dy	100-380	
	1-4 wk	99-310	
	1-12 mo	102-264	
	1-5 yr	105-269	
	6-10 yr	94-241	
	11-15 yr	83-213	
	16-20 yr	80-210	
	21-50 yr	70-204	
TSH (mIU/mL)	Cord	<2.5-17.4	TSH surge peaks from 80-90 mIU/mL in term newborn by 30 min after birth. Values after 1 wk are within adult normal range. Elevated values suggest primary hypothyroidism, whereas suppressed values are the best indicator of hyperthyroidism.
	1-3 dy	<2.5-13.3	
	1-4 wk	0.6-10.0	
	1-12 mo	0.6-6.3	
	1-15 yr	0.6-6.3	
	16-50 yr	0.2-7.6	
TBG (mg/dL)	Cord	0.7-4.7	
	1-3 dy	—	
	1-4 wk	0.5-4.5	
	1-12 mo	1.6-3.6	
	1-5 yr	1.3-2.8	
	6-20 yr	1.4-2.6	
	21-50 yr	1.2-2.4	

From Fisher DA. The thyroid. In Rudolf AM, editor. Pediatrics. Norwalk, Conn: Appleton & Lange; 1991 and LaFranchi SH, Pediatr Clin North Am 1979; 26(1):33-51.

RIA, radioimmunoassay; *RU,* resin uptake; T_3, triiodothyronine; T_4, thyroxine; *TBG,* thyroxine-binding globulin; *TSH,* thyroid-stimulating hormone.

9

ENDOCRINOLOGY

and demonstrate a reduction of urine volume and decreased fluid intake in response to exogenous vasopressin. Patients with nephrogenic DI have no significant change in fluid intake or urine volume or specific gravity. Continued fluid intake associated with decreased output and increased specific gravity suggests psychogenic DI.

4. **Dexamethasone suppression test (DST)**

TABLE 9-20

SERUM T$_4$ (mcg/dL) IN PRETERM AND TERM INFANTS

	Birthweight		
Age (days)	VLBW	LBW	Term
1-3	7.9 ± 3.3	11.4 ± 2.5	12 ± 1.9
4-6	6.5 ± 2.9	9.9 ± 2.5	11 ± 2.5
7-10	6.3 ± 3.0	9.5 ± 2.3	
11-14	5.7 ± 2.8	9.2 ± 2.1	
15-28	7.0 ± 2.5	9.1 ± 2.3	
29-56	7.8 ± 2.5	9.3 ± 3.3	

From Frank JE et al. J Pediatr 1996; 128(4):548-555.
LBW, Low birth weight: 1500-2499 g; Term: 2500-5528 g; *VLBW,* very low birth weight: 400-1499 g.

TABLE 9-21

MEAN STRETCHED PENILE LENGTH (cm)

Age	Mean ± SD	−2.5 SD
Birth		
30 wk gestation	2.5 ± 0.4	1.5
34 wk gestation	3.0 ± 0.4	2.0
Full term	3.5 ± 0.4	2.5
0-5 mo	3.9 ± 0.8	1.9
6-12 mo	4.3 ± 0.8	2.3
1-2 yr	4.7 ± 0.8	2.6
2-3 yr	5.1 ± 0.9	2.9
3-4 yr	5.5 ± 0.9	3.3
4-5 yr	5.7 ± 0.9	3.5
5-6 yr	6.0 ± 0.9	3.8
6-7 yr	6.1 ± 0.9	3.9
7-8 yr	6.2 ± 1.0	3.7
8-9 yr	6.3 ± 1.0	3.8
9-10 yr	6.3 ± 1.0	3.8
10-11 yr	6.4 ± 1.1	3.7
Adult	13.3 ± 1.6	9.3

From Feldman KW, Smith DW. J Pediatr 1975; 86:395 and Lee PA et al: Johns Hopkins Med J 1980; 146:156-163.
Measured from pubic ramus to tip of glans while traction is applied along length of phallus to point of increased resistance.
SD, standard deviation.

a. Dexamethasone suppresses secretion of ACTH by the normal pituitary, decreasing endogenous production of cortisol and excretion of 17-hydroxycorticosteroids (17-OHCS) and 17-ketosteroids. It is useful in determining the etiology of glucocorticoid or androgen overproduction.

b. Method: Give dexamethasone PO for 3 days (low dose: 1.25 mg/m^2/day; high dose: 3.75 mg/m^2/day divided every 6 hours) and collect 24-hour urine for 17-OHCS.

c. Interpretation: In normal patients, low-dose DST causes 17-OHCSs to fall to <1 mg/m^2/day. In CAH, 17-OHCS levels are suppressed only by

TABLE 9-22
TESTICULAR SIZE

Tanner Stage (Genital)	Length (cm) (Mean ± SD)	Volume (mL)
I	2.0 ± 0.5	2
II	2.7 ± 0.7	5
III	3.4 ± 0.8	10
IV	4.1 ± 1.0	20
V	5.0 ± 0.5	29

Testicular volume of >4 mL or a long axis >2.5 cm is evidence that pubertal testicular growth has begun.

SD, standard deviation.

the high-dose DST. 17-OHCS levels are not suppressed even with the high-dose DST in ectopic ACTH production, adrenocortical carcinoma, and some hypothalamic tumors. Incomplete suppression of 17-ketosteroids suggests that the patient has entered puberty. Markedly increased, nonsuppressible 17-ketosteroids suggest the presence of an androgen-producing tumor.

5. **Gonadotropin-releasing hormone (GnRH) stimulation test**
a. The GnRH stimulation test measures pituitary LH and FSH reserve. It is helpful in the differential diagnosis of precocious or delayed sexual development.
b. Method: Give 100 mcg of synthetic GnRH (Factrel) SC, and measure LH and FSH levels at 0 and 40 minutes.
c. Interpretation: Prepubertal children should show no or minimal increase in LH and FSH in response to GnRH. A rise of LH into the adult range occurs in central precocious puberty. See Table 9-3 for normal gonadotropin values.

6. **Urinary 17-ketosteroids**
a. Measurement of urinary 17-ketosteroid levels reveals some end products of androgen metabolism. It is most useful in evaluation of androgen excess.
b. Method: Collect and refrigerate 24-hour urine specimen.
c. Interpretation (see Table 9-12 for normal values).
   (1) Increased in CAH (it may take 1 to 2 weeks for 17-ketosteroids to rise above the normally high newborn levels), virilizing adrenal tumors, androgen-producing gonadal tumors, Cushing's syndrome, and stressful illness.
   (2) Decreased in Addison's disease, anorexia nervosa, and panhypopituitarism.

7. **Urinary 17-hydroxycorticosteroids (17-OHCS)**
a. 17-OHCS measures approximately one third of end products of cortisol metabolism. It is most useful in evaluation of cortisol excess.
b. Method: Collect a 24-hour urine specimen. Refrigerate during collection and process immediately (17-OHCS are destroyed at room temperature).

c. Interpretation (see Table 9-13 for normal values).
  (1) Increased in Cushing's syndrome, stressful illness, obesity, hyperthyroidism, and 11-hydroxylase deficiency.
  (2) Decreased in malnutrition, pituitary disorders involving ACTH, Addison's disease, administration of exogenous corticosteroids, liver disease, hypothyroidism, and newborn period (as a result of decreased glucuronidation).
  (3) Urinary free cortisol (see Table 9-11) can also be measured, eliminating some of the nonspecificity of 17-OHCS measurement. Interpretation is similar to that for 17-OHCS.

8. Human chorionic gonadotropin (hCG) stimulation test
a. An hCG test measures capacity for testosterone biosynthesis. It is useful in differentiation of cryptorchidism (undescended testes) from anorchia (absent testes).
b. Method: Give 1000 U of hCG IV/IM for 3 days and measure serum testosterone and dihydrotestosterone on day 0 and day 4.
c. Interpretation: Testosterone level >100 ng/dL in response to hCG stimulation is evidence for adequate testosterone biosynthesis. In cryptorchidism, testosterone rises to adult levels after hCG administration; in anorchia there is no rise.

REFERENCES

1. Report of the Expert Committee on the Diagnosis and Classification of Diabetes Mellitus. Diabetes Care 1999; 22 (Suppl 1):S5-19.
2. American Diabetes Association. Consensus statement: type 2 diabetes in children. Diabetes Care 2000; 22(12):381.
3. Pinhas-Hamiel O, Zeitler P. Type 2 diabetes: Not just for grownups anymore. Contemp Pediatr 2001; 18(1):102-125.
4. American Diabetes Association. Hyperglycemic crises in patients with diabetes mellitus. Diabetes Care 2001; 24(1):154-161.
5. Fisher DA. The thyroid. In Rudolf AM, editor. Pediatrics. Norwalk, Conn: Appleton & Lange; 1991.
6. LaFranchi SH. Hyperthyroidism. Pediatr Clin North Am 1979; 26(1):33-51.
7. Frank JE, et al. Thyroid function in very low birth weight infants: effects on neonatal hypothyroidism screening. J Pediatr 1996; 128(4):548-555.
8. Orth DN, Kovacs WJ. The adrenal cortex. In Wilson JD, editor. Williams' textbook of endocrinology. Philadelphia: WB Saunders; 1998.
9. American Academy of Pediatrics, Section on Endocrinology and Committee on Genetics. Technical report: congenital adrenal hyperplasia. Pediatrics 2000; 106(6):1511-1518.
10. Levine LS. Congenital adrenal hyperplasia. Pediatr Rev 2000; 21(5):159-170.
11. Reeves WB, Bichet DG, Andreoli TE. Posterior pituitary and water metabolism. In Wilson JD, editor. Williams' textbook of endocrinology. Philadelphia: WB Saunders; 1998.
12. Plotnik L. Growth, growth hormone, and pituitary disorders. In McMillan J, editor. Oski's pediatrics principles and practice. Philadelphia: Lippincott Williams & Wilkins; 1999.
13. MacGillivray MH. The basics for the diagnosis and management of short stature: a pediatric endocrinologist's approach. Pediatr Ann 2000; 29(9):570-575.
14. Styne DM. New aspects in the diagnosis and treatment of pubertal disorders. Pediatr Endocrinol 1997; 44(2):505-529.
15. Root AW. Precocious puberty. Pediatr Rev 2000; 21(1):10-19.
16. Rosen DS, Foster C. Delayed puberty. Pediatr Rev 2001; 22(9):309-314.
17. American Academy of Pediatrics, Committee on Genetics, Sections on Endocrinology and Urology. Evaluation of newborn with developmental anomalies of the external genitalia. Pediatrics 2000; 106(1):138-142.

FLUIDS AND ELECTROLYTES

Dominique Foulkes, MD

I. MAINTENANCE REQUIREMENTS

A. CALORIC EXPENDITURE METHOD

The caloric expenditure method is based on the understanding that water and electrolyte requirements more accurately parallel caloric expenditure than body weight or body surface area (BSA). This method is effective for all ages, types of body habitus, and clinical states.

1. **Determine the child's standard basal caloric (SBC) expenditure** as approximated by resting energy expenditure (REE) (see Table 20-1).

2. **Adjust caloric expenditure needs by various factors** (e.g., fever, activity) as described on p. 435.

3. For each 100 calories metabolized in 24 hours, the average patient will need 100 to 120 mL H_2O, 2 to 4 mEq Na^+, and 2 to 3 mEq K^+, as seen in Table 10-1.

B. HOLLIDAY-SEGAR METHOD

The Holliday-Segar method estimates caloric expenditure in fixed weight categories; it assumes that for each 100 calories metabolized, 100 mL of H_2O will be required. Fluid rates can be adjusted based on clinical state (e.g., fever, tachypnea). This method is not suitable for neonates <14 days old; generally, it overestimates fluid needs in neonates compared with the caloric expenditure method (Table 10-2).

C. BODY SURFACE AREA METHOD

The BSA method is based on the assumption that caloric expenditure is proportional to BSA (Table 10-3). It should not be used for children <10 kg. See p. 450 for BSA nomogram and conversion formula.

TABLE 10-1

AVERAGE WATER AND ELECTROLYTE REQUIREMENTS PER 100 CALORIES PER 24 HOURS

Clinical State	H_2O (ml)	Na^+ (mEq)	K^+ (mEq)
Average patient receiving parenteral fluids*	100-120	2-4	2-3
Anuria	45	0	0
Acute CNS infections and inflammation	80-90	2-4	2-3
Diabetes insipidus	Up to 400	Var	Var
Hyperventilation	120-210	2-4	2-3
Heat stress	120-240	Var	Var
High-humidity environment	80-100	2-4	2-3

CNS, Central nervous system; *Var*, variable requirement.
*Adequate maintenance solution: Dextrose 5% to 10% (as needed) in 0.2% NaCl + 20 mEq/L KCl or KAcetate.

HOLLIDAY-SEGAR METHOD

Body Weight	Water		Electrolytes (mEq/100 mL H_2O)
	mL/kg/day	mL/kg/hr	
First 10 kg	100 ÷ 24 hr/day	≈4	Na^+ 3
Second 10 kg	50 ÷ 24 hr/day	≈2	Cl^- 2
Each additional kg	20 ÷ 24 hr/day	≈1	K^+ 2

EXAMPLE: 8-YEAR-OLD WEIGHING 25 KG

mL/kg/day		mL/kg/hr	
100 (for 1st 10 kg) × 10 kg = 1000 mL/day		4 (for 1st 10 kg) × 10 kg = 40 mL/hr	
50 (for 2nd 10 kg) × 10 kg = 500 mL/day		2 (for 2nd 10 kg) × 10 kg = 20 mL/hr	
20 (per add'l kg) × 5 kg = 100 mL/day		1 (per add'l 1 kg) × 5 kg = 5 mL/hr	
25 kg 1600 mL/day		25 kg 65 mL/hr	

STANDARD VALUES FOR USE IN BODY SURFACE AREA METHOD

H_2O	1500 mL/m²/24 hr
Na^+	30-50 mEq/m²/24 hr
K^+	20-40 mEq/m²/24 hr

From Finberg L, Kravath RE, Fleishman AR. Water and electrolytes in pediatrics. Philadelphia: WB Saunders; 1982 and Hellerstein S. Pediatr Rev 1993; 14(3):103-115.

II. DEFICIT THERAPY

The most precise method of assessing fluid deficit is based on pre-illness weight, calculated as follows:

$$\text{Fluid deficit (L)} = \text{Pre-illness weight (kg)} - \text{Illness weight (kg)}$$

$$\% \text{ Dehydration} = \frac{\text{Pre-illness weight} - \text{Illness weight}}{\text{Pre-illness weight}} \times 100\%$$

If this is not available, clinical observation may be used, as described below.

A. CLINICAL ASSESSMENT (Table 10-4)

1. Hypotonic (hyponatremic) dehydration

a. Serum Na^+ <130 mEq/L.

b. Implies excess Na^+ loss.

2. Isotonic (isonatremic) dehydration

a. Serum Na^+ 130 to 150 mEq/L.

b. Implies proportional losses of Na^+ and free water (FW).

3. Hypertonic (hypernatremic) dehydration

a. Serum Na^+ >150 mEq/L.

b. Implies excess FW loss.

c. The skin may appear thick and doughy, with normal turgor, and children may be excessively irritable on examination.

B. GENERAL GUIDELINES FOR DEFICIT CALCULATION

1. Intracellular fluid (ICF) and extracellular fluid (ECF) compartments

a. Estimate of percent dehydration from extracellular and intracellular compartments related to duration of illness (Table 10-5).

TABLE 10-4

CLINICAL OBSERVATIONS IN DEHYDRATION*

Examination	Older child: 3% (30 mL/kg) Infant: 5% (50 mL/kg)	6% (60 mL/kg) 10% (100 mL/kg)	9% (90 mL/kg) 15% (150 mL/kg)
Dehydration	Mild	Moderate	Severe
Skin turgor	Normal	Tenting	None
Skin (touch)	Normal	Dry	Clammy
Buccal mucosa/lips	Moist	Dry	Parched/cracked
Eyes	Normal	Deep set	Sunken
Tears	Present	Reduced	None
Fontanelle	Flat	Soft	Sunken
CNS	Consolable	Irritable	Lethargic/obtunded
Pulse rate	Normal	Slightly increased	Increased
Pulse quality	Normal	Weak	Feeble/impalpable
Capillary refill	Normal	≈2 sec	>3 sec
Urine output	Normal	Decreased	Anuric

Modified from Behrman RE, Kliegman RM, Arvin AM. Nelson textbook of pediatrics, 16th ed. Philadelphia: WB Saunders; 2000 and Oski FA. Principles and practice of pediatrics, 3rd ed. Philadelphia: JB Lippincott; 1999.

CNS, Central nervous system.

*For the same degree of dehydration, clinical symptoms are generally worse for hyponatremic dehydration than for hypernatremic dehydration.

TABLE 10-5

PERCENT OF DEFICIT FROM EXTRACELLULAR AND INTRACELLULAR COMPARTMENTS

Duration of Illness	% Deficit From ECF	% Deficit From ICF
<3 days	80	20
≥3 days	60	40

TABLE 10-6

INTRACELLULAR AND EXTRACELLULAR FLUID COMPOSITION

	Intracellular (mEq/L)	Extracellular (mEq/L)
Na^+	20	135-145
K^+	150	3-5
Cl^-	—	98-110
HCO_3^-	10	20-25
PO_4^{3-}	110-115	5
Protein	75	10

b. Normal ICF and ECF composition (Table 10-6).

c. Electrolyte deficit (from ECF and ICF losses).

(1) Na^+ deficit is the amount of Na^+ that was lost from the Na^+-containing ECF compartment during the dehydration period (see Table 10-5):

Na^+ deficit (mEq) =
Fluid deficit (L) × Proportion from ECF × Na^+ concentration (mEq/L) in ECF

Intracellular Na^+ is negligible as a proportion of total; therefore it can be disregarded.

    (2) K^+ deficit is the amount of K^+ that was lost from the K^+-containing ICF compartment during the dehydration period (see Table 10-5):

K^+ deficit (mEq) =
Fluid deficit (L) × Proportion from ICF × K^+ concentration (mEq/L) in ICF

2. Electrolyte deficits (in excess of ECF/ICF electrolyte losses)
a. Formula

$$\text{mEq required} = (CD - CP) \times fD \times wt$$

where:
    CD = concentration desired (mEq/L)
    CP = concentration present (mEq/L)
    fD = distribution factor as fraction of body weight (L/kg)
    wt = baseline weight before illness (kg)
b. Apparent distribution factor (fD)
    (1) HCO_3^-: 0.4-0.5
    (2) Cl^-: 0.2-0.3
    (3) Na^+: 0.6-0.7
3. FW deficit in hypernatremic dehydration: Calculation is based on the amount of FW required to decrease the serum Na^+ by 1 mEq/L and is based on the patient's actual serum Na^+.[1] An estimate of FW needed to decrease the serum Na^+ by 1 mEq/L is 4 mL/kg (or 3 mL/kg if Na^+ >170, because less FW is required to decrease serum Na^+ at higher concentrations).

C. OVERVIEW OF PARENTERAL REHYDRATION
1. Phase I (emergency) management: If the patient is hemodynamically unstable, phase I should be carried out regardless of the type of dehydration (isotonic, hypotonic, or hypertonic) suspected.
a. Symptomatic dehydration or shock requires one or more boluses of 20 mL/kg isotonic fluid (i.e., lactated Ringer's [LR] or 0.9% normal saline [NS]) in the first 30 minutes.
b. Consider giving colloid (e.g., albumin), blood, or plasma (10 mL/kg) if there is no response after two 20-mL/kg boluses of isotonic fluid, or if there is acute blood loss.
c. For seizures caused by hyponatremia, as an initial estimate give 10 to 12 mL/kg of 3% NaCl over 60 minutes. Alternatively, to calculate the volume of 3% NaCl needed to raise the serum Na^+ by X mEq/L[2], compute the following:

    Amount of 3% NaCl (mL) = [X mEq/L × Body weight (kg)] × 0.6 L/kg

where X = (125 mEq/L - actual serum [Na]) to initially raise the serum Na+ rapidly to 125 mEq/L.
2. Phase II deficit (replacement, maintenance, and ongoing losses).
a. Calculate deficit volume using percent dehydration (including FW deficit in hypernatremic dehydration).

b. Calculate electrolyte deficit (including excess deficit in hyponatremic dehydration).

c. Calculate maintenance fluids and electrolytes.

d. Give half of the replacement therapy in addition to maintenance needs over the first 8 hours and the second half over the next 16 hours.

NOTE: This may be different in case of hypernatremic dehydration.

e. Take into consideration ongoing losses, such as continued diarrhea, excessive urinary losses, and surgical or enteral drains.[3]

3. Sample calculations

a. See Tables 10-7 to 10-9.

b. Maintenance calculations based on Holliday-Segar method (see Table 10-2).

4. Special considerations

a. In hypernatremic dehydration, half of the FW deficit and all of the solute deficit can be replaced over 24 hours (see Table 10-9). NOTE: **Avoid dropping the serum Na^+ >15 mEq/L per 24 hours to minimize the risk of cerebral edema.** Thus for total Na^+ corrections of >30 (i.e., serum Na^+ >175), FW deficit replacement should be spread over >48 hours. Follow serum Na^+ level at least every 4 hours initially.[3]

TABLE 10-7

ISONATREMIC DEHYDRATION CALCULATIONS*

Example: 7-kg infant with 10% dehydration (≥3 days). Serum Na^+ = 137. Illness weight = 6.3 kg.

	H_2O (mL)	Na^+ (mEq)	K^+ (mEq)
Maintenance	700	21	14
DEFICIT	700		
$0.6 \times 0.7\ L \times 145 =$		61	—
$0.4 \times 0.7\ L \times 150 =$		—	42
24-HOUR TOTAL	1400	82	56
FLUID SCHEDULE			
First 8 hr ⅓ maintenance	233	7	5
+ ½ deficit	350	31	21
FIRST 8-HR TOTAL	583	38	26

Exact calculations: 583 mL/8 hr = 73 mL/hr; 38 mEq Na^+/0.583 L = 65 mEq/L; 26 mEq K^+/0.583 L = 45 mEq/L)

Next 16 hr ⅔ maintenance	467	14	9
+ ½ deficit	350	30	21
NEXT 16-HR TOTAL	817	44	30

Exact calculations: 817 mL/16 hr = 51 mL/hr; 44 mEq Na^+/0.817 L = 54 mEq/L; 30 mEq K^+/0.817 L = 37 mEq/L)

A convenient fluid for this patient would be D_5 ½ NS + 40 mEq/L KCl or potassium acetate to run at 75 mL/hr for the first 8 hours and the same fluid at 50 mL/hr over the next 16 hours.

*In the absence of hypokalemia, 20 to 30 mEq/L of potassium is commonly used and is usually adequate; monitor carefully for hyperkalemia and adequate urine output if high concentrations of potassium are used. Potassium infusion rates should not exceed 1.0 mEq/kg/hr. If rate exceeds 0.5 mEq/kg/hr, the patient should be placed on a cardiorespiratory monitor.

TABLE 10-8

HYPONATREMIC DEHYDRATION CALCULATIONS*

Example: 7-kg infant with 10% dehydration (≥3 days). Serum Na^+ = 115. Illness weight = 6.3 kg.

		H_2O (mL)	Na^+ (mEq)	K^+ (mEq)
Maintenance		700	21	14
DEFICIT		700		
Na^+	0.6×0.7 L $\times 145$		61	—
Excess Na^+ deficit	$(135-115) \times 0.6 \times 7$		84	—
K^+	0.4×0.7 L $\times 150$		—	42
24 HR TOTAL		1400	166	56
FLUID SCHEDULE				
First 8 hr	⅓ maintenance	233	7	5
	+ ½ deficit	350	73	21
	FIRST 8-HR TOTAL	583	80	26

Exact calculations: 583 mL/8 hr = 73 mL/ hr; 80 mEq Na^+/0.583 L = 137 mEq/L ; 26 mEq K^+/0.583 L = 45 mEq/L

Next 16 hr	⅔ maintenance	467	14	9
	+ ½ deficit	350	72	21
	NEXT 16-HR TOTAL	817	86	30

Exact calculations: 817 mL/16 hr = 51 mL/hr; 86 mEq Na^+/0.817 L = 105 mEq/L; 30 mEq K^+/0.817 L = 37 mEq/L

A convenient fluid for this patient would be D_5NS + 40 mEq/L KCl or potassium acetate to run at 75 mL/hr for the first 8 hours and D_5 ½ NS and 40 mEq/L KCl or potassium acetate at 50 mL/hr over the next 16 hours.

*In the absence of hypokalemia, 20 to 30 mEq/L of potassium is commonly used and is usually adequate; monitor carefully for hyperkalemia and adequate urine output if high concentrations of potassium are used. Potassium infusion rates should not exceed 1.0 mEq/kg/hr. If rate exceeds 0.5 mEq/kg/hr, the patient should be placed on a cardiorespiratory monitor.

b. Rapid correction of hyponatremia may be associated with central pontine myelinolysis. Rapid increases in serum Na^+ level should therefore be reserved for symptomatic patients only. In asymptomatic patients, the target rate of rise should not exceed 2 to 4 mEq/L every 4 hours, or about 10 to 20 mEq/L in 24 hours.

5. Probable deficits of water and electrolytes in severe dehydration (Table 10-10).

6. Ongoing losses

a. Use Table 10-11 to estimate ongoing electrolyte losses for various body fluids.

b. Significant losses should be measured and may require replacement every 6 to 8 hours. Because of the wide range of normal values, specific analyses are suggested in individual cases.

D. ORAL REHYDRATION THERAPY

1. Applications of oral rehydration therapy (ORT)

a. Indications: Mild to moderate dehydration.

b. Contraindications: Shock, severe dehydration, intractable vomiting, >10 mL/kg/hr stool losses, coma, acute abdomen, or severe gastric distention.

TABLE 10-9

HYPERNATREMIC DEHYDRATION CALCULATIONS
Example: 7-kg infant with 10% dehydration (≥3 days).
Serum Na^+ = 155. Illness weight = 6.3 kg.

	H_2O (mL)	Na^+ (mEq)	K^+ (mEq)
24-hr maintenance	700	21	14
DEFICIT			
Free water 4 mL/kg × 7 kg × (155-145)	280		
Solute fluid	420		
0.6 × 0.42 × 145		37	—
0.4 × 0.42 × 150		—	25
24-HOUR TOTAL	1400	58	39
FLUID SCHEDULE			
First 24 hr 24-hr maintenance	700	21	14
½ Free-water deficit	140	—	—
Solute fluid deficit	420	37	25
FIRST DAY TOTAL	1260	58	39

Calculations: 1260 mL/24hr = 53 mL/hr; 58 mEq Na^+/1.26 L = 46 mEq/L; 39 mEq K^+/1.26 L = 31 mEq/L)

An appropriate initial fluid for this patient would be D_5 ¼ NS with 30 mEq/L KCl or potassium acetate to run at 50 mL/hr for the first 24 hours. Follow serum Na^+ and adjust fluid composition and rate based on clinical response. The second half of the free-water deficit may be replaced subsequently over the next 24 hours, or more rapidly depending on the rate of decline of serum Na^+ (avoid decline of >15 mEq/L in 24 hours).

10

TABLE 10-10

DEFICITS OF WATER AND ELECTROLYTES IN SEVERE DEHYDRATION

Condition	H_2O (mL/kg)	Na^+ (mEq/kg)	K^+ (mEq/kg)	Cl^- (mEq/kg)
DIARRHEAL DEHYDRATION				
Hyponatremic [Na+]* <130 mEq/L	100-120	10-15	8-15	10-12
Isotonic [Na+]* = 130-150 mEq/L	100-120	8-10	8-10	8-10
Hypernatremic [Na+]* >150 mEq/L	100-120	2-4	0-6	0-3
PYLORIC STENOSIS	100-120	8-10	10-12	10-12
DIABETIC KETOACIDOSIS	100	8	6-10	6

From Hellerstein S. Pediatr Rev 1993; 14(3):103-115.
*[Na] refers to the serum or plasma sodium concentration.

c. In patients with severe dehydration, intravenous (IV) therapy (starting with isotonic 20-mL/kg boluses) should be used initially until pulse, blood pressure, and level of consciousness return to normal. At that time, oral rehydration can often be safely instituted.

2. **Technique**
a. If the patient is vomiting, give 5 to 10 mL of oral rehydration fluid (using

FLUIDS AND ELECTROLYTES

TABLE 10-11

ELECTROLYTE COMPOSITION OF VARIOUS BODY FLUIDS

Fluid	Na+ (mEq/L)	K+ (mEq/L)	Cl− (mEq/L)
Gastric	20-80	5-20	100-150
Pancreatic	120-140	5-15	90-120
Small bowel	100-140	5-15	90-130
Bile	120-140	5-15	80-120
Ileostomy	45-135	3-15	20-115
Diarrhea	10-90	10-80	10-110
Burns*	140	5	110
Sweat			
Normal	10-30	3-10	10-35
Cystic fibrosis	50-130	5-25	50-110

From Behrman RE, Kliegman RM, Arvin AM. Nelson textbook of pediatrics, 16th ed. Philadelphia: WB Saunders; 2000.

*3-5 g/dL of protein may be lost in fluid from burn wounds.

TABLE 10-12

ORAL REHYDRATION SOLUTIONS

	CHO (g/dL)	Na+ (mEq/L)	K+ (mEq/L)	Cl− (mEq/L)	Base (mEq/L)	mOsm/kg H_2O
Ceralyte	4	70	20	60	30	220
Infalyte	3	50	25	45	30	200
Naturalyte	2.5	45	20	35	48	265
Pedialyte	2.5	45	20	35	30	250
Rehydralyte	2.5	75	20	65	30	310
WHO/UNICEF ORS*	2	90	20	80	30	310

From Snyder J. Semin Pediatr Infect Dis 1994; 5:231.

CHO, Carbohydrate.

*Available from Jianas Bros. Packaging Co., 2533 SW Boulevard, Kansas City, MO 64108.

a syringe, teaspoon, or cup) every 5 to 10 minutes, and gradually increase amount as tolerated. Monitor this phase of rehydration closely.

b. Occasionally (<5% of cases), severe vomiting may necessitate IV fluids. Small amounts of vomiting should not warrant abandoning oral rehydration. Measure amount of fluid lost through vomiting when possible.

3. **Deficit replacement**

a. Mild dehydration: 50 mL/kg oral rehydration solution (ORS) over 4 hours.

b. Moderate dehydration: 100 mL/kg ORS over 4 hours.[4]

4. **For a list of ORS,** see Table 10-12.

5. **Commonly consumed fluids and their approximate electrolyte composition** can be found in Table 10-13. **NOTE: These fluids are not recommended for rehydration.**

6. Maintenance phase

TABLE 10-13					

APPROXIMATE ELECTROLYTE COMPOSITION OF COMMONLY CONSUMED FLUIDS (NOT RECOMMENDED FOR ORT)*

	CHO (g/dL)	Na^+ (mEq/L)	K^+ (mEq/L)	Cl^- (mEq/L)	HCO_3^- (mEq/L)	mOsm/kg H_2O
Apple juice	11.9	0.4	26	—	—	700
Coca-Cola	10.9	4.3	0.1	—	13.4	656
Gatorade	5.9	21	2.5	17	—	377
Ginger ale	9	3.5	0.1	—	3.6	565
Milk	4.9	22	36	28	30	260
Orange juice	10.4	0.2	49	—	50	654

From Behrman RE, Kliegman RM, Arvin AM. Nelson textbook of pediatrics, 16th ed. Philadelphia: WB Saunders; 2000.

CHO, carbohydrate.

*Values vary slightly depending on source.

10

FLUIDS AND ELECTROLYTES

a. Goal: Provide usual diet in addition to replacing ongoing losses.
b. Breast-fed infants should resume breast-feeding ad lib, and formula-fed infants should resume their regular formula.
c. Children should continue with their regular diet (there is no role for bowel rest).
  (1) Foods to encourage
    (a) Complex carbohydrates (rice, baked potatoes, noodles, crackers, toast, cereals that are not high in simple sugars).
    (b) Soups (clear broths with rice, noodles, or vegetables).
    (c) Yogurt, vegetables (without butter), fresh fruits (not canned in syrup).
  (2) Foods to minimize
    (a) Foods that are high in fat or simple sugars (fried foods, juices, sodas).
    (b) Plain water should not be the only source of oral fluid.
d. Replacement of ongoing losses: Regardless of the degree of dehydration, give approximately 10 mL/kg (or about 120 mL in older children) of rehydration solution for each diarrheal stool.
e. As a general rule, pharmacologic agents should not be used to treat acute diarrhea.[4] Probiotic agents are undergoing study in children, and may shorten the course of acute diarrheal illness.[5]

III. SERUM ELECTROLYTE DISTURBANCES
A. POTASSIUM
1. Hypokalemia
a. Etiologies and laboratory data (Table 10-14).
b. Clinical manifestations: Skeletal muscle weakness or paralysis, ileus, and cardiac dysrhythmias.[3,6] Electrocardiogram (ECG) changes include delayed depolarization, with flat or absent T waves and, in extreme cases, U waves.

TABLE 10-14

CAUSES OF HYPOKALEMIA

Decreased Stores			
	Normal BP		
Hypertension	Renal	Extrarenal	Normal Stores
Renovascular disease	RTA	Skin losses	Metabolic alkalosis
Excess renin	Fanconi syndrome	GI losses	↑ Insulin
Excess mineralocorticoid	Bartter syndrome	High CHO diet	Leukemia
Cushing syndrome	DKA	Enema abuse	β₂ catecholamines
	Antibiotics	Laxative abuse	Familial hypokalemic periodic paralysis
	Diuretics	Anorexia nervosa	
	Amphotericin B	Malnutrition	

LABORATORY DATA

↑ Urine K⁺	↑ Urine K⁺	↓ Urine K⁺	↑ Urine K⁺

CHO, Carbohydrate; *DKA,* diabetic ketoacidosis; *GI,* gastrointestinal; *RTA,* renal tubular acidosis.

c. Laboratory tests to consider:
  (1) Blood: Electrolytes, with blood urea nitrogen/creatinine (BUN/Cr), creatine phosphokinase (CPK), glucose, renin, arterial blood gas (ABG), cortisol.
  (2) Urine: Urinalysis, K⁺, Na⁺, Cl⁻, osmolality, 17-ketosteroids.
  (3) Other: ECG.
d. Management: Rapidity of treatment should be proportional to severity of symptoms.
  (1) Acute: Calculate electrolyte deficit and replace with potassium acetate or potassium chloride. See Formulary for dosage information. Enteral replacement is safer when feasible, with less risk of iatrogenic hyperkalemia. Follow serum K⁺ closely.
  (2) Chronic: Calculate daily requirements and replace with potassium chloride or potassium gluconate. See Formulary for dosage information.

2. Hyperkalemia

a. See Table 10-15 for etiologies of hyperkalemia, and Table 10-16 for clinical manifestations.
b. Management
  (1) Mild to moderate (K⁺ = 6 to 7): Goal is to enhance excretion of K⁺.
    (a) Place patient on cardiac monitor. Eliminate K⁺ from diet and parenteral fluids.
    (b) Na⁺ polystyrene resin (Kayexalate) by mouth (PO) every 6 hours or as a retention enema over 4 to 6 hours. See Formulary for dosage information.
  (2) Severe (K⁺ >7): Goal is to move K⁺ into cells acutely.
    (a) Regular insulin, 0.1 U/kg IV with D₂₅W as 2 mL/kg (0.5 g/kg) over 30 minutes. Repeat dose in 30 to 60 minutes, or begin

TABLE 10-15

CAUSES OF HYPERKALEMIA

Increased Stores		Normal Stores
Increased Urine K+	Decreased Urine K+	
Transfusion with aged blood	Renal failure	Cell lysis syndromes
	Hypoaldosteronism	Leukocytosis (>100 K/mm³)
Exogenous K+ (e.g., salt substitutes)	Aldosterone insensitivity	Thrombocytosis (>750 K/mm³)
	↓Insulin	Metabolic acidosis*
Spitzer syndrome	K+-sparing diuretics	Blood drawing (hemolyzed sample)
	Congenital adrenal hyperplasia	Type IV RTA
		Rhabdomyolysis/crush injury
		Malignant hyperthermia
		Theophylline intoxication

*For every 0.1-unit reduction in arterial pH, there is an approximately 0.2-0.4 mEq/L increase in plasma K+.

TABLE 10-16

CLINICAL MANIFESTATIONS OF K+ DISTURBANCES

Serum K+	ECG Changes	Other Symptoms
~2.5	AV conduction defect, prominent U wave, ventricular dysrhythmia, ST segment depression	Apathy, weakness, paresthesias
~7.5	Peaked T waves	Weakness, paresthesias
~8.0	Loss of P wave, widening of QRS	—
~9.0	ST segment depression, further widening of QRS	Tetany
~10	Bradycardia, sine wave QRS-T, first-degree AV block, ventricular dysrhythmias, cardiac arrest	—

From Feld LG, Kaskel FJ, Schoeneman MJ. Adv Pediatr 1988; 35:497-535.
AV, Atrioventricular; *ECG,* electrocardiogram.

    infusion of $D_{25}W$ 1 to 2 mL/kg/hr with regular insulin 0.1 U/kg/hr. Monitor glucose hourly.

   (b) $NaHCO_3$ 1 to 2 mEq/kg IV given over 5 to 10 minutes. May be used even in the absence of acidosis.

   (c) With onset of ECG changes, urgent reversal of membrane effects is required. Give calcium gluconate (10%) 100 mg/kg per dose (1 mL/kg per dose) over 3 to 5 minutes. May repeat in 10 minutes (does not lower serum K+ concentration). Note that calcium gluconate solution is not compatible with $NaHCO_3$. Flush lines between infusions.

   (d) Dialysis is recommended if these measures are unsuccessful.

B. SODIUM

1. Hyponatremia

TABLE 10-17

HYPONATREMIA*

Decreased Weight		Increased or Normal Weight
Renal Losses	Extrarenal Losses	
CAUSE		
Na⁺-losing nephropathy	GI losses	Nephrotic syndrome
Diuretics	Skin losses	Congestive heart failure
Adrenal insufficiency	Third spacing	SIADH
	Cystic fibrosis	Acute/chronic renal failure
		Water intoxication
		Cirrhosis
		Excess salt-free infusions
LABORATORY DATA		
↑Urine Na⁺	↓Urine Na⁺	↓Urine Na⁺†
↑Urine volume	↓Urine volume	↓Urine volume
↓Specific gravity	↑Specific gravity	↑Specific gravity
↓Urine osmolality	↑Urine osmolality	↑Urine osmolality
MANAGEMENT		
Replace losses	Replace losses	Restrict fluids
Treat cause	Treat cause	Treat cause

GI, Gastrointestinal; *SIADH,* syndrome of inappropriate antidiuretic hormone secretion.

*Hyperglycemia and hyperlipidemia cause spurious hyponatremia.

†Urine Na⁺ may be appropriate for level of Na⁺ intake in patients with SIADH and water intoxication.

a. Etiologies (Table 10-17).
b. Factitious etiologies
   (1) Hyperlipidemia: Na⁺ ↓ by 0.002 × lipid (mg/dL).
   (2) Hyperproteinemia: Na⁺ ↓ by 0.25 × [protein (g/dL) - 8].
   (3) Hyperglycemia: Na⁺ ↓ 1.6 mEq/L for each 100-mg/dL rise in glucose.
c. Clinical manifestations: Na⁺ ≤120 mEq/L is often symptomatic (seizure, shock, lethargy).[3,6] If the change was less acute or chronic over several months, the patient may be relatively asymptomatic.
d. For hyponatremia secondary to syndrome of inappropriate antidiuretic hormone (SIADH), the principal treatment is fluid restriction until Na⁺ levels normalize. Use hypertonic NaCl for refractory seizures. See p. 236 and previous section for management of hyponatremic dehydration.

2. Hypernatremia
a. Etiologies and management (Table 10-18).
b. Clinical manifestations: Predominantly neurologic symptoms: lethargy, weakness, altered mental status, irritability, and seizures.[3,6] Additional symptoms may include muscle cramps, depressed deep tendon reflexes, and respiratory failure.

C. CALCIUM
1. Hypocalcemia
a. Etiologies: Hypoparathyroidism (decreased parathyroid hormone [PTH] levels or ineffective PTH response), vitamin D deficiency, hyperphospha-

TABLE 10-18		
HYPERNATREMIA		
Decreased Weight		
Renal Losses	Extrarenal Losses	Increased Weight
CAUSE		
Nephropathy	GI losses	Exogenous Na$^{+\dagger}$
Diuretic use	Respiratory losses*	Mineralocorticoid excess
Diabetes insipidus	Skin losses	Hyperaldosteronism
Postobstructive diuresis		
Diuretic phase of ATN		
LABORATORY DATA		
↑ Urine volume	↓ Urine volume	Relative ↓ urine volume
↑ Urine Na$^+$	↓ Urine Na$^+$	Relative ↓ urine Na$^+$
↓ Specific gravity	↑ Specific gravity	Relative ↑ specific gravity
MANAGEMENT		
Replace FW losses based on calculations in text and treat cause. Consider a natriuretic agent if there is increased weight.		

ATN, Acute tubular necrosis; *FW,* free water; *GI,* gastrointestinal.

*This cause of hypernatremia is usually secondary to free water loss, so that the fractional excretion of sodium may be decreased or normal.

$\dagger$Exogenous Na$^+$ administration will cause an increase in the fractional excretion of sodium.

temia (i.e., secondary to excessive use of sodium phosphate enemas), pancreatitis, malabsorption states (malnutrition), drug therapy (anticonvulsants), hypomagnesemia, and maternal hyperparathyroidism if patient is a neonate.

b. Clinical manifestations of tetany: Neuromuscular irritability with weakness, paresthesias, fatigue, cramping, altered mental status, seizures, laryngospasm, and cardiac dysrhythmias.[3,6] ECG changes include prolonged QT interval. Clinically, hypocalcemia may be detected by carpopedal spasm after arterial occlusion of an extremity for 3 minutes (Trousseau's sign) or muscle twitching with percussion of the facial nerve (Chvostek's sign).

c. Laboratory data
   (1) Blood: Ca^{2+} (total and ionized); also consider phosphate, alkaline phosphatase, Mg^{2+}, total protein, albumin (a change in serum albumin of 1 g/dL changes total serum Ca^{2+} in the same direction by 0.8 mg/dL), BUN, Cr, PTH, pH (acidosis increases ionized calcium, whereas alkalosis decreases it), 25-OH vitamin D.
   (2) Urine: Consider Ca^{2+}, phosphate, Cr.
   (3) Other: ECG; also consider chest radiograph (to visualize thymus), and ankle and wrist films for rickets.[2]

d. Management
   (1) Treat the underlying disease.
   (2) Chronic: Consider use of oral supplements of calcium carbonate, calcium gluconate, calcium glubionate, or calcium lactate. See Formulary for dosage information.

10

FLUIDS AND ELECTROLYTES

    (3) Acute symptomatic: Consider use of IV forms, such as calcium gluconate, calcium gluceptate, or calcium chloride (cardiac arrest dose). See Formulary for dosage information.

        (a) Significant hyperphosphatemia should be corrected before correction of hypocalcemia because soft tissue calcification may occur if total $[Ca^{2+}] \times [PO_4^{3-}] > 80$ (see p. 248).

        (b) Symptoms of hypocalcemia that are refractory to Ca^{2+} supplementation may be caused by hypomagnesemia.

2. Hypercalcemia

a. Etiologies: Hyperparathyroidism, vitamin D intoxication, excessive exogenous calcium administration, malignancy, prolonged immobilization, diuretics (thiazides), Williams syndrome, granulomatous disease (i.e., sarcoidosis), hyperthyroidism, milk-alkali syndrome.

b. Clinical manifestations[3,6]: Weakness, irritability, lethargy, seizures, coma, abdominal cramping, anorexia, nausea, vomiting, polyuria, polydipsia, renal calculi, and pancreatitis. ECG changes include shortened QT interval.

c. Laboratory data

    (1) Blood: Ca^{2+} (total and ionized); also consider phosphate, alkaline phosphatase, total protein, albumin, BUN, Cr, PTH, and vitamin D.

    (2) Urine: Consider Ca^{2+}, phosphate, Cr.

    (3) Other: ECG; also consider kidney, ureter, bladder (KUB) radiograph and renal ultrasound (for renal calculi).[2]

d. Management

    (1) Treat the underlying disease.

    (2) Hydrate to increase urine output and Ca^{2+} excretion. If glomerular filtration rate (GFR) and blood pressure (BP) are stable, give NS with maintenance K^+ at two to three times maintenance rate until Ca^{2+} is normalized.

    (3) Diuresis with furosemide.

    (4) Consider hemodialysis for severe or refractory cases.

    (5) Steroids may be indicated in malignancy, granulomatous disease, and vitamin D toxicity to decrease vitamin D and Ca^{2+} absorption. Consult appropriate specialists before administering steroids for these conditions.

    (6) Severe or persistently elevated Ca^{2+}: Give calcitonin or bisphosphonate in consultation with an endocrinologist.

D. MAGNESIUM

1. Hypomagnesemia

a. Etiologies: Increased urinary losses (diuretic use, renal tubular acidosis, hypercalcemia, chronic adrenergic stimulants, chemotherapy), increased gastrointestinal losses (malabsorption syndromes, severe malnutrition, diarrhea, vomiting, short bowel syndromes, enteric fistulas), endocrine etiologies (diabetes mellitus, PTH disorders, hyperaldosterone states), and decreased intake (i.e., prolonged parenteral fluid therapy with

Mg^{2+}-free solutions). May be associated with neonatal hypocalcemic tetany.

b. Clinical manifestations[3,6]: Anorexia, nausea, weakness, malaise, depression, nonspecific psychiatric symptoms, hyperreflexia, carpopedal spasm, clonus, and tetany. ECG changes include both atrial and ventricular ectopy and torsades de pointes.

c. Laboratory data: Mg^{2+} and Ca^{2+} (total and ionized); consider evaluation for renal or gastrointestinal losses or endocrine etiologies outlined above.

d. Management

    (1) Acute: Give magnesium sulfate. See Formulary for dosing and side effects.

    (2) Chronic: Magnesium oxide or magnesium sulfate.[2] See Formulary for dosing.

2. Hypermagnesemia

a. Etiologies: Renal failure, excessive administration (e.g., eclampsia/preeclampsia states, status asthmaticus, cathartics, enemas, administration of magnesium for phosphate binding in renal failure). Neonates born prematurely after tocolysis with magnesium sulfate are at high risk for respiratory sequelae, but serum magnesium levels tend to normalize within 72 hours.

b. Clinical manifestations[3,6]: Depressed deep tendon reflexes, lethargy, confusion, and, in extreme cases, respiratory failure.

c. Laboratory data: Mg^{2+}, BUN, Cr, and Ca^{2+}.

d. Management

    (1) Stop supplemental Mg^{2+}.

    (2) Diuresis.

    (3) Give Ca^{2+} supplements such as calcium chloride (use cardiac arrest doses), calcium gluceptate, or calcium gluconate. See Formulary for dosing.

    (4) Dialysis if life-threatening levels are present.

E. PHOSPHATE

1. Hypophosphatemia

a. Etiologies: Starvation; protein-energy malnutrition; malabsorption syndromes; intracellular shifts associated with respiratory or metabolic alkalosis, the treatment of diabetic ketoacidosis, and the administration of corticosteroids; increased renal losses (i.e., renal tubular defects, diuretic use); vitamin D-deficient and vitamin D-resistant rickets; and very-low-birthweight (VLBW) infants when intake does not meet demand.

b. Clinical manifestations[3,6]: Becomes symptomatic only at very low levels (<1.0 mg/dL) with irritability, paresthesias, confusion, seizures, apnea in VLBW infants, and coma.

c. Laboratory data

    (1) Blood: Phosphate, Ca^{2+} (total and ionized), electrolytes including BUN/Cr (follow for low K$^+$, Mg^{2+}, Na$^+$); consider vitamin D, PTH.

    (2) Urine: Consider Ca^{2+}, phosphate, Cr, pH.

10

FLUIDS AND ELECTROLYTES

d. Management
   (1) Insidious onset of symptoms: Give oral potassium phosphate or sodium phosphate. See Formulary for dosing.
   (2) Acute onset of symptoms: Give IV potassium phosphate or sodium phosphate. See Formulary for dosing.

2. Hyperphosphatemia

a. Etiologies: Hypoparathyroidism (but rarely occurs in the absence of renal insufficiency), reduction of GFR to <25% (may occur at smaller reductions of GFR in neonates), excessive administration of phosphate (PO, IV, or enemas), and use of cytotoxic drugs to treat malignancies.

b. Clinical manifestations[3,6]: Symptoms of the resulting hypocalcemia. See pp. 244-246.

c. Laboratory data
   (1) Blood: Phosphate, Ca^{2+} (ionized and total), electrolytes including BUN/Cr; consider CBC, vitamin D, PTH, ABG.
   (2) Urine: Consider Ca^{2+}, phosphate, Cr, urinalysis.

d. Management
   (1) Restrict dietary phosphate.
   (2) Give phosphate binders (calcium carbonate, aluminum hydroxide; use with caution in renal failure). See Formulary for dosing.
   (3) For cell lysis (with normal renal function), give an NS bolus and IV mannitol. See p. 506 for management of tumor lysis syndrome.
   (4) If patient has poor renal function, consider dialysis.

IV. ACID-BASE DISTURBANCES

A. ANION GAP

The anion gap (AG) represents anions other than bicarbonate and chloride required to balance the positive charge of Na^+. Clinically it is calculated as follows:

$$AG = Na^+ - (Cl^- + CO_2)$$

(Normal: 12 mEq/L ± 2 mEq/L)

B. METABOLIC ACIDOSIS WITH NORMAL ANION GAP (HYPERCHLOREMIC METABOLIC ACIDOSIS)

1. Gastrointestinal loss of bicarbonate

a. Diarrhea (secretory).
b. Fistula or drainage of the small bowel or pancreas.
c. Surgery for necrotizing enterocolitis.
d. Ureteral sigmoidostomy or ileal loop conduit.
e. Ileoileal pouch.
f. Use of anion exchange resins in presence of renal impairment.

2. Renal tubular acidosis, especially Type II (see Table 18-1, p. 399).

3. Other causes

a. Administration of HCl, NH_4Cl, arginine, or lysine hydrochloride.
b. Hyperalimentation.
c. Dilutional acidosis.

C. METABOLIC ACIDOSIS WITH INCREASED ANION GAP

1. Increased acid production (noncarbonic acid)

a. Increased β-hydroxybutyric acid and acetoacetic acid production
   (1) Insulin deficiency (diabetic ketoacidosis).
   (2) Starvation or fasting.
   (3) Ethanol intoxication.
b. Increased lactic acid production
   (1) Tissue hypoxia.
   (2) Sepsis.
   (3) Exercise.
   (4) Ethanol ingestion.
   (5) Systemic diseases (e.g., leukemia, diabetes mellitus, cirrhosis, pancreatitis).
   (6) Inborn errors of metabolism (IEMs) (carbohydrates, urea cycle, amino acids, organic acids).
c. Increased short-chain fatty acids (acetate, propionate, butyrate, D-lactate) from colonic fermentation.
   (1) Viral gastroenteritis.
   (2) Other causes of carbohydrate malabsorption.
d. Other acute intoxications
   (1) Methanol intoxication.
   (2) Ethylene glycol intoxication.
   (3) Paraldehyde intoxication.
   (4) Salicylate/ NSAID intoxication.
e. Increased sulfuric acid

2. Decreased acid excretion: Acute and chronic renal failure.[7]

D. METABOLIC ALKALOSIS

1. Volume contraction with H^+ loss.

a. Vomiting.
b. Gastric suction.
c. Diuretic therapy.

2. Increased urinary H^+ excretion (i.e., thiazide and loop diuretics).

V. SERUM OSMOLALITY

1. Defined as the number of particles per liter. May be approximated by:

$$2[Na^+] + \frac{\text{Glucose (mg/dL)}}{18} + \frac{\text{BUN (mg/dL)}}{2.8}$$

2. Normal range: 275 to 295 mOsm/L.

VI. PARENTERAL FLUID COMPOSITION (Table 10-19)

FLUIDS AND ELECTROLYTES

10

TABLE 10-19
COMPOSITION OF FREQUENTLY USED PARENTERAL FLUIDS

Liquid	CHO (g/100 mL)	Protein* (g/100 mL)	cal/L	Na$^+$ (mEq/L)	K$^+$ (mEq/L)	Cl$^-$ (mEq/L)	HCO$_3$$^{-†}$ (mEq/L)	Ca^{2+} (mEq/L)	mOsm/L
D$_5$W	5	—	170	—	—	—	—	—	252
D$_{10}$W	10	—	340	—	—	—	—	—	505
NS (0.9% NaCl)	—	—	—	154	—	154	—	—	308
½ NS (0.45% NaCl)	—	—	—	77	—	77	—	—	154
D$_5$ ¼ NS (0.225% NaCl)	5	—	170	34	—	34	—	—	329
3% NaCl	—	—	—	513	—	513	—	—	1027
8.4% sodium bicarbonate (1 mEq/mL)	—	—	—	1000	—	—	1000	—	2000
Ringer's	0-10	—	0-340	147	4	155.5	—	≈4	
Lactated Ringer's	0-10	—	0-340	130	4	109	28	3	273
Amino acid 8.5% (Travasol)	—	8.5	340	3	—	34	52	—	880
Plasmanate	—	5	200	110	2	50	29	—	
Albumin 25% (salt poor)	—	25	1000	100-160	—	<120	—	—	300
Intralipid‡	2.25	—	1100	2.5	0.5	4.0	—	—	258-284

CHO, Carbohydrate; *HCO$_3$*, bicarbonate; *NS*, normal saline.
*Protein or amino acid equivalent.
†Bicarbonate or equivalent (citrate, acetate, lactate).
‡Values are approximate; may vary from lot to lot. Also contains <1.2% egg-phosphatides.

REFERENCES

1. Segar WE: Parenteral fluid therapy. Curr Probl Pediatr 1972; 3(2):3-40.
2. Fleisher G, Ludwig S. Textbook of pediatric emergency medicine. Baltimore: Williams & Wilkins; 2000.
3. Barkin R. Pediatric emergency medicine, 2nd ed. St Louis: Mosby; 1997.
4. American Academy of Pediatrics Practice Parameter: The management of acute gastroenteritis in young children. Pediatrics 1996; 97:424-431.
5. Saavedra J. Probiotics and infectious diarrhea. Am J Gatroenterology 2000; 95:S16-18.
6. Feld LG, Kaskel FJ, Schoeneman MJ. The approach to fluid and electrolyte therapy in pediatrics. Adv Pediatr 1988; 35:497-535.
7. Hanna J, Scheinman J, Chan J. The kidney in acid-base balance. Pediatr Clin North Am 1995; 42(6):1365.

10

FLUIDS AND ELECTROLYTES

GASTROENTEROLOGY

Samina H. Taha, MD

11

I. WEBSITES

www.aap.org (American Academy of Pediatrics)
www.naspgn.org (North American Society for Pediatric Gastroenterology and Nutrition)
www.acg.gi.org (American College of Gastroenterology)

II. GASTROINTESTINAL EMERGENCIES

A. GASTROINTESTINAL BLEEDING

1. Initial evaluation (Fig. 11-1)
a. Assess airway, breathing, and circulation (ABCs) and hemodynamic stabilization (i.e., pallor, tachycardia, delayed capillary refill).
b. Perform physical examination, looking for evidence of bleeding.
c. Verify bleeding with rectal examination and/or Hemoccult testing of stool or emesis. Obtain baseline laboratory tests. Consider the following additional laboratory studies: complete blood count (CBC) with platelets, prothrombin time/partial thromboplastin time (PT/PTT), blood type and crossmatch, reticulocyte count, blood smear, blood urea nitrogen/creatinine (BUN/Cr), electrolytes, and a panel to assess for disseminated intravascular coagulation (DIC). Consider gastric lavage to differentiate upper from lower gastrointestinal (GI) bleeding and to assess for ongoing bleeding.
d. Provide specific therapy based on assessment and site of bleeding.
e. Begin initial fluid resuscitation with normal saline (NS) or lactated Ringer's (LR) solution. Consider transfusion if there is continued bleeding, symptomatic anemia, and/or a hematocrit level <20%.
2. For a differential diagnosis of GI bleeding, see Table 11-1

B. ACUTE ABDOMEN[1]

1. Differential diagnosis
a. GI source: Appendicitis, pancreatitis, intussusception, malrotation with volvulus, inflammatory bowel disease (IBD), gastritis, bowel obstruction, mesenteric lymphadenitis, irritable bowel syndrome, abscess, hepatitis, perforated ulcer, Meckel's diverticulitis, cholecystitis, choledocholithiasis, constipation, gastroenteritis.
b. Renal source: Henoch-Schönlein purpura (HSP), urinary tract infection (UTI), pyelonephritis, nephrolithiasis.
c. Gynecologic source: Ectopic pregnancy, ovarian cyst/torsion, pelvic inflammatory disease (PID).
d. Oncologic source: Wilms' tumor, neuroblastoma.
e. Other sources: Pneumonia, sickle cell anemia, diabetic ketoacidosis (DKA), juvenile rheumatoid arthritis (JRA).
2. Diagnosis
a. History: Course and characterization of pain, diarrhea, melena, hematochezia, fever, last oral intake, menstrual history, vaginal

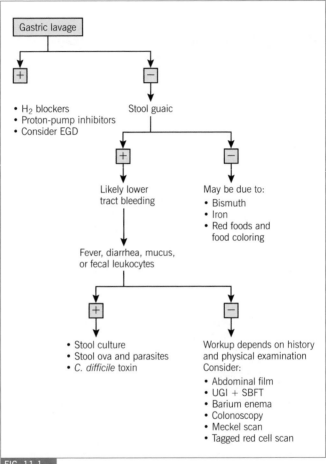

Evaluation of GI bleeding. May use gastrostomy (G tube) if present; use with caution if esophageal varices suspected. *EGD*, Esophagogastroduodenoscopy; *SBFT*, small bowel follow-through; *UGI*, upper GI.

    discharge/bleeding, urinary symptoms, and respiratory symptoms. Also assess past GI history, travel history, and diet.

b. Physical examination
   (1) General: Vital signs, toxicity, rashes, arthritis, jaundice.
   (2) Abdominal: Moderate to severe abdominal tenderness on palpation, rebound/guarding, rigidity, masses, change in bowel sounds.

TABLE 11-1

DIFFERENTIAL DIAGNOSIS OF GI BLEEDING*

	Upper GI Bleed	Lower GI Bleed
Newborns	**Swallowed maternal blood**	**Anal fissure**
	Hemorrhagic gastritis	**Allergic proctocolitis**
	Stress ulcer	**Infectious diarrhea**
	Idiopathic	Hirschsprung's disease
	Coagulopathy	Necrotizing enterocolitis
	Gastric outlet obstruction	Volvulus
	Gastric volvulus	Stress ulcer
	Pyloric stenosis	Vascular malformation
	Antral/pyloric webs	GI duplication
Infants	**Epistaxis**	**Anal fissure**
	Gastritis	**Infectious diarrhea**
	Esophagitis	**Allergic proctocolitis**
	Stress ulcer	**Meckel's diverticulum**
	Gastric/duodenal ulcer	Intussusception
	Foreign bodies	GI duplication
	Gastric volvulus	Peptic ulcer
	Esophageal varices	Foreign body
Children	**Epistaxis**	**Anal fissure**
	Tonsillitis/sinusitis	**Infectious diarrhea**
	Gastritis	Polyp
	Mallory-Weiss tear	Hemorrhoids
	Gastric/duodenal ulcer	Inflammatory bowel disease
	Medications	Henoch-Schonlein purpura
	Tumors	Meckel's diverticulum
	Hematologic disorders	Peptic ulcer
	Esophageal varices	Hemolytic uremic syndrome
	Munchausen by proxy	Vascular malformations

From Mezoff AG, Preud Homme DL. Contemp Pediatr 1994; 11:60-92.
*In order of frequency, most common in bold.

  (3) Rectal: Include testing for occult blood.
  (4) Pelvic: Discharge, masses, adnexal/cervical motion tenderness.
3. **Studies**
a. Radiology: First obtain plain abdominal radiographs to assess for obstruction, constipation, free air, gallstones, or kidney stones, and chest radiographs to check for pneumonia. Then consider abdominal/pelvic ultrasonography, abdominal spiral computed tomography (CT) with contrast (include rectal contrast for appendicitis evaluation), other contrast studies, and endoscopy.
b. Laboratory: Electrolytes, chemistry panel, CBC, liver and kidney function tests, coagulation studies, blood type and screen/crossmatch, urinalysis, amylase, lipase, gonorrhea/chlamydia cultures (or ligase chain reaction [LCR]/probes), beta-human chorionic gonadotropin (β-hCG), erythrocyte sedimentation rate (ESR), C-reactive protein (CRP).

4. Management

a. Immediate: Patient should be placed on nothing by mouth (NPO) status. Begin rehydration. Consider nasogastric decompression, serial abdominal examinations, surgical/gynecological/GI evaluation as indicated, pain control (may confound examination), and antibiotics as indicated.

b. Definitive: Surgical or endoscopic exploration as warranted.

III. VOMITING

See Table 11-2 for evaluation of vomiting.

TABLE 11-2

EVALUATION OF VOMITING

Type	Etiology	Evaluation
Typically bilious	Obstruction	• Review feeding and
	Intussusception	medication history
	Malrotation ± volvulus	• NG/OG tube for
	Pancreatitis	decompression if GI
	Intestinal dysmotility	obstruction is suspected
	Peritoneal adhesions	• If bilious and/or
	Incarcerated inguinal hernia	hematemesis, consider
	Intestinal atresia, stenosis	surgical consultation
	Superior mesenteric artery	• Serum electrolytes, CBC
	syndrome	• Plain abdominal film with
	Incarcerated inguinal hernia	upright or cross-table lateral
Typically nonbilious	Overfeeding	views to rule out
	GERD	obstruction, free air
	Milk-protein sensitivity	• Abdominal ultrasound if
	Infection	pyloric stenosis is suspected
	Peptic disease	• Upper GI series to rule out
	Drugs	pyloric stenosis, obstruction,
	Electrolyte imbalance	anomalies, evaluate GI
	Eating disorders	motility
	Necrotizing enterocolitis	• Neurologic evaluation and
	Metabolic abnormality	imaging
	Pyloric stenosis	• Consider feeding
	CNS lesion	modifications ± medications
	Esophageal/gastric atresia,	if GERD is suspected
	stenosis	• Avoid antiemetics unless
	Hirschsprung's disease	specific, benign etiology is
	Annular pancreas	identified
	Web	
Either bilious	Ileus	
or nonbilious	Appendicitis	

Modified from Saavedra J. Gastroenterology. In Seidel H et al. Primary care of the newborn. 2001; 119-120 and Murray K et al. Vomiting. Pediatr Rev 1998; 19(10):337-341.

IV. EVALUATION OF LIVER FUNCTION TESTS (LFTs)

1. **Study results suggestive of liver cell injury:** Aspartate aminotransferase (AST), alanine aminotransferase (ALT), lactate dehydrogenase (LDH), and NH_3.
2. **Study results suggestive of cholestasis:** Increased bilirubin, urobilinogen, γ-glutamyltransferase (GGT), alkaline phosphatase, 5'-nucleotidase, serum bile acids.
3. **Tests of synthetic function:** Albumin, prealbumin, PT, activated partial prothrombin time (aPTT), cholesterol. Elevated NH_3 is evidence of decreased ability to detoxify ammonia. See Table 11-3 for evaluation and interpretation of LFTs.

NOTE: See Chapter 15 for hepatitis immunization recommendations.

V. HYPERBILIRUBINEMIA[2,3]

Bilirubin is the product of hemoglobin metabolism. There are two forms: direct (conjugated) and indirect (unconjugated). Hyperbilirubinemia is usually the result of increased hemoglobin load, reduced hepatic uptake, reduced hepatic conjugation, or decreased excretion. Direct hyperbilirubinemia is defined as direct bilirubin >15% of total bilirubin >2 mg/dL. See Box 11-1 for differential diagnosis of hyperbilirubinemia. Also refer to Chapter 17 for evaluation and treatment of newborn jaundice.

VI. DIARRHEA

Usual stool output is 10 g/kg/day in children and 200 g/day in adults. *Diarrhea* is increased water in stool, resulting in increased stool frequency or loose consistency. *Chronic diarrhea* is diarrhea lasting more than 14 days. *Acute diarrhea* is most commonly of an infectious, usually viral, etiology. A bacterial etiology is more common in bloody diarrhea; it is usually secretory or dysenteric. See Tables 11-4 and 11-5 for general treatment information.

The etiology of diarrhea may be **infectious** or **malabsorptive**, and the mechanism is osmotic or secretory. In **osmotic** diarrhea, stool volume depends on diet and decreases with fasting (fecal Na^+ <60 mosmol/L). In **secretory** diarrhea, stool volume is increased and does not vary with diet (fecal Na^+ >60 mosmol/L).

Oral rehydration therapy (ORT) is almost always successful and should be attempted with an appropriate oral rehydration solution in cases of mild to moderate dehydration. See Chapter 10 for calculation of deficit and maintenance fluid requirements and oral rehydration composition. Breast-feeding should continue, and a regular diet should be restarted as soon as the patient is rehydrated. Parenteral hydration is indicated in severe dehydration, hemodynamic instability, or failure of ORT.

Text continued on p. 263

11

GASTROENTEROLOGY

TABLE 11-3

EVALUATION OF LIVER FUNCTION TESTS

Enzyme	Source	Increased	Decreased	Comments
AST/ALT	Liver	Hepatocellular injury	Vitamin B_6 deficiency	ALT more specific than AST for liver
	Heart	Rhabdomyolysis	Uremia	AST > ALT in hemolysis
	Skeletal muscle	Muscular dystrophy		AST/ALT >2 in 90% of alcohol disorders
	Pancreas	Hemolysis		in adults
	RBCs	Liver cancer		
	Kidney			
Alkaline phosphatase	Liver	Hepatocellular injury	Low phosphate	Highest in cholestatic conditions
	Osteoblasts	Bone growth, disease, trauma	Wilson's disease	Must be differentiated from bone source
	Small intestine	Pregnancy	Zinc deficiency	
	Kidney	Familial	Hypothyroidism	
	Placenta		Pernicious anemia	

GGT	Bile ducts	Estrogen therapy	Not found in bone
	Renal tubules	Artificially low in	Increased in 90% primary liver disease
	Pancreas	hyperbilirubinemia	Biliary obstruction
	Small intestine		Intrahepatic cholestasis
	Brain		Induced by alcohol
			Specific for hepatobiliary disease in
			nonpregnant patient
5'-NT	Liver cell membrane	Cholestasis	Specific for hepatobiliary disease in
	Intestine		nonpregnant patient
	Brain		
	Heart		
	Pancreas		
NH₃	Bowel	Hepatic disease secondary to urea	Converted to urea in liver
	Bacteria	cycle dysfunction	
	Protein metabolism	Hemodialysis	
		Valproic acid therapy	
		Urea cycle enzyme deficiency	
		Organic acidemia and carnitine	
		deficiency	

Alk phos, Alkaline phosphatase; *AST/ALT,* aspartate aminotransferase/alanine aminotransferase; *GGT,* γ-glutamyl transpeptidase; *5'-NT,* 5'-nucleotidase; *RBCs,* red blood cells.

GASTROENTEROLOGY

11

BOX 11-1

DIFFERENTIAL DIAGNOSIS OF HYPERBILIRUBINEMIA

INDIRECT HYPERBILIRUBINEMIA

Transient Neonatal Jaundice
Physiologic jaundice
Breast-feeding jaundice
Breast milk jaundice
Reabsorption of extravascular blood
Polycythemia

Hemolytic Disorders
Blood group incompatibility
Hemoglobinopathies
Red cell membrane disorders
Microangiopathies
Red cell enzyme deficiencies
Autoimmune disease

Enterohepatic Recirculation
Hirschsprung's disease
Cystic fibrosis
Ileal atresia
Pyloric stenosis

Disorders of Bilirubin Metabolism
Crigler-Najjar syndrome
Gilbert syndrome
Hypothyroidism
Hypoxia
Acidosis

Miscellaneous
Sepsis
Dehydration
Hypoalbuminemia
Drugs

DIRECT HYPERBILIRUBINEMIA

Biliary Obstruction
Biliary atresia
Paucity of intrahepatic bile ducts (Alagille)
Choledochal cyst
Inspissated bile syndrome
Fibrosing pancreatitis
Primary sclerosing cholangitis
Gallstones
Neoplasm

Infection
Sepsis
Urinary tract infection
Cholangitis

Infection—cont'd
Liver abscess
Viral hepatitis
Herpes simplex virus
Varicella-zoster virus
Syphilis
Toxoplasmosis
Tuberculosis
Leptospirosis
Histoplasmosis
Toxocariasis

Metabolic Disorders
Alpha 1-antitrypsin deficiency
Cystic fibrosis
Galactosemia
Galactokinase deficiency
Wilson's disease
Hereditary fructose intolerance
Niemann-Pick disease
Glycogen storage disease
Dubin-Johnson syndrome
Rotor syndrome

Chromosomal Abnormalities
Turner syndrome
Trisomy 18
Trisomy 21

Drugs
Aspirin
Acetaminophen
Iron
Isoniazid
Vitamin A
Erythromycin
Sulfonamides
Oxacillin
Rifampin
Ethanol
Steroids
Tetracycline
Methotrexate

Miscellaneous
Neonatal hepatitis syndrome
Parenteral alimentation
Reye's syndrome

TABLE 11-4

TREATMENT RECOMMENDATIONS FOR BACTERIAL ENTERIC INFECTIONS

Organism	Clinical Syndrome	Treatment Recommendations	Therapy*
Salmonella	Diarrhea	No treatment, can prolong carriage	Amoxicillin
	Invasive disease or:	Treatment recommended: length of treatment depends on site of	TMP/SMZ
	<3 months of age	infection; relapses are common, and retreatment recommended	Third-generation
	Malignancy		cephalosporin
	Hemoglobinopathy		
	Immunosuppressed		
	Chronic GI disease		
	Severe colitis		
Shigella	Diarrhea or dysentery	Treatment shortens duration of signs and symptoms, eliminates organism from feces, prevents spread of organism	TMP/SMZ
Yersinia	Noninvasive diarrhea	Treatment in normal host does not have established benefit	TMP/SMZ
	Septicemia and infection other than GI tract	Treatment recommended	Third-generation cephalosporin
Campylobacter	Diarrhea or dysentery	Treatment shorten's duration of illness; prevents relapse	Erythromycin
Escherichia coli EHEC (O157) (enterohemorrhagic)†	HUS	Antimicrobial therapy does not appear to prevent progression to HUS and routine antibiotics are discouraged	
EPEC (enteropathogenic)	Diarrhea	Nonabsorbable oral antibiotics	Gentamycin/Neomycin
	Chronic carriage	Absorbable oral antibiotics	TMP/SMZ
ETEC (enterotoxigenic)	Diarrhea	Disease usually self-limited and no treatment recommended	
EIEC (enteroinvasive)	Diarrhea	Treatment recommended	

HUS, Hemolytic uremic syndrome; *TMP/SMZ*, trimethoprin/sulfamethoxazole.
*Definitive therapy should be based on culture sensitivities.
†From Wong S et al. N Engl J Med 2000: 342(26):1930-1936.

GASTROENTEROLOGY **11**

TABLE 11-5

TREATMENT OF PARASITIC ENTERIC INFECTIONS

Organism	Clinical Syndrome	Treatment Recommendations	Antiparasitic
Giardia lamblia	Asymptomatic carriage	No treatment unless household member with: Pregnancy Cystic fibrosis Hypogammaglobulinemia	Metronidazole
	Diarrhea	Symptomatic disease should be treated	Metronidazole Furazolidone
Amebae	Asymptomatic	Treatment recommended for all infection	Paromomycin
	Diarrhea/dysentery Extraintestinal	Treatment recommended for all infection	Metronidazole followed by iodoquinol

VII. CONSTIPATION AND ENCOPRESIS

Constipation is the failure to evacuate the lower colon regularly and is defined clinically as painful passage of stools with hard consistency. There is a wide variation in normal stooling patterns from several times daily to weekly. Encopresis is the leakage of stool around impaction. This occurs with chronic constipation, in which there is a loss of sensation in the distended rectal vault.

A. DIFFERENTIAL DIAGNOSIS OF NONFUNCTIONAL CONSTIPATION

1. **Neurologic** (e.g., Hirschsprung's disease, spinal pathology, botulism).
2. **Obstructive** (e.g., anal ring, small left colon, meconium ileus, mass).
3. **Endocrine/metabolic** (e.g., collagen vascular disease, hypothyroidism).
4. **Medicinal** (e.g., opiates, iron, tricyclic antidepressants, chemotherapy agents).

B. COMPLICATIONS

1. Abdominal pain.
2. Rectal fissures, ulcers, and prolapse.
3. UTI, urinary incontinence, ureteral obstruction.
4. Stasis syndrome with bacterial overgrowth.
5. Social isolation.

C. TREATMENT OF FUNCTIONAL CONSTIPATION: LONG-TERM BEHAVIORAL MODIFICATION ALONG WITH MEDICATION

The goal of treatment of functional constipation is weaning of medication once normal colorectal sensation and stooling patterns have been established. The three stages of treatment include:

1. **Disimpaction (2 to 5 days):** Enemas may be attempted at home once daily for 2 to 5 days. Prolonged use may result in hypophosphatemia and hypocalcemia. Refractory constipation may require colonic lavage with isotonic polyethylene glycol-electrolyte solution (see Formulary for dosage). This can be given at home or via nasogastric (NG) tube in the hospital.
   a. Enema (see Formulary for dosage)
      (1) Mineral oil
      (2) Hypertonic phosphate
      (3) Milk and molasses 50:50 mix up to 6 oz maximum.
   b. Oral/nasogastric (see Formulary for dosage)
      (1) Mineral oil: Use with caution in patients younger than 1 year of age and in those with neurologic impairment because of risk of aspiration.
      (2) Magnesium citrate
      (3) Polyethylene glycol: Also available for outpatient use (Miralax): In adults, dissolve 17 g in 8 oz water once daily for up to 2 weeks.
      (4) Sodium phosphate oral solution (Fleet Phospho-Soda)
2. **Sustained evacuation (usually 3 to 12 months):** This stage restores normal colorectal tone and requires habitual toilet use with positive rewards and behavioral therapy. Initial diet should be low in fiber, with a transition to a high-fiber diet once disimpaction has occurred.

11

GASTROENTEROLOGY

Medications include lubricants, hyperosmolar sugars, and stimulants. These medications can also be used for mild constipation. See Formulary for specific dosages. Generic names of medications follow:

a. Fiber supplements: Barley malt, cellulose, psyllium, polycarbophil.

b. Lubricants: Mineral oil, surfactant.

c. Hyperosmolar sugars: Fructose/sorbitol (prune juice); lactulose (do not use in patients younger than 6 months).

d. Laxatives and stool softeners: Magnesium hydroxide, senna, diphenylmethane, docusate sodium, bisacodyl, glycerin.

3. **Gradually wean from medications.**

VIII. MISCELLANEOUS TESTS

A. OCCULT BLOOD

1. **Purpose:** To screen for the presence of blood through detection of heme in stool.

2. **Method:** Smear a small amount of stool on the test areas of an occult blood test card and allow to air dry. Apply developer as directed.

3. **Interpretation:** A blue color resembling that of the control indicates the presence of heme. Brisk transit of ingested red meat and inorganic iron may yield a false-positive result. Screening for the presence of blood in gastric aspirates or vomitus should be performed using Gastroccult, not stool Hemoccult cards.

B. D-XYLOSE TEST

1. **Purpose:** To screen for small bowel malabsorption by measuring the amount of D-xylose absorbed after an oral load. Unreliable in patients with edema, renal disease, delayed gastric emptying, severe diarrhea, rapid transit time, or small bowel bacterial overgrowth.

2. **Method:** Have infants fast for 4 to 6 hours, older children for 8 hours. Give a 14.5 g/m^2 (maximum 25 g) oral load of D-xylose as a 10% water solution. Ensure adequate urine output using supplementary oral or intravenous (IV) fluid, collect all urine for 5 hours, and send for quantitation. Alternatively, send serum specimens for D-xylose concentration before the load and 30, 60, 90, and 120 minutes after the load.

3. **Interpretation (urine)**

a. Children >6 months old

   (1) 5 hours urinary excretion of <15% of the oral load suggests malabsorption.

   (2) 15% to 24% is indeterminate.

   (3) >25% is normal.

b. Infants <6 months old: 5 hours urinary excretion <10% suggests malabsorption.

4. **Interpretation (serum):** Failure of the serum level to exceed 25 mg/dL in any of the postabsorptive specimens suggests malabsorption.

C. TESTS FOR FAT MALABSORPTION: QUANTITATIVE FECAL FAT

1. **Purpose:** To screen for fat malabsorption by quantitating fecal fat excretion.

2. **Method:** Patient should be on a normal diet (35% fat) with the amount of calories and fat ingested recorded for 2 days before the test and during the test itself. Collect and freeze all stools passed within 72 hours, and send to the laboratory for determination of total fecal fatty acid content.

3. Interpretation

a. Total fecal fatty acid excretion of >5 g fat/24 hours may suggest malabsorption.

NOTE: **Results will vary with amount of fat ingested and normal values have not been established for children <2 years old.**

b. The coefficient of absorption (CA) is a more accurate indicator of malabsorption and does not vary with fat intake:

$$CA = (g \text{ fat ingested} - g \text{ fat excreted})/(g \text{ fat ingested}) \times 100$$

NOTE: **Quantitative fecal fat is recommended over qualitative methods (e.g., staining with Sudan III), which depend on spot checks and are thus unreliable for diagnosing fat malabsorption.**

REFERENCES

1. Moir CR. Abdominal pain in infants and children. Mayo Clin Proc 1996; 71(10):984-989.
2. Provisional Committee for Quality Improvement and Subcommittee on Hyperbilirubinemia Practice Parameter. Management of hyperbilirubinemia in the healthy term newborn. Pediatrics 1994; 94: 558-565.
3. Gartner L. Neonatal jaundice. Pediatr Rev 1994; 15(11):422-431.

11

GASTROENTEROLOGY

GENETICS

Vivian V. Pearson, MD

When evaluating any child for a genetic disorder, one of the most valuable tools is the three-generation pedigree. For each family member, note age, gender, and medical status or cause of death. Specifically ask about family history of neonatal or childhood deaths, mental retardation, developmental delay, birth defects, seizure disorders, known genetic disorders, ethnicity, consanguinity, infertility, miscarriages, and stillbirths.

I. NEWBORN METABOLIC SCREEN

12

All states screen for phenylketonuria and hypothyroidism; for a list of screening tests and number of states that use each test, see Table 12-1. Tandem mass spectrometry is currently available to screen for disorders of amino, organic, and fatty acid metabolism. Only a few states have implemented tandem mass spectrometry at the time of this publication; however, that number is expected to increase.[1]

A. TIMING

1. **Screen after at least 24 hours of normal protein and lactose feeding.** Formula-fed infants may not have a diagnostic abnormality before 36 hours of age. Breast-fed infants may not have a diagnostic abnormality before 48 to 72 hours of age.

2. **Recommendations from the American Academy of Pediatrics:**

   a. Screen all infants before hospital discharge. For normal term infants, screen as close as possible to hospital discharge.

   b. All infants should be screened by 7 days of age.

   c. If first screen is before 24 hours of age, re-screen by 14 days of age.

NOTE: **Many geneticists recommend re-screening at 3 days of age if the first screen is before 24 hours of age.**

B. MANAGEMENT OF POSITIVE SCREENING RESULTS

See Table 12-1.[2-5]

II. INBORN ERRORS OF METABOLISM: ABNORMALITIES OF BIOCHEMICAL PATHWAYS

Inborn errors of metabolism (IEMs) may present any time from the neonatal period to adulthood. Although these disorders are often thought of as rare, when considered collectively, they represent significant treatable causes of morbidity and mortality.[6-10]

A. PRESENTATIONS

1. **Neonatal onset:** Often presents with anorexia, lethargy, vomiting, and/or seizures. Symptoms often develop at 24 to 72 hours of age. One in five sick full-term neonates with no risk factors for infection will have metabolic disease.

2. **Late onset (>28 days old):** Some IEMs characteristically present late, whereas others present beyond the newborn period if the defect is partial.

TABLE 12-1
NEWBORN METABOLIC SCREENS AND INITIAL MANAGEMENT OF ABNORMAL RESULTS

Disease (Number of States That Conduct Screen†)	Normal Value	Abnormal Values and Responses*			Definitive Tests
		Clinical Evaluation‡ Repeat Screen Within 48 Hours	Clinical Evaluation‡ Send Definitive Test Telephone Contact With Referral Center	Clinical Evaluation Send Definitive Test Immediate Transfer to Referral Center	
Phenylketonuria (51)	Phe <2	Phe 2-6	Phe 6-12	Phe >12	Plasma amino acids (Phe, Tyr), biopterins
Hypothyroidism (51)					
Term infant ≤1 wk old	T_4 within 2 SD of mean; TSH <30 mcIU/mL	T_4 >2 SD below mean; TSH <100 mcIU/mL	T_4 >2 SD below mean; TSH >100 mcIU/mL *Start levothyroxine after drawing tests*	—	T_4, free T_4, TSH; thyroid-binding globulin or T_3 resin uptake
Term infant >1 wk old	T_4 within 2 SD of mean; TSH <30 mcIU/mL	T_4 >2 SD below mean; TSH <50 mcIU/mL	T_4 >2 SD below mean; TSH >50 mcIU/mL *Start levothyroxine after drawing tests*	—	T_4, free T_4, TSH; thyroid-binding globulin or T_3 resin uptake
Galactosemia§(48) (sugar in mg/dL) Note: sugar = galactose + gal-1-P	Beutler FST nl, sugar <10	Beutler FST nl and sugar 10-40 **or** Beutler FST abnl and sugar <10 *Check urine reducing subs; if positive, remove lactose from diet, contact referral center*	Beutler FST abnl and sugar ≥or Beutler FST nl and sugar >40 *Check urine reducing subs; remove lactose from diet*	—	Galactose-1-P uridyltransferase; galactokinase; UDP gal-4-epimerase; galactose; galactose-1-phosphate

Hemoglobinopathy (47)	Hemoglobin electrophoresis	See Chapter 13	—	—	—
Biotinidase deficiency (22)	Colorimetric biotinidase assay nl	Colorimetric biotinidase assay abnl	—	—	Plasma biotinidase RIA, urine organic acids
Congenital adrenal hyperplasia (22)	Enzyme (17-OHP) immunoassay nl	Immunoassay abnl	—	—	Quantitative plasma 17-OHP
Maple syrup urine disease§ (21)	Leu <2	Leu 2-4 *Check urine ketones; if positive, transfer to referral center*	Leu 4-8 *Restrict protein to 1.5 g/kg/day; check urine ketones; if positive, transfer to referral center*	Leu >8	Plasma amino acids
Homocystinuria (14)	Methionine <2 mg/dL	>2 mg/dL *transfer to referral center*	—	—	Plasma amino acids (Met), plasma homocysteine
Cystic fibrosis (6)	Immunoreactive trypsin test 70-140 mcg/mL	>140 mcg/mL Second test at 30 days of age; if >80 mcg/dL, use confirmatory test	—	—	Sweat test or DNA analysis

Modified from American Academy of Pediatrics. Pediatrics 2000; 106:383-427; American Academy of Pediatrics, Committee on Genetics. Pediatrics 1996; 98:473-501; Council of Regional Networks for Genetic Services. J Pediatr 2000; (suppl)137:S1-S46; and Elsas LJ. Newborn screening. In Rudolph AM, Hoffman JIE, Rudolph CD, editors. Rudolph's pediatrics, 20th ed. Norwalk, Conn: Appleton & Lange; 1996.

Note: Other tests used in <5 states include human immunodeficiency virus (HIV), MCAD, toxoplasmosis, G6PD, and tandem mass spectrometry (for >30 disorders).[1]

Nl, Normal; abnl, abnormal.

*Disease-specific responses in italics.

†Number of states screened includes 50 states and Washington DC.

‡More aggressive interventions should be taken if clinical evaluation is worrisome.

§Maple syrup urine disease and galactosemia can be rapidly fatal if untreated; err on the side of aggressive evaluation and treatment.

GENETICS

12

BOX 12-1

LABORATORY TESTS FOR INBORN ERRORS OF METABOLISM

INITIAL TESTS

Complete blood count with differential

Serum electrolytes (calculate anion gap)

Blood glucose

Aspartate aminotransferase (AST)

Alanine aminotransferase (ALT)

Total and direct bilirubin

Blood gas

Plasma ammonium

Plasma lactate

Urine dipstick: pH, ketones, glucose, protein, bilirubin

Urine odor (see Table 12-4)

Urine-reducing substances (Clinitest tablet [Ames Co.], identifies all reducing
  substances in urine; see Box 12-2)

FURTHER TESTING IF WORK-UP IS SUSPICIOUS

Plasma amino acids

Quantitative plasma carnitine

Urine organic acids

If lactate level is elevated, serum pyruvate and repeat lactate level

---

a. Typical symptoms: Vomiting, respiratory distress, and changes in mental status, including confusion, lethargy, irritability, aggressive behavior, hallucinations, seizures, and coma.

b. Symptoms are usually brought on by intercurrent illness, prolonged fast, dietary indiscretion, or any process causing increased catabolism.

B. EVALUATION OF SUSPECTED METABOLIC DISEASE

1. **For laboratory tests recommended to detect IEMs,** see Box 12-1. For sample collection requirements, see Table 12-2.

2. **If the initial evaluation is suspicious for metabolic disease, obtain further testing as listed in Box 12-1 and consult a geneticist.** Early diagnosis and appropriate therapy are essential for preventing irreversible brain damage and death.

C. DIFFERENTIAL DIAGNOSIS

A differential diagnosis is based on predominant signs and symptoms.

1. **Interpretation of initial laboratory findings** (Table 12-3).

2. **Differential diagnosis of hyperammonemia** (Fig. 12-1).

3. **Differential diagnosis of recurrent hypoglycemia** (see section E, Recurrent Hypoglycemia, p. 274).

4. **Abnormal urine odors** (Table 12-4).

5. **Positive urine reducing substances** (Box 12-2).

D. GENERAL ACUTE MANAGEMENT OF INBORN ERRORS OF METABOLISM

1. Stop dietary sources of protein.

TABLE 12-2

SAMPLE COLLECTION

Specimen	Volume (mL)	Tube*	Handling
Plasma ammonium	1-3	Green top	On ice; immediate transport to laboratory; levels rise rapidly on standing
Plasma amino acids†	1-3	Green top	On ice; if must store, spin down, separate plasma and freeze
Plasma carnitine	1-3	Green top	On ice
Acylcarnitine profile	Saturate newborn screen filter paper with blood		Dry and mail to reference laboratory
Lactate	3	Gray top	On ice
Karyotype	3	Green top	Room temperature
Very-long-chain fatty acids	3	Purple top	Room temperature
White blood cells for enzymes/DNA	3	Purple top	Room temperature
Urine organic acids	5-10	—	Deliver immediately or freeze
Urine amino acids	5-10	—	Deliver immediately or freeze
Skin biopsy		Tissue culture medium or patient's plasma	Refrigerate; do not freeze

*Additives in tubes: purple, K3EDTA; green, lithium heparin; gray, potassium oxalate and sodium fluoride.
†Obtain after a 3-hour fast.

12

GENETICS

2. **Start intravenous (IV) fluids:** D_{10} at 1.5 to 2 times maintenance dose delivers 10 to 15 mg/kg/min of glucose to stop catabolism. (A catabolic state results in an endogenous protein load.) Add Na^+/K^+ based on the degree of dehydration and electrolyte levels. In severe dehydration, give a normal saline (NS) bolus in addition to D_{10} at 1.5 to 2 times the maintenance dose to stop catabolism.
3. Provide HCO_3^- replacement for severe acidosis (pH <7.1) only.
4. **In cases of hyperammonemia, the following experimental drugs may be used. They should only be used in consultation with a geneticist because overdoses may be lethal**: sodium benzoate 250 mg/kg (5.5 g/m^2) IV, sodium phenylacetate 250 mg/kg (5.5 g/m^2) IV, and arginine-HCl (10% solution) 6 mL/kg (12 g/m^2) IV. Give these doses as a bolus over 90 minutes. Repeat the same doses over 24 hours as a mainte-

TABLE 12-3

DIFFERENTIAL DIAGNOSIS OF SUSPECTED METABOLIC DISEASE

Deficient pathway	Amino acid metabolism	Urea cycle	Carbohydrate metabolism	Fatty acid oxidation	Organic acid metabolism	Energy metabolism
Example	Maple syrup urine disease	OTC deficiency	Glycogen storage disease type I	Medium-chain acyl-coA dehydrogenase deficiency	Methylmalonic acidemia	Pyruvate dehydrogenase complex deficiency
Test						
Blood pH	Acidic	Alkaline	Acidic	Variable	Acidic	Acidic
Anion gap	↑	Normal	↑	±	↑	↑
Ketones	↑	Negative	↑	Inappropriately low	↑	– or ↑
Lactate	Normal	Normal	↑	Slight ↑	Normal or ↑	Markedly ↑
Glucose	Variable	Normal	↓	→	Normal or ↑	± or →
NH$_4^+$	Normal or slight ↑	Markedly ↑	Normal	Moderate ↑	Normal or ↑	± or ↑
FTT	Yes	Yes	Yes	No	Yes	Yes
Developmental delay	Yes	Yes	No	No	Yes	Yes
Neurologic signs	Lethargy to coma, hypertonia	Irritable, combative, coma, hypotonia	Hypoglycemic seizures	Lethargy to coma	Lethargy to coma, hypotonia	Lethargy to coma, hypotonia

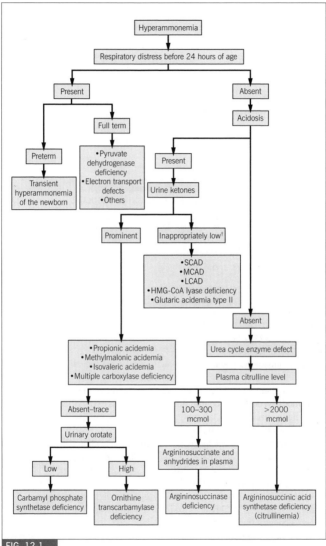

FIG. 12-1

Differential diagnosis of hyperammonemia. Dagger indicates hypoglycemia present when symptomatic. *HMG-CoA,* Hydroxymethylglutaryl-CoA; *LCAD,* long-chain acyl-CoA dehydrogenase; *MCAD,* medium-chain acyl-CoA dehydrogenase; *SCAD,* short-chain acyl-CoA dehydrogenase.

TABLE 12-4	
UNUSUAL URINE ODORS	
Disease	Odor
ACUTE DISEASE	
Maple syrup urine disease	Maple syrup, burned sugar
Isovaleric acidemia	Cheesy or sweaty feet
Multiple carboxylase deficiency	Cat's urine
3-OH,3-methyl glutaryl-CoA lyase deficiency	Cat's urine
NONACUTE DISEASE	
Phenylketonuria	Musty
Hypermethioninemia	Rancid butter, rotten cabbage
Trimethylaminuria	Fishy

BOX 12-2

DISORDERS ASSOCIATED WITH A POSITIVE URINE-REDUCING SUBSTANCES TEST

Galactose: Galactosemia, galactokinase deficiency, severe liver disease
Fructose: Hereditary fructose intolerance, essential fructosuria
Glucose: Diabetes mellitus, renal tubular defects
p-Hydroxyphenylpyruvic acid: Tyrosinemia
Xylose: Pentosuria

---

nance dose. Ondansetron may be used to decrease nausea and vomiting associated with these drugs. (Benzoate and phenylacetate are substrates for alternate pathways of nitrogen excretion; arginine supplementation allows continued operation of the urea cycle in defects in which the block is proximal to arginine.)

5. **If the patient's condition is unresponsive to above management, hemodialysis should be initiated.** Hemodialysis is often required in neonates because of their inherently catabolic state. Exchange transfusion should not be used.

6. **Long-term therapy** will likely include protein restriction, citrulline supplementation, and oral sodium phenylbutyrate (Buphenyl).

E. RECURRENT HYPOGLYCEMIA

Recurrent hypoglycemia may result from endocrine disorders or IEMs, including defects in gluconeogenesis, glycogen breakdown (glycogen storage diseases), and fatty acid oxidation, or toxic impairment of gluconeogenesis (organic acidemias).

1. **Laboratory evaluation:** If the patient is stable, the following tests should be performed before giving glucose:

a. Blood gas.

b. Electrolytes.

c. Chemistry panel.

d. Gray-top glucose.

e. Plasma lactate.

f. Insulin, growth hormone, and cortisol. Consider C peptide if exogenous insulin is suspected.

g. Plasma amino acids, acylcarnitine profile, quantitative carnitine levels, and urine for ketones should also be studied, but samples may be obtained after giving glucose.

2. **Glycogen storage disease types I and III**

a. Presentation: Hepatomegaly, symptomatic hypoglycemia.

   (1) Type I (glucose-6-phosphatase deficiency [G6PD]) typically presents at 1 to 2 months of age with prominent hepatomegaly; the patient is symptomatic with fasting >3 hours.

   (2) Type III (glycogen debrancher deficiency) often presents at >6 months of age, when trying to get a child to sleep through the night; the patient is symptomatic with fasting for 8 to 12 hours.

b. Laboratory findings: Hypoglycemia and lactic acidemia after a short fast; elevated aspartate aminotransferase (AST), alanine aminotransferase (ALT), cholesterol, uric acid (type I only), and lactate at baseline.

c. Definitive diagnosis: Liver biopsy for enzyme assay.

d. Therapy: Frequent feedings, nocturnal nasogastric feedings; uncooked cornstarch.

3. **Fatty acid oxidation defects:** Defects of the carnitine cycle or of β-oxidation: short-, medium-, long-, and very-long-chain acyl-CoA dehydrogenase deficiency, abbreviated as SCAD, MCAD, LCAD, and VLCAD, respectively. For each chain length there is a corresponding hydroxyacyl-CoA dehydrogenase deficiency: SCHAD, MCHAD, LCHAD, and VLCHAD, respectively.

a. Presentation: Change in mental status, emesis, or seizures after a prolonged fast or at time of increased caloric need; hepatomegaly; in some defects cardiomyopathy, dysrhythmias, or skeletal muscle weakness are present.

b. Laboratory findings: Hypoglycemia with inappropriately low ketones is the hallmark. Also noted are moderately elevated liver function tests (LFTs) and ammonia, low total carnitine, and mild metabolic acidosis. Different defects have characteristic patterns on organic acid, acylcarnitine, and acylglycine analyses.

c. Therapy

   (1) Acute: See pp. 270-271, 274; carnitine supplementation.

   (2) Chronic: Carnitine supplementation, avoidance of fasting, IV fluid with D_{10} if unable to maintain oral (PO) intake as a result of illness.

III. NEURODEGENERATIVE DISORDERS: ABNORMALITIES OF ORGANELLE FUNCTION

NOTE: Many other neurodegenerative disorders exist; an exhaustive list is beyond the scope of this chapter.

A. LYSOSOMAL DISORDERS

Lysosomal disorders (e.g., the mucopolysaccharidoses) include neurodegeneration with systemic storage resulting from lysosomal enzyme defects (e.g., Hurler, Hunter, Scheie, Sanfilippo, and Sly syndromes).

12

GENETICS

1. **Presentation:** Hepatosplenomegaly, corneal clouding (except Hunter syndrome), dysostosis multiplex, coarse features, neurologic deterioration.
2. **Laboratory findings:** Inclusion bodies on peripheral blood smear, positive urine mucopolysaccharide (MPS) spot; characteristic findings on eye examination and skeletal survey.
3. **Definitive diagnosis:** Assay of skin fibroblasts for specific lysosomal hydrolases.
4. **Therapy:** Experimental therapy with exogenous enzyme; bone marrow transplantation may provide some enzyme activity but cannot reverse brain damage.

B. PEROXISOMAL DISORDERS

Peroxisomal disorders include Refsum syndrome, X-linked adrenoleukodystrophy (ALD), Zellweger syndrome, and others.

1. **Presentation:** Seizures, loss of milestones, loss of white matter on magnetic resonance imaging (MRI) scans. There is progressive neurodegeneration, and eventually death.
2. **Laboratory findings:** Elevated very-long-chain fatty acids, pipecolic acid, phytanic acid, and plasmalogens.
3. **Definitive diagnosis:** Enzyme assays in cultured skin fibroblasts and microscopy of peroxisomes.
4. **Therapy:** Treat adrenal insufficiency if present; provide vitamin K. Research protocols include dietary lipid therapy, bone marrow transplant, and immunosuppression.

V. DYSMORPHOLOGY

The suspicion for many syndromes and chromosomal anomalies is often raised by major or minor anomalies noted on physical examination. The most common anomalies and commonly used diagnostic tests are listed here. More complete information can be found in reference works by Hall, Froster-Iskenius, Allandon[11] and Jones.[12] In addition to well-known syndromes, many rare genetic disorders are listed in reference works.[12,13] Searching the Online Mendelian Inheritance in Man (OMIM) website, *www3.ncbi.nlm.nih.gov/omim*, with a free text search of patient findings may lead to a more complete diagnostic differential.

A. PHYSICAL EXAMINATION

1. **Head:** Hypotelorism; hypertelorism (for inner and outer canthal distance charts see Pirneck EK et al[14]); abnormal palpebral fissure length and angle[11] or epicanthal folds; long, short, or flat philtrum; ear pits or tags; low-set or posteriorly rotated ears; micrognathia; retrognathia.
2. **Skeletal:** Fifth-digit clinodactyly, syndactyly, polydactyly. Rhizomelic shortening (shortening of proximal long bones) is typical of conditions such as achondroplasia. Proportionate dwarfism is characteristic of growth hormone deficiency. Upper:lower segment ratio (Fig. 12-2) is low in Marfan syndrome.

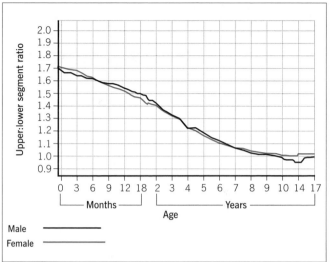

FIG. 12-2

Normal upper:lower segment ratio by age. The lower segment equals distance from pubic symphysis to floor. Ratio equals upper segment/lower segment = [height – lower segment]/lower segment.

B. STRUCTURAL DIAGNOSTIC TESTS

1. Brain MRI.
2. **Ophthalmologic examination** for optic atrophy, coloboma, cataracts, retinal abnormalities, lens subluxation, or corneal abnormalities.
3. Echocardiogram.
4. **Abdominal ultrasound** for polysplenia or asplenia, absent or horseshoe kidney, ureteral or bladder defects, and abdominal situs.
5. **Skeletal survey** for abnormalities of bone length or structure.

C. GENETIC DIAGNOSTIC TESTS

1. **Karyotype:** Detects abnormal numbers of chromosomes and deletions, duplications, translocations, and inversions large enough to be seen by light microscopy. For indications, see section VII.
2. **Fluorescence in situ hybridization (FISH):** Hybridization of a fluorescently tagged DNA probe to chromosomes allows detection of submicroscopic deletions and duplications. FISH assays are commonly available for the following syndromes: Williams (7q11), Prader-Willi and Angelman (15q11), Miller-Dieker (17p13.3), Smith-Magenis (17p11.2), velocardiofacial and DiGeorge (22q11). Telomere deletions and many other genetic disorders are also testable by FISH. For a complete, updated online list of genetic diagnostic tests, see *www.geneclinics.org*.

3. **Deoxyribonucleic acid (DNA) analysis:** Many monogenic disorders now have DNA tests available. Contact your laboratory or *www.genetests.org* for a list of those available.

VI. COMMON SYNDROMES

For more information on common syndromes and other chromosomal abnormalities and syndromes, see *Smith's recognizable patterns of human malformation, 5th ed,* by Jones.[12]

A. TRISOMY 21 (INCIDENCE: 1:660)

1. **Features:** Presence of 6 of the following 10 cardinal features in the neonate is highly suggestive of the diagnosis of trisomy 21: hypotonia, poor Moro reflex, hyperflexibility, excess skin on back of the neck, flat facies, slanted palpebral fissures, anomalous auricles, pelvic dysplasia, dysplasia of the midphalanx of the fifth finger, and a single transverse palmar (Simian) crease.
2. **Associated findings:** Mental retardation (100%), hearing loss (75%), eye disease (60%), serous otitis media (50% to 70%), cardiac defects (50%), thyroid disease (15%), gastrointestinal (GI) atresias (12%), atlantoaxial instability (12%), and leukemia (1%).
3. **Testing:** Karyotype for diagnosis, echocardiogram, yearly thyroid function tests, LFTs, complete blood count (CBC), and audiologic evaluation; radiographs of the atlantooccipital junction and ophthalmologic examination by 3 to 5 years of age.[15]
4. **Natural history:** Growth charts for children with trisomy 21 appear on pp. 451-454. Approximately 50% of those with congenital heart defects survive to age 30; 80% of those without congenital heart defects survive to age 30.

B. TRISOMY 18 (INCIDENCE: 1:3000, WITH 3:1 FEMALE PREDOMINANCE)

1. **Features:** Clenched hand, with index finger overlapping third and fifth finger overlapping fourth, intrauterine growth retardation (IUGR), decreased fetal activity, low-arch dermal ridge pattern, inguinal or umbilical hernia, cardiac defects, prominent occiput, low-set ears, micrognathia, rocker bottom feet.
2. **Testing:** Karyotype with FISH analysis allows results within 24 to 48 hours.
3. **Natural history:** Apnea, severe failure to thrive; 50% die by 1 week, 90% by 1 year; profound mental retardation in survivors.

C. TRISOMY 13 (INCIDENCE: 1:5000)

1. **Features:** Holoprosencephaly, polydactyly, scalp skin defects, seizures, deafness, microcephaly, sloping forehead, cleft lip, cleft palate, retinal anomalies, microphthalmia, abnormal ears, single umbilical artery, inguinal hernia, omphalocele, cardiac defects, urinary tract malformations.
2. **Testing:** Karyotype with FISH analysis allows results within 24 to 48 hours.

3. **Natural history:** 44% die within 1 month; >70% die by 1 year; profound mental retardation in survivors.

D. TURNER SYNDROME—45,X (INCIDENCE: 1:5000)

1. **Features:** Short female with broad chest, wide-spaced nipples, webbed neck, congenital lymphedema.
2. **Associated findings:** Gonadal dysgenesis (90%), renal anomalies (60%), cardiac defects (20%), most commonly coarctation of the aorta, hearing loss (50%).
3. **Testing:** Karyotype for diagnosis. Baseline echocardiogram, renal ultrasound; blood pressure (BP), hearing, and scoliosis screen with each examination; thyroid function tests and echocardiogram every 1 to 2 years.[16]
4. **Natural history:** Infertility, normal lifespan, mean IQ 90, short stature. Growth charts for girls with Turner syndrome appear on p. 455.

E. FRAGILE X (INCIDENCE: 1:1500 MALES)

1. **Features:** Boys: Mild to profound mental retardation (6% of boys with mental retardation), cluttered speech, autism (60%), macrocephaly, large ears, prognathism, postpubertal macroorchidism, tall stature. Phenotype most prominent in boys; girls may have only learning disabilities (0.3% of girls have mental retardation).
2. **Testing:** Karyotype of lymphocytes cultured in folate-deficient medium reveals nonstaining gap present at Xq27.3, site of a CGG expansion. The number of CGG repeats correlates with disease severity. DNA analysis is also possible and is recommended for females.
3. **Natural history:** Normal lifespan.

F. MARFAN SYNDROME (INCIDENCE 2 TO 3:10,000)

1. **Features:** There are major and minor diagnostic criteria involving the skeletal, ocular, cardiovascular, and pulmonary systems, and skin or integument. Features include but are not limited to tall stature, low upper:lower segment ratio (see Fig. 12-2), arachnodactyly, joint laxity, scoliosis, pectus excavatum or carinatum, lens subluxation, glaucoma, retinal detachment, dilation with or without dissecting aneurysm of ascending aorta, mitral valve prolapse, lumbosacral dural ectasia by computed tomography (CT) or MRI scans, and inguinal and/or femoral hernias.
2. **Testing:** Slit lamp examination, echocardiogram, genetic evaluation. Diagnosis is made clinically and requires major criteria in at least two different organ systems and involvement of a third organ system. For a complete list of criteria, see Scriver et al[8] and De Paepe et al.[17]
3. **Natural history:** Patients with aortic root dilation >2 standard deviations (SDs) above the mean should be treated with atenolol and followed with a yearly echocardiogram. Significant aortic root dilation requires surgical repair. With corrective surgery, mean age of survival approaches normal life span; this is significantly lower in patients with untreated vascular complications.[18]

12

GENETICS

VII. GENETIC CONSULTATION

A. INDICATIONS FOR REFERRAL

1. Known or suspected hereditary disorder.
2. **Major physical anomalies,** unusual body proportions, short stature, dysmorphic features.
3. Major organ malformation.
4. **Developmental delay or mental retardation;** learning disabilities in females who have brothers with mental retardation.
5. Complete or partial blindness or hearing loss.
6. **Deterioration of motor or speech abilities** in a previously thriving child.
7. Maternal exposure to drugs, alcohol, or radiation during pregnancy.
8. Strong family history of cancer.
9. Failure to thrive if routine evaluation is unrevealing.

B. INDICATIONS FOR PRENATAL COUNSELING

1. Genetic disorder or birth defect in one partner.
2. Known carrier of a genetic disorder.
3. Previous child with known or suspected genetic disorder.
4. Maternal age ≥35 years.
5. Family history of known or suspected chromosomal anomaly.
6. Multiple early miscarriages or stillbirths.
7. Member of an ethnic group known to have a high incidence of a specific genetic disorder.

C. INDICATIONS FOR KARYOTYPE

1. **Two major** *OR* **one major and two minor malformations** (include small for gestational age and mental retardation as major).
2. Features of a specific chromosomal syndrome.
3. At risk for familial chromosomal aberration.
4. Ambiguous genitalia.
5. **More than two spontaneous abortions or infertility** (karyotype both partners).
6. Girls with short stature.

REFERENCES

1. American College of Medical Genetics/American Society of Human Genetics Test and Technology Transfer Committee Working Group. Tandem mass spectrometry in newborn screening. Genet Med 2000; 2:267-269.
2. American Academy of Pediatrics. A report from the Newborn Screening Task Force. Pediatrics 2000; 106:383-427.
3. American Academy of Pediatrics, Committee on Genetics. Neonatal screening fact sheets. Pediatrics 1996; 98:473-501.
4. Council of Regional Networks for Genetic Services. US newborn screening system guidelines II: follow-up of children, diagnosis, management, and evaluation. J Pediatr 2000; (suppl)137: S1-S46.
5. Elsas LJ. Newborn screening. In Rudolph AM, Hoffman JIE, Rudolph CD, editors. Rudolph's pediatrics, 20th ed. Norwalk, Conn: Appleton & Lange; 1996.
6. Epstein CJ, assoc. ed. Genetic disorders and birth defects. In Rudolph AM, Hoffman JIE, Rudolph CD, editors. Rudolph's pediatrics, 20th ed. Norwalk, Conn: Appleton & Lange; 1996.
7. Fernandes J, Sauderbray J-M, Vanden Berghe G. Inborn metabolic diseases, 3rd ed. Berlin: Springer-Verlag; 2000.

8. Scriver CR et al. The molecular and metabolic bases of inherited disease, 8th ed. New York: McGraw-Hill; 2001.
9. Seashore M, Wappner R. Genetics in primary care and clinical medicine. Norwalk, Conn: Appleton & Lange; 1996.
10. Seidel HM, Rosenstein BJ, Pathak A. Primary care of the newborn, 3rd ed. St Louis: Mosby; 2001.
11. Hall JG, Froster-Iskenius UG, Allanson JE. Handbook of normal physical measurements. Oxford, England: Oxford Medical Publications; 1989.
12. Jones K. Smith's recognizable patterns of human malformation, 5th ed. Philadelphia: WB Saunders; 1997.
13. Gorlin R, Cohen M, Levin L. Syndromes of the head and neck, 3rd ed. New York: Oxford University Press; 1990.
14. Pirnick EK et al. Interpupillary distance in a normal black population. Clin Genet 1999; 55: 182-191.
15. American Academy of Pediatrics, Committee on Genetics. Health supervision for children with Down syndrome. Pediatrics 1994; 93:855-859.
16. American Academy of Pediatrics, Committee on Genetics. Health supervision for children with Turner syndrome. Pediatrics 1995; 96:1166-1173.
17. De Paepe A et al. Revised diagnostic criteria for the Marfan syndrome. Am J Med Genet 1996; 62:417.
18. American Academy of Pediatrics, Committee on Genetics. Health supervision of children with Marfan syndrome. Pediatrics 1996; 98:978-982.

12

GENETICS

HEMATOLOGY

Michelle Hudspeth, MD and Heather Symons, MD

I. WEBSITES

www.bloodline.net
www.bloodjournal.org
www.sicklecelldisease.org

II. ANEMIA

A. GENERAL EVALUATION

Anemia is defined by age-specific norms (Fig. 13-1 and Table 13-1). Evaluation includes the following:

1. **Complete history:** Includes melena, hematochezia, blood loss, fatigue, pica, medication exposure, growth and development, nutritional history, ethnic background, and family history of anemia, splenectomy, or cholecystectomy.
2. **Physical examination:** Includes pallor, jaundice (including scleral icterus), glossitis, tachypnea, tachycardia, cardiac murmur, hepatosplenomegaly, and signs of systemic illness.
3. **Initial laboratory tests:** May include a complete blood count (CBC) with red blood cell (RBC) indices, reticulocyte count, blood smear, stool for occult blood, urinalysis, and serum bilirubin.

B. DIAGNOSIS

Anemias may be categorized as macrocytic, microcytic, or normocytic. Table 13-2 gives a differential diagnosis of anemia based on RBC production and cell size. Note that normal ranges for hemoglobin and mean corpuscular volume (MCV) are age dependent.

C. EVALUATION OF SPECIFIC CAUSES OF ANEMIA

1. **Iron deficiency anemia:** Hypochromic/microcytic anemia with a low reticulocyte count and an elevated red cell distribution width (RDW).
   a. Serum ferritin reflects total body iron stores after 6 months of age and is the first value to fall in iron deficiency. Ferritin is an acute phase reactant, and it may be falsely elevated with inflammation or infection. See Chapter 24 for normal ferritin values.
   b. Other indicators include low serum iron and/or transferrin levels and an elevated total iron-binding capacity (TIBC). See Chapter 24 for normal iron, transferrin, and TIBC values.
   c. Free erythrocyte protoporphyrin (FEP) accumulates when the conversion of protoporphyrin to heme is blocked. FEP is elevated in iron deficiency, plumbism, and erythrocyte protoporphyria. Levels >300 mcg/dL are generally found only with lead intoxication.
   d. Iron therapy (see Formulary for dosage information) should result in an increased reticulocyte count in 2 to 3 days and an increase in hematocrit (HCT) after 1 to 4 weeks of therapy. Iron stores are generally repleted with 3 months of therapy.
2. **Hemolytic anemia:** Rapid RBC turnover. Etiologies include congenital

TABLE 13-1

AGE-SPECIFIC BLOOD CELL INDICES

Age	Hb (g%)[a]	HCT (%)[a]	MCV (fL)[a]	MCHC (g/% RBC)[a]	Reticulocytes	WBCs (×10³/mm³)[b]	Platelets (10³/mm³)[b]
26-30 wk gestation[c]	13.4 (11)	41.5 (34.9)	118.2 (106.7)	37.9 (30.6)	—	4.4 (2.7)	254 (180-327)
28 wk	14.5	45	120	31.0	(5-10)	—	275
32 wk	15.0	47	118	32.0	(3-10)	—	290
Term[d] (cord)	16.5 (13.5)	51 (42)	108 (98)	33.0 (30.0)	(3-7)	18.1 (9-30)[e]	290
1-3 dy	18.5 (14.5)	56 (45)	108 (95)	33.0 (29.0)	(1.8-4.6)	18.9 (9.4-34)	192
2 wk	16.6 (13.4)	53 (41)	105 (88)	31.4 (28.1)		11.4 (5-20)	252
1 mo	13.9 (10.7)	44 (33)	101 (91)	31.8 (28.1)	(0.1-1.7)	10.8 (4-19.5)	
2 mo	11.2 (9.4)	35 (28)	95 (84)	31.8 (28.3)			
6 mo	12.6 (11.1)	36 (31)	76 (68)	35.0 (32.7)	(0.7-2.3)	11.9 (6-17.5)	
6 mo-2 yr	12.0 (10.5)	36 (33)	78 (70)	33.0 (30.0)	—	10.6 (6-17)	(150-350)

2-6 yr	12.5 (11.5)	37 (34)	81 (75)	34.0 (31.0)	(0.5-1.0)	8.5 (5-15.5)	(150-350)
6-12 yr	13.5 (11.5)	40 (35)	86 (77)	34.0 (31.0)	(0.5-1.0)	8.1 (4.5-13.5)	(150-350)
12-18 yr							
Male	14.5 (13)	43 (36)	88 (78)	34.0 (31.0)	(0.5-1.0)	7.8 (4.5-13.5)	(150-350)
Female	14.0 (12)	41 (37)	90 (78)	34.0 (31.0)	(0.5-1.0)	7.8 (4.5-13.5)	(150-350)
Adult							
Male	15.5 (13.5)	47 (41)	90 (80)	34.0 (31.0)	(0.8-2.5)	7.4 (4.5-11)	(150-350)
Female	14.0 (12)	41 (36)	90 (80)	34.0 (31.0)	(0.8-4.1)	7.4 (4.5-11)	(150-350)

Data from Forestier F et al. Pediatr Res 1986; 20:342; Oski FA, Naiman JL. Hematological problems in the newborn infant. Philadelphia: WB Saunders; 1982; Nathan D, Oski FA. Hematology of infancy and childhood. Philadelphia: WB Saunders; 1998; Matoth Y, Zaizov R, Varsano I. Acta Paediatr Scand 1971; 60:317; and Wintrobe MM. Clinical hematology. Baltimore: Williams and Wilkins; 1999.

Hb, hemoglobin.

[a]Data are mean (−2 SD).

[b]Data are mean (±2 SD).

[c]Values are from fetal samplings.

[d]<1 mo, capillary hemoglobin exceeds venous: 1 hr: 3.6 g difference; 5 dy: 2.2 g difference; 3 wk: 1.1 g difference.

[e]Mean (95% confidence limits).

13

HEMATOLOGY

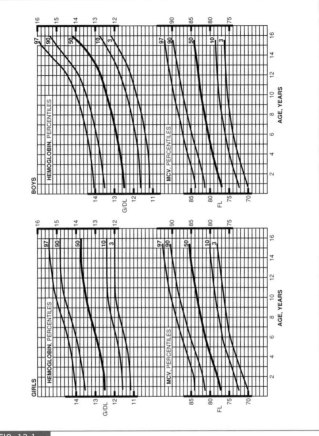

FIG. 13-1

Hemoglobin and mean corpuscular volume by age. *(From Dallman PR, Siimes MA. J Pediatr 1979; 94:26.)*

membranopathies, hemoglobinopathies, enzymopathies, metabolic defects, and immune-mediated destruction. Useful studies include the following:

a. Reticulocyte count: Usually elevated and indicates increased production of RBCs to compensate for increased destruction. **Corrected reticulocyte count (CRC)**: Corrected for differences in HCT, CRC is an indicator of erythropoietic activity. A CRC >1.5 suggests increased RBC production as a result of hemolysis or blood loss.

$$CRC = \% \text{ Reticulocytes} \times \text{Patient HCT/Normal HCT}$$

TABLE 13-2
CLASSIFICATION OF ANEMIA

Reticulocyte Count	Microcytic Anemia	Normocytic Anemia	Macrocytic Anemia
Low	Iron deficiency	Chronic disease	Folate deficiency
	Lead poisoning	RBC aplasia (TEC, infection, drug induced)	Vitamin B_{12} deficiency
	Chronic disease	Malignancy	Aplastic anemia
	Aluminum toxicity	Juvenile rheumatoid arthritis	Congenital bone marrow dysfunction
	Copper deficiency	Endocrinopathies	(Diamond-Blackfan or Fanconi syndromes)
	Protein malnutrition	Renal failure	Drug induced
			Trisomy 21
			Hypothyroidism
Normal	Thalassemia trait	Acute bleeding	Dyserythropoietic anemia I, III
	Sideroblastic anemia	Hypersplenism	Active hemolysis
		Dyserythropoietic anemia II	—
High	Thalassemia syndromes	Antibody-mediated hemolysis	
	Hemoglobin C disorders	Hypersplenism	
		Microangiopathy (HUS, TTP, DIC, Kasabach-Merritt)	
		Membranopathies (spherocytosis, elliptocytosis)	
		Enzyme disorders (G6PD, pyruvate kinase)	
		Hemoglobinopathies	

From Nathan D, Oski FA. Hematology of infancy and childhood. Philadelphia: WB Saunders; 1988.
DIC, Disseminated intravascular coagulation; *G6PD,* glucose-6-phosphate dehydrogenase; *HUS,* hemolytic uremic syndrome; *TEC,* transient erythroblastopenia of childhood; *TTP,* thrombotic thrombocytopenic purpura.

HEMATOLOGY

13

b. Increased plasma aspartate aminotransferase (AST) and lactate dehydrogenase (LDH) from release of intracellular enzymes.

c. Haptoglobin: Binds free hemoglobin; decreased with intravascular and extravascular hemolysis.

d. Direct Coombs' test (DCT): Tests for the presence of antibody on patient RBCs. Can be falsely negative if affected cells have already been destroyed or antibody titer is low.

e. Glucose-6-phosphate dehydrogenase (G6PD) assay: Used to diagnose G6PD deficiency, an X-linked disorder. May be normal immediately after a hemolytic episode, as older, more enzyme-deficient cells have been lysed. See Chapter 28 for a list of oxidizing drugs.

f. Osmotic fragility test: Useful in diagnosis of hereditary spherocytosis.

g. Heinz body preparation: Precipitated hemoglobin within RBCs; present in unstable hemoglobinopathies and during oxidative stress (e.g., G6PD deficiency).

3. Red cell aplasia: Normocytic or macrocytic, low reticulocyte count, variable platelet and white blood cell (WBC) counts. Bone marrow aspiration evaluates RBC precursors in the marrow to look for bone marrow dysfunction, neoplasm, or specific signs of infection. May not be necessary for the diagnosis of transient erythroblastopenia of childhood (TEC) or aplastic crisis.

a. Acquired aplasias
   (1) Infectious causes, including parvovirus in children with rapid RBC turnover (infects RBC precursors), Epstein-Barr virus (EBV), cytomegalovirus (CMV), human herpes virus 6 (HHV-6), or human immunodeficiency virus (HIV).
   (2) TEC: Occurs from age 6 months to 4 years, with >80% of cases presenting after 1 year of age with a normal or slightly low MCV and low reticulocyte count. There is usually spontaneous recovery within 4 to 8 weeks.
   (3) Exposures (drugs, radiation, chemicals).

b. Congenital aplasias (macrocytic), including the following:
   (1) Fanconi's anemia: An autosomal recessive disorder, Fanconi's anemia usually presents before 10 years of age, and may present with pancytopenia. Patients may have absent thumbs, renal anomalies, microcephaly, or short stature. Chromosomal fragility studies may be diagnostic.
   (2) Diamond-Blackfan-Oski syndrome: An autosomal recessive pure RBC aplasia, this syndrome presents in the first year of life. It is associated with congenital anomalies in one third of cases, including triphalangeal thumb, short stature, and cleft lip.

c. Aplastic anemia (macrocytic).

III. HEMOGLOBINOPATHIES

A. HEMOGLOBIN ELECTROPHORESIS

Hemoglobin electrophoresis involves separation of hemoglobin variants based on molecular charge and size. All positive sickle preparations and solubility tests for sickle hemoglobin (e.g., Sickledex) should be confirmed with electrophoresis or isoelectric focusing (a component of the mandatory newborn screen in many states). See Table 13-3 for interpretation of neonatal hemoglobin electrophoresis patterns.

B. SICKLE CELL ANEMIA

Sickle cell anemia is caused by a genetic defect in β-globin present in 1 in 500 African-Americans; 8% of African-Americans are carriers.

1. **Diagnosis:** Often made on newborn screen with hemoglobin electrophoresis. The sickle preparation and Sickledex are both rapid tests that are positive in all sickle hemoglobinopathies (e.g., sickle trait [AS], sickle cell anemia [SS], sickle-C [SC], sickle β-thalassemia [Sβ-thal]). False negative test results may be seen in neonates and other patients with a high percentage of fetal hemoglobin.

2. **Complications:** A hematologist should generally be consulted.[1]

a. Fever (temperature ≥38.6° C).

   (1) Evaluation: Complete history and physical examination, CBC with differential, reticulocyte count, and blood cultures. Consider urine

---

TABLE 13-3

NEONATAL HEMOGLOBIN (Hb) ELECTROPHORESIS PATTERNS*

FA	Fetal Hb and adult normal Hb; the normal newborn pattern.
FAV	Indicates the presence of both HbF and HbA. However, an anomalous band (V) is present, which does not appear to be any of the common Hb variants.
FAS	Indicates fetal Hb, adult normal HbA and HbS, consistent with benign sickle cell trait.
FS	Fetal and sickle HbS without detectable adult normal HbA. Consistent with homozygous sickle Hb genotype (S/S) or sickle β-thalassemia, with manifestations of sickle cell anemia during childhood.
FC†	Designates the presence of HbC without adult normal HbA. Consistent with clinically significant homozygous HbC genotype (C/C), resulting in a mild hematologic disorder presenting during childhood.
FSC	HbS and HbC present. This heterozygous condition could lead to the manifestations of sickle cell disease during childhood.
FAC	HbC and adult normal HbA present, consistent with benign HbC trait.
FSAA₂	Heterozygous HbS/β-thalassemia, a clinically significant sickling disorder.
FAA₂	Heterozygous HbA/β-thalassemia, a clinically benign hematologic condition.
F†	Fetal HbF is present without adult normal HbA. Although this may indicate a delayed appearance of HbA, it is also consistent with homozygous β-thalassemia major, or homozygous hereditary persistence of fetal HbF.
FV†	Fetal HbF and an anomalous Hb variant (V) are present.
AF	May indicate prior blood transfusion. Submit another filter paper blood specimen when the infant is 4 mo of age, at which time the transfused blood cells should have been cleared.

*Hemoglobin variants are reported in order of decreasing abundance; for example, FA indicates more fetal than adult hemoglobin.
†Repeat blood specimen should be submitted to confirm the original interpretation.

culture, lumbar puncture, blood type and cross-match, chest radiograph, and other cultures if clinically indicated.

(2) Treatment: Prompt administration of intravenous (IV) antibiotics (i.e., high-dose, third-generation cephalosporin). Consider additional coverage with vancomycin if there is suspicion of meningitis. Consider adding clindamycin if penicillin-resistant pneumococcus is suspected, or if patient appears ill. Admit patient if he or she is <3 years old, is toxic in appearance, if there is concern about laboratory results, or if there is evidence of additional acute complications. In older children, use an antibiotic with a long half-life (e.g., ceftriaxone) if patient is treated as an outpatient, and reevaluate within 24 hours. If considering outpatient care, patient must have a home phone, and family must be reliable.

b. Vasoocclusive crisis:
   (1) Commonly presents as dactylitis in children <2 years old, and as unifocal/multifocal pain in children >2 years.
   (2) Treatment: Initially, attempt to control pain with oral analgesics (e.g., nonsteroidal antiinflammatory drugs [NSAIDs], narcotics) and hydration at home. Consider hospital admission if there is inadequate pain control with oral medications, or if additional complications are present. If hospitalized for IV analgesia, also treat with IV fluids, incentive spirometry, and close monitoring for additional complications. Patient-controlled analgesia (PCA) pumps with parenteral narcotics and parenteral NSAIDs (i.e., ketorolac) can be useful in the hospitalized patient (see Formulary and Chapter 27 for choice of analgesics, dosing, and weaning).

c. Acute chest syndrome:
   (1) Defined as a new pulmonary infiltrate and some combination of fever, cough, chest pain, tachypnea, dyspnea, or hypoxemia.
   (2) Treatment: Hospital admission, oxygen, incentive spirometry, bronchodilators, antibiotics (an appropriate combination of a cephalosporin, and/or clindamycin/vancomycin, with the addition of a macrolide if atypical pneumonia is suspected), analgesia, and optimization of fluid status. Consider simple transfusion for moderately severe illness, partial exchange transfusion for severe or rapidly progressive disease. An A-a gradient (see p. 526) can be useful to quantify severity of disease. A chest radiograph, CBC, reticulocyte count, blood type and screen, and blood culture should also be obtained. To avoid hyperviscosity and potential worsening of the clinical condition, avoid increasing to Hgb >10 g/dL or hematocrit >30%. Treatment with high-dose dexamethasone has been proposed, although this still remains a controversial therapeutic agent, and rebound pain with weaning may occur.[2] Pulmonary function tests (PFTs) may be helpful in both acute and chronic management.

d. Splenic sequestration:
   (1) Defined as an acute illness with an Hgb level 2 g/dL or more below the patient's baseline value, with an acutely enlarged spleen. May be associated with leukopenia and thrombocytopenia.
   (2) Treatment: Serial abdominal examinations, close monitoring of all vital signs, fluid resuscitation, and RBC transfusion (10 mL/kg) for Hgb <4.5 g/dL with signs of cardiovascular compromise. May need to repeat RBC transfusion. In severe cases, exchange transfusion may be necessary. With recovery after all transfusions, autotransfusion may occur, resulting in a large increase in Hgb and risk of congestive heart failure. Therefore the goal of transfusion should be hemodynamic stability, and posttransfusion Hgb should not exceed 8 g/dL.
e. Aplastic crisis:
   (1) Defined as an acute illness, with Hgb below patient's baseline value and substantially decreased reticulocyte count (often <1%). It is usually self-limited, and frequently follows viral infections, especially parvovirus B19. Patients should be isolated given the risk to pregnant health care workers.
   (2) Treatment: Hospital admission, close monitoring of all vital signs, intravenous fluids, and packed RBC transfusion with small aliquots for symptomatic anemia (i.e., 5 to 6 mL/kg over 3 to 4 hours) to avoid fluid overload.
f. Additional complications include priapism, cerebrovascular accident (CVA), transient ischemic attack (TIA), gallbladder disease, and avascular necrosis.
3. Health maintenance: Ongoing consultation and clinical involvement with a pediatric hematologist and/or sickle cell program are essential.
a. Pneumococcal vaccine: Heptavalent protein-conjugate vaccine should be provided according to routine childhood schedule. A 23-valent polysaccharide vaccine should be provided after 2 years of age, with a booster after 3 to 5 years (see p. 322, Table 15-6).
b. Begin prophylaxis with penicillin as soon as diagnosis is made; prophylaxis may be discontinued by age 5 if patient has had no prior severe pneumococcal infections or splenectomy and has documented pneumococcal vaccinations.
c. Consider supplementation with folic acid.
d. An annual ophthalmologic examination should be performed after 10 years of age.
e. An annual transcranial Doppler examination should be performed between ages 2 and 16 years in patients with SS disease to screen for high risk of CVA.
f. Closely follow growth, development, and school performance.
C. THALASSEMIAS
Thalassemias are defects in α- or β-globin production. It can be difficult to distinguish between α- and β-thalassemia minor and iron deficiency. The

Mentzer index is useful. An MCV/RBC level >13.5 suggests iron deficiency; <11.5 is suggestive of thalassemia minor.

1. **α-Thalassemia minor** (two-gene deletion) occurs in 1.5% of African-Americans and is common in Southeast Asians. Hemoglobin electrophoresis will be normal (except in a neonate in whom there will be some HbA2 and 1% to 2% HbBarts [γ4]).

2. **β-Thalassemia** is found throughout the Mediterranean, Middle East, India, and Southeast Asia. Electrophoresis in β-thalassemia minor will show 3% to 8% HbA2 and may show 2% to 4% fetal hemoglobin. See Table 13-3 for interpretation of neonatal hemoglobin electrophoresis.

3. **There are many other abnormal hemoglobins,** including unstable forms and those with variations in oxygen affinity.

IV. NEUTROPENIA
DEFINITION
Neutropenia is defined as an absolute neutrophil count <1500/mm^3, although neutrophil counts vary with age (Table 13-4). Severe neutropenia is defined as an absolute neutrophil count <500. See Box 13-1 for a differential diagnosis of neutropenia. Children with significant neutropenia are at risk of bacterial and fungal infections. Granulocyte colony-stimulating factor (G-CSF) may be indicated. See Formulary for dosage information. Transient neutropenia secondary to viral illness rarely causes significant morbidity. For management of fever and neutropenia in oncology patients, see Chapter 21.

V. THROMBOCYTOPENIA
A. DEFINITION
Thrombocytopenia is defined as a platelet count <150,000/mm^3 (see Table 13-1). Clinically significant bleeding is unlikely with platelet counts >20,000/mm^3 in the absence of other complicating factors.
B. DIFFERENTIAL DIAGNOSIS
1. **Idiopathic thrombocytopenic purpura (ITP):** ITP is a diagnosis of exclusion; it can be acute or chronic. WBC count and hemoglobin levels are normal. Hemorrhagic complications are rare with platelet counts >20,000/ mm^3. Many patients require no therapy. Treatment options include Rh (D) immune globulin (useful only in Rh-positive patients), intravenous immune globulin (see p. 310 for IVIG dosing), or corticosteroids (i.e., prednisone 2 mg/kg/day). Splenectomy or chemotherapy may be considered in chronic cases. Platelet transfusions are not generally helpful, but are necessary in life-threatening bleeding.

2. **Platelet alloimmunization:** A common cause of thrombocytopenia in newborns. Transplacental maternal antibodies (usually against PLA-1 antigen) cause fetal platelet destruction and in-utero bleeding. If severe, a transfusion of maternal platelets will be more effective in raising the

TABLE 13-4

AGE-SPECIFIC LEUKOCYTE DIFFERENTIAL

Age	Total Leukocytes* Mean (range)	Neutrophils† Mean (range)	Neutrophils† %	Lymphocytes Mean (range)	Lymphocytes %	Monocytes Mean	Monocytes %	Eosinophils Mean	Eosinophils %
Birth	18.1 (9-30)	11 (6-26)	61	5.5 (2-11)	31	1.1	6	0.4	2
12 hr	22.8 (13-38)	15.5 (6-28)	68	5.5 (2-11)	24	1.2	5	0.5	2
24 hr	18.9 (9.4-34)	11.5 (5-21)	61	5.8 (2-11.5)	31	1.1	6	0.5	2
1 wk	12.2 (5-21)	5.5 (1.5-10)	45	5.0 (2-17)	41	1.1	9	0.5	4
2 wk	11.4 (5-20)	4.5 (1-9.5)	40	5.5 (2-17)	48	1.0	9	0.4	3
1 mo	10.8 (5-19.5)	3.8 (1-8.5)	35	6.0 (2.5-16.5)	56	0.7	7	0.3	3
6 mo	11.9 (6-17.5)	3.8 (1-8.5)	32	7.3 (4-13.5)	61	0.6	5	0.3	3
1 yr	11.4 (6-17.5)	3.5 (1.5-8.5)	31	7.0 (4-10.5)	61	0.6	5	0.3	3
2 yr	10.6 (6-17)	3.5 (1.5-8.5)	33	6.3 (3-9.5)	59	0.5	5	0.3	3
4 yr	9.1 (5.5-15.5)	3.8 (1.5-8.5)	42	4.5 (2-8)	50	0.5	5	0.3	3
6 yr	8.5 (5-14.5)	4.3 (1.5-8)	51	3.5 (1.5-7)	42	0.4	5	0.2	3
8 yr	8.3 (4.5-13.5)	4.4 (1.5-8)	53	3.3 (1.5-6.8)	39	0.4	4	0.2	2
10 yr	8.1 (4.5-13.5)	4.4 (1.5-8.5)	54	3.1 (1.5-6.5)	38	0.4	4	0.2	2
16 yr	7.8 (4.5-13.0)	4.4 (1.8-8)	57	2.8 (1.2-5.2)	35	0.4	5	0.2	3
21 yr	7.4 (4.5-11.0)	4.4 (1.8-7.7)	59	2.5 (1-4.8)	34	0.3	4	0.2	3

From Dallman PR. In Rudolph AM, editor. Pediatrics, 20th ed. New York: Appleton-Century-Crofts; 1996.

*Numbers of leukocytes are × 10^3/mm³; ranges are estimates of 95% confidence limits; percents refer to differential counts.

†Neutrophils include band cells at all ages and a small number of metamyelocytes and myelocytes in the first few days of life.

13

HEMATOLOGY

BOX 13-1

DIFFERENTIAL DIAGNOSIS OF CHILDHOOD NEUTROPENIA

ACQUIRED	CONGENITAL
Infection	Cyclic neutropenia
Immune	Severe congenital neutropenia (Kostmann
Hypersplenism	syndrome)
Vitamin B_{12}, folate, copper deficiency	Chronic benign neutropenia of childhood
Drugs or toxic substances	Schwachman syndrome
Aplastic anemia	Fanconi syndrome
Malignancies or preleukemic	Metabolic disorders (amino acidopathies,
disorders	glycogenosis)
Ionizing radiation	Osteopetrosis

---

platelet count than random donor platelets. Diagnosis may be confirmed as follows:
a. A mixing study of maternal or neonatal plasma and paternal platelets.
b. Absence of maternal PLA-1 antigen.
c. A mixing study with patient plasma and a panel of known minor platelet antigens.
3. **Other causes of thrombocytopenia** include microangiopathic hemolytic anemias, such as disseminated intravascular coagulation (DIC) and hemolytic-uremic syndrome (HUS), infection causing marrow suppression, malignancy, HIV, drug-induced thrombocytopenia, marrow infiltration, cavernous hemangiomas (Kasabach-Merritt syndrome), thrombocytopenia with absent radii syndrome (TAR), thrombosis, hypersplenism, and other rare inherited disorders (e.g., Wiskott-Aldrich syndrome).

VI. COAGULATION[3] (FIGS. 13-2 AND 13-3)

A. TESTS OF COAGULATION

An incorrect anticoagulant:blood ratio will give inaccurate results. See Table 13-5 for normal hematologic values.
1. **Activated partial thromboplastin time (aPTT):** Measures intrinsic system; requires factors V, VIII, IX, X, XI, XII, fibrinogen, and prothrombin. May be prolonged in heparin administration, hemophilia, von Willebrand's disease (VWD), DIC, and the presence of circulating inhibitors (e.g., lupus anticoagulants or other antiphospholipid antibodies).
2. **Prothrombin time (PT):** Measures extrinsic pathway; requires fibrinogen, prothrombin, and factors V, VII, and X. May be prolonged in deficiencies of vitamin K-associated factors, malabsorption, liver disease, DIC, warfarin administration, and circulating inhibitors.
3. **Bleeding time (BT):** Evaluates clot formation, including platelet number and function, and von Willebrand's factor (vWF). Performed at patient bedside. Always assess the platelet number and check for a history

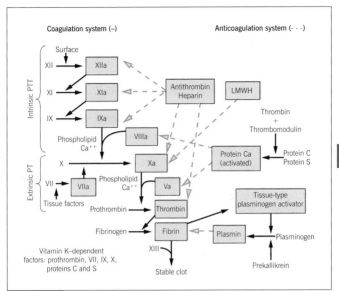

FIG. 13-2

Coagulation cascade. *(Modified from Rosenberg RD, Bauer KA. Hosp Pract 1986; 21(3):131).*

13

HEMATOLOGY

of ingestion of platelet inhibitors, such as NSAIDs, before a bleeding time test.

B. HYPERCOAGULABLE STATES

Hypercoagulable states present clinically as venous or arterial thrombosis.

1. **Congenital or genetic thrombotic risks:** Carefully assess family history for stroke, thrombosis, spontaneous abortion, and obstetric complications.

a. Natural anticoagulants: Decreased levels of protein C, protein S, antithrombin III, or activated protein C resistance (i.e., factor V Leiden).

   (1) Protein C or protein S deficiency: A hereditary, autosomal dominant disorder. In homozygous form, it presents as neonatal purpura fulminans. Heterozygotes have a threefold to sixfold increased risk of venous thrombosis.

   (2) Antithrombin III deficiency: Hereditary, autosomal dominant disorder. Homozygotes die in infancy; heterozygotes have increased risk of thrombosis.

   (3) Activated protein C resistance (factor V Leiden): 2% to 5% of Caucasians are heterozygotes (fivefold to tenfold risk of venous thrombosis); 1 in 1000 are homozygotes (an eightyfold to 100-fold venous thrombosis risk).

TABLE 13-5

AGE-SPECIFIC COAGULATION VALUES

Coagulation Tests	Preterm Infant 30-36 wk, Day of Life #1	Term Infant, Day of Life #1	1-5 yr	6-10 yr	11-16 yr	Adult
PT (sec)	15.4 (14.6-16.9)	13.0 (10.1-15.9)	11 (10.6-11.4)	11.1 (10.1-12.1)	11.2 (10.2-12.0)	12 (11.0-14.0)
INR	—	—	1.0 (0.96-1.04)	1.0 (0.91-1.11)	1.02 (0.93-1.10)	1.10 (1.0-1.3)
aPTT (sec)	108 (80-168)	42.9 (31.3-54.3)	30 (24-36)	31 (26-36)	32 (26-37)	33 (27-40)
Fibrinogen (g/L)	2.43 (1.50-3.73)	2.83 (1.67-3.09)	2.76 (1.70-4.05)	2.79 (1.57-4.0)	3.0 (1.54-4.48)	2.78 (1.56-4.0)
Bleeding time (min)	—	—	6 (2.5-10)	7 (2.5-13)	5 (3-8)	4 (1-7)
Thrombin time (sec)	14 (11-17)	12 (10-16)	—	—	—	10
II (U/mL)	0.45 (0.20-0.77)	0.48 (0.26-0.70)	0.94 (0.71-1.16)	0.88 (0.67-1.07)	0.83 (0.61-1.04)	1.08 (0.70-1.46)
V (U/mL)	0.88 (0.41-1.44)	0.72 (0.43-1.08)	1.03 (0.79-1.27)	0.90 (0.63-1.16)	0.77 (0.55-0.99)	1.06 (0.62-1.50)
VII (U/mL)	0.67 (0.21-1.13)	0.66 (0.28-1.04)	0.82 (0.55-1.16)	0.85 (0.52-1.20)	0.83 (0.58-1.15)	1.05 (0.67-1.43)
VIII (U/mL)	1.11 (0.50-2.13)	1.00 (0.50-1.78)	0.90 (0.59-1.42)	0.95 (0.58-1.32)	0.92 (0.53-1.31)	0.99 (0.50-1.49)
vWF (U/mL)	1.36 (0.78-2.10)	1.53 (0.50-2.87)	0.82 (0.47-1.04)	0.95 (0.44-1.44)	1.00 (0.46-1.53)	0.92 (0.50-1.58)
IX (U/mL)	0.35 (0.19-0.65)	0.53 (0.15-0.91)	0.73 (0.47-1.04)	0.75 (0.63-0.89)	0.87 (0.59-1.22)	1.09 (0.55-1.63)
X (U/mL)	0.41 (0.11-0.71)	0.40 (0.12-0.68)	0.88 (0.58-1.16)	0.75 (0.55-1.01)	0.79 (0.50-1.17)	1.06 (0.70-1.52)
XI (U/mL)	0.30 (0.08-0.52)	0.38 (0.10-0.66)	0.97 (0.56-1.50)	0.86 (0.52-1.20)	0.74 (0.50-0.97)	0.97 (0.67-1.27)
XII (U/mL)	0.38 (0.10-0.66)	0.53 (0.13-0.93)	0.93 (0.64-1.29)	0.92 (0.60-1.40)	0.81 (0.34-1.37)	1.08 (0.52-1.64)
PK (U/mL)	0.33 (0.09-0.57)	0.37 (0.18-0.69)	0.95 (0.65-1.30)	0.99 (0.66-1.31)	0.99 (0.53-1.45)	1.12 (0.62-1.62)

HMWK (U/mL)	0.49 (0.09-0.89)	0.54 (0.06-1.02)	0.98 (0.64-1.32)	0.93 (0.60-1.30)	0.91 (0.63-1.19)	0.92 (0.50-1.36)
XIIIa (U/mL)	0.70 (0.32-1.08)	0.79 (0.27-1.31)	1.08 (0.72-1.43)	1.09 (0.65-1.51)	0.99 (0.57-1.40)	1.05 (0.55-1.55)
XIIIs (U/mL)	0.81 (0.35-1.27)	0.76 (0.30-1.22)	1.13 (0.69-1.56)	1.16 (0.77-1.54)	1.02 (0.60-1.43)	0.97 (0.57-1.37)
D-Dimer	—	—	—	—	—	Positive titer ≥ 1:8
FDPs	—	—	—	—	—	Borderline titer = 1:25-1:50; Positive titer > 1:50
COAGULATION INHIBITORS						
ATIII (U/mL)	0.38 (0.14-0.62)	0.63 (0.39-0.97)	1.11 (0.82-1.39)	1.11 (0.90-1.31)	1.05 (0.77-1.32)	1.0 (0.74-1.26)
α_2-M (U/mL)	1.10 (0.56-1.82)	1.39 (0.95-1.83)	1.69 (1.14-2.23)	1.69 (1.28-2.09)	1.56 (0.98-2.12)	0.86 (0.52-1.20)
C_1-Inh (U/mL)	0.65 (0.31-0.99)	0.72 (0.36-1.08)	1.35 (0.85-1.83)	1.14 (0.88-1.54)	1.03 (0.68-1.50)	1.0 (0.71-1.31)
α_2-AT (U/mL)	0.90 (0.36-1.44)	0.93 (0.49-1.37)	0.93 (0.39-1.47)	1.00 (0.69-1.30)	1.01 (0.65-1.37)	0.93 (0.55-1.30)
Protein C (U/mL)	0.28 (0.12-0.44)	0.35 (0.17-0.53)	0.66 (0.40-0.92)	0.69 (0.45-0.93)	0.83 (0.55-1.11)	0.96 (0.64-1.28)
Protein S (U/mL)	0.26 (0.14-0.38)	0.36 (0.12-0.60)	0.86 (0.54-1.18)	0.78 (0.41-1.14)	0.72 (0.52-0.92)	0.81 (0.60-1.13)
FIBRINOLYTIC SYSTEM						
Plasminogen (U/mL)	1.70 (1.12-2.48)	1.95 (1.60-2.30)	0.98 (0.78-1.18)	0.92 (0.75-1.08)	0.86 (0.68-1.03)	0.99 (0.7-1.22)
TPA (ng/mL)	—	—	2.15 (1.0-4.5)	2.42 (1.0-5.0)	2.16 (1.0-4.0)	4.90 (1.40-8.40)
α_2-AP (U/mL)	0.78 (0.4-1.16)	0.85 (0.70-1.00)	1.05 (0.93-1.17)	0.99 (0.89-1.10)	0.98 (0.78-1.18)	1.02 (0.68-1.36)
PAI (U/mL)	—	—	5.42 (1.0-10.0)	6.79 (2.0-12.0)	6.07 (2.0-10.0)	3.60 (0-11.0)

Data from Andrew M et al: *Blood* 1987; 70:165-172; Andrew M et al. *Blood* 1988; 72:1651-1657; and Andrew M et al. *Blood* 1992; 8:1998-2005.
α_2-AP, α_2-Antiplasmin; α_2-AT, α_2-antitrypsin; α_2-M, α_2-macroglobulin; ATIII, antithrombin III; HMWK, high-molecular-weight kininogen; PAI, plasminogen activator inhibitor; PK, prekallikrein; TPA, tissue plasminogen activator; VIII, factor VIII procoagulant.

13

HEMATOLOGY

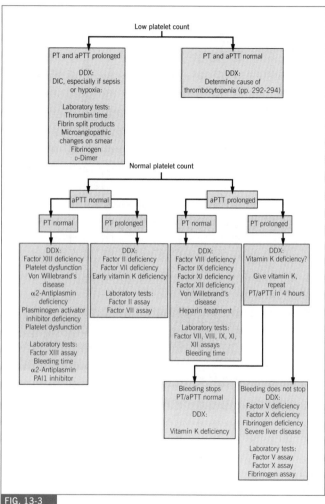

FIG. 13-3

Differential diagnosis of bleeding disorders.

b. Homocystinemia: Increased levels of homocystine associated with venous and arterial thromboses.

c. Others include prothrombin mutation (G20210A), plasminogen abnormalities, and dysfibrinogenemia.

2. **Acquired thrombotic risks**

a. Endothelial damage: Indwelling vascular catheter, hypertension, surgery, smoking, diabetes, hyperlipidemia, and oral contraceptives.

b. Hyperviscosity: Macroglobulinemia, sickle cell disease, and polycythemia.

c. Platelet activation: Essential thrombocytosis, oral contraceptives, and heparin-associated thrombocytopenia.

d. Antiphospholipid syndromes: Venous or arterial thrombosis and spontaneous abortions. Occurs commonly in patients with systemic lupus erythematosus (SLE) or malignancies, and may occur transiently after a viral infection or during pregnancy. Characterized by prolonged aPTT, antiphospholipid and/or anticardiolipin antibody detection, and prolonged dilute Russell's viper venom time (dRVVT). False positive RPR may occur.

e. Other: Includes procoagulant factors such as drugs (e.g., L-asparaginase), malignancies, liver disease, renal disease, nephrotic syndrome, infection, inflammatory disease, diabetes, paroxysmal nocturnal hemoglobinuria, lp(a), increased factor VIII, and increased factor XI.

3. **Laboratory evaluation**

a. Exclude common acquired causes as discussed previously. Initial laboratory screening includes PT, aPTT, circulating anticoagulants; dRVVT; factor V Leiden polymerase chain reaction (PCR) or activated protein C resistance assay; PCR for prothrombin 20210 mutation; activity assays for antithrombin III, protein C, and protein S; and total plasma homocysteine levels. Extended evaluation should include alpha-1-antiplasmin, methyltetrahydrofolate reductase deficiency, plasminogen, and PAI-1.

b. The identification of one risk factor, such as an indwelling vascular catheter, does not preclude the search for others, especially when accompanied by a family history of thrombosis.

4. **Treatment of thromboses**

a. Heparin therapy: For deep venous thrombus or pulmonary embolus.

  (1) Loading dose: 50 to 75 U/kg IV over 30 minutes to 1 hour, followed by maintenance continuous infusion of heparin at 28 U/kg/hr if patient is <1 year old, or 20 U/kg/hr if ≥1 year old.

  (2) Obtain aPTT level 6 hours after loading dose and adjust per Table 13-6. Goal is aPTT at 1.5 to 2.5 times baseline aPTT.

  (3) Heparin may be reversed with protamine (see Formulary for dosage information).

b. Low-molecular-weight heparin (LMWH)[4]: LMWH (or enoxaparin) may be useful in children, although it is less studied and more costly than heparin. LMWH has more specific anti-Xa activity, a longer half-life, and a more predictable dose:efficacy ratio.

13

HEMATOLOGY

TABLE 13-6		
ADJUSTMENT AND MONITORING OF HEPARIN THERAPY		
aPTT Control Ratio	Rebolus/Dose Interruption	Heparin Infusion Adjustment
<1.2 ×	Repeat original load	Increase by 5 U/kg/hr
1.2-1.4 ×	Repeat half original load	Increase by 3 U/kg/hr
1.5-2.5 ×	None	No change
2.6-3.2 ×	None	Decrease by 3 U/kg/hr
3.3-4.0 ×*	Stop infusion, recheck aPTT in 1 hr Restart infusion when aPTT is in or is projected to be in therapeutic range	Decrease by 5 U/kg/hr
4.0-5.0 ×*	Stop infusion, recheck aPTT in 2 hr Restart infusion when aPTT is in or is projected to be in therapeutic range	Decrease by 7 U/kg/hr
>5.0 ×*	Stop infusion; call hematologist on call immediately	

From The Johns Hopkins Hospital laboratory guidelines, 10/98.

NOTE: Draw aPTT 6 hr after bolus dose, and repeat 6-8 hr after every dose adjustment. Repeat daily during stable dosing period. Check platelet count every third day until heparin is discontinued.

*Make sure sample not drawn from heparinized line.

    (1) Dose depends on preparation. See Formulary for enoxaparin dosage information.

    (2) Monitor LMWH therapy by following anti-Xa activity. Therapeutic range is 0.5 to 1.0 U/mL for full anticoagulation and 0.2 to 0.4 U/mL for prophylactic dosing.

 c. Warfarin may be used for long-term anticoagulation, although it carries significant risk for morbidity and mortality. Patient must receive heparin while initiating warfarin therapy secondary to hypercoagulability from decreased protein C and S levels.

    (1) Warfarin is usually administered orally at a loading dose for 2 to 3 days, followed by a daily dose sufficient to maintain the PT INR (international normalized ratio) in the desired range, usually two to three times baseline. See Formulary for warfarin dosing. Infants often require higher daily doses of warfarin. In all patients, levels should be measured every 1 to 2 weeks (Table 13-7).

    (2) Warfarin efficacy is greatly affected by dietary intake of vitamin K.

    (3) Warfarin is protein bound, and many drugs alter the therapeutic level. Concomitant medicines should be carefully reviewed.

    (4) Warfarin effect can be reversed with the administration of vitamin K or fresh frozen plasma (FFP). Vitamin K dosing for elevated INR is still controversial. Actual dosage recommendations are only present in the adult literature.

      (a) INR above desired range and <5: Hold the next warfarin dose and readjust subsequent dosages.

      (b) INR 5-9: Evaluate for risk of bleeding. If low risk, hold the next one to two doses. If high risk, consider also giving a low dose of vitamin K orally (1 to 2.5 mg for adults).

TABLE 13-7

ADJUSTMENT AND MONITORING OF WARFARIN TO MAINTAIN AN INR BETWEEN 2 AND 3*

I. Day 1:	If the baseline INR is 1.0-1.3:
	Dose = 0.2 mg/kg orally

II. Loading Days 2 to 4: If the INR is:

INR	Action
1.1-1.3	Repeat initial loading dose
1.4-1.9	50% of initial loading dose
2.0-3.0	50% of initial loading dose
3.1-3.5	25% of initial loading dose
>3.5	Hold until INR <3.5, then restart at 50% less than previous dose

III. Maintenance Oral Anticoagulation Dose Guidelines

INR	Action
1.1-1.4	Increase by 20% of dose
1.5-1.9	Increase by 10% of dose
2.0-3.0	No change
3.1-3.5	Decrease by 10% of dose
>3.5	Hold until INR <3.5, then restart at 20% less than the previous dose

*Onset of action of warfarin is 36-72 hours, peak effects in 5-7 days. Because of this long half-life, avoid making dose adjustments with excessive frequency.

   (c) INR >9: Vitamin K is generally recommended. If there is low
       risk for bleeding, give vitamin K orally (3 to 5 mg for adults).
       If there is high risk for bleeding, give vitamin K orally or IV
       and FFP.
   (d) INR ≥20, or life-threatening bleeding: Give vitamin K IV (10 mg
       for adults) and FFP. Repeat every 12 hours as needed.[5]
 d. Consult a hematologist for thrombolytic therapy.
NOTE: Children receiving anticoagulation therapy should be protected from
trauma. Intramuscular injections are contraindicated. The use of
antiplatelet agents and arterial punctures should be avoided.

C. BLEEDING DISORDERS (see Fig. 13-3)
1. **Disorders of platelet number or function.**
2. **Inherited abnormalities of coagulation factors**
 a. Factor VIII deficiency (hemophilia A; X-linked disorder): prolonged aPTT,
    reduced factor VIII activity. PT and BT are normal. Treat with factor VIII
    concentrate. Recombinant factor VIII is preferred to reduce risk of
    infection. The factor level is usually raised by 2% per 1 unit of factor
    VIII/kg (see Table 13-8 for desired level). Factor may need to be redosed
    based on the clinical scenario. The first dose has a shorter half-life, and
    a second dose, if needed, is given after 4 to 8 hours. Thereafter, the
    half-life is approximately 8 to 12 hours, and subsequent doses are
    usually dosed every 12 hours. Continuous infusion is often required for
    surgical patients, usually with a 50-U/kg loading dose, followed by 3 to
    4 U/kg/hr.

Units of factor VIII = Weight (kg) × Desired % replacement × 0.5

b. Factor IX deficiency (hemophilia B, Christmas disease; X-linked): Laboratory studies include a prolonged aPTT and low factor IX activity. Treat with factor IX concentrate. The factor level is usually raised by 1% for each unit of factor IX concentrate/kg; it has a half-life of 18 to 24 hours. As with factor VIII, a second dose, if needed, should be given at a shorter interval. Recombinant factor IX has a shorter half-life; consider evaluation of in vivo factor survival in each patient.

c. Von Willebrand's disease: The vWF binds platelets to subendothelial surfaces and carries factor VIII. Typical vWD type I is characterized by a prolonged BT and normal platelet count. The aPTT is mildly or moderately prolonged, and there is decreased ristocetin cofactor activity. Factor VIII and vWF levels are decreased in type 1 disease, but may be normal in variants with dysfunctional vWF.

(1) In patients with a proven response to desmopressin acetate (DDAVP), bleeding or minor surgical procedures may be treated with DDAVP, intravenously over 20 to 30 minutes, or intra-nasally (see Formulary for dosage information).
Note: **DDAVP may be contraindicated in vWD type IIb because it may exacerbate thrombocytopenia.**

(2) For more severe disease or patients with dysfunctional vWF, the treatment of choice is Humate P (heat-inactivated vWF-enriched concentrate: 40 mcg/kg), a similar product containing active vWF, or cryoprecipitate; note the associated infectious risks of these pooled blood products. Concentrates are preferred because they are virally inactivated.

(3) Aminocaproic acid, 100 mg/kg IV or by mouth (PO) every 4 to 6 hours (up to 24 g/day); may be useful for treatment of oral bleeding and as prophylaxis for dental extractions.

3. **Acquired coagulation factor abnormalities**

a. DIC: Characterized by a prolonged PT and aPTT, decreased fibrinogen and platelets, increased fibrin degradation products, and D-dimers. Treatment includes identifying and treating the underlying disorder. Replacement of depleted coagulation factors with FFP may be necessary in severe cases, specifically in cases of symptomatic bleeding; 10 to 15 mL/kg will raise the clotting factors by about 20%. Fibrinogen, if depleted, can be given as cryoprecipitate. Platelet transfusions may also be necessary.

TABLE 13-8

DESIRED FACTOR REPLACEMENT IN HEMOPHILIA

Bleeding Site	Desired Level (%)
Joint or simple hematoma	20-40
Simple dental extraction	50
Major soft tissue bleed	80-100
Serious oral bleeding	80-100
Head injury	100+
Major surgery (dental, orthopedic, other)	100+

b. Liver disease: The liver is the major site of synthesis for factors V, VII, IX, X, XI, XII, XIII, prothrombin, plasminogen, fibrinogen, proteins C and S, and ATIII. Treatment with FFP and platelets may be needed, but this will increase hepatic protein load. Vitamin K should be given to patients with liver disease and clotting abnormalities (see Formulary for dosage information).

c. Vitamin K deficiency: Factors II, VII, IX, X, protein C, and protein S are vitamin K dependent. Early vitamin K deficiency may present with isolated prolonged PT because factor VII has the shortest half-life.

d. Hemolytic-uremic syndrome/thrombotic thrombocytopenic purpura (HUS/TTP): Characterized by the triad of microangiopathic hemolytic anemia, uremia, and thrombocytopenia, HUS/TTP is often triggered by bacterial enteritis, especially caused by *Escherichia coli* O157:H7, although there are a variety of causes. HUS does not typically include coagulation abnormalities, such as those seen in DIC. TTP includes the triad of HUS in addition to fever and CNS changes, and is more common in older adolescents and adults.

VII. BLOOD COMPONENT REPLACEMENT

A. BLOOD VOLUME

Blood volume requirements are age-specific (Table 13-9).

B. BLOOD PRODUCT COMPONENTS

1. **RBCs:** The decision to transfuse RBCs should be made with consideration of clinical symptoms and signs, the degree of cardiorespiratory or CNS disease, the cause and course of anemia, and options for alternative therapy, noting the risks of transfusion-associated infections and reactions.

a. Packed RBC (PRBC) transfusion: Concentrated RBCs, with HCT of 55% to 70%. A typed and cross-matched blood product is preferred when possible; O-negative (or O-positive) blood may be used if transfusion cannot be delayed. O-negative is preferred for females of child-bearing age to reduce risks of Rh sensitization.

b. Unless rapid replacement is required for acute blood loss or shock, infuse no faster than 2 to 3 mL/kg/hr (generally 10 mL/kg aliquots over 4 hours) to avoid congestive heart failure. A rule of thumb in severe compensated anemia is to give an 'X' mL/kg aliquot, where

TABLE 13-9
APPROXIMATE BLOOD VOLUME

Age	Total Blood Volume (mL/kg)	Age	Total Blood Volume (mL/kg)
Preterm infants	90-105	4-6 yr	80-86
Term newborns	78-86	7-18 yr	83-90
1-12 mo	73-78	Adults	68-88
1-3 yr	74-82		

From Nathan D, Oski FA. Hematology of infancy and childhood. Philadelphia: WB Saunders; 1998.

13

HEMATOLOGY

X = hemoglobin (mg/dL); that is, if Hb = 5, transfuse 5 mL/kg over 4 hours.

$$\text{Volume of PRBCs (mL)} = \text{EBV (mL)} \times \frac{\text{Desired HCT} - \text{Actual HCT}}{\text{HCT of PRBCs}}$$

where EBV is the estimated blood volume and HCT of pRBCs is usually 55% to 70%.

  c. Leukocyte-poor PRBCs
    (1) Filtered RBCs: 99.9% of WBCs removed from product; used for CMV-negative patients to reduce risk of CMV transmission. Also reduces likelihood of a nonhemolytic febrile transfusion reaction.
    (2) Washed RBCs: 92% to 95% of white cells removed from product. Similar advantages to leukocyte-poor filtered RBCs. Although filtered leukocyte-poor blood is now more commonly used, washing may be helpful if a patient has preexisting antibodies to blood products (e.g., patients who have complete IgA deficiency or a history of urticarial transfusion reactions).
  d. Irradiated blood products
    (1) Many blood products (PRBCs, platelet preparations, leukocytes, FFP, and others) contain viable lymphocytes capable of proliferation and engraftment in the recipient, causing graft-versus-host disease (GVHD). Irradiation with 1500 cGy before transfusion may prevent GVHD, but does not prevent antibody formation against donor white cells. Engraftment is most likely in young infants, immunocompromised patients, or patients receiving blood from first-degree relatives.
    (2) Indications: Intensive chemotherapy, leukemia, lymphoma, bone marrow transplantation, solid organ transplantation, known or suspected immune deficiencies, intrauterine transfusions, and transfusions in neonates.
  e. CMV-negative blood: Obtained from donors who test negative for CMV. May be given to neonates or other immunocompromised patients, including those awaiting organ or marrow transplant who are CMV-negative.
2. **Platelets:** Indicated to treat severe or symptomatic thrombocytopenia.
  a. Single-donor product: Preferred over pooled concentrate for patients with antiplatelet antibodies.
  b. Leukocyte-poor: Use if there is a history of significant acute, febrile platelet transfusion reactions.
  c. Usually give 4 U/m^2, or approximately 10 mL/kg of normally concentrated platelet product. The platelet count is raised by 10,000 to 15,000/mm^3 by giving 1 U/m^2. For infants and children, 10 mL/kg will increase the platelet count by approximately 50,000/mm^3. Hemorrhagic complications are rare with platelet counts >20,000/mm^3. A platelet count >50,000/mm^3 is advisable for minor procedures such as lumbar puncture; >100,000/mm^3 is advisable for major surgery or intracranial

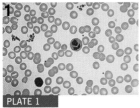

PLATE 1

Normal smear. Round RBCs with central pallor about one third of the cell's diameter, scattered platelets, occasional white blood cells.

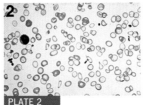

PLATE 2

Iron deficiency. Hypochromic/microcytic RBCs, poikilocytosis, plentiful platelets, occasional ovalocytes, and target cells. Basophilic stippling may also be present, as in lead intoxication and β-thalassemia.

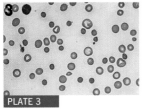

PLATE 3

Spherocytosis. Microspherocytes a hallmark (densely stained RBCs with no central pallor).

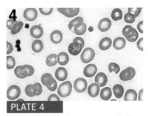

PLATE 4

Basophilic stippling as a result of staining of ribosomal complexes containing RNA throughout the cell; seen with heavy metal intoxication, thalassemia, pyrimidine 5'-nucleotidase deficiency, iron deficiency, and other states associated with ineffective erythropoiesis.

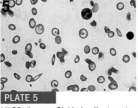

PLATE 5

HbSS disease. Sickled cells, target cells, hypochromia, poikilocytosis, Howell-Jolly bodies, nucleated RBCs common (not shown).

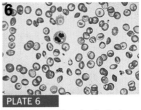

PLATE 6

HbSC disease. Target cells, "oat cells," poikilocytosis; sickle forms rarely seen.

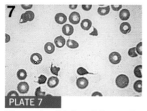

PLATE 7

Microangiopathic hemolytic anemia. RBC fragments, anisocytosis, polychromasia, decreased platelets.

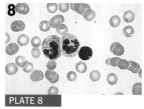

PLATE 8

Toxic granulations. Prominent dark blue primary granules; commonly seen with infection and other toxic states, such as Kawasaki's disease.

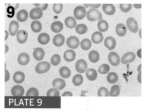

PLATE 9

Howell-Jolly body. Small, dense nuclear remnant in an RBC; suggests splenic dysfunction or asplenia.

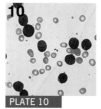

PLATE 10

Leukemic blasts showing large nucleus:cytoplasm ratio.

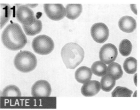

PLATE 11

Polychromatophilia. Diffusely basophilic because of RNA staining; seen with early release of reticulocytes from the marrow.

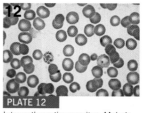

PLATE 12

Intraerythrocytic parasites. Malaria.

operation. Peak posttransfusion concentration is reached 45 to 60 minutes after transfusion. Platelet products should not be refrigerated because this promotes premature platelet activation and clumping.

3. **FFP:** Contains all clotting factors except platelets. Used in severe clotting factor deficiencies with active bleeding or to reverse the effects of warfarin. Also may replace anticoagulant factors (antithrombin III, protein C, protein S). Used in treatment of DIC, vitamin K deficiency with active bleeding, or TTP. The usual amount is 10 to 15 mL/kg; repeat doses as needed. In TTP plasma exchange is often preferred.

4. **Cryoprecipitate:** Enriched for factor VIII (5 to 10 U/mL), vWF, and fibrinogen. Useful for children with factor VIII, fibrinogen, or vWF deficiency in the context of active bleeding. Concentrates are preferred because of viral inactivation.

5. **Monoclonal factor VIII:** Highly purified factor, derived from pooled human blood.

6. **Recombinant factor VIII or IX:** Highly purified, with less infectious risk than pooled human products. There is a risk of inhibitor formation, as with other products.

C. PARTIAL PRBC EXCHANGE TRANSFUSION

A partial PRBC exchange transfusion may be indicated for sickle cell patients with acute chest syndrome, stroke, intractable pain crisis, or refractory priapism. Replace with Sickledex-negative cells. Goal is to reduce percent HbSS to <40%. Follow HCT carefully during transfusion to avoid hyperviscosity, maintaining HCT <35%. To calculate the volume of PRBC needed for a double PRBC volume exchange, use the following equation:

$$\frac{\text{EBV (mL)} \times \text{Patient HCT} \times 2}{\text{HCT of PRBC (55\% to 70\%)}}$$

where EBV is the estimated blood volume in milliliters and is age-dependent (see Table 13-9).

D. COMPLICATIONS OF TRANSFUSIONS

1. Acute transfusion reactions

a. Acute hemolytic reaction: Most often the result of blood group incompatibility. Signs and symptoms include fever, chills, tachycardia, hypotension, and shock. Treatment includes immediate cessation of blood transfusion and institution of supportive measures. Laboratory findings include DIC, hemoglobinuria, and positive Coombs' test.

b. Febrile nonhemolytic reaction: Usually the result of host antibody response to donor leukocyte antigens, common in previously transfused patients. Symptoms include fever, chills, and diaphoresis. Stop transfusion and evaluate as described below. Prevention includes premedication with antipyretics, antihistamines, and corticosteroids; and, if necessary, use of leukocyte-poor PRBCs (see p. 304).

c. Urticarial reaction: Reaction to donor plasma proteins. Stop transfusion immediately; treat with antihistamines, and epinephrine and steroids

if there is respiratory compromise (see also treatment of anaphylaxis, pp. 8-9). Use washed or filtered RBCs with the next transfusion.
  d. Evaluation of acute transfusion reaction
    (1) Patient's urine: Test for hemoglobin.
    (2) Patient's blood: Confirm blood type, screen for antibodies, and repeat DCT on pretransfusion and posttransfusion sera.
    (3) Donor blood: Culture for bacteria.
2. **Delayed transfusion reaction:** Minor blood group antigen incompatibility. Occurs 3 to 10 days after transfusion. Symptoms include fatigue, jaundice, and dark urine. Laboratory findings include anemia, a positive Coombs' test, new RBC antibodies, and hemoglobinuria.
3. **Transmission of infectious diseases:** There is a low incidence of transmission of infectious disease at present because of vigilance in blood product screening.[6] Data from 1955 to 1999 estimate the risk of transmitting infection as follows: HIV, 1 in 676,000; human T-cell leukemia/lymphoma virus, 1 in 641,000; hepatitis B, 1 in 63,000; hepatitis C, 1 in 127,000; parvovirus, 1 in 10,000. CMV may also be transmitted by blood products.
4. **Sepsis:** Sepsis occurs with products that are contaminated with bacteria, particularly platelets, as they are stored at room temperature.

VIII. INTERPRETATION OF BLOOD SMEAR

See Plates 1 to 12 on insert following p. 304. Examine the smear in an area where the RBCs are nearly touching but do not overlap.
1. **RBCs:** Examine RBC size, shape, and color.
2. **WBCs:** A rough estimation of the WBC count can be made by looking at the smear under high power (100× magnification with a 10× objective and 10× lens). Every one white cell per high-powered field correlates with approximately 500/mm^3.
3. **Platelets:** A rough approximation is one platelet/oil immersion field corresponds to 10,000 to 15,000/mm^3. Platelet clumps usually indicate >100,000 platelets/mm^3.

REFERENCES

1. Shafer F. Mid-Atlantic sickle-cell disease consortium. In Press.
2. Bernini JC et al. Beneficial effect of intravenous dexamethasone in children with mild to moderately severe acute chest syndrome complicating sickle cell disease. Blood 1998; 92(9): 3082-3089.
3. Rosenberg RD, Bauer KA. New insights into hypercoagulable states. Hosp Pract 1986; 21(3):131.
4. Massicotte P et al. Low-molecular-weight heparin in pediatric patients with thrombotic disease: a dose finding study. J Pediatr 1996; 128:313-318.
5. Hirsh J et al. Fifth ACCP Consensus Conference on antithrombotic therapy. Chest 1998; 114(5): 439S-769S.
6. American Academy of Pediatrics. 2000 Red book: report of the committee on infectious diseases, 25th ed. Elk Grove Village, Ill: American Academy of Pediatrics; 2000.

IMMUNOLOGY

Michelle Hudspeth, MD and Heather Symons, MD

Michelle Hudspeth, MD and Heather Symons, MD

I. WEBSITES
www.primaryimmune.org.

II. INDICATIONS FOR PRIMARY IMMUNODEFICIENCY EVALUATION
See Table 14-1.

III. EVALUATION OF A SUSPECTED IMMUNODEFICIENCY
See Table 14-2.

14

IV. IMMUNE GLOBULIN (INTRAVENOUS AND INTRAMUSCULAR)[1,2]

A. GENERAL INFORMATION
1. Separated from pooled human plasma by alcohol fractionation. Intravenous immune globulin (IVIG) then modified for IV administration.
2. Protein content is ≥95% IgG but contains trace amounts of IgA and IgM.
3. Standard dosing provides immediate antibody levels with a half-life of 3 to 4 weeks.

B. INTRAVENOUS IMMUNE GLOBULIN (IVIG)
1. **Availability:** As 5% to 12% solutions (50 to 120 mg/mL).
2. Indications
a. Antibody deficiency disorders (replacement therapy).
   (1) Dosage: 400 to 600 mg/kg IV per month.
   (2) Determine optimal frequency and dose of IVIG by monitoring clinical

---

TABLE 14-1

INDICATIONS FOR PRIMARY IMMUNODEFICIENCY EVALUATION

	Indications
Family history	Positive for early unexplained death, sepsis, recurrent infections, or specific immunodeficiency diagnoses
Frequency of infection	Elevated frequency of documented infections including pneumonia, sepsis, osteomyelitis, meningitis
Chronicity of infection	Persistent sinusitis and otitis media, bronchiectasis, recurrent abscesses
Severity of infection	Sepsis or meningitis, especially if recurrent or severe
Complication of infection	Present (e.g., mastoiditis complicating otitis media)
Site of infection	Unusual sites (e.g., liver or brain abscess)
Infecting organism	Opportunistic, recurrent, or unusual pathogens (e.g., *Aspergillus, Serratia, Nocardia, Burkholderia cepacia*)
Response to therapy	Poor response or recurring infection after antimicrobial discontinuation
Other signs	Failure to thrive, dermatitis, recurrent diarrhea, history of autoimmune disease

Modified from Zitelli BJ, Davis HW. Atlas of pediatric physical diagnosis. Philadelphia: Mosby; 1997.

TABLE 14-2

EVALUATION OF A SUSPECTED IMMUNODEFICIENCY

Suspected Abnormality	Clinical Findings	Initial Tests	More Advanced Tests
Antibody (e.g., X-linked agamma-globulinemia, IgA deficiency)	Sinopulmonary and systemic infections (pyogenic bacteria)	Immunoglobulin levels (IgG, IgM, IgA)	B-cell enumeration
	Enteric infections (enterovirus, other viruses, Giardia sp.)	Antibody titers to protein antigens (diphtheria, tetanus)	Immunofixation
	Autoimmune disease (ITP, hemolytic anemia, IBD)	Antibody titers to polysaccharide antigens (≥2-yr-old child) before and after immunization (pneumococcal polysaccharide vaccine)	IgG subclass levels
Cell-mediated immunity (e.g., DiGeorge syndrome)	Pneumonia (pyogenic bacteria, fungi, Pneumocystis carinii, viruses)	Total lymphocyte counts	T-cell enumeration and subsets (CD3, CD4, CD8)
	Gastroenteritis (viruses, Giardia sp. Cryptosporidium sp.)	HIV ELISA/Western blot	In vitro T-cell proliferation to mitogens, antigens, or allogeneic cells
	Dermatitis/mucositis (fungi)	Delayed-type hypersensitivity skin test (Candida sp., tetanus toxoid, mumps, Trichophyton sp.)	Chest radiograph for thymic hypoplasia
			FISH 22 for DiGeorge syndrome
Antibody and cell-mediated immunity (e.g., severe combined	See above	See above	See above
			ADA assay

Defect	Clinical Presentation	Diagnostic Tests
immunodeficiency, ataxia telangiectasia, Wiskott-Aldrich syndrome, common variable immunodeficiency, hyper-IgM syndrome)		Alpha-fetoprotein Platelet count/size
Phagocytosis (chronic granulomatous disease, leukocyte adhesion deficiency, Chediak-Higashi syndrome)	Cutaneous infections, abscesses, lymphadenitis (staphylococci, enteric bacteria, fungi, mycobacteria), poor wound healing	WBC/neutrophil count and morphology Nitroblue tetrazolium (NBT) test Chemotactic assay Phagocytic and bacterial assay
Spleen	Bacteremia/hematogenous infection (pneumococcus, other streptococci, Neisseria sp.)	Peripheral blood smear for Howell-Jolly bodies Hemoglobin electrophoresis (HbSS) Technetium-99 spleen scan
Complement	Bacterial sepsis, autoimmune disease (lupus, glomerulonephritis), angioedema, pyogenic infection, encapsulated bacterial infections (i.e., Neisseria sp.)	CH50 (total hemolytic complement) Alternative pathway assays Individual component assays

From Rosen FS, Cooper MD, Wedgewood R. N Engl J Med 1995; 333(7):431-440 and Shyur SD, Hill HR. J Pediatr 1996; 129(1):8-24.
ADA, Adenosine deaminase; *ELISA,* enzyme-linked immunosorbent assay; *FISH,* fluorescent in situ hybridization; *HIV,* human immunodeficiency virus; *IBD,* inflammatory bowel disease; *ITP,* idiopathic thrombocytopenic purpura; *WBC,* white blood cell.

14

IMMUNOLOGY

response and IgG trough levels. IgG trough levels ideally are >500 mg/dL over the initial pretreatment level.

b. Idiopathic thrombocytopenic purpura (ITP)

   (1) Initial therapy for acute ITP: 0.8 to 1 g/kg IV in one or two doses.

   (2) See p. 292.

c. Kawasaki disease

   (1) Dose: 2 g/kg IV as a single dose over 10 to 12 hours, or 400 mg/kg daily on four consecutive days. Should be started within first 10 days of illness.

   (2) Treatment should include aspirin. See pp. 166-168.

d. Pediatric human immunodeficiency virus (HIV) infection.

   (1) Dose: 400 mg/kg every 28 days.

   (2) May be indicated in HIV-positive children with humoral immunodeficiency, including patients with the following:

      (a) Hypogammaglobulinemia.

      (b) Recurrent serious bacterial infections.

      (c) Failure to form antibodies to common antigens.

      (d) High risk for measles, defined as absence of detectable antibody after two doses of vaccine and living in high-prevalence area.

      (e) HIV-associated thrombocytopenia (dose: 500 to 1000 mg/kg/day for 3 to 5 days).

      (f) Chronic bronchiectasis (dose: 600 mg/kg per month).

e. Bone marrow transplantation: May reduce incidence of infection and death; does not decrease incidence of graft-versus-host disease (GVHD).

f. Parvovirus B19 infection: Treatment of chronic parvovirus B19 infection in an immunodeficient patient appears to be effective and should be considered.

C. INTRAMUSCULAR IMMUNE GLOBULIN (IMIG)

1. **Availability:** As 15% to 18% solution.

2. **Indications**

a. Hepatitis A prophylaxis (see p. 326).

b. Measles prophylaxis (see p. 334).

3. **Precautions:** IMIG preparations should never be given intravenously because they contain IgG aggregates, which may cause anaphylactoid reactions.

D. SPECIFIC IMMUNE GLOBULINS

1. **Hyperimmune globulins:** Prepared from donors known to have high antibody titers to antigens from specific sources. *Examples:* Those used in infectious diseases include hepatitis B (HBIG), rabies (RIG), tetanus (TIG), varicella-zoster (VZIG), cytomegalovirus (CMV-IVIG), respiratory syncytial virus immune globulin (RSV-IVIG), and RhO (D) immune globulin (RhO[D]IVIG).

2. **Monoclonal antibody preparations** include palivizumab (Synagis), which is a humanized monoclonal antibody against RSV (see Formulary for dosage information).

E. ADVERSE REACTIONS

1. **IVIG and IMIG (systemic symptoms occur in 1% to 15% of patients):** High fever, hemodynamic changes (hypertension, hypotension, tachycardia), hypersensitivity reactions (urticaria, bronchospasm, anaphylaxis).

2. **IVIG**

a. May cause less serious systemic reactions (headache, myalgia, fever, chills, nausea, and vomiting), often related to infusion rate. Decreasing the rate of infusion can alleviate symptoms. Prophylaxis with antihistamines, antipyretics, and/or IV hydrocortisone can prevent or reduce symptoms.

b. Aseptic meningitis.

c. Acute renal failure.

3. **IMIG:** May cause local discomfort, bleeding, or acrodynia with repeated use.

4. **Immune globulin and all other blood products containing IgA:** Relatively contraindicated in patients with complete IgA deficiency because they may rarely develop anti-IgA antibodies, which can cause anaphylaxis. Because systemic reactions are very rare, routine screening for IgA deficiency is not recommended. Specific brands of IVIG with very low levels of IgA are available.

14

IMMUNOLOGY

V. IMMUNOLOGIC REFERENCE VALUES

A. **SERUM IgG, IgM, IgA, AND IgE LEVELS** (Table 14-3)

B. **LYMPHOCYTE ENUMERATION** (Table 14-4)

C. **SERUM IgG SUBCLASS LEVELS** (Table 14-5)

D. **SERUM COMPLEMENT LEVELS** (Table 14-6)

TABLE 14-3

SERUM IgG, IgM, IgA, AND IgE LEVELS*

Age	IgG (mg/dL)	IgM (mg/dL)	IgA (mg/dL)	IgE (IU/ml)
Cord blood (term)	1121 (636-1606)	13 (6.3-25)	2.3 (1.4-3.6)	0.22 (0.04-1.28)
1 mo	503 (251-906)	45 (20-87)	13 (1.3-53)	
6 wk				0.69 (0.08-6.12)
2 mo	365 (206-601)	46 (17-105)	15 (2.8-47)	
3 mo	334 (176-581)	49 (24-89)	17 (4.6-46)	0.82 (0.18-3.76)
4 mo	343 (196-558)	55 (27-101)	23 (4.4-73)	
5 mo	403 (172-814)	62 (33-108)	31 (8.1-84)	
6 mo	407 (215-704)	62 (35-102)	25 (8.1-68)	2.68 (0.44-16.3)
7-9 mo	475 (217-904)	80 (34-126)	36 (11-90)	2.36 (0.76-7.31)
10-12 mo	594 (294-1069)	82 (41-149)	40 (16-84)	
1 yr	679 (345-1213)	93 (43-173)	44 (14-106)	3.49 (0.80-15.2)
2 yr	685 (424-1051)	95 (48-168)	47 (14-123)	3.03 (0.31-29.5)
3 yr	728 (441-1135)	104 (47-200)	66 (22-159)	1.80 (0.19-16.9)
4-5 yr	780 (463-1236)	99 (43-196)	68 (25-154)	8.58 (1.07-68.9)[†]
6-8 yr	915 (633-1280)	107 (48-207)	90 (33-202)	12.89 (1.03-161.3)[‡]
9-10 yr	1007 (608-1572)	121 (52-242)	113 (45-236)	23.6 (0.98-570.6)[§]
14 yr				20.07 (2.06-195.2)
Adult	994 (639-1349)	156 (56-352)	171 (70-312)	13.2 (1.53-114)

From Kjellman NM, Johansson SG, Roth A. Clin Allergy 1976; 6:51-59; Jolliff CR et al. Clin Chem 1982; 28:126-128; and Zetterström O, Johansson SG. Allergy 1981; 36(8):537-547.

*Numbers in parentheses are the 95% confidence intervals (CIs).

[†]IgE data for 4 yr.

[‡]IgE data for 7 yr.

[§]IgE data for 10 yr.

TABLE 14-4

NUMBERS OF T CELLS AND B CELLS*

Age	CD3 (total T cells) (%)[†]	CD4 (T-helper) (%)[†]	CD8 (T-suppressor/cytotoxic) (%)[†]	CD4/CD8 Ratio[†]	CD19 (B cells) (%)[‡]
Neonatal	0.6-5.0 (28-76)	0.4-3.5 (17-52)	0.2-1.9 (10-41)	1.0-2.6	0.04-1.1 (5-22)
1 wk-2 mo	2.3-7.0 (60-85)	1.7-5.3 (41-68)	0.4-1.7 (9-23)	1.3-6.3	0.6-1.9 (4-26)
2-5 mo	2.3-6.5 (48-75)	1.5-5.0 (33-58)	0.5-1.6 (11-25)	1.7-3.9	0.6-3.0 (14-39)
5-9 mo	2.4-6.9 (50-77)	1.4-5.1 (33-58)	0.6-2.2 (13-26)	1.6-3.8	0.7-2.5 (13-35)
9-15 mo	1.6-6.7 (54-76)	1.0-4.6 (31-54)	0.4-2.1 (12-28)	1.3-3.9	0.6-2.7 (15-39)
15-24 mo	1.4-8.0 (39-73)	0.9-5.5 (25-50)	0.4-2.3 (11-32)	0.9-3.7	0.6-3.1 (17-41)
2-5 yr	0.9-4.5 (43-76)	0.5-2.4 (23-48)	0.3-1.6 (14-33)	0.9-2.9	0.2-2.1 (14-44)
5-10 yr	0.7-4.2 (55-78)	0.3-2.0 (27-53)	0.3-1.8 (19-34)	0.9-2.6	0.2-1.6 (10-31)
10-16 yr	0.8-3.5 (52-78)	0.4-2.1 (25-48)	0.2-1.2 (9-35)	0.9-3.4	0.2-0.6 (8-24)
Adult	0.7-2.1 (55-83)	0.3-1.4 (28-57)	0.2-0.9 (10-39)	1.0-3.6	0.1-0.5 (6-19)

From Comans-Bitter WM et al. J Pediatr 1996; 130(3):388-393.

*Absolute counts (× 10⁹/L).

[†]Normal values (5th to 95th percentile).

[†]Normal values (5th to 95th percentile).

[‡]Normal values (25th to 75th percentile). Values in parentheses 5th to 95th percentile for adult data.

14

IMMUNOLOGY

TABLE 14-5

SERUM IgG SUBCLASS LEVELS*

Age (yr)	IgG1 (mg/dL)	IgG2 (mg/dL)	IgG3 (mg/dL)	IgG4 (mg/dL)[†]
0-1	340 (190-620)	59 (30-140)	39 (9-62)	19 (6-63)
1-2	410 (230-710)	68 (30-170)	34 (11-98)	13 (4-43)
2-3	480 (280-830)	98 (40-240)	28 (6-130)	18 (3-120)
3-4	530 (350-790)	120 (50-260)	30 (9-98)	32 (5-180)
4-6	540 (360-810)	140 (60-310)	39 (9-160)	39 (9-160)
6-8	560 (280-1120)	150 (30-630)	48 (40-250)	81 (11-620)
8-10	690 (280-1740)	210 (80-550)	85 (22-320)	42 (10-170)
10-13	590 (270-1290)	240 (110-550)	58 (13-250)	60 (7-530)
13-adult	540 (280-1020)	210 (60-790)	58 (14-240)	60 (11-330)

From Schur PH. Ann Allergy 1987; 58:89-96, 99.
*Numbers in parentheses are the 95% CIs.
†10% of individuals appear to have absent IgG4 levels.

TABLE 14-6

SERUM COMPLEMENT LEVELS*

Age	C3 (mg/dL)	C4 (mg/dL)
Cord blood (term)	83 (57-116)	13 (6.6-23)
1 mo	83 (53-124)	14 (7.0-25)
2 mo	96 (59-149)	15 (7.4-28)
3 mo	94 (64-131)	16 (8.7-27)
4 mo	107 (62-175)	19 (8.3-38)
5 mo	107 (64-167)	18 (7.1-36)
6 mo	115 (74-171)	21 (8.6-42)
7-9 mo	113 (75-166)	20 (9.5-37)
10-12 mo	126 (73-180)	22 (12-39)
1 yr	129 (84-174)	23 (12-40)
2 yr	120 (81-170)	19 (9.2-34)
3 yr	117 (77-171)	20 (9.7-36)
4-5 yr	121 (86-166)	21 (13-32)
6-8 yr	118 (88-155)	20 (12-32)
9-10 yr	134 (89-195)	22 (10-40)
Adult	125 (83-177)	28 (15-45)

Modified from Jolliff CR et al. Clin Chem 1982; 28:126-128.
*Numbers in parentheses are the 95% confidence intervals (CIs).

REFERENCES

1. American Academy of Pediatrics. 2000 Red book: report of the Committee on Infectious Diseases, 25th ed. Elk Grove Village, Ill: The Academy; 2000.
2. Thampakkul S, Ballow M. Replacement with intravenous immune serum globulin therapy in patients with antibody immune deficiency. Immunol Clin North Am 2001; 21(1):165.

IMMUNOPROPHYLAXIS

Irene Moff, MD

I. SOURCES OF INFORMATION

A. PRINTED SOURCES

American Academy of Pediatrics. *2000 Red Book: Report of the Committee on Infectious Diseases,* 25th ed. Elk Grove Village, Ill: The Academy, 2000.

Updated Recommended Childhood Vaccination Schedule is published each January in *Pediatrics* and *Morbidity and Mortality Weekly Report.*

Current issues of *Morbidity and Mortality Weekly Report.*

Vaccine package inserts.

B. ELECTRONIC/TELEPHONE SOURCES

State health departments.

The voice information system from the Centers for Disease Control and Prevention (CDC) can provide telephone consultation and send printed material on vaccines. Phone number: (800) 232-SHOT.

The CDC: http://www.cdc.gov.

The American Academy of Pediatrics (AAP): http://www.aap.org.

The Vaccine Adverse Event Reporting System (VAERS) provides a mechanism for reporting health effects that occur after immunization that may be related to the vaccine. To submit a report or for questions, call 1-800-822-7967 or access their web page at http://www.vaers.org.

General vaccine information and safety: http://www.vaccinesafety.edu and http://www.immunize.org.

II. IMMUNIZATION SCHEDULES

A. RECOMMENDED CHILDHOOD IMMUNIZATION SCHEDULE
(Fig. 15-1)

B. CATCH-UP IMMUNIZATION SCHEDULES

1. **Lapsed immunizations:** Resume immunization schedule as if the usual interval had elapsed. Repeating doses is not indicated.

2. **Catch-up immunization schedules:** See Tables 15-1 and 15-2.

a. *Haemophilus influenzae* type b (Hib): See p. 325.

b. Pneumococcus conjugate vaccine (PCV7): See Table 15-3.

C. MINIMUM AGE FOR INITIAL VACCINATION AND MINIMUM INTERVALS BETWEEN DOSES OF VARIOUS VACCINES
(Table 15-4)

15

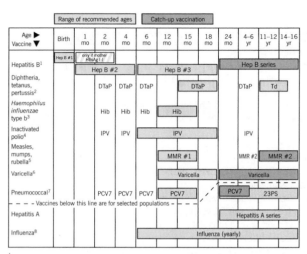

Age ► Vaccine ▼	Birth	1 mo	2 mo	4 mo	6 mo	12 mo	15 mo	18 mo	24 mo	4–6 yr	11–12 yr	14–16 yr
				Range of recommended ages		**Catch-up vaccination**						
Hepatitis B[1]	Hep B #1	only if mother HBsAg (-)									Hep B series	
		Hep B #2				Hep B #3						
Diphtheria, tetanus, pertussis[2]			DTaP	DTaP	DTaP		DTaP			DTaP	Td	
Haemophilus influenzae type b[3]			Hib	Hib	Hib	Hib						
Inactivated polio[4]			IPV	IPV		IPV				IPV		
Measles, mumps, rubella[5]						MMR #1				MMR #2	MMR #2	
Varicella[6]						Varicella				Varicella		
Pneumococcal[7]			PCV7	PCV7	PCV7	PCV7			PCV7	23PS		
Hepatitis A										Hepatitis A series		
Influenza[8]						Influenza (yearly)						

– – – Vaccines below this line are for selected populations – – –

[1]All infants should receive the first dose of hepatitis B vaccine soon after birth and before hospital discharge; the first dose may also be given by age 2 months if the infant's mother is HBsAg-negative. Only monovalent hepatitis B vaccine can be used for the birth dose.

[2]The fourth dose of DTaP may be administered as early as 12 mo of age if 6 mo have elapsed since the third dose and if the child is unlikely to return at age 15–18 mo. Td is recommended at 11–12 yr of age if at least 5 yr have elapsed since the last dose of DTaP. Subsequent routine Td boosters are recommended every 10 yr.

[3]If PRP-OMP is administered at 2 and 4 mo of age, a dose at 6 mo is not required. DTaP/Hib combination products *should not be* used for primary immunization in infants at 2, 4, or 6 mo of age until FDA approved for these ages.

[4]An all-IPV schedule is recommended for routine childhood polio vaccination in the United States. All children should receive four doses of IPV at ages 2 mo, 4 mo, 6–18 months, and 4–6 yr. OPV is acceptable in special circumstances: children of parents who do not accept the number of injections, late initiation of immunization that would require an unacceptable number of injections, and imminent travel to polio-endemic areas. OPV remains the vaccine of choice for mass immunization campaigns to control outbreaks caused by wild poliovirus.

[5]The second dose of MMR is recommended routinely at 4–6 yr of age but may be administered during any visit, provided at least 4 weeks have elapsed since the first dose. Those who have not previously received the second dose should complete the schedule by the 11–12 yr visit.

[6]Varicella vaccine is recommended at any visit for susceptible children ≥1 yr of age. Susceptible persons ≥13 yr of age should receive two doses given at least 4 weeks apart.

[7]The heptavalent pneumococcal conjugate vaccine (PCV7) is recommended for all children ages 2–23 mo. It is also recommended for certain children ages 24–59 mo. Pneumococcal polysaccharide vaccine (23PS) is recommended in addition to PCV7 for certain high-risk groups (see p. 335 for further information).

[8]Influenza vaccine is recommended annually for certain high-risk children ≥ 6 mo (see pp. 327, 329-330) and can be administered to all others wishing to obtain immunity.

FIG. 15-1

Recommended childhood immunization schedule, United States, 2002. Dark bars indicate vaccines to be given if previous recommended doses were missed or given earlier than the recommended minimum age. Most recent recommendations can be found on the CDC or AAP websites (see p. 315). *(Modified from the CDC Advisory committee on Immunization Practices, www.cdc.gov/nip/acip.)*

TABLE 15-1

RECOMMENDED IMMUNIZATION SCHEDULES FOR CHILDREN <7 YEARS NOT IMMUNIZED IN THE FIRST YEAR OF LIFE

Recommended Time/Age	Immunizations	Comments
First visit	DTaP, Hib, HBV, MMR, IPV, PCV7	Hib and PCV7 not needed if immunocompetent child ≥5 yr May combine DTaP and Hib after 15 mo
Interval after first visit		
1 mo	DTaP, HBV, Var	
2 mo	DTaP, Hib, IPV, PCV7	Second dose of Hib indicated only if 1st dose given at <15 mo Second dose of PCV7 indicated if child <2 yr
≥8 mo	DTaP, HBV, IPV	IPV and HBV are not given if third doses previously given
4-6 yr (at or before school entry)	DTaP, IPV, MMR	DTaP not necessary if fourth dose given after fourth birthday. IPV not necessary if third dose given after fourth birthday.

Modified from American Academy of Pediatrics. 2000 Red book: report of the Committee on Infectious Diseases, 25th ed. Elk Grove Village, Ill: The Academy; 2000.

TABLE 15-2

RECOMMENDED IMMUNIZATION SCHEDULES FOR CHILDREN 7-12 YEARS NOT IMMUNIZED IN THE FIRST YEAR OF LIFE

Recommended Time/Age	Immunizations	Comments
First visit	HBV, MMR, Td, IPV	—
Interval after first visit		
2 mo	HBV, MMR, Var, Td, IPV	—
8-14 mo	HBV, Td, IPV	IPV, HBV not needed if third doses given earlier

NOTE: Varicella vaccine can be administered to susceptible children any time after 12 mo of age. Unimmunized children who lack a reliable history of chickenpox should be immunized before their thirteenth birthday. Children >12 yr require two doses of varicella vaccine.
Modified from American Academy of Pediatrics. 2000 Red book: report of the Committee on Infectious Diseases, 25th ed. Elk Grove Village, Ill: The Academy; 2000.

TABLE 15-3

CATCH-UP IMMUNIZATION SCHEDULE FOR PCV7 IN PREVIOUSLY UNVACCINATED CHILDREN

Age at First Dose	Primary Series	Booster Dose*
2-6 mo	3 doses, 6-8 wk apart	1 dose at 12-15 mo of age
7-11 mo	2 doses, 6-8 wk apart	1 dose at 12-15 mo of age
12-23 mo	2 doses, 6-8 wk apart	
≥24 mo	1 dose	

Modified from American Academy of Pediatrics Committee on Infectious Diseases. Pediatrics 2000; 106(2):362-366.
*Booster doses to be given at least 6 to 8 weeks after the final dose of the primary series.

TABLE 15-4

MINIMUM AGE FOR INITIAL VACCINATION AND MINIMUM INTERVAL BETWEEN VACCINE DOSES, BY TYPE OF VACCINE

Vaccine	Minimum Age for First Dose[a]	Minimum Interval from Dose to Dose		
		1 to 2[a]	2 to 3[a]	3 to 4
DTaP[b]	6 wk	1 mo	1 mo	6 mo
Hib (primary series)				
HbOC	6 wk	1 mo	1 mo	2 mo[c]
PRP-T	6 wk	1 mo	1 mo	2 mo[c]
PRP-OMP	6 wk	1 mo	2 mo[c]	—
PCV7	6 wk	1 mo[d]	1 mo[d]	2 mo[d]
IPV	6 wk	1 mo	1 mo	1 mo[e]
MMR	12 mo[f]	1 mo	—	—
HBV	Birth	1 mo	2 mo[g]	—
Varicella	12 mo	1 mo[h]	—	—

Modified from Atkinson W et al: Epidemiology and prevention of vaccine-preventable diseases: the pink book, 6th ed. Atlanta: National Immunization Program, Centers for Disease Control and Prevention; 2000.

[a]These minimum acceptable ages and intervals may not correspond with the optimal recommended ages and intervals for vaccination. See Fig. 15-1.

[b]The total number of doses of diphtheria and tetanus toxoids should not exceed six each before the seventh birthday. If the fourth dose is given after the fourth birthday, the fifth (booster) dose is not needed.

[c]The booster dose of Hib vaccine recommended after the primary vaccination series should be administered no earlier than 12 mo of age.

[d]See Table 15-3 for recommendations of number of doses at different ages.

[e]If the third dose is given after the fourth birthday, the fourth (booster) dose is not needed.

[f]Although the age for measles vaccination may be as young as 6 mo in outbreak areas where cases are occurring in children <1 yr of age, children initially vaccinated before the first birthday should be revaccinated at 12-15 mo of age, and an additional dose of vaccine should be administered at the time of school entry or according to local policy. Doses of MMR or other measles-containing vaccine should be separated by at least 1 mo.

[g]This final dose is recommended at least 4 mo after the first dose and no earlier than 6 mo of age.

[h]A second dose of varicella is indicated only in children ≥13 yr.

III. IMMUNIZATION GUIDELINES

A. VACCINE INFORMED CONSENT

Vaccine information statements (VISs) can be obtained from local health departments, the CDC, the AAP, and vaccine manufacturers. For vaccines that do not currently have VISs, the CDC produces "important information" statements.

B. VACCINE ADMINISTRATION

1. **Volume/dose:** Unless otherwise specified, all pediatric immunization doses are 0.5 mL.
2. **Preferred sites** of administration of intramuscular (IM) and subcutaneous (SC) vaccines follow:
a. Less than 18 months old: Anterolateral thigh.
b. Toddlers: Anterolateral thigh or deltoid (deltoid preferred if large enough).
c. Adolescents and young adults: Deltoid.

3. Route
a. IM: Deep into muscle to avoid tissue damage from adjuvants, usually with a 22- to 25-gauge needle, ⅞- to 1-inch long in infants and toddlers and 1 to 2 inches long in adolescents and young adults.
b. SC: Into pinched skinfold with a 23- to 25-gauge needle ⅝- to ¾-inch long.
4. **Simultaneous administration:** Routine childhood vaccines, including live viral vaccines, are safe and effective when administered simultaneously at different sites, generally 1 to 2 inches apart. Otherwise, the interval between administration of live viral vaccines should be >1 month.

C. MISCONCEPTIONS REGARDING VACCINE ADMINISTRATION
Vaccines may be given despite the presence of the following:
1. Mild acute illness, regardless of fever.
2. Low-grade fever.
3. Convalescent phase of illness.
4. Recent exposure to infectious disease.
5. Mild to moderate local reaction to previous dose of vaccine (soreness, redness, swelling).
6. Current antimicrobial therapy.
7. Prematurity (see also pp. 320-321).
8. Malnutrition.
9. Allergy to penicillin or other antibiotic (except anaphylactic reaction to neomycin or streptomycin).
10. Pregnancy of mother or another household contact (except varicella vaccine may be deferred if there is a pregnant, varicella-susceptible household contact).
11. Breast-feeding.
12. Unimmunized household contact.

D. EGG ALLERGIES
1. Measles/mumps/rubella (MMR) vaccine can be given to children with egg allergies without prior skin testing (see p. 333 for details).
2. Skin testing with yellow fever vaccine is recommended before administration in children with a history of immediate hypersensitivity reaction (e.g., anaphylaxis or generalized urticaria) to eggs.
3. Immediate hypersensitivity reaction to eggs is a contraindication to influenza vaccine. Less severe or local manifestations of allergy to egg are not contraindications to influenza vaccine.

IV. IMMUNOPROPHYLAXIS GUIDELINES FOR SPECIAL HOSTS
A. IMMUNOCOMPROMISED HOSTS
1. Congenital immunodeficiency disorders
a. Live bacterial and live viral vaccines are generally contraindicated. See the AAP's *Red Book* for details regarding individual immunodeficiencies.
b. Inactivated vaccines should be given according to the routine schedule. Immune response may vary and may be inadequate.

15

IMMUNOPROPHYLAXIS

c. Immunoglobulin (IG) therapy may be indicated.

d. Household contacts: Immunize according to the routine childhood immunization schedule. A yearly influenza vaccine is recommended.

2. **Known or suspected human immunodeficiency virus (HIV) disease**

a. Inactivated vaccines should be given according to the routine immunization schedule (see Fig. 15-1).

b. MMR vaccine should be given to asymptomatic or mildly symptomatic patients with $CD4^+$ T-lymphocyte counts ≥15%. Immunize at 12 months of age; administer the second dose as soon as 1 month later to ensure early seroconversion.

c. Varicella vaccine should be considered in asymptomatic or mildly symptomatic patients with $CD4^+$ T-lymphocyte counts ≥25%. Give two doses 3 months apart.

d. 23-valent pneumococcal polysaccharide vaccine (23PS) is recommended at 2 and 5 years, in addition to the routine PCV7 vaccines.

e. Influenza: Immunize all patients at the start of the influenza season as early as 6 months of age and yearly thereafter.

3. **Oncology patients:** See Table 15-5.

4. **Functional or anatomic asplenia** (including sickle cell disease)

a. Penicillin prophylaxis: See Chapter 13, p. 291.

b. Pneumococcal vaccine

   (1) Children ≤5 years at diagnosis: Table 15-6.

   (2) Children >5 years at diagnosis: Immunization with a single dose of PCV7 or 23PS is acceptable. If both vaccines are given, their administration should be separated by 6 to 8 weeks. A second dose of 23PS may be given in 5 years. Data are insufficient for the most effective combination of the pneumococcal vaccines in older children.

c. Meningococcal vaccine at 2 years of age or at diagnosis if ≥2 years old.

d. Ensure that Hib series is completed; children ≥5 years who never received Hib immunization should receive one dose.

e. Children ≥2 years undergoing elective splenectomy should receive one or both of the pneumococcal vaccines and the meningococcal vaccine at least 2 weeks before surgery to ensure optimal immune response. Children <2 years should receive PCV7 before surgery.

B. CORTICOSTEROID ADMINISTRATION

Only live viral and live bacterial vaccines are potentially contraindicated (see Table 15-7 for details).

C. PATIENTS TREATED WITH IG OR OTHER BLOOD PRODUCTS

See AAP's *Red Book* for suggested intervals between immunoglobulin or blood product administration and MMR or varicella immunization.

D. PRETERM INFANTS

Immunize according to chronologic age using regular vaccine dosage.

1. **Hepatitis B virus (HBV):** Initiation of HBV vaccine may be delayed for

TABLE 15-5	
IMMUNIZATION FOR ONCOLOGY PATIENTS*	
Vaccine	Indications and Comments
DTaP	Indicated for incompletely immunized children <7 yr, even during active chemotherapy
Td	Indicated 1 yr after completion of therapy in children ≥7 yr
Hib	Indicated for incompletely immunized children if <7 yr
HBV	Indicated for incompletely immunized children
23PS	Indicated for asplenic patients
PCV7	Indicated for incompletely immunized children <5 yr
Meningococcus	Consider in asplenic patients
IPV	Indicated for incompletely immunized children; IPV also recommended for all household contacts requiring immunization to reduce the risk of vaccine-associated polio
MMR	Contraindicated until child is in remission and finished with all chemotherapy for 3-6 mo; may need to reimmunize after chemotherapy if titers have fallen below protective levels
Influenza	Defer in active chemotherapy; may give as early as 3-4 wk after remission and off chemotherapy if during influenza season; peripheral granulocyte and lymphocyte counts should be >1000/mm^3; should also be given to household contacts of children with cancer
Varicella	Consider immunizing children who have remained in remission and have finished chemotherapy for >1 yr; with absolute lymphocyte count of >700/mm^3 and platelet count of >100,000/mm^3 within 24 hr of immunization; check titers of previously immunized children to verify protective levels of antibodies

*Immune reconstitution is slower for oncology patients who have received bone marrow transplants. See CDC: MMWR 2000; 49(No. RR-10): 1-147 for vaccine schedule.

infants of hepatitis B surface antigen (HBsAg)–negative mothers until the child is >2 kg or 2 months of age, whichever is earlier.

2. **Influenza:** Give each fall to children >6 months with chronic lung disease. Household contacts should also receive influenza vaccine.

E. PREGNANCY

Live virus vaccines are generally contraindicated during pregnancy. Influenza vaccine should be given to all women who will be >14 weeks' gestation during the influenza season. Influenza vaccine is considered safe at any stage of pregnancy. Pregnant women not immunized, or incompletely immunized against tetanus should receive Td to prevent neonatal tetanus. Pregnant women not immunized, or incompletely immunized against polio should receive the inactivated poliomyelitis vaccine (IPV). When indicated, hepatitis A virus (HAV) and HBV vaccines may be given to pregnant women. Pneumococcal vaccines should be deferred during pregnancy, although 23PS has been administered safely.

15

IMMUNOPROPHYLAXIS

TABLE 15-6

RECOMMENDATIONS FOR PNEUMOCOCCAL IMMUNIZATION WITH PCV7 OR 23PS VACCINE FOR CHILDREN AT HIGH RISK OF PNEUMOCOCCAL DISEASE

Age	Previous Doses	Recommendations
≤23 mo	None	PCV7 as in Table 15-3
24-59 mo	1-3 doses of PCV7	1 booster dose of PCV7 at least 6-8 wk after last dose of PCV7
		First dose of 23PS vaccine at 24 mo, at least 6-8 wk after last dose of PCV7
		Second dose of 23PS vaccine, 3-5 yr after first dose of 23PS vaccine
24-59 mo	4 doses of PCV7	First dose of 23PS vaccine at 24 mo, at least 6-8 wk after last dose of PCV7
		Second dose of 23PS vaccine, 3-5 yr after first dose of 23PS vaccine
24-59 mo	None	Two doses of PCV7 6-8 wk apart
		First dose of 23PS vaccine, 6-8 wk after last dose of PCV7
		Second dose of 23PS vaccine, 3-5 yr after first dose of 23PS vaccine
24-59 mo	1 dose of 23PS	Two doses of PCV7, 6-8 wk apart, beginning at least 6-8 wk after last dose of 23PS vaccine
		One dose of 23PS vaccine, 3-5 yr after first dose of 23PS vaccine

Modified from Centers for Disease Control and Prevention. MMWR 2000; 49(No. RR-10):1-147.

TABLE 15-7

LIVE VIRUS IMMUNIZATION FOR PATIENTS RECEIVING CORTICOSTEROID THERAPY

Steroid Dose	Recommended Guidelines
Topical or inhaled therapy or local injection of steroids	Live virus vaccines may be given unless there is clinical evidence of immunosuppression; if suppressed, wait 1 mo after cessation of therapy to give live vaccines
Physiologic maintenance doses of steroids	Live virus vaccines may be given
Low-dose steroids (<2 mg/kg/day prednisone or equivalent, or <20 mg/day if >10 kg)	Live virus vaccines may be given
High-dose steroids (≥2 mg/kg/day prednisone or equivalent, or 20 mg/day if >10 kg)	
• Duration of therapy <14 days	May give live virus vaccines immediately after cessation of therapy
• Duration of therapy ≥14 days	Do not give live virus vaccines until therapy has been discontinued for 1 mo
Children with immunosuppressive disorders receiving steroid therapy	Live virus vaccines are contraindicated, except in children with HIV who are not severely immunocompromised

Modified from American Academy of Pediatrics. 2000 Red book: report of the Committee on Infectious Diseases, 25th ed. Elk Grove Village, Ill: The Academy; 2000.

V. IMMUNOPROPHYLAXIS GUIDELINES FOR SPECIFIC DISEASES

A. DIPHTHERIA/TETANUS/PERTUSSIS VACCINES AND TETANUS IMMUNOPROPHYLAXIS

1. Description
   a. DTaP: Diphtheria and tetanus toxoids combined with acellular pertussis vaccine; preferred formulation for children <7 years.
   b. DT: Diphtheria and tetanus toxoids without pertussis vaccine; use in children <7 years in whom pertussis vaccine is contraindicated.
   c. Td: Tetanus toxoid with one third to one sixth the dose of diphtheria toxoid of other preparations; use in individuals ≥7 years.
   d. DTP: Diphtheria and tetanus toxoids combined with whole-cell pertussis vaccine; no longer marketed in the United States.

2. Indications
   a. Routine: See Fig. 15-1.
   b. Tetanus prophylaxis in wound management: See Table 15-8.
   c. Unimmunized pregnant women: Two doses of Td 4 weeks apart; the second dose should be ≥2 weeks before delivery.
   d. Pregnant women who have not completed a primary series: Give Td as soon as possible.

3. Contraindications
   a. General contraindication: Anaphylactic reaction to vaccine or vaccine constituent.
   b. Contraindication to pertussis vaccine: Encephalopathy not attributable to another cause within 7 days of a prior dose of pertussis vaccine. Use DT for remaining doses in series.

4. Precautions
   a. General precaution: Moderate or severe acute illness regardless of fever.
   b. The following adverse events after a prior dose of pertussis vaccine are considered precautions to subsequent doses.
      (1) Convulsion, with or without fever within 3 days.

15

IMMUNOPROPHYLAXIS

TABLE 15-8

INDICATIONS FOR TETANUS PROPHYLAXIS

Prior Tetanus Toxoid Doses	Clean, Minor Wounds		All Other Wounds	
	Tetanus Vaccine[a]	TIG	Tetanus Vaccine[a]	TIG
Unknown or <3	Yes	No	Yes	Yes
≥3, last <5 yr ago	No	No	No	No[b]
≥3, last 5-10 yr ago	No	No	Yes	No[b]
≥3, last >10 yr ago	Yes	No	Yes	No[b]

Modified from American Academy of Pediatrics. 2000 Red book: report of the Committee on Infectious Diseases, 25th ed. Elk Grove Village, Ill: The Academy; 2000.

TIG, tetanus immune globulin: 250 U IM. Equine tetanus antitoxin, TAT, may be substituted if TIG unavailable (3000-5000 U IM after sensitivity testing of patient).

[a]Vaccine choice for child <7 yr old is DTaP (DT if pertussis is contraindicated). For child ≥7 yr, Td is the vaccine of choice.

[b]Any child with HIV infection or who is within the first year after bone marrow transplantation should receive TIG for any tetanus-prone wound regardless of vaccination status.

    (2) Persistent, inconsolable crying for ≥3 hours within 48 hours.

    (3) Collapse or shock-like state (hypotonic-hyporesponsive episode) within 48 hours.

    (4) Temperature ≥40.5° C not explained by another cause within 48 hours.

5. Children with neurologic disorders

a. Seizures

    (1) Poorly controlled or new-onset seizures: Defer pertussis immunization until seizure disorder is well controlled and progressive neurologic disorder is excluded; then use DTaP and antipyretics for 24 hours after immunization.

    (2) Personal or family history of febrile seizures: Use DTaP and antipyretics for 24 hours after immunization.

b. Known or suspected progressive neurologic disorder: Defer pertussis immunization until diagnosis and treatment are established and neurologic condition is stable. Progressive disorders may merit permanent deferral of pertussis immunization. Reconsider pertussis immunization at each visit. Use DT if pertussis vaccine is permanently deferred.

Note: Children <1 year with neurologic disorders necessitating temporary deferment of pertussis vaccine should not receive DT because the risk of diphtheria and tetanus is low in the first year of life. After the first birthday, initiate either DT or DTaP immunization as clinically indicated previously.

6. Side effects

a. Minor side effects within 3 days: Erythema (26% to 39%), swelling (15% to 30%), pain (4% to 11%), fever >38.3° C (3% to 5%), anorexia (19% to 25%), vomiting (7% to 13%), drowsiness (40% to 47%), fussiness (14% to 19%).

b. Moderate to severe side effects: Anaphylaxis (1/50,000); seizures, persistent crying >3 hours, hypotonic-hyporesponsive episode, temperature ≥40.5° C (rare).

7. Administration: DTaP, DT, and Td are all given in a dose of 0.5 mL IM.

8. Special considerations

a. Pertussis exposure: Immunize all unimmunized or partially immunized close contacts <7 years.

    (1) Give fourth dose of DTaP if third dose was given >6 months prior.

    (2) Give booster dose of DTaP if last dose was given >3 years prior and child is <7 years old.

b. Chemoprophylaxis for all household and other close contacts: Treat with erythromycin to limit secondary transmission regardless of immunization status. Estolate preparation may be better tolerated (see Formulary). Azithromycin, clarithromycin, and trimethoprim-sulfamethoxazole are possible alternatives, but their efficacy is unproven.

Note: The total number of DT and DTaP immunizations should not exceed six by the fourth birthday.

B. HAEMOPHILUS INFLUENZAE TYPE B IMMUNOPROPHYLAXIS

1. **Description:** The four licensed vaccines consist of a capsular polysaccharide antigen (PRP) conjugated to a carrier. It is not necessary to use the same formulation for the entire series. Vaccines do not confer protection against the disease associated with the carrier (e.g., PRP-T does not protect against tetanus). Routine use of these vaccines has led to a 99% decline in invasive Hib disease in infants and young children.

a. **PRP-OMP:** Conjugated to outer membrane protein of *Neisseria meningitidis*; requires only two doses in primary series; children without prior DTaP vaccine may respond better to PRP-OMP than to other formulations.

b. **HbOC:** Conjugated to mutant diphtheria toxin.

c. **PRP-T:** Conjugated to tetanus toxoid.

2. **Indications**

a. Routine: See Fig. 15-1.

b. Children not immunized against Hib before 7 months of age: Give all doses 2 months apart (1 month acceptable to accelerate immunization). If initiating Hib immunization at 7 to 11 months, give three doses; at 12 to 14 months, give two doses; and at 15 to 59 months, give one dose. Immunization is not necessary for immunocompetent children ≥60 months.

c. Unimmunized children >15 months with underlying conditions predisposing to invasive Hib disease (e.g., IgG2 deficiency, HIV) require two doses of vaccine.

d. Children undergoing splenectomy may benefit from an additional dose 7 to 10 days before procedure, even if series was previously completed.

e. Children with invasive Hib disease at age <24 months: Begin Hib immunization 1 month after acute illness and continue as if previously unimmunized.

NOTE: **Consider immunologic workup for children who contract invasive Hib disease after completing the immunization series.**

3. **Contraindication:** Anaphylactic reaction to vaccine or vaccine constituent.

4. **Precaution:** Moderate or severe acute illness regardless of fever.

5. **Side effects:** Local pain, redness, and swelling in 25% of recipients; frequency of fever and irritability when Hib is given with DTaP are the same as for DTaP alone.

6. **Administration:** Dose is 0.5 mL IM; PRP-T and HbOC may be given SC in patients with coagulation disorders.

7. **Special considerations:** Consider prophylactic rifampin to selected household and child care contacts of children with invasive Hib disease; see AAP's *Red Book* for details.

C. HEPATITIS A VIRUS IMMUNOPROPHYLAXIS

1. **Description:** Hepatitis A (HAV) vaccine is an inactivated adsorbed vaccine; two brands are available, both with pediatric and adult formulations. It is licensed only for children ≥2 years.

15

IMMUNOPROPHYLAXIS

2. Indications
a. Children living in regions of elevated hepatitis A rates (consult local public health authority). See Fig. 15-1 for schedule.
b. Travelers to or residents of endemic areas.
c. After exposure to HAV if future exposure is likely.
d. Military personnel.
e. Homosexual or bisexual men.
f. Users of illicit injection drugs.
g. Patients with clotting factor disorders.
h. Patients with chronic liver disease, including HBV or hepatitis C (HCV).
i. Persons at risk of occupational exposure.
j. Immunocompromised individuals may be immunized, although efficacy is not established in immunocompromised children.
k. Consider use in staff of institutions with ongoing or recurrent outbreaks.
3. **Contraindication:** Anaphylactic reaction to vaccine or vaccine constituent.
4. **Precaution:** Moderate or severe acute illness regardless of fever.
5. **Side effects:** Local reactions include induration, redness, swelling (18%); headache (12%); fever (6%); fatigue, malaise, anorexia, nausea (1% to 10%). No serious adverse events have been reported.
6. **Administration:** See Table 15-9 for dose and schedule; give IM.
7. Special considerations
a. Preexposure immunoprophylaxis for travelers
   (1) HAV vaccine is preferred for travelers ≥2 years old; a single dose usually provides adequate immunity if time does not allow further doses before travel.
   (2) IG, given IM, is protective for up to 5 months; see AAP's *Red Book* for dosing.
b. Postexposure immunoprophylaxis
   (1) IG 0.02 mL/kg IM is 80% to 90% effective in preventing symptomatic infection if given within 2 weeks of exposure. Maximum dose per site is 3 mL for infants and small children and 5 mL for large children and adults.
   (2) Also give HAV vaccine if ≥2 years old and future exposure is likely.

TABLE 15-9					
RECOMMENDED DOSAGES AND SCHEDULES FOR HAV VACCINES					
Age (yr)	Vaccine	Antigen	Volume (mL)	No. of Doses	Schedule
2-18	Havrix (SB)	720 ELU	0.5	2	Initial and 6-12 mo later
	Vaqta (Merck)	25 U	0.5	2	Initial and 6-18 mo later
≥19	Havrix (SB)	1440 ELU	1.0	2	Initial and 6-12 mo later
	Vaqta (Merck)	50 U	1.0	2	Initial and 6-12 mo later

Modified from American Academy of Pediatrics. 2000 Red book: report of the Committee on Infectious Diseases, 25th ed. Elk Grove Village, Ill: The Academy; 2000.
SB, SmithKline Beecham; *ELU,* enzyme-linked immunoassay units; *U,* antigen units.

Studies suggest that HAV vaccine alone may be effective for postexposure prophylaxis, but data are insufficient to recommend alone.

D. HEPATITIS B VIRUS IMMUNOPROPHYLAXIS

1. Description

a. Hepatitis B immune globulin (HBIG): Prepared from plasma containing high-titer anti-HBsAg antibodies and negative for antibodies to HIV and HCV. *Dose:* Infants, 0.5 mL IM; older children, 0.06 mL/kg IM.

b. HBV vaccine: Adsorbed HBsAg produced recombinantly. Different recombinant vaccines may be used interchangeably.

2. Indications

a. Routine: See Fig. 15-1.

b. Infants of mothers who are HBsAg positive or indeterminate: See Fig. 15-2.

3. Contraindication: Anaphylactic reaction to vaccine, baker's yeast, or another vaccine constituent.

4. Precaution: Moderate or severe acute illness regardless of fever.

5. Side effects: Pain at injection site or fever >37.7° C in 1% to 6%; immediate hypersensitivity reaction is very rare.

6. Administration

a. See Table 15-10 for dose; give IM.

b. An alternate two-dose regimen is approved for vaccination of adolescents ages 11 to 15 years. The dose is 10 mcg (1 mL) IM given a minimum of 4 months apart. The adverse effects are similar to the three-dose regimen.

7. Special considerations: See Table 15-11 for HBV prophylaxis after percutaneous exposure to blood.

E. INFLUENZA VACCINE AND CHEMOPROPHYLAXIS

1. Description

a. Inactivated influenza vaccines are produced in embryonated eggs.

b. Vaccines contain three viral strains (usually two type A and one type B), based on expected prevalent influenza strains for the upcoming winter.

c. Preparations

   (1) Inactivated whole virus vaccine from intact purified virus particles; should not be used in children <13 years.

   (2) Split-virus vaccines: Licensed for children >6 months.

      (a) Subvirion: Inactivated whole virus vaccine with denatured viral lipid membrane.

      (b) Purified surface antigen vaccine.

   (3) A nasally administered live, attenuated vaccine is under consideration for licensure by the U.S. Food and Drug Administration (FDA) at the time of publication and will potentially be available in 2002.

2. Indications

a. High-risk children

   (1) Asthma and other chronic pulmonary diseases.

   (2) Hemodynamically significant cardiac disease.

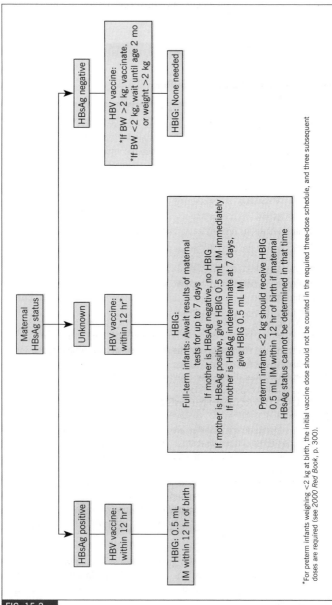

FIG. 15-2

Management of neonates born to mothers with unknown or positive HbsAg status. *BW,* Birth weight. *(Modified from American Academy of Pediatrics. 2000 Red book: report of the Committee on Infectious Diseases, 25th ed. Elk Grove Village, Ill: The Academy; 2000.)*

TABLE 15-10
RECOMMENDED DOSE FOR HBV VACCINES

Patient Group	Recombivax HB Dose (mcg)[a]	Engerix-B Dose (mcg)[b]
Up to 19 yr	5	10
11-15 yr[c]	10[c]	—
≥20 yr	10	20
Patients undergoing dialysis and other immunosuppressed adults	40	40

Modified from American Academy of Pediatrics. 2000 Red book: report of the Committee on Infectious Diseases, 25th ed. Elk Grove Village, Ill: The Academy; 2000.
[a]Recombivax HB is available from Merck & Co. in pediatric, adult, and dialysis patient formulations.
[b]Engerix-B is available from SmithKline Beecham in a single formulation.
[c]May use alternative 2-dose regimen 6 months apart.

TABLE 15-11
HBV PROPHYLAXIS AFTER PERCUTANEOUS EXPOSURE TO BLOOD

	HBsAg Status of Source of Blood		
Exposed Person	Positive	Negative	Unknown
Unimmunized	HBIG Start vaccine series	Start vaccine series	Start vaccine series If source known to be high risk, treat as if HbsAg positive
Immunized			
Known responder	No treatment	No treatment	No treatment
Known nonresponder	HBIG Start vaccine series	Start vaccine series	Start vaccine series If source known to be high risk, treat as if HBsAg positive
Response unknown	Test exposed person for anti-HBs If <10 mIU/mL, give HBIG, reimmunize If ≥10 mIU/mL, no treatment	No treatment	Test exposed person for anti-HBs If <10 mIU/mL, reimmunize If ≥10 mIU/mL, no treatment

Modified from American Academy of Pediatrics. 2000 Red book: report of the Committee on Infectious Diseases, 25th ed. Elk Grove Village, Ill: The Academy; 2000.

15

IMMUNOPROPHYLAXIS

(3) Immunosuppressive disorders and therapy.
(4) HIV infection.
(5) Sickle cell anemia and other hemoglobinopathies.
(6) Diseases requiring long-term aspirin therapy.
(7) Chronic renal disease.
(8) Chronic metabolic disease, including diabetes mellitus.

   b. Close contacts of high-risk children and adults
     (1) Household contacts.
     (2) Health care workers.
   c. Consider immunization for other high-risk persons
     (1) Pregnant women who will be in their second or third trimester during influenza season.
     (2) International travel to areas with influenza outbreaks.
     (3) Institutional settings, including colleges and other residential facilities.

3. Contraindication: Anaphylactic reaction to vaccine, vaccine constituent, chicken, or eggs.

4. Precaution: Moderate or severe acute illness regardless of fever.

5. Side effects
   a. Fever 6 to 24 hours after immunization in children <2 years; rare in children >2 years.
   b. Local reactions uncommon in children <13 years; 10% in children ≥13 years.
   c. Side effects and immunogenicity are similar for whole and split-virus vaccines in children >12 years.
   d. Guillain-Barré syndrome (GBS): Influenza immunization has been associated with GBS in approximately 1 per million persons ≥45 years of age; GBS has not been associated with influenza immunization in children.

6. Administration
   a. Administer during the fall in preparation for winter influenza season.
   b. Dosage and schedule: See Table 15-12; give IM.

7. Special considerations
   a. Children receiving chemotherapy have poor seroconversion rates until chemotherapy is discontinued for 3 to 4 weeks and absolute neutrophil and lymphocyte counts are >1000/mm^3.
   b. Immunization may be delayed in patients on prolonged high-dose steroids (equivalent to 2 mg/kg/day or >20 mg/day of prednisone) until dose is decreased, only if time allows before the influenza season.
   c. Chemoprophylaxis for influenza A and B[1].

TABLE 15-12

INFLUENZA VACCINE DOSAGE AND SCHEDULE

Age	Vaccine Type	Volume (mL)	Number of Doses
6-35 mo	Split virus only	0.25	1 or 2*
3-8 yr	Split virus only	0.5	1 or 2*
9-12 yr	Split virus only	0.5	1
>12 yr	Whole or split virus	0.5	1

Modified from American Academy of Pediatrics. 2000 Red book: report of the Committee on Infectious Diseases, 25th ed. Elk Grove Village, Ill: The Academy; 2000.

*Two doses, at least 1 mo apart, are recommended for children ≤8 yr receiving influenza vaccine for the first time.

(1) Amantadine and rimantadine are approved for prophylaxis of influenza A in children ≥12 months. Amantadine is also approved for treatment of influenza in children ≥12 months.
   (a) Indications
      (i) High-risk children immunized after influenza is present in the community: Give for 2 weeks after immunization.
      (ii) Unimmunized individuals providing care to high-risk individuals.
      (iii) Immunodeficient individuals unlikely to have protective response to vaccine.
      (iv) Individuals at high risk for influenza infection with contraindication to vaccine.
   (b) Chemoprophylaxis is not a substitute for immunization and does not interfere with the immune response to the vaccine.
(2) Zanamivir and oseltamivir have recently been approved for treating uncomplicated acute illness caused by influenza.
   (a) Oseltamivir was recently approved for prophylaxis of influenza A and B in ages ≥13 years. A new formulation was approved for treating influenza in children ≥12 months of age.
   (b) Zanamivir is approved for use in children ≥7 years of age. The FDA is currently reviewing its potential as a prophylactic medication.

F. LYME IMMUNOPROPHYLAXIS

1. **Description:** Recombinant vaccine against the *Borrelia burgdorferi* outer surface protein A (rOspA), an antigen expressed by the Lyme spirochete in the tick midgut. The tick ingests host antibody, killing the organism in the tick and aborting human infection. NOTE: **As of the time of publication, the Lyme vaccine has been removed from the U.S. market.**

2. Indications
a. Currently licensed only for persons between 15 and 70 years of age.
b. Highest rates of transmission occur in northeast and north central United States, but risk varies even within townships and counties. Check with local public health authorities to identify areas of high risk for disease transmission.
c. Consider vaccination in the following persons:
   (1) Patients >15 years of age who reside, work, or play in high or moderate risk areas during the transmission season (typically April through July) and who have frequent or prolonged exposure to tick habitats (e.g., woods, thick brush, overgrown grassy areas).
   (2) Patients >15 years of age who reside in high to moderate risk areas during the transmission season and who have tick exposure that is neither frequent nor prolonged. In these cases, the vaccine is of uncertain benefit.
   (3) Those with a history of previous *uncomplicated* Lyme arthritis who are at continued risk.

3. Contraindications

a. The rOspA vaccine is not recommended for the following groups because safety and efficacy have not been established:

(1) Children <15 years of age.

(2) Pregnant women.

(3) Persons with immunodeficiency, musculoskeletal disease (e.g., rheumatoid arthritis, joint pain, diffuse musculoskeletal pain), second- or third-degree heart block, chronic joint or neurologic illness related to Lyme disease.

b. Persons with treatment-resistant Lyme arthritis should not be vaccinated because this condition is associated with increased reactivity to the OspA antigen used in the vaccine.

4. Side effects: Pain at the injection site (24%); local redness and swelling (<2%); myalgias, influenza-like illness, fever or chills in ≤3%.

5. Administration

a. Dose is 0.5 mL (30 mcg) rOspA IM.

b. Three doses given at 0, 1, and 12 months are recommended. For optimal protection, doses should be timed so that the second and third doses are given several weeks before the start of Lyme transmission season (usually in April).

c. Vaccine efficacy: For the LYMErix rOsp-A vaccine, protection against clinical Lyme disease was 49% after two doses and 76% after three doses. The duration of protective immunity is unknown, but data suggest that boosters beyond the third dose may be needed.

6. Special considerations

a. The risk of Lyme disease is greatly reduced by the use of tick repellents (e.g., those containing DEET), protective clothing (long-sleeve shirts and long pants, tucking pant legs into socks), and checking for and removing ticks. Transmission of disease requires 24 to 48 hours of tick attachment.

b. Early detection of Lyme disease is important because timely and correct antibiotic therapy nearly always results in a prompt cure.

c. Postexposure antibiotic prophylaxis in children with tick bites is not recommended.

d. Care providers should be aware that vaccine-induced antibodies to OspA antigen routinely cause falsely positive enzyme-linked immunosorbent assay (ELISA) results for Lyme disease. Careful interpretation of Western immunoblotting can usually discriminate between *B. burgdorferi* infection and rOspA immunization because most patients do not develop anti-OspA antibodies after natural infection.

G. MEASLES/MUMPS/RUBELLA IMMUNOPROPHYLAXIS

1. Description

a. MMR: Combined vaccine composed of live, attenuated viruses. Measles and mumps vaccines are grown in chick embryo cell culture; rubella vaccine is prepared in human diploid cell culture.

b. Monovalent measles, rubella, and measles/rubella (MR) formulations are available.

c. IG: Intramuscular IG and intravenous IG (IGIV) preparations contain similar concentration of measles antibody.

2. **Indications**

a. Routine: See Fig. 15-1.

b. Screen all women of child-bearing age for susceptibility. People are considered susceptible to rubella unless they have documentation of one dose of rubella-containing vaccine or serologic evidence of immunity. If susceptible, immunize with one dose of MMR unless pregnant.

3. **Contraindications**

a. Anaphylactic reaction to prior MMR, MR, or monovalent immunization.

b. Anaphylactic neomycin or gelatin allergy.

c. Immunocompromised states: See p. 319.

d. Pregnant women or women considering pregnancy within 3 months.

4. **Precautions**

a. Moderate or severe acute illness regardless of fever.

b. If a hypersensitivity reaction occurs after the first dose of vaccine, consider skin testing or checking antibody titers to determine if a second dose is needed.

c. Children with a history of thrombocytopenia may develop transient thrombocytopenia after immunization, but the vaccine benefits outweigh the risks.

d. See AAP's *Red Book* for suggested intervals between IG or blood product administration and immunization.

5. **Misconceptions:** The following are not contraindications to MMR administration:

a. Anaphylactic reaction to eggs: Consider observing patient for 90 minutes after vaccine administration. Skin testing is not predictive of hypersensitivity reaction and therefore is not recommended.

b. Allergy to penicillin.

c. Exposure to measles.

d. History of seizures: There is a slightly increased risk of seizure after immunization. Temperature should be followed and treated with antipyretics.

6. **Side effects**

a. Minor side effects 7 to 12 days after immunization: Fever to 39.4° C lasting 1 to 5 days (5% to 15%); transient rash (5%).

b. Moderate to severe side effects: Febrile seizures (rare); transient thrombocytopenia (1 in 25,000 to 1 in 40,000) 2 to 3 weeks after immunization; encephalitis and encephalopathy (<1 in 1 million).

7. **Administration**

a. Dose is 0.5 mL SC.

b. Immunize >2 weeks before planned administration of IG.

c. Purified protein derivative (PPD) testing may be done on the day of immunization; otherwise postpone PPD 4 to 6 weeks because of suppression of response.

8. Special considerations

a. Measles postexposure immunoprophylaxis.
   (1) Persons are susceptible to measles unless they have documentation of physician-diagnosed measles, have laboratory evidence of immunity, or had two doses of measles-containing vaccine after 12 months of age.
   (2) Vaccine prevents or modifies disease if given within 72 hours of exposure.
   (3) Immune globulin (IG) prevents or modifies disease if given within 6 days of exposure. Dosage is as follows:
      (a) Standard dose IG for children and pregnant women: 0.25 mL/kg (maximum dose 15 mL) IM.
      (b) High-dose IG for immunocompromised children: 0.5 mL/kg (maximum dose 15 mL) IM. Not required if IGIV received within 3 weeks before exposure.
   (4) Household contacts
      (a) Vaccine should be given to those with one prior dose of vaccine (do not require IG).
      (b) If contact is ≥5 months old and unimmunized, or <5 months old and mother is susceptible, IG should be given at time of exposure and measles vaccine should be given 5 months later. Two doses of measles-containing vaccine are still required after 12 months of age.
   (5) Community outbreak: Vaccine should be given to susceptible contacts ≥6 months old.
   (6) Immunocompromised individuals should receive IG.
   (7) Susceptible pregnant women should receive IG.

b. Rubella postexposure immunoprophylaxis: IG may modify rubella disease but does not prevent congenital rubella syndrome; therefore it is not recommended for exposed pregnant women.

H. MENINGOCOCCUS IMMUNOPROPHYLAXIS

1. Description: Quadrivalent serogroup-specific vaccine made from purified capsular polysaccharide antigen from groups A, C, Y, and W-135. Immunogenicity of serogroup antigens varies with age of child. No vaccine is available for group B because of poor immunogenicity.

2. Indications

a. High-risk children ≥2 years of age include the following:
   (1) Functional or anatomic asplenia.
   (2) Terminal complement or properdin deficiencies.

b. Possible adjunct to postexposure chemoprophylaxis in an outbreak setting.

c. Consider in college freshmen, particularly those living in dormitories or residence halls.

d. Travelers to endemic or hyperendemic areas.

3. **Contraindication:** Anaphylactic reaction to vaccine or vaccine constituent.
4. **Precaution:** Moderate or severe acute illness regardless of fever.
5. **Side effect:** Localized erythema for 1 to 2 days occurs infrequently.
6. **Administration:** Dose is 0.5 mL SC.
7. **Postexposure chemoprophylaxis:** Antibiotics should be given to exposed household, child care, and nursery school contacts within 24 hours of primary case diagnosis. Individuals with potential contact with oral secretions of infected patient should also receive chemoprophylaxis.
a. Rifampin is the drug of choice (see Chapter 26 for dosage information).
b. Ciprofloxacin (500 mg single dose) may be given to persons ≥18 years.
c. Ceftriaxone (125 mg single dose in children ≤12 years, 250 mg single dose in children >12 years) may be more efficacious than rifampin in reducing nasal carriage when exposed to group A meningococci.

I. PNEUMOCOCCUS IMMUNOPROPHYLAXIS

1. Description
a. PCV7: Pneumococcal conjugate vaccine includes seven purified capsular polysaccharides of *Streptococcus pneumoniae,* each coupled to a variant of diphtheria toxin. Serotypes are 4, 9V, 14, 19F, 23F, 18C, and 6B, which account for over 80% of bacteremia and meningitis and over 60% of acute otitis media (AOM) among children <6 years old.
b. 23PS: Purified capsular polysaccharide includes antigen from 23 serotypes of *S. pneumoniae*. 23PS is not approved for use in children <2 years.
c. Nine-valent and 11-valent conjugate vaccines may become available in the near future.

2. Indications
a. Routine: See Fig. 15-1.
b. See Table 15-3 for catch-up schedule for previously unvaccinated children ages 7 to 24 months.
c. See Table 15-6 for an immunization schedule of high-risk children ages 24 to 59 months, including those with the following conditions:
   (1) Sickle cell disease, functional or anatomic asplenia.
   (2) HIV infection.
   (3) Congenital immune deficiency.
   (4) Chronic renal insufficiency, including nephrotic syndrome.
   (5) Immunosuppression, including malignant neoplasms, leukemias, lymphomas, and Hodgkin's disease, and solid organ transplantation (guidelines for the use of pneumococcal vaccines for children who have received bone marrow transplants are currently undergoing revision).
   (6) Chronic cardiac disease.
   (7) Chronic pulmonary disease (including asthma treated with high-dose oral corticosteroid therapy).
   (8) Cerebrospinal fluid (CSF) leaks.
   (9) Diabetes mellitus.

15

IMMUNOPROPHYLAXIS

d. Consider immunization in the following children:
(1) All children ages 24 to 35 months.
(2) Children ages 36 to 59 months attending out-of-home care.
(3) Children ages 36 to 59 months who are of American Indian, Alaska Native, or African American descent.

3. **Contraindication:** Anaphylactic reaction to vaccine or vaccine constituent.

4. **Precautions**

a. Moderate or severe acute illness regardless of fever.

b. Generally defer during pregnancy because effect on the fetus is unknown; consider in mothers at high risk of severe pneumococcal disease.

5. **Side effects:** Pain and erythema at injection site (common); fever, fussiness, drowsiness, decreased appetite (less common); severe systemic reactions such as anaphylaxis (rare).

6. **Administration**

a. Dose of PCV7 is 0.5 mL IM.

b. Dose of 23PS is 0.5 mL IM or SC.

c. Concurrent administration of PCV7 and 23PS vaccines is not recommended. Either vaccine may be given concurrently with other vaccines in a separate syringe at a separate injection site.

d. Give vaccine 2 weeks or more before elective splenectomy, chemotherapy, radiotherapy, or immunosuppressive therapy; or give 3 months after chemotherapy or radiotherapy.

7. **Special considerations**

a. Passive immunoprophylaxis with IGIV is recommended for some children with congenital or acquired immune deficiencies.

b. See functional or anatomic asplenia, p. 320.

J. POLIOMYELITIS IMMUNOPROPHYLAXIS

1. **Description**

a. IPV: Trivalent enhanced-potency vaccine of formalin-inactivated poliovirus types 1, 2, and 3 grown in human diploid or Vero cells.

b. OPV: No longer available in the United States. Children who have received the appropriate number of doses of OPV in other countries should be considered adequately immunized.

2. **Indications**

a. Routine: See Fig. 15-1.

b. Unimmunized or partially immunized individuals who are at imminent risk of exposure to poliovirus (dose interval may be 4 weeks).

3. **Contraindications:** Anaphylaxis to vaccine, vaccine constituent, streptomycin, polymyxin B, or neomycin.

4. **Precautions**

a. Moderate or severe acute illness, regardless of fever.

b. Although there is no convincing evidence of adverse effects, immunization during pregnancy should be avoided for reasons of theoretical risk.

5. **Side effects:** No serious side effects have been associated with use of the IPV vaccine.
6. **Administration:** Dose is 0.5 mL SC.

K. RABIES IMMUNOPROPHYLAXIS (Table 15-13)

1. **Description**
   a. Human diploid cell vaccine (HDCV): Inactivated rabies virus grown in human diploid cell culture.
   b. Rhesus diploid cell vaccine, rabies vaccine adsorbed (RVA): Inactivated rabies virus grown in rhesus monkey fetal lung cell culture; adsorbed to aluminum salt.
   c. Human rabies immune globulin (RIG): Antirabies IG prepared from plasma of donors hyperimmunized with rabies vaccine.

2. **Indications**
   a. Preexposure prophylaxis: Indicated for high-risk groups, including veterinarians, animal handlers, laboratory workers, children living in high-risk environments, those traveling to high risk areas, spelunkers.
      (1) Three injections of vaccine on days 0, 7, and 21 or 28.
      (2) Rabies serum antibody titers should be followed at 6-month intervals for those at continuous risk and at 2-year intervals for those with risk of frequent exposure; give booster doses only if titers are nonprotective.
   b. Postexposure prophylaxis (see Table 15-13).

TABLE 15-13

RABIES POSTEXPOSURE PROPHYLAXIS

Animal Type	Evaluation and Disposition of Animal	Postexposure Prophylaxis Recommendations
Dogs, cats, ferrets	Healthy and available for 10 days observation	Do not begin prophylaxis unless animal develops symptoms of rabies
	Rabid or suspected rabid	Immediate immunization and RIG; euthanize animal and test brain
	Unknown (escaped)	Consult public health officials
Skunk, raccoon, bat,* fox, most other carnivores	Regard as rabid unless animal is euthanized and brain is negative for rabies by fluorescein antibody test	Immediate immunization and RIG†
Livestock, rodents, rabbit, other mammals	Consider individually	Consult public health officials; these bites rarely require treatment

Modified from American Academy of Pediatrics. 2000 Red book: report of the Committee on Infectious Diseases, 25th ed. Elk Grove Village, Ill: The Academy; 2000.
*In the case of direct contact between a human and a bat, consider prophylaxis even if a bite, scratch, or mucous membrane exposure is not apparent.
†Treatment may be discontinued if animal fluorescent antibody is negative.

15

IMMUNOPROPHYLAXIS

3. **Contraindication:** Anaphylactic reaction to vaccine or vaccine constituent.

NOTE: **If a patient has a serious allergic reaction to HDCV, RVA may be used instead.**

4. **Precaution:** Moderate or severe acute illness regardless of fever.
5. **Side effects (HDCV):** Local reactions (pain, erythema, swelling) in 25%, mild systemic reactions (headache, nausea, abdominal pain, muscle aches, dizziness) in 20%, neurologic illness similar to GBS or focal central nervous system (CNS) disorder (1 in 150,000), immune complex–like reaction (generalized urticaria, arthralgia, arthritis, angioedema, nausea, vomiting, fever, and malaise) 2 to 21 days after immunization, rare in primary series, 6% after booster dose.
6. **Administration:** Dose is 1 mL IM for HDCV and RVA.
7. **Postexposure prophylaxis**
a. General wound management
   (1) Clean immediately with soap and water.
   (2) Avoid suturing wound unless indicated for functional reasons.
   (3) Consider tetanus prophylaxis and antibiotics if indicated.
b. Indications: See Table 15-13. Infectious exposures include bites, scratches, or contamination of open wound or mucous membrane with infectious material of a rabid animal or human.

NOTE: **Report all patients suspected of rabies infection to public health authorities.**

c. Administration
   (1) Vaccine and RIG should be given jointly except in previously immunized patients (no RIG required).
   (2) Vaccine for postexposure prophylaxis
      (a) Either IM HDCV or RVA may be used, particularly if patient has severe allergy to one type; do not use intradermal HDCV.
      (b) Deltoid muscle except infants.
      (c) Routine serologic testing not indicated.
      (d) Unimmunized: 1 mL IM on days 0, 3, 7, 14, and 28.
      (e) Previously immunized: 1 mL IM on days 0 and 3. Do not give RIG.
   (3) RIG: Dose is 20 IU/kg. Infiltrate around the wound and give remainder IM.

L. RESPIRATORY SYNCYTIAL VIRUS (RSV) IMMUNOPROPHYLAXIS

1. **Description**
a. No vaccine is available.
b. Palivizumab (monoclonal RSV-IG): Humanized mouse monoclonal IgG to RSV, recombinantly produced for IM administration.
c. Polyclonal RSV-IGIV: IG pooled from donors with high serum titers of RSV-neutralizing antibody, for IV administration. Provides some protection against other respiratory viruses.
2. **Indications**
a. Infants and children <2 years with chronic lung disease (CLD) who

require oxygen within the 6 months before the RSV season. Palivizumab is preferred.

b. Infants <32 weeks' estimated gestational age (EGA) at birth who do not have CLD may benefit from prophylaxis with palivizumab.
   (1) EGA ≤28 weeks: Consider until 12 months of age.
   (2) EGA 29 to 32 weeks: Consider until 6 months of age.

c. Infants born between 32 and 35 weeks gestation with underlying conditions that predispose them to respiratory complications may benefit from prophylaxis. Because of the large number of patients in this group, prophylaxis should be administered on a case-by-case basis.

d. Children with severe immunodeficiency may benefit from RSV-IGIV, although its use has not been evaluated in randomized trials.

3. **Contraindications:** RSV-IGIV is contraindicated in cyanotic congenital heart disease. Palivizumab is also not recommended for children with cyanotic congenital heart disease. However, those with CLD or prematurity who meet the above criteria and who also have asymptomatic acyanotic heart disease (ventricular septal defect, patent ductus arteriosus) may benefit from palivizumab.

4. **Side effects**

a. Palivizumab: Side effects are comparable to placebo.

b. RSV-IGIV
   (1) Fever in 6% (2% in placebo group).
   (2) 8% of children with CLD required extra diuretics around the time of administration.

5. **Administration:** Give RSV-IGIV or palivizumab at onset of RSV season and then monthly during the RSV season. Consult the local health department for the optimal schedule.

a. Palivizumab: Dose is 15 mg/kg IM monthly.

b. Polyclonal RSV-IGIV: Dose is 15 mL/kg (750 mg/kg) IV monthly. Must defer MMR and varicella vaccines for 9 months after the last dose.

M. VARICELLA IMMUNOPROPHYLAXIS

1. **Description**

a. Vaccine: Cell-free live attenuated varicella virus vaccine.

b. Varicella-zoster immune globulin (VZIG): Prepared from plasma-containing high-titer antivaricella antibodies.

2. **Indications**

a. Routine: See Fig. 15-1.

b. Aim to immunize before the thirteenth birthday because two doses are needed after that time.

c. Serologic evaluation is optional before vaccination in healthy persons ≥13 years of age but unlikely to be cost effective. Children <13 years do not require serologic evaluation.

3. **Contraindications**

a. Anaphylactic reaction to vaccine, neomycin, or gelatin.

b. Patients with altered immunity: See p. 319.

c. Pregnancy.

15

IMMUNOPROPHYLAXIS

4. Precautions

a. Moderate to severe illness regardless of fever.

b. Patients on salicylate therapy. There is a theoretical risk of Reye syndrome after varicella immunization, although no cases have been reported. There is a known risk of developing Reye syndrome in children receiving long-term salicylate therapy who acquire the wild type virus.

c. Recent blood product or IG administration. Defer 9 months after RSV-IGIV and 5 months after all other blood products.

d. Family history of immunodeficiency.

5. Misconceptions: Vaccine **may** be given in the following circumstances:

a. Certain children with acute lymphoblastic leukemia in remission >1 year may be immunized under a research protocol. Approval must be obtained by the appropriate institutional review board.

b. Household contacts of immunocompromised hosts: If a rash develops in the immunized child, avoid direct contact if possible.

c. Household contacts of pregnant women.

6. Side effects

a. Local reaction, 20% to 35%; mild varicelliform rash within 5 to 26 days of vaccine administration, 3% to 5%; zosterlike illness, 18 cases per 100,000 person-years.

b. Vaccine rash often very mild, but patient may be infectious; reversion to wild-type virus has not been reported.

7. Administration

a. Dose is 0.5 mL SC.

b. May give simultaneously with MMR; otherwise, allow at least 1 month between MMR and varicella vaccines.

c. Do not give for 5 months after VZIG; do not give concurrently.

d. Avoid salicylates for 6 weeks after vaccine administration if possible.

8. Postexposure prophylaxis

a. Indications: VZIG should be administered within 96 hours of exposure to individuals who are at high risk for severe varicella and who have had a significant exposure (see below). Repeat VZIG every 3 weeks if exposure is ongoing or repeated.

   (1) Individuals at high risk for severe varicella include the following:

      (a) Immunocompromised individuals without a history of varicella.

      (b) Susceptible pregnant women.

      (c) Newborn infant with onset of varicella in mother from 5 days before to 2 days after delivery (even if mother received VZIG during pregnancy).

      (d) Hospitalized preterm infant who was born at <28 weeks gestation or who weighs <1000 g, regardless of maternal history.

      (e) Hospitalized preterm infant who was born at ≥28 weeks gestation to a susceptible mother.

   (2) Significant exposures include the following:

      (a) Household contact.

      (b) Face-to-face indoor play.

(c) Onset of varicella in the mother of a newborn from 5 days before to 2 days after delivery.

(d) Hospital exposures: Roommate, face-to-face contact with infectious individual, visit by contagious individual, or intimate contact with person with active zoster lesions.

NOTE: **For VZIG recipients, incubation period may be up to 28 days instead of 21 days.**

b. VZIG dose is 12.5 U/kg IM (maximum dose 625 U; minimum dose 125 U). Do not give IV. Local discomfort is common.

c. Varicella vaccine should be administered to susceptible children (except those with significant immune compromise as per p. 320) within 72 hours after varicella exposure. If the child was exposed at the same time as the index case, the vaccine may not protect against the disease.

REFERENCE

1. Centers for Disease Control and Prevention. Guidelines for preventing opportunistic infections among hematopoietic stem cell transplant recipients: recommendations of CDC, the Infectious Disease Society of America, and the American Society of Blood and Marrow Transplantation. MMWR 2000; 49(No. RR-10):1-147.

15

IMMUNOPROPHYLAXIS

MICROBIOLOGY AND INFECTIOUS DISEASE

Laurel Bell, MD and Shilpa Hattangadi, MD

I. MICROBIOLOGY

A. COLLECTION OF SPECIMENS

1. **Preparation:** Proper specimen collection is essential to minimize contamination. Clean venipuncture site with 70% isopropyl ethyl alcohol. Apply tincture of iodine or 10% povidone-iodine and allow to dry for at least 1 minute. Clean blood culture bottle injection site with alcohol only.
2. **Collection:** Obtain 1 to 2 mL for a neonate, 2 to 3 mL for an infant, 3 to 5 mL for a child, and 10 to 20 mL for an adolescent.

B. RAPID MICROBIOLOGIC IDENTIFICATION OF COMMON AEROBIC BACTERIA (Fig. 16-1)

C. CHOOSING APPROPRIATE ANTIBIOTIC BASED ON SENSITIVITIES

1. Definitions[1,2]
   a. Minimum inhibitory concentration (MIC): The lowest concentration of an antimicrobial agent that prevents visible growth after an 18- to 24-hour incubation period.
   b. Minimum bactericidal concentration (MBC): The lowest concentration of an antimicrobial agent that kills >99.9% of organisms, as measured by subculturing to antibiotic-free media after 18- to 24-hour incubation.
2. **Common pitfalls:** See Table 16-1 for clinically significant, common discrepancies between in vitro (laboratory reported) and in vivo antibiotic sensitivity profiles.

II. INFECTIOUS DISEASE

A. FEVER EVALUATION AND MANAGEMENT GUIDELINES (Figs. 16-2 and 16-3)

B. COMMON PEDIATRIC INFECTIONS: GUIDELINES FOR INITIAL MANAGEMENT (Table 16-2)

C. CONGENITAL INFECTIONS

1. **Intrauterine infections:** TORCH infections (**T**oxoplasmosis; **O**thers such as syphilis, varicella-zoster,* and other viruses; **R**ubella; **C**ytomegalovirus [CMV]; and **H**erpes simplex virus [HSV*]) often present in the neonate with similar findings: intrauterine growth retardation (IUGR), microcephaly, hepatosplenomegaly, rash, central nervous system [CNS] manifestations, early jaundice, and low platelets.[5] Table 16-3 helps differentiate possible infections based on frequency of symptoms. Initial evaluation of a neonate depends on level of suspicion and severity of

Text continued on p. 354

---

*HSV and varicella-zoster virus (VZV) usually present as perinatal infections, and rarely as an intrauterine infection. See p. 355 for descriptions.

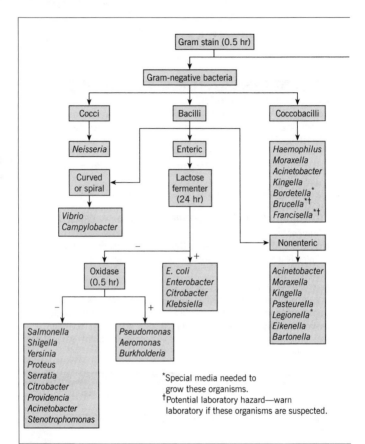

FIG. 16-1

Algorithm demonstrating identification of aerobic bacteria. Numbers in parentheses indicate the time required for the tests.

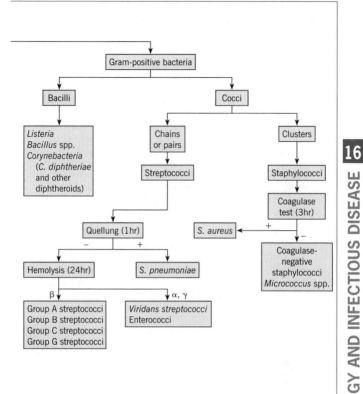

TABLE 16-1

COMMON PITFALLS BETWEEN IN VITRO AND IN VIVO ANTIBIOTIC
SENSITIVITY PROFILES

Bacteria	Pitfall
Staphylococci	If a Staphylococcus is more than two dilutions more sensitive to a first-generation cephalosporin than to a "staphylococcal penicillin" (e.g., oxacillin), suspect that the organism is methicillin-resistant *Staphylococcus aureus*, and consider using vancomycin rather than cephalosporins or other β-lactams.[2]
Salmonella	Despite in vitro susceptibility to aminoglycosides, salmonella are not susceptible in vivo to this class of antibiotics.
Enterobacter spp. Citrobacter spp. *Pseudomonas aeruginosa* Serratia spp. Providencia spp.	All are inducibly resistant to all cephalosporins; therefore cephalosporins should not be used as sole treatment for invasive or serious infections caused by these organisms. Because β-lactamase inhibitors are potent inducers of cephalosporin resistance, and they do not overcome resistance in these organisms, β-lactamase inhibitors should not be used.[3]
Pseudomonas and related species: *P. aeruginosa* Acinetobacter spp. *Burkholderia cepacia* *Stenotrophomonas maltophilia*	Burkholderia and Stenotrophomonas are resistant to aminoglycosides and often are only susceptible to TMP-SMX, the drug of choice in most cases for these organisms. *P. aeruginosa* and Acinetobacter spp, on the other hand, are usually susceptible to aminoglycosides, but resistant to TMP-SMX (despite reported in vitro susceptibility).
Enterococci	Intrinsic resistance to most antibiotic classes necessitates double-agent therapy for synergy and bacterial killing in the treatment of invasive infections. Recommended therapy is ampicillin (vancomycin if ampicillin-resistant). Add an aminoglycoside (preferably gentamicin; streptomycin also active) for serious invasive infections. Other antibiotics with activity against enterococci include amoxicillin, penicillin, piperacillin, and imipenem. Vancomycin-resistant enterococcus (VRE) is usually *Enterococcus faecium*, though rarely *E. faecalis*. Linezolid is active against most enterococcal isolates, including VRE. Quinupristin/dalfopristin (Synercid) is active against most *E. faecium*, including VRE, but not against *E. faecalis*. The following antibiotics are **not** clinically active against enterococci: all cephalosporins, antistaphylococcal penicillins (e.g., oxacillin), macrolides, clindamycin, and quinolones.

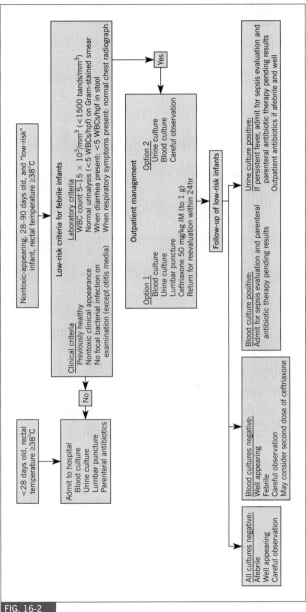

FIG. 16-2

Algorithm for the management of a previously healthy infant <90 days of age with a fever without localizing signs. *hpf,* High-power field. This algorithm is a suggested, but not exhaustive approach to management. *(Modified from Baraff LJ et al. Ann Emerg Med 2000; 36(6):602-614.)*

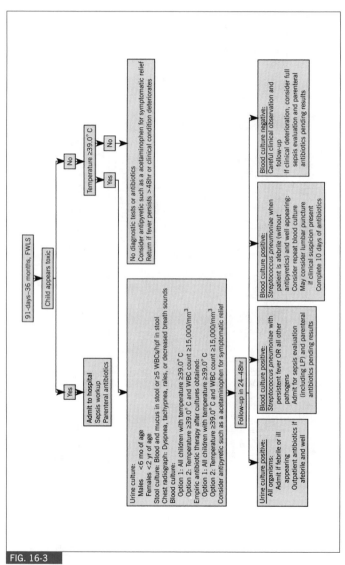

FIG. 16-3

Algorithm for the management of a previously healthy child 91 days to 36 months of age with a fever without localizing signs (FWLS). This algorithm is a suggested, but not exhaustive approach to management. *(Modified from Baraff LK et al. Pediatrics 1993; 92:5-9.)*

TABLE 16-2
COMMON PEDIATRIC INFECTIONS: GUIDELINES FOR INITIAL MANAGEMENT

Infectious Syndrome	Usual Etiology	Suggested Empiric Therapy	Suggested Length of Therapy/Comments
Bacteremia (outpatient)	Streptococcus pneumoniae, Haemophilus influenzae, Neisseria meningitidis, Escherichia coli, Salmonella	Empiric: Ceftriaxone.	7-10 days (longer for some pathogens). Occult bacteremia with susceptible S. pneumoniae may be treated with amoxicillin if afebrile, well, and without focal complications.
Bites			
Human	Streptococci, Staphylococcus aureus, Staphylococcus epidermidis, anaerobes, Eikenella corrodens	PO: Amoxicillin/clavulanate. Alt: TMP/SMX + clindamycin. IV: Ampicillin/sulbactam.	5-7 days. Cleaning, irrigation, and debridement most important. Assess tetanus immunization status, risk of hepatitis B and HIV. Antibiotic prophylaxis routinely used for human bites.
Dog/cat	Human bite pathogens plus Pasteurella multocida	Same.	7-10 days. Assess tetanus immunization status, risk of rabies. Antibiotic prophylaxis for all cat bites and selected dog bites.
Cellulitis	GAS, S. aureus	PO: Cephalexin. If penicillin allergic, clindamycin or macrolide. IV: Oxacillin. Alt: Clindamycin.	3 days after acute inflammation resolves (usually 7-10 days).
Conjunctivitis			
Neonatal	Chlamydia trachomatis	PO: Erythromycin, other macrolides.	14 days. Topical ineffective in preventing pneumonia.
	Neisseria gonorrhoeae	IM/IV: Ceftriaxone, cefotaxime.	Localized to eye: Single dose. Disseminated: 7 days of parenteral therapy.
Suppurative	S. pneumoniae, H. influenzae, S. aureus	Ophthalmic; erythromycin or bacitracin/polymyxin B, or polymyxin B/TMP.	5 days. Ointments preferred for infants or young children and eyedrops for older children and adolescents.

cont'd

16

MICROBIOLOGY AND INFECTIOUS DISEASE

TABLE 16-2

COMMON PEDIATRIC INFECTIONS: GUIDELINES FOR INITIAL MANAGEMENT—cont'd

Infectious Syndrome	Usual Etiology	Suggested Empiric Therapy	Suggested Length of Therapy/Comments
Gastroenteritis			
Community acquired	Viruses, *Escherichia coli*	Antibiotic therapy strongly discouraged because of increased risk of hemolytic-uremic syndrome occurring in patients with *E. coli* O157:H7 treated with antibiotics.[4]	Primary treatment: fluid and electrolyte replacement.
	Salmonella	Cefotaxime or ceftriaxone.	10-14 days for infants <6 mo, toxicity or immunocompromised status. Antibiotics generally not indicated otherwise.
	Shigella	TMP/SMX. Alt: Cefixime.	5 days.
	Yersinia	TMP/SMX, aminoglycosides, cefotaxime, tetracycline (>8 yr).	Usually no antibiotic therapy is recommended except with bacteremia, extraintestinal infections, or immunocompromised hosts.
Nosocomial	*Clostridium difficile*	Metronidazole.	7 days. Community organisms unlikely after 72 hr of hospitalization.
Mastoiditis (acute)	*S. pneumoniae, Streptococcus pyogenes, S. aureus, H. influenzae*	Oxacillin plus cefotaxime or ceftriaxone. Alt: Amoxicillin/clavulanic acid.	10 days.
Meningitis			
Neonate <1 mo	GBS, Enterobacteriaceae, *Listeria monocytogenes*	Ampicillin and cefotaxime. Alt: Ampicillin and gentamicin	14-21 days for GBS and *Listeria*. 21 days for Enterobacteriaceae (cefotaxime, aminoglycoside).

1-3 mo	GBS, S. pneumoniae, H. influenzae, N. meningitidis, Enterobacteriaceae	Ampicillin and cefotaxime.	10-14 days for S. pneumoniae, 7 days for N. meningitidis, 7-10 days for H. influenzae.
Infants >3 mo and children	S. pneumoniae, N. meningitidis, H. influenzae, neonatal pathogens	Cefotaxime or ceftriaxone. Vancomycin should be also added empirically for possible penicillin-resistant S. pneumoniae, until susceptibility is known.	Dexamethasone before antibiotics recommended for infants and children >6 wk with Hib meningitis. Dexamethasone treatment is otherwise controversial. See Red Book[8] for chemoprophylaxis recommendations for contacts of meningococcal and Hib disease.
Orbital cellulitis	S. pneumoniae, H. influenzae, Moraxella catarrhalis, S. aureus, GAS, anaerobes	Cefotaxime or ceftriaxone plus clindamycin.	10 days. Monitor for cavernous thrombosis.
Osteomyelitis	S. aureus, GAS	Semisynthetic penicillin (oxacillin, nafcillin). Alt: Clindamycin.	4-6 wk.
<5 yr	Add Hib	Add cefotaxime.	
Foot puncture	Add Pseudomonas	Add ceftazidime.	
Sickle cell disease	Add Salmonella	Add cefotaxime.	
Otitis media (acute)	S. pneumoniae, H. influenzae (nontypeable), M. catarrhalis	Firstline: Amoxicillin or high-dose amoxicillin (80-100 mg/kg/day). Alt for penicillin allergy: Cefuroxime, cefdinir, cefprozil, azithromycin. Persistent otitis media: Amoxicillin/clavulanic acid, cefuroxime, or ceftriaxone (IM/IV).	5-10 days. For persistent otitis media (at 2-3 days' follow-up) despite antibiotic therapy, consider tympanocentesis (see p. 72). Short course 5-7 days for >2 yr old without language or hearing deficit.
Otitis externa (uncomplicated)	Pseudomonas, Enterobacteriaceae, Proteus	Eardrops: Polymyxin B/neomycin/hydrocortisone. Alt: Ofloxacin drops.	7-10 days.

cont'd

16

MICROBIOLOGY AND INFECTIOUS DISEASE

TABLE 16-2
COMMON PEDIATRIC INFECTIONS: GUIDELINES FOR INITIAL MANAGEMENT—cont'd

Infectious Syndrome	Usual Etiology	Suggested Empiric Therapy	Suggested Length of Therapy/Comments
Periorbital cellulitis (preseptal)	Associated with sinusitis: See sinusitis	IV: Oxacillin + cefotaxime. PO: Amoxicillin/clavulanate.	10-14 days.
	Associated with skin lesion: See cellulitis		
	Hematogenous (<2 yr): See bacteremia		
Pharyngitis	GAS	PO: Penicillin VK. IM: Benzathine penicillin G × 1 dose. Alt: Erythromycin, cephalexin.	10 days. TMP/SMX **not** effective. 10 days.
Pneumonia			
Neonatal	E. coli, GBS, S. aureus, Listeria monocytogenes	Ampicillin + gentamicin or ampicillin + cefotaxime.	10-21 days. Blood cultures indicated. Effusions should be drained, Gram's stain of fluid obtained.
3 wk-4 mo	Chlamydia trachomatis	Erythromycin. Alt: Clarithromycin.	10 days.
Infant/child (6 wk-4 yr) Lobar	S. pneumoniae	PO: Amoxicillin. Alt: Clindamycin. IV: Cefuroxime, ceftriaxone, cefotaxime.	7-10 days.
Atypical	Bordetella pertussis	Erythromycin (estolate preparation preferred) or clarithromycin.	14 days. Chemoprophylaxis indicated for close contacts.
	Respiratory viruses	No antibiotics indicated.	
	Influenza	Zanamivir or oseltamivir	Reduces symptoms notably if given within 36 hours after onset of symptoms.

≥4 yr			
Lobar	S. pneumoniae	PO: Amoxicillin. Alt: Erythromycin. IV: Cefuroxime, ceftriaxone, or cefotaxime PLUS PO/IV macrolide. Clarithromycin. Azithromycin.	7-10 days. 10 days. 5 days.
Atypical	Mycoplasma pneumoniae or Chlamydia pneumoniae	Erythromycin, clarithromycin, azithromycin, or tetracycline (>8 yr).	14-21 days (5 days if using azithromycin).
	Influenza	Zanamivir or oseltamivir.	See comments above.
Septic arthritis			
<5 yr	S. aureus, GBS, Hib	See osteomyelitis.	3-4 wk IV. May switch to PO after response.
>5 yr	S. aureus, GAS		Aspiration of affected joint recommended.
Adolescent	Add Neisseria gonorrhoeae	See p. 365.	
Sinusitis			
Acute	S. pneumoniae, H. influenzae, M. catarrhalis	See otitis media.	10-14 days.
Chronic	Add S. aureus, anaerobes	Amoxicillin/clavulanate or cefpodoxime.	21 days.
UTI			
Uncomplicated	E. coli, Proteus Enterococci	PO: TMP/SMX, cefixime. IV: Cefixime, cefotaxime **or** ampicillin and gentamicin.	7-21 days (cystitis vs. pyelonephritis and age dependent).
Abnormal host/ urinary tract	Add Pseudomonas	Ceftazidime.	14-21 days. Parenteral until afebrile ×24 hr.
Ventriculoperitoneal shunt, infected	S. epidermidis, S. aureus, Enterobacteriaceae	Vancomycin + cefotaxime or ceftriaxone. Add aminoglycoside for Enterobacteriaceae. Consider adding rifampin.	21 days. Shunt removal or revision may be necessary.

Alt, Alternative; GAS, group A streptococci; GBS, group B streptococci; Hib, Haemophilus influenzae type b; TMP/SMX, trimethoprim-sulfamethoxazole.

MICROBIOLOGY AND INFECTIOUS DISEASE

16

TABLE 16-3

FREQUENCY OF CLINICAL FINDINGS IN INFANTS WITH CONGENITAL INFECTIONS

Clinical Findings	Rubella	Toxoplasma	CMV	Syphilis	HSV
Intrauterine growth retardation	+++	±	++	++	±
Reticuloendothelial system					
Jaundice	+	++	+++	+++	+
Hepatitis	±	+	+++	+++	+
Hepatosplenomegaly	+++	++	+++	+++	+
Anemia	+	+++	++	+++	−
Thrombocytopenia	++	±	+++	++	+
Disseminated intravascular coagulation	−	−	±	−	++
Adenopathy	++	++	−	++	−
Dermal erythropoiesis	+	−	+	−	−
Skin rash	−	+	−	++	+++
Bone abnormalities	++	−	±	++	−
Eye					
Cataracts	++	±	±	±	−
Retinopathy	++	+++	+	±	+++
Microphthalmia	+	±	±	−	±
Central nervous system					
Microcephaly	+	+	++	−	±
Meningoencephalitis	++	+++	+++	++	+++
Brain calcification	±	++	++	−	+
Hydrocephalus	−	++	±	±	++
Hearing defect	+++	+	+++	+	−
Pneumonitis	++	+	±	+	±
Cardiovascular					
Myocarditis	+	±	±	±	−
Congenital defect	+++	−	−	−	−

From McMillan JA et al, editors. Oski's pediatrics: principles and practice, 3rd ed. Lippincott Williams and Wilkins; 1999.

±, rare; +, 5% to 20%; ++, 20% to 50%; +++, more than 50%; □, prominent feature of particular infection; *CMV,* cytomegalovirus; *HSV,* herpes simplex virus.

clinical findings.[6] Consider head CT or head ultrasound (intracerebral calcifications), long bone films (metaphyseal abnormalities), ophthalmologic examination (keratoconjunctivitis and chorioretinitis), brainstem evoked responses for hearing evaluation, blood, urine and cerebrospinal fluid (CSF) evaluation (cultures, serology, counts) as part of initial investigation. See Table 16-4 for specific diagnostic criteria and therapy for the most common intrauterine infections.

2. **Group B streptococcal (GBS) infection**
a. Presentation
(1) Early-onset disease (<7 days old): respiratory distress, apnea, shock, pneumonia, and meningitis.

     (2) Late-onset disease (1 week to 3 months): Bacteremia, meningitis, osteomyelitis, septic arthritis, and cellulitis.

b. Maternal intrapartum antibiotic prophylaxis (IAP): The chemoprophylaxis regimen is ampicillin or penicillin; use clindamycin if patient is allergic to penicillin. IAP is recommended for women with vaginal/anorectal screening cultures positive for GBS at 3 to 37 weeks gestation, or one or more of the following risk factors:

     (1) Previous infant with invasive disease.

     (2) GBS bacteriuria during pregnancy.

     (3) Delivery at <37 weeks gestation.

     (4) Ruptured membranes for >18 hours.

     (5) Intrapartum temperature >38° C (100.4° F).

     (6) Unknown GBS status.

c. Management of neonates: Fig. 16-4 shows the management of neonates born to mothers for whom intrapartum prophylaxis of GBS is indicated.

d. Treatment of neonatal GBS disease: Benzylpenicillin or ampicillin, plus an aminoglycoside (usually gentamicin). Duration of therapy depends on extent of disease.

3. Perinatal viral infections

a. Varicella-zoster: If a mother develops varicella from 5 days before to 2 days after delivery, varicella infection in the infant can be fatal. Neonates usually look well at birth, then develop vesicles between 3 to 10 days of life. Dissemination can result in pneumonitis, encephalitis, purpura fulminans, widespread bleeding, hypotension, and death. If mother develops varicella more than 5 days before delivery and infant's gestational age is more than 28 weeks, severity of disease tends to be milder secondary to transplacental transfer of antibody.[9] See Table 16-4 for diagnosis and treatment.

b. Herpes simplex virus: Neonatal infections with HSV are often severe, with high mortality and morbidity rates despite therapy. HSV infection can present as (1) disseminated disease with lung and severe liver disease, (2) localized CNS infection, or (3) disease localized to skin, eye, mouth (SEM). Initial symptoms can occur any time in the first 4 weeks of life. Disseminated disease often occurs in the first week of life. CNS disease presents latest, often in the second or third week of life.[8] See Table 16-4 for diagnosis and treatment.

c. Enterovirus: Neonates that develop enterovirus infections can develop severe disease with major systemic manifestations (hepatic necrosis, myocarditis, encephalitis, pneumonia, necrotizing enterocolitis [NEC], and disseminated intravascular coagulation [DIC]) mimicking overwhelming bacterial infection. Death is typically caused by hepatic failure or myocarditis.[7] See Table 16-4 for diagnosis and treatment.

4. Hydrops fetalis: Infectious causes of hydrops account for 8% of all cases; the most common causes of nonimmune hydrops fetalis are parvovirus B19, CMV, HSV, *Toxoplasmosis gondii,* and *Treponema pallidum.* Less common agents include enterovirus, adenovirus, rubella,

TABLE 16-4

DIAGNOSTIC CRITERIA AND THERAPY FOR COMMON INTRAUTERINE AND PERINATAL INFECTIONS

Disease	Diagnostic Criteria	Therapy
Cytomegalovirus (CMV)	CMV IgM from serum, CMV culture and early antigen from urine between 2 days and 1 week of age.	Treatment of symptomatic infants with ganciclovir is under investigation.
Enterovirus	Cultures from throat, stool, rectal swab; CSF for culture and PCR.	IVIG Pleconaril is an orally active agent that promises safe and effective treatment of severe enteroviral illness in neonates and other age groups.[7] It is currently available on a compassionate care basis from the manufacturer, Viropharma in Exton, PA (610) 217-7541 or www.questions@viropharma.com.
Hepatitis B	Check maternal HepBsAg status. If a HepBsAg positive mother is also HepBeAg positive, infant has a 90% chance of acquiring chronic hepatitis B infection if not given appropriate prophylaxis.	See Chapter 15 for initial management. To monitor success of efforts to prevent perinatal transmission of HBV, obtain HepBsAg and anti-HBs 1-3 months after completion of Hep B series (series should be at birth, 1 mo, 6 mo). If HepBsAg is negative on follow-up, but anti-HBs concentration is <10 mIU/mL, infant should repeat vaccine series (0, 1, and 6 mo) with testing of anti-HBs 1 mo after series.
Hepatitis C	Check maternal HepC antibody status. If possible check infant's HepC Ab status at 1 yr of age. If symptomatic, however, and earlier diagnosis needed, HCV PCR or HCV RNA can be checked at 1-2 mo of age.	No therapy until HCV status ascertained at 1 yr of life. Treatment with interferon α and ribavirin is under investigation.
Herpes simplex virus (HSV)	HSV culture of blood, urine, stool, CSF, and skin vesicles. Also HSV surface cultures from conjunctiva, nasopharynx, mouth and rectum. Surface cultures obtained before 24-48 hr of life may indicate colonization from intrapartum exposure, without infection. Positive cultures obtained from any of these sites >48 hr after birth indicate viral replication suggestive of infection.[8]	Parenteral acyclovir 45-60 mg/kg/day divided by Q8 hours for 14 days if only SEM disease; give 60 mg/kg/day for 21 days if CNS or disseminated disease. Infants with ocular involvement should also get topical ophthalmologic drug (1%-2% trifluridine, 1% iododeoxyuridine, or 3% vidarabine).

HIV	See Section E, p. 359.
Parvovirus	Parvovirus PCR and IgM antibody from serum.	Intrauterine blood transfusions may be indicated in selected cases. Infant treatment is supportive.
Rubella	Rubella virus can usually be obtained from nasal specimens. Throat swabs, blood, urine, and CSF can also yield virus. Check serum for rubella IgM.[9] Knowledge of maternal rubella immune status at onset of pregnancy is the most helpful piece of information. If checked late in pregnancy, infection early in pregnancy cannot be excluded.	Postexposure prophylaxis with immunoglobulin is not routinely recommended. Mothers with nonimmune status should be vaccinated in the immediate postpartum period, even if breast-feeding.
Syphilis	See pp. 358-359.	
Toxoplasmosis	*Prenatal diagnosis:* A definitive diagnosis can be made by detecting either the parasite in fetal blood or amniotic fluid, or documenting *Toxoplasmosis gondii* IgM or IgA antibody in fetal blood. *T. gondii* DNA by PCR from amniotic fluid also can be valid. *Postnatal diagnosis:* Attempts should be made to isolate *T. gondii* from placenta, umbilical cord, or assay for *T. gondii* by PCR from peripheral blood, CSF, and amniotic fluid. A positive IgM or IgA within 6 mo of life, or persistently positive IgG titers beyond 1 yr of life can also be diagnostic.	Treatment indicated for chorioretinitis or significant organ damage. Pyrimethamine in combination with sulfadiazine is synergistic against *T. gondii.*
Varicella (VZV)	Direct fluorescent antigen (DFA) from vesicle scraping is rapid and sensitive. VZV PCR from body fluid or tissue is also very sensitive. Virus may be cultured from vesicle base during first 3-4 days of eruption, but it can be difficult to distinguish VZV from HSV.	*Maternal:* Acyclovir may be beneficial during pregnancy. VZIG after exposure for susceptible pregnant women is recommended. *Infant:* VZIG immediately if maternal rash develops between 5 days before and 2 days after birth. Acyclovir if neonate develops varicella.

16

MICROBIOLOGY AND INFECTIOUS DISEASE

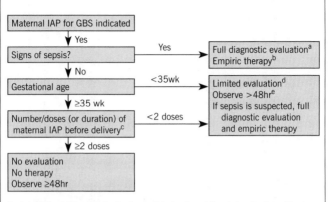

a Includes CBC and differential, blood culture, and chest radiograph if respiratory symptoms. A lumbar puncture is performed at the discretion of the physician.
b Duration of therapy will vary depending on results of blood culture and CSF findings (if obtained), as well as on the clinical course of the infant. *If* laboratory results and clinical course are unremarkable, duration may be as short as 48–72hr.
c Applies to penicillin or ampicillin chemoprophylaxis.
d CBC and differential, blood culture.
e Does not allow early discharge.

FIG. 16-4

Empiric management of neonate born to a mother who received intrapartum antimicrobial prophylaxis (IAP) to prevent early onset GBS disease. This algorithm is a suggested but not exclusive approach to management. *(From American Academy of Pediatrics, Committee on Infectious Diseases and Committee on Fetus and Newborn. Pediatrics 1997; 99:493.)*

polio, influenza B, respiratory syncytial virus (RSV), *Listeria*, *Leptospira*, *Trypanosoma cruzii*, *Chlamydia*, and *Ureaplasma ureolyticum*.[10] Specific serology or cultures for the more common etiologic agents is indicated when hydrops is identified by ultrasound. See respective sections for appropriate diagnostic work-up.

5. Congenital syphilis
a. Testing during pregnancy: All pregnant women should be screened with a nontreponemal antibody test (Venereal Disease Research Laboratory [VDRL] test or Rapid Plasma Reagin [RPR] test) early in pregnancy and preferably again at delivery. In areas of high prevalence and in patients considered high risk, a test early in the third trimester is also indicated. Positive screening for RPR or VDRL should be confirmed with a treponemal antibody test (FTA). If there is evidence of infection, treatment is indicated, and serologies (RPR or VDRL titers) should be followed to assess effectiveness of therapy.

b. Evaluation of infants
   (1) No newborn should be discharged from the hospital without determining the mother's serologic status for syphilis. Testing of cord blood or infant serum is not adequate for screening.
   (2) An infant should be evaluated for congenital syphilis if he or she is born to a mother who has a positive nontreponemal test, confirmed by a positive treponemal test, and who has one or more of the following:
       (a) Was not treated.
       (b) Had treatment but course was poorly documented.
       (c) Received inadequate doses or duration of treatment.
       (d) Was treated with nonpenicillin regimen (e.g., erythromycin).
       (e) Was treated less than 1 month before delivery.
       (f) Had insufficient serologic follow-up to ensure that she responded appropriately to treatment by demonstrating a fourfold or greater decrease in titers in 3 months after course of treatment.
   (3) Further evaluation of infants with the preceding conditions should include the following:
       (a) Physical examination (e.g., rash [vesiculobullous], hepatomegaly, generalized lymphadenopathy, persistent rhinitis).
       (b) Quantitative nontreponemal test on infant's serum. (Cord blood not adequate).
       (c) Examine CSF for protein, cell count, and VDRL test. CSF VDRL is specific but NOT sensitive. (Do not perform RPR or FTA-ABS test [fluorescent treponemal antibody absorption] on CSF.)
       (d) Radiologic studies: Long bone films for diaphyseal periostitis, osteochondritis.
       (e) If available, antitreponemal IgM via a testing method recognized by the CDC either as a standard or provisional method.
       (f) Other tests as clinically indicated (e.g., chest radiograph, complete blood count [CBC], liver function tests [LFTs]).
   (4) Guide for interpretation of the syphilis serology of mothers and their infants[8] (Table 16-5).
   (5) Treatment of neonates with proven or possible congenital syphilis (Table 16-6): Follow nontreponemal serologic tests at 3, 6, and 12 months after treatment. See Table 16-7 for guidance in interpreting follow-up serology.
   (6) Treatment of syphilis (postneonatal) (Table 16-8).

D. SELECTED SEXUALLY TRANSMITTED DISEASES
1. Pelvic inflammatory disease (PID) (Table 16-9).
2. Therapy for chlamydia, gonorrhea, and PID (Table 16-10).

E. HUMAN IMMUNODEFICIENCY VIRUS (HIV) AND ACQUIRED IMMUNODEFICIENCY SYNDROME (AIDS)
For the most recent information on the diagnosis and management of children with HIV infection, check the recommendations at **http://www.hivatis.org/.**

TABLE 16-5				

GUIDE FOR INTERPRETATION OF THE SYPHILIS SEROLOGY OF MOTHERS AND THEIR INFANTS

Nontreponemal Test (e.g., VDRL, RPR, ART)		Treponemal Test (e.g., MHA-TP, FTA-ABS)		
Mother	Infant	Mother	Infant	Interpretation*
−	−	−	−	No syphilis or incubating syphilis in the mother and infant
+	+	−	−	No syphilis in mother (false-positive nontreponemal test with passive transfer to infant)†
+	+ or −	+	+	Maternal syphilis with possible infant infection; or mother treated for syphilis during pregnancy; or mother with latent syphilis and possible infection of infant‡
+	+	+	+	Recent or previous syphilis in the mother; possible infection in infant
−	−	+	+	Mother successfully treated for syphilis before or early in pregnancy; or mother with Lyme disease, yaws, or pinta (i.e., false-positive serology)†

Modified from Pickering LK, editor. 2000 Red book: report of the Committee on Infectious Diseases, 25th ed. Elk Grove Village, Ill: American Academy of Pediatrics; 2000.

ART, automated reagin test; *MHA-TP,* microhemagglutination test for *T. pallidum.*

*Table presents a guide and not the definitive interpretation of serologic tests for syphilis in mothers and their newborns. Other factors that should be considered include the timing of maternal infection, the nature and timing of maternal treatment, quantitative maternal and infant titers, and serial determination of nontreponemal test titers in both mother and infant.

†False positive nontreponemal reagin tests can occur with acute bacterial or viral infections, early HIV infection, vaccination, and a variety of autoimmune diseases. Some illnesses (e.g., systemic lupus erythematosus) can also give false positive treponemal tests. Other spirochetal illnesses (relapsing fever, yaws, pinta, leptospirosis, rat bite fever) can also yield both positive nontreponemal and treponemal tests. Lyme disease gives a false ⊕ FTA-ABS, but a negative nontreponemal test.[2]

‡Mothers with latent syphilis may have nonreactive nontreponemal tests.

1. **Counseling and testing:** Legal requirements vary by state. Counseling includes informed consent for testing, implications of positive test results, and prevention of transmission. All pregnant women should be offered counseling and testing, regardless of risk factors, so they can make an informed decision regarding therapy aimed at reducing transmission to their infants. When maternal HIV status has not been determined before or immediately after delivery, newborns should undergo HIV testing after counseling and consent of the mother (unless state law allows testing without consent).

2. **Diagnosis of HIV in children**

TABLE 16-6

TREATMENT OF NEONATES WITH PROVEN OR POSSIBLE CONGENITAL SYPHILIS

Clinical Status	Antimicrobial Therapy[a]
Proven or highly probable disease[b]	Aqueous crystalline penicillin G 50,000 U/kg/dose IV Q12hr for the first week, then Q8hr for a total course of 10-14 days[c,d]
Asymptomatic, normal CSF and radiologic examination—maternal treatment history:	
• None, inadequate penicillin treatment,[e] undocumented, failed, or reinfected	Aqueous crystalline penicillin G IV for 10-14 days[c,d] (see dosing above) **or** Clinical, serologic follow-up and benzathine penicillin G 50,000 U/kg IM, single dose[f]
• Adequate therapy but given <1 mo before delivery, mother's response to treatment not demonstrated by a fourfold decrease in titer of a nontreponemal serologic test, or erythromycin therapy	Clinical, serologic follow-up and benzathine penicillin G 50,000 U/kg IM, single dose[f]

Modified from Pickering LK, editor. 2000 Red book: report of the Committee on Infectious Diseases, 25th ed. Elk Grove Village, Ill: American Academy of Pediatrics; 2000.

[a]See Chapter 26 for further drug information.

[b]Proven or probable disease if:
1) Physical or radiologic evidence of active disease.
2) Infant's nontreponemal titer is at least four times higher than the mother's titer.
3) CSF VDRL is reactive or CSF cell count and/or protein is abnormal.
4) Positive antitreponemal IgM test.
5) Placenta or umbilical cord is positive for treponemes organisms using specific fluorescent antibody staining.

[c]If more than 1 day of therapy is missed, the entire course should be restarted.

[d]Alternatively, some experts recommend procaine penicillin G 50,000 U/kg IM daily for 10-14 days, but CSF levels may be inadequate.

[e]Mother's penicillin dose unknown, undocumented, or inadequate **or** lack of fourfold or greater decrease in nontreponemal antibody titer in mother.

[f]Some experts recommend aqueous crystalline penicillin G as for proven or highly probably disease (see text). Other experts would follow the infant without giving antibiotic therapy if both clinical and serologic follow-up can be ensured.

TABLE 16-7

INTERPRETATION OF SYPHILIS SEROLOGY AFTER TREATMENT OF SUSPECTED CONGENITAL SYPHILIS

Actual Congenital Syphilis Infection Status	Rapid Plasma Reagin (RPR)	Fluorescent Treponemal Antibody (FTA)	Comments
Not congenitally infected	Titers decrease fourfold by 3 mo; negative by 6 mo	Negative by 12-18 mo	Both RPR and FTA are waning passive maternal antibodies
Congenitally infected and successfully treated	Same as above	Long-lasting positive (may be lifelong)	—
Congenitally infected but *not* successfully treated	Increase or less than fourfold decrease by 3 mo	Long-lasting positive (may be life long)	Needs complete re-evaluation and treatment for syphilis

TREATMENT FOR SYPHILIS (POSTNEONATAL)

Type or Stage	Firstline Drug and Dosage	Alternatives
Congenital syphilis (diagnosed >4 wk of age)	Aqueous crystalline penicillin 200,000-300,000 U/kg/24 hr IV Q6hr × 10-14 days	—
Early acquired syphilis of <1 yr duration	Benzathine benzylpenicillin 50,000 U/kg (maximum 2.4 × 10^6 U) IM × 1 dose	Tetracycline 500 mg PO Q6hr × 14 days (for >8 yr) **or** Doxycycline 4 mg/kg/24 hr (maximum 200 mg) PO Q12hr × 14 days (for >8 yr).
Syphilis of >1 yr duration (late syphilis)	Benzathine benzylpenicillin 50,000 U/kg (maximum 2.4 × 10^6 U) IM every wk × 3 successive weeks **(Note: Must examine CSF to exclude asymptomatic neurosyphilis)**	Tetracycline 500 mg PO Q6hr × 28 days (for >8 yr) **or** Doxycycline 4 mg/kg/24 hr (maximum 200 mg) PO Q12hr × 28 days (for >8 yr).
Neurosyphilis	Aqueous crystalline benzylpenicillin 200,000-300,000 U/kg/day IV Q4-6hr (maximum 4 × 10^6 U IV Q4hr) × 10-14 days; may be followed by benzathine penicillin 50,000 U/kg/dose (maximum 2.4 × 10^6 U) IM every week × 3 wk	Aqueous procaine benzylpenicillin 2.4 × 10^6 U IM Q24hr × 10-14 days + probenecid 500 mg PO Q6hr × 10-14 days; may be followed by benzathine penicillin 50,000 U/kg/dose (maximum 2.4 × 10^6 U) IM every week × 3 wk. (If penicillin allergic, especially if <9 yr, consider penicillin desensitization and administration in an appropriate setting. Also patient should be managed in consultation with a specialist.)

Modified from Pickering LK, editor. 2000 Red book: report of the Committee on Infectious Diseases, 25th ed. Elk Grove Village, Ill: American Academy of Pediatrics; 2000.

a. Infected child:
   (1) Child <18 months is considered HIV infected if he or she:
      (a) Has positive results on two separate determinations (excluding cord blood) from one or more of the following HIV detection tests:
         (i) HIV culture.
         (ii) HIV polymerase chain reaction (PCR).
         (iii) HIV antigen (p24).
      (b) Meets criteria for AIDS diagnosis based on 1987 AIDS surveillance case definition (from revision of the Centers for Disease Control and Prevention [CDC] surveillance case definition for AIDS[11]).

TABLE 16-9
DIAGNOSIS OF PELVIC INFLAMMATORY DISEASE

Etiology	Diagnostic Criteria	Diagnostic Techniques	Admission Criteria
1. *Neisseria gonorrhea* 2. *Chlamydia trachomatis* 3. Lower genital tract flora (*Hemophilus influenzae*, gram-negative rods, anaerobes, *Streptococcus agalactiae*)	Minimal criteria (all of the following): 1. Lower abdominal tenderness 2. Adnexal tenderness 3. Cervical motion tenderness 4. Absence of other etiology Additional criteria (one or more of the following): 1. Fever greater than 38.3° C 2. Abnormal cervical or vaginal discharge 3. Elevated erythrocyte sedimentation rate (ESR) 4. Elevated C-reactive protein (CRP) 5. Laboratory confirmation of infection with *N. gonorrhea* or *C. trachomatis* Other: 1. Endometriosis 2. Tuboovarian abscess (TOA)	*Chlamydia trachomatis* 1. *Definitive:* Tissue culture (only acceptable method for evaluation of child abuse). 2. *Presumptive:* Antigen detection through fluorescent staining with DNA probe, enzyme immunoassay (EIA), or monoclonal antibody (DFA); polymerase chain reaction (PCR) and ligase chain reaction (LCR) can be used on urine or cervical samples; DNA probe not reliable on bloody specimens; serologies not available. *Neisseria gonorrhea* 1. *Definitive:* Tissue culture (selective media with carbon dioxide incubation for transport). 2. *Presumptive:* Gram-negative intracellular diplococci on smear, or EIA or DNA probe of specimen; PCR or LCR may be used on urine or cervical sample.	1. Cannot exclude diagnosis of surgical abdomen (such as appendicitis) 2. Presence of tuboovarian abscess 3. Pregnancy 4. Immunodeficiency 5. Inability to tolerate or follow outpatient oral regimen 6. Failure to respond to oral antibiotic therapy 7. Clinical follow-up cannot be arranged (especially in adolescents)

MICROBIOLOGY AND INFECTIOUS DISEASE

16

TABLE 16-10

THERAPY FOR CHLAMYDIA, GONORRHEA, AND PELVIC INFLAMMATORY DISEASE

Type or Stage	Firstline Drug and Dosage	Alternatives
CHLAMYDIA TRACHOMATIS INFECTION		
Urethritis, cervicitis, or proctitis	Doxycycline 100 mg PO bid × 7 days (if > 9 yr) **or** Azithromycin 1 g PO × 1 dose	Erythromycin base 500 mg PO qid × 7 days **or** Erythromycin ethylsuccinate 800 mg PO qid × 7 days **or** Ofloxacin 300 mg PO bid × 7 days (if >18 yr)
Infection in pregnancy	Erythromycin base 500 mg PO qid × 7 days **or** Amoxicillin 500 mg PO tid × 7 days	Erythromycin base 250 mg PO qid × 14 days **or** Erythromycin ethylsuccinate 400 mg PO qid × 14 days, **or** Azithromycin 1 g PO × 1 dose
Neonatal ophthalmia	Erythromycin base 50 mg/kg/24 hr PO or IV ÷ qid × 14 days	Topical treatment is ineffective.
Neonatal pneumonia	Erythromycin base 50 mg/kg/24 hr PO or IV ÷ qid × 14 days	—
GONORRHEA*		
Newborns		
Sepsis, arthritis, meningitis, scalp abscess	Ceftriaxone 25-50 mg/kg/24 hr IV/IM Q24hr × 7 days (10-14 days if meningitis) **or** Cefotaxime 50 mg/kg/24 hr IV/IM Q12hr × 7 days (10-14 days if meningitis)	—
Neonatal ophthalmia	Ceftriaxone 25-50 mg/kg (maximum 125 mg) IV/IM × 1 dose plus saline irrigation **or** Cefotaxime 100 mg/kg per dose IM/IV × 1 dose	All infants should receive silver nitrate, tetracycline, or erythromycin ointment instilled into each eye within 1 hr of birth. **Note:** All infants with GC conjunctivitis should be evaluated for possible sepsis/disseminated disease and the need to be treated for a longer time.
Prepubertal children who weigh <100 lb (45 kg)		
Uncomplicated urethritis, vulvovaginitis, proctitis, or pharyngitis	Ceftriaxone 125 mg IM × 1 dose	Spectinomycin 40 mg/kg (maximum 2 g) IM × 1 dose.
Bacteremia, peritonitis, or arthritis	Ceftriaxone 50 mg/kg/24 hr (maximum 1 g) IM/IV Q24hr × 7-10 days	—

Children who weigh ≥100 lb (45 kg) and ≥9 yr

Condition	Treatment	Alternative
Uncomplicated endocervicitis or urethritis	Ceftriaxone 125 mg IM × 1 dose **or** Cefixime 400 mg PO × 1 dose **or** Ciprofloxacin 500 mg PO × 1 dose (if >18 yr) **PLUS** Ofloxacin 400 mg PO × 1 dose (if >18 yr) **or** Azithromycin 1 g PO × 1 dose **or** Doxycycline 100 mg PO bid × 7 days	Spectinomycin 40 mg/kg (maximum 2 g) IM × 1 dose.
Pharyngitis	Same as uncomplicated endocervicitis or urethritis therapy	—
Disseminated gonococcal infections	Ceftriaxone 1 g/24 hr IV/IM Q24hr × 7 days	Cefotaxime or ceftizoxime 3 g IV Q8hr × 7 days. For persons allergic to β-lactam drugs: Spectinomycin 2 g IM Q12hr × 7 days **or** Ciprofloxacin 1 g/24 hr IV Q12hr **or** Ofloxacin 800 mg IV Q12hr.
Bacteremia or arthritis	Ceftriaxone 50 mg/kg/day (maximum dose 2 g) IM or IV Q24hr × 10-14 days	
PID		
Inpatient	Cefoxitin 2 g IV Q6hr **or** Cefotetan 2 g IV Q12hr **plus** Doxycycline 100 mg IV/PO Q12hr If clinical improvement after 24 hrs follow with: Doxycycline 100 mg PO Q12hr **or** Clindamycin 450 mg PO Q6hr (for total of 14 days).	Clindamycin 900 mg IV Q8hr **plus** Gentamicin 2 mg/kg loading dose **plus** Gentamicin 1.5 mg/kg IV Q8hr Same
Outpatient	Doxycycline 100 mg PO bid × 14 days **plus** Cefoxitin 2 g IM × 1 dose and probenicid 1 g PO × 1 dose **or** Ceftriaxone 250 mg IM × 1 dose	(>18 years) Ofloxacin 400 mg PO bid × 14 days **plus** Clindamycin 450 mg PO qid **or** Metronidazole 500 mg PO bid × 14 days —

From Centers for Disease Control and Prevention. MMWR 1998; 47(RR-1).
*Therapy should include treatment for presumed concomitant chlamydial infection.

16

MICROBIOLOGY AND INFECTIOUS DISEASE

(2) A child >18 months is considered HIV infected if he or she:
   (a) Is HIV antibody positive by repeated reactive enzyme immuno-assay (EIA) and confirmatory test (e.g., Western blot or immuno-fluorescence assay [IFA]).
   (b) Meets any of the test criteria for a child <18 months.
b. Perinatally exposed child: A child is considered exposed when he or she does not meet the aforementioned criteria and:
   (1) Is HIV seropositive by EIA and confirmatory test (e.g., Western blot or IFA) and is 18 months old at the time of the test.
   (2) Has unknown antibody status but was born to a mother known to be infected with HIV.
c. Seroreverter: A child who was born to an HIV-infected mother and who:
   (1) Has been documented as HIV antibody negative (i.e., two or more negative EIA tests performed at ≥6 to 18 months of age or one negative EIA test after 18 months of age) or
   (2) Has had at least two negative HIV virologic tests from separate specimens (both performed at >1 month and one at >4 months), or
   (3) Has no other laboratory evidence of infection and
   (4) Has not had an AIDS-defining condition.
3. **Pediatric HIV immunologic categories** (Table 16-11)
4. **Guidelines for prophylaxis against first episode of opportunistic infections** (Table 16-12)
5. **Management of perinatal HIV exposure:** Recommendations provided are current at the time of publication; check the recent recommendations for most current therapy at **www.hivatis.org/**.
a. Prevention of vertical transmission: Use of antiretroviral therapy during pregnancy, during delivery, and in the newborn dramatically reduces HIV transmission. Bottle-feeding of formula is also recommended to reduce transmission through breast milk.
   (1) Pregnancy: All HIV-infected women should be offered antiretroviral therapy for their own health, consistent with the standards of non-pregnant adults. Additionally, zidovudine should be offered, in addition to the patient's own regimen, to reduce the risk of transmission of HIV to her newborn. The following regimen was shown to reduce transmission: zidovudine (ZDV) 100 mg orally (PO) 5 times per 24 hr initiated at 14 to 34 weeks gestation and continued throughout pregnancy (established to be effective in women who do not otherwise have clinical indications for ZDV therapy). Many experts use 200 mg PO three times per day (TID) or 300 mg PO twice daily (BID), extrapolated from data on other adult populations. Higher viral loads have been associated with increased risk of transmission. Elective Cesarean section (before onset of labor or membrane rupture) has been shown to decrease transmission for women not receiving antiretroviral therapy or with high viral loads.
   (2) Labor: During labor, intravenous (IV) ZDV in a loading dose of 2 mg/kg over 1 hour, followed by continuous infusion of 1 mg/kg/hour

TABLE 16-11

1994 REVISED PEDIATRIC HIV CLASSIFICATION SYSTEM: IMMUNOLOGIC CATEGORIES BASED ON AGE-SPECIFIC CD4+ LYMPHOCYTE COUNT AND PERCENT

	Age of Child		
Immunologic Category	<12 mo No./mcL (%)	1-5 yr No./mcL (%)	6-12 yr No./mcL (%)
1: No suppression	≥1500 (≥25)	≥1000 (≥25)	≥500 (≥25)
2: Moderate suppression	750-1499 (15-24)	500-999 (15-24)	200-499 (15-24)
3: Severe suppression	<750 (<15)	<500 (<15)	<200 (<15)

From Centers for Disease Control and Prevention. MMWR 1994; 43(RR-12).

until delivery. Consider adding nevirapine (NVP) for high-risk situations such as high viral load in mother, no prenatal care, or break in baby's skin.

(3) Newborn: For the newborn, ZDV 2 mg/kg/dose PO every 6 hours (or 1.5 mg/kg/dose IV every 6 hours until tolerating PO) for first 6 weeks of life, beginning 8 to 12 hours after birth. For premature infants (<34 weeks) use 2 mg/kg/dose PO (1.5 mg/kg/dose IV) every 12 hours initially, then increase to 2 mg/kg/dose PO every 8 hours at 2 weeks if gestational age >30 weeks, or at 4 weeks if gestational age <30 weeks. In high-risk situations in which the mother received intrapartum NVP, give a single dose of 2 mg/kg to the neonate at 48 to 72 hours of life. In high-risk situation in which the mother did not receive intrapartum NVP, give one dose of 2 mg/kg/dose PO immediately after birth, and a second dose at 48 to 72 hours of life. For high-risk situations, also consider adding lamivudine (3TC) therapy to ZDV for 1 week at 2 mg/kg/dose PO BID. Monitor ZDV toxicity with CBCs at each blood draw because the main toxicity is anemia.

b. Ongoing management of indeterminate infants

(1) *Pneumocystis carinii* pneumonia (PCP) prophylaxis with trimethoprim-sulfamethoxazole (TMP/SMX) should be initiated for all HIV-exposed infants at 4 to 6 weeks of life. PCP prophylaxis should be continued until clinical status excludes HIV infection. Dose is 75 mg/m^2/dose of TMP PO BID for 3 consecutive days per week. For infected infants, refer to Table 16-12.

(2) HIV diagnostic tests (DNA PCR or viral culture) should be obtained on the infant between birth and 2 weeks of life (cord blood should not be used), at 1 to 2 months, and again at 3 to 6 months to determine infection status. A positive test should be immediately repeated for confirmation of infection. If all tests are negative, the infant should be tested for HIV antibody at 12 and 18 months of age to document disappearance of the antibody.

(3) Clinical monitoring: Infants should be evaluated at routine well-child

TABLE 16-12
PROPHYLAXIS FOR FIRST EPISODE OF OPPORTUNISTIC DISEASE IN HIV-INFECTED INFANTS AND CHILDREN

Pathogen	Indication	Preventive Regimens	
		First Choice	Alternatives
STRONGLY RECOMMENDED AS STANDARD OF CARE			
Pneumocystis carinii	HIV-infected or HIV-indeterminate infants 4-6 wk → 12 mo of age HIV-children 1-5 yr with CD4+ count <500 mcL or CD4+ percent <15% HIV-infected children 6-12 yr with CD4+ count <200 mcL or CD4+ percent <15%	TMP/SMX 150/750 mg/m²/day in two divided doses PO 3×/week on consecutive days. Acceptable alternative dosage schedules: Single dose PO 3×/week on consecutive days. Two divided doses PO every day. Two divided doses PO 3×/week on alternate days.	Aerosolized pentamidine (children ≥5 yr) 300 mg every mo via Respirgard II nebulizer; dapsone (children ≥1 mo) 2 mg/kg (maximum 100 mg) PO every day; IV pentamidine 4 mg/kg Q2-4 wk.
Mycobacterium tuberculosis			
Isoniazid sensitive	Tuberculin skin test reaction ≥5 mm **or** prior positive TST result without treatment **or** contact with case of active tuberculosis	Isoniazid 10-15 mg/kg (maximum 300 mg) PO **or** IM every day × 12 mo) **or** 20-30 mg/kg (maximum 900 mg) PO BIW × 12 mo.	Rifampin 10-20 mg/kg (maximum 600 mg) PO or IV every day × 12 mo.
Isoniazid resistant	Same as above; high probability of exposure to isoniazid-resistant tuberculosis	Rifampin 10-20 mg/kg (maximum 600 mg) PO **or** IV every day × 12 mo.	Uncertain.
Multidrug (isoniazid and rifampin) resistant	Same as above; high probability of exposure to multidrug-resistant tuberculosis	Choice of drug requires consultation with public health authorities.	None.

Mycobacterium avium complex	For children <1 yr, CD4+ count <750/mcL 1-2 yr, CD4+ count <500/mcL 2-6 yr, CD4+ count <75/mcL ≥6 yr, CD4+ count <50/mcL	Clarithromycin 7.5 mg/kg (maximum 500 mg) PO bid **or** azithromycin 20 mg/kg (maximum 1200 mg) PO once weekly.	*Children <6 yr:* Rifabutin 5 mg/kg PO every day when suspension becomes available *Children ≥6 yr:* Rifabutin 300 mg PO every day; azithromycin, 5 mg/kg (maximum 250 mg) PO every day.
Varicella-zoster virus	Significant exposure to varicella with no history of chickenpox or shingles	VZIG 1 vial (1.25 mL)/10 kg (maximum 5 vials) IM, administered ≤96 hr after exposure, ideally within 48 hr.	None.
GENERALLY RECOMMENDED			
Toxoplasma gondii*	IgG antibody to Toxoplasma and severe immunosuppression	TMP/SMX 150/750 mg/m²/day in 2 divided doses PO every day.	*Dapsone (children ≥1 mo):* 2 mg/kg or 15 mg/m² (maximum 25 mg) PO every day **plus** pyrimethamine 1 mg/kg PO every day **plus** leucovorin 5 mg PO every 3 days.
NOT RECOMMENDED FOR MOST PATIENTS; INDICATED FOR USE ONLY IN UNUSUAL CIRCUMSTANCES			
Cryptococcus neoformans	Severe immunosuppression	Fluconazole 3-6 mg/kg PO every day.	Itraconazole 2-5 mg/kg PO Q12-24hr.
Histoplasma capsulatum	Severe immunosuppression, endemic geographic area	Itraconazole 2-5 mg/kg PO Q12-24hr.	None.
Cytomegalovirus (CMV)†	CMV antibody positivity and severe immunosuppression	Children 6-12 yr: Oral ganciclovir under investigation.	None.

From Centers for Disease Control and Prevention. MMWR 1997; 46(RR-12).

BIW, Twice a week; *TMP/SMX,* trimethoprim-sulfamethoxazole.

*Protection against *Toxoplasma* is provided by the preferred anti-*Pneumocystis* regimens. Pyrimethamine alone probably provides little, if any, protection.

†Data on oral ganciclovir are still being evaluated; durability of effect is unclear. Acyclovir is not protective against CMV.

MICROBIOLOGY AND INFECTIOUS DISEASE

16

visits for signs and symptoms of HIV infection. In addition to HIV diagnostic tests, the following monitoring tests are recommended: CBC and T-cell subsets at birth to 2 weeks, 1 to 2 months, and 4 to 6 months. Any suspicious clinical or laboratory findings merit careful and close follow-up.

6. **Management of HIV-infected infants and children**
NOTE: **Primary care physicians are encouraged to participate in the care and management of HIV-infected children in consultation with specialists who have expertise in the care of such children. Knowledge about antiretroviral therapy is changing, and in areas where enrollment into clinical trials is possible, it should be encouraged.**
   a. Criteria for initiation of antiretroviral therapy
      (1) Initiation of antiretroviral therapy depends on virologic, immunologic, and clinical status.
      (2) All HIV-infected infants, 12 months of age, regardless of immunologic, virologic, or clinical status, should be started on antiretroviral therapy.
      (3) Antiretroviral therapy should be initiated in children with evidence of immune suppression as indicated by CD4 lymphocyte absolute number or percentage in Immunologic Category 2 or 3 (see Table 16-11).
      (4) Therapy should be initiated in any child with clinical symptoms related to HIV infection.
      (5) For asymptomatic HIV-infected children >1 year of age with normal immune status, consideration should be given to initiating therapy.
   b. Antiretroviral regimen: For the most recent recommendations, refer to **http://www.hivatis.org/.** Data suggest the use of combination therapy for initial and ongoing therapy (except chemoprophylaxis in an exposed infant as previously listed; if an infant is identified as HIV infected while receiving prophylaxis, therapy should be changed to combination therapy).
   c. Clinical and laboratory monitoring in HIV-infected children: Immune status, viral load, and evidence of HIV progression and drug toxicity should be monitored on a regular basis (about every 3 months). Careful attention to routine aspects of pediatric care, such as growth, development, and vaccines, is essential.
7. **Immunizations in HIV-infected or HIV-exposed infants and children:** Specific guidelines are discussed on p. 320. In general, live viral (e.g., oral poliovirus vaccine [OPV]) and live bacterial (e.g., Bacillus Calmette-Guérin [BCG]) vaccines should not be given. The measles/mumps/rubella (MMR) and varicella vaccines may be administered under certain circumstances. Pneumococcal vaccine at 2 years of age (or conjugated pneumococcal series starting at 2 months of age) and yearly influenza immunization, starting at 6 months of age, are also recommended.

F. TUBERCULOSIS

1. **Recommended tuberculosis testing**

a. Tuberculin skin test (TST) recommendations (from American Academy of Pediatrics. *2000 Red Book,* Chicago: The Academy: 2000): BCG immunization is not a contraindication to tuberculin skin testing.

  (1) Immediate testing

    (a) Contacts of people with confirmed or suspected infectious tuberculosis (contact investigation); includes contacts of persons incarcerated in the last 5 years.

    (b) Children with clinical or radiographic findings of tuberculosis.

    (c) Children emigrating from or with history of travel to endemic countries (e.g., Asia, the Middle East, Africa, Latin America); contacts of people indigenous to these countries.

  (2) Annual testing (initial TST is at the time of diagnosis or circumstance, beginning as early as age 3 months)

    (a) HIV-infected children or those living in a household with HIV-infected people.

    (b) Incarcerated adolescents.

  (3) Testing every 2-3 years: Children exposed to the homeless, HIV-infected people, nursing home residents, institutionalized or incarcerated adolescents or adults, illicit drug users, and migrant farm workers.

  (4) Testing at 4 to 6 and 11 to 16 years of age:

    (a) Children of immigrants (with unknown TST status) from endemic countries (continued personal exposure by travel to endemic areas and contact with people from the endemic areas are indications for repeat TST).

    (b) Children without specific risk factors residing in high-prevalence areas (may vary within each region of country).

  (5) Children at increased risk of progression of infection to disease: Medical conditions such as diabetes mellitus, chronic renal failure, malnutrition, and congenital or acquired immunodeficiencies (immunodeficiency itself may increase risk of progression to severe disease, so if exposure is likely, immediate and periodic tuberculin skin testing should be considered; TST should always be performed before initiation of immunosuppressive therapy).

b. Standard tuberculin skin test is the Mantoux test. The tine test (MPT) is no longer recommended.

  (1) Inject 5 tuberculin units (5TU) of purified protein derivative (0.1 mL) intradermally on the volar aspect of the forearm to form a 6- to 10-mm weal. Results of skin testing (positive or negative) should be read 48 to 72 hours later by qualified medical personnel.

  (2) Definition of positive Mantoux test (regardless of whether BCG has been previously administered). See Table 16-13.

2. **Drug therapy**

TABLE 16-13

POSITIVE CONDITIONS FOR TUBERCULIN SKIN TESTING (TST)

Induration >5 mm	Children in close contact with known or suspected contagious cases of tuberculosis
	Children suspected to have tuberculosis based on clinical or radiographic findings
	Children with immunosuppressive conditions (including HIV infection)
Induration >10 mm	Children at increased risk of dissemination based on young age (<4 yr) or other medical conditions (cancer, diabetes mellitus, chronic renal failure, or malnutrition)
	Children with increased exposure: those born in or whose parents who were born in endemic countries; those with travel to endemic countries; those exposed to HIV-infected adults, homeless persons, illicit drug users, nursing home residents, incarcerated or institutionalized persons, or migrant farm workers
Induration >15 mm	Children 4 yr or older without above risk factors

From Pickering LK, editor: 2000 Red book: report of the Committee on Infectious Diseases, 25th ed. Elk Grove Village, Ill: American Academy of Pediatrics; 2000.

a. Prophylaxis
  (1) Indications
    (a) Children with positive tuberculin tests but no evidence of clinical disease.
    (b) Recent contacts, especially HIV-infected children, of people with infectious tuberculosis, even if tuberculin test and clinical evidence are not indicative of disease.
  (2) Recommendations (see Chapter 26 for specific doses) (Table 16-14).
b. Treatment for active tuberculosis disease (for details, see Pickering LH, editor. *2000 Red Book.* Chicago: American Academy of Pediatrics; 2000) (see Table 16-14).

G. OTHER IMPORTANT INFECTIONS

1. Lyme disease

a. Presentation
  (1) Early localized disease: Clinical manifestations appear between 3 and 32 days after tick bite and include erythema migrans (annular rash at site of bite, target lesion with clear or necrotic center), fever, headache, myalgia, malaise.
  (2) Early disseminated disease: Appears some 3 to 10 weeks after the tick bite and includes secondary erythema migrans with multiple, smaller target lesions, cranioneuropathy (especially facial nerve palsy), systemic symptoms as previously listed, and lymphadenopathy; 1% may develop carditis with heart block or aseptic meningitis.

(3) Late disease: Intermittent, recurrent symptoms occur 2 to 12 months from initial tick bite and include pauciarticular arthritis affecting large joints (7% of those untreated), peripheral neuropathy, encephalopathy.

b. Transmission: Disease is caused by spirochete *Borrelia burgdorferi*. Inoculation occurs via a deer tick, Ixodes scapularis or Ixodes pacificus. After a bite from an infected deer tick, the spirochete disseminates systemically through the blood and lymphatics. Of note, transmission of *B. burgdorferi* from infected ticks requires a prolonged time (24 to 48 hours) of tick attachment. Lyme disease is endemic in New England and has a high occurrence on the East coast, but it has been reported in 48 states. April to October is the peak season.

c. Diagnosis: Most cases of Lyme disease can be diagnosed clinically by the characteristic erythema migrans rash or arthritis. Serologic confirmation of diagnosis is with immunoassays for *B. burgdorferi*-specific IgM, which peaks at 3 to 6 weeks after disease onset, and with *B. burgdorferi*-specific IgG, which rises weeks to months after symptoms appear and persists. False-positive results of these assays are frequent as a result of cross-reactivity with viral infections, other spirochetal infections (except syphilis), and autoimmune diseases. Western blot assays should be used to confirm positive results. Lyme disease–specific antibodies can be isolated from CSF in patients with CNS involvement.

d. Treatment: Therapy depends on the stage of disease. Antibiotic prophylaxis is not routinely recommended for ticks attached <24 to 48 hours. For early localized disease, doxycycline for 14 to 21 days is the treatment of choice for patients ≥8 years of age. Amoxicillin is recommended for younger children. Early disseminated and late-onset disease can both be treated by the same oral regimen as early disease but for an extended period of 21 to 28 days. Of note, when facial palsy is present, therapy is effective only at preventing late stages of disease and does not affect the duration of paralysis. Disease resulting in carditis, persistent or recurrent arthritis (<2 months), and/or meningitis or encephalitis should be treated with a parenteral regimen of either ceftriaxone or penicillin for 14 to 21 days.

2. **Mycoplasma**

a. Presentation
  (1) Pneumonia: Malaise, fever, occasional headache, cough, and widespread rales.
  (2) Systemic: Aseptic meningitis, encephalitis, cerebellar ataxia, myocarditis, or arthritis.

b. Diagnosis: Pneumonia is usually diagnosed by clinical presentation and/or chest radiograph showing most commonly bilateral diffuse infiltrates. Cold agglutinins, with titers greater than 1:64 are very specific, but not sensitive. The bedside agglutination test is equivalent to cold agglutination titers of >1:64. Mycoplasma IgM is not well stan-

TABLE 16-14

RECOMMENDED TREATMENT REGIMENS FOR DRUG-SUSCEPTIBLE TUBERCULOSIS IN INFANTS, CHILDREN, AND ADOLESCENTS

Infection or Disease Category	Regimen*	Remarks
Asymptomatic infection (positive skin test, no disease)	Prophylaxis	If daily therapy is not possible, therapy twice a week may be used for 6-9 mo. HIV-infected children should be treated for 12 mo.
Isoniazid susceptible	6-9 mo of isoniazid Q24hr	Also indicated for contacts of people with infectious tuberculosis, even if tuberculin test is negative, including all children <4 yr with household TB contacts.
Isoniazid resistant	6-9 mo of rifampin Q24hr	Repeat TST 12 wk after contact with TB is broken; if negative (in normal host), may discontinue prophylaxis; if positive (and no evidence of TB disease), complete prophylactic regimen.
Isoniazid/rifampin resistant*	Consultation with a tuberculosis specialist	For management of neonates born to mothers with evidence of TB infection, see 2000 Red Book.[8]
Pulmonary	**6 mo regimens** 2 mo of isoniazid, rifampin, and pyrazinamide Q24hr, followed by 4 mo of isoniazid and rifampin daily **or** 2 mo of isoniazid, rifampin, and pyrazinamide daily, followed by 4 mo of isoniazid and rifampin twice a week	If possible drug resistance is a concern, another drug (ethambutol or streptomycin) is added to the initial three-drug therapy until drug susceptibilities are determined. Drugs can be given 2 or 3 times/wk under direct observation in the initial phase if nonadherence is likely.

9 mo alternative regimens (for hilar adenopathy only):

9 mo of isoniazid and rifampin Q24hr **or** 1 mo of isoniazid and rifampin Q24hr, followed by 8 mo of isoniazid and rifampin twice a week	Regimens consisting of 6 mo of isoniazid and rifampin Q24hr, and 1 mo of isoniazid and rifampin Q24hr, followed by 5 mo of isoniazid and rifampin twice a week, have been successful in areas where drug resistance is rare.
Extrapulmonary: meningitis, disseminated (miliary), bone/joint disease	
2 mo of isoniazid, rifampin, pyrazinamide, and streptomycin once a day, followed by 10 mo of isoniazid and rifampin Q24hr (12 mo total) **or**	Streptomycin is given with initial therapy until drug susceptibility is known.
2 mo of isoniazid, rifampin, pyrazinamide, and streptomycin Q24hr, followed by 10 mo of isoniazid and rifampin twice a week (12 mo total)	For patients who may have acquired tuberculosis in geographic areas where resistance to streptomycin is common: capreomycin (15-30 mg/kg/day) or kanamycin (15-30 mg/kg/day) may be used instead of streptomycin.
Other (e.g., cervical lymphadenopathy)	See Pulmonary.

Modified from Pickering LK, editor. 2000 Red book: report of the Committee on Infectious Diseases, 25th ed. Elk Grove Village, Ill: American Academy of Pediatrics; 2000.
*Duration of therapy is longer in HIV-infected persons, and additional drugs may be indicated.

16

MICROBIOLOGY AND INFECTIOUS DISEASE

dardized, and IgG (showing rising titers) is performed, but is not routinely necessary. Mycoplasma PCR is available in some institutions.

c. Treatment: Usually macrolides; however, doxycycline and fluoroquinolones are also effective.

H. FUNGAL/YEAST INFECTIONS

1. **Place specimen** (nail or skin scrapings, biopsy specimens, fluids from tissues or lesions) **in 10% KOH on glass slide to look for hyphae, pseudohyphae.**

2. **Germ tube screen of yeast** (3 hours) for *Candida albicans*: all germ tube–positive yeast are *C. albicans*, but not all *C. albicans* are germ tube–positive.

3. **Common community-acquired fungal infections, etiology, and treatment** are listed in Table 16-15.

I. EXPOSURES TO BLOOD-BORNE PATHOGENS AND POSTEXPOSURE PROPHYLAXIS (PEP)

1. HIV[12]

a. Risk of occupational transmission of HIV

   (1) Needle sticks: Three infections for every 1000 exposures (0.3%). Risk is greater when the exposure involves a larger volume of blood and/or higher titer of HIV, as in a deep injury, visible blood on the

TABLE 16-15
COMMON COMMUNITY-ACQUIRED FUNGAL INFECTIONS

Disease	Usual Etiology	Suggested Therapy	Suggested Length of Therapy
Tinea capitis (ringworm of scalp)	*Trichophyton tonsurans, Microsporum canis*	Oral griseofulvin: Give with fatty foods. Fungal shedding decreased with 1%-2.5% selenium sulfide shampoo. Alt: Terbinafine.	4-6 wk or 2 wk after clinical resolution.
Tinea corporis/ pedis (ringworm of body/feet)	*Trichophyton rubrum, Trichophyton mentagrophytes, Microsporum canis*	Topical antifungal (miconazole, clotrimazole). Terbinafine.	4 wk. 2 wk.
Oral candidiasis (thrush)	*Candida albicans, Candida tropicalis*	Nystatin suspension or troches.	3 days after clinical resolution.
Candidal skin infections (intertriginous)	*Candida albicans*	Topical nystatin, miconazole, clotrimazole.	3 days after clinical resolution.
Tinea unguium (ringworm of nails)		Terbinafine or itraconazole or fluconazole	6 weeks 3 months 3-6 months

device causing the injury, a device previously used in the source patient's vein/artery, or a source patient in the late stages of HIV infection.

(2) Mucous membrane exposure: One infection for every 1000 exposures (0.1%). The risk may be higher when the exposure involves a larger volume of blood and a higher titer of HIV, prolonged skin contact, extensive surface area of exposure, or skin integrity that is visibly compromised.

b. Prophylaxis

(1) Optimally, PEP should be initiated within 1 to 2 hours of exposure.

(2) Basic 4-week regimen of two drugs (zidovudine [ZVD] and lamivudine [3TC]; 3TC and stavudine [d4T]; or didanosine [ddI] and d4T) for most exposures, and addition of a third drug for exposures with higher risk of transmission.

(3) Use of ZDV alone as PEP is no longer recommended.

(4) For most recent recommendations, refer to CDC guidelines. **The CDC's postexposure prophylaxis hotline (open 24 hr/day) is 888-448-4911.**

2. **Hepatitis B:** Recommendations for hepatitis B prophylaxis after percutaneous exposure to blood that contains (or might contain) HBsAg includes hepatitis B immune globulin (HBIG) and initiation of hepatitis B vaccine series. For details, see the Chapter 15.

J. INFECTIOUS DISEASES IN INTERNATIONALLY ADOPTED CHILDREN

For more information see **www.cdc.gov/travel/other/adoption.htm.**

REFERENCES

1. Nelson JD. Pocket book of pediatric antimicrobial therapy. Baltimore: Williams & Wilkins; 1995.
2. Mandell GL, Bennett JE, Dolin R. Principles and practice of infectious disease. New York: Churchill Livingstone; 1995.
3. Sanders WE, Sanders CC. Inducible β-lactamases: clinical and epidemiologic implications for use of newer cephalosporins. Rev Infect Dis 1988; 10:830.
4. Wong CS et al. The risk of hemolytic-uremic syndrome after antibiotic treatment of Escherichia coli o157:H7 infections. New Engl J Med 2000; 342:1930.
5. Gomella TA. Neonatology: management, procedures, on-call problems, diseases and drugs. Nowalk, Conn: Appleton & Lange; 1999.
6. McMillan JA et al (editors). Oski's pediatrics: principles and practice. 3rd ed. Philadelphia: Lippincott Williams and Wilkins; 1999.
7. Robart HA et al. Treatment of potentially life-threatening enterovirus infections with pleconaril. Clin Infect Dis 2000; 32:228.
8. Pickering LK, editor. *2000 Red book: report of the Committee on Infectious Diseases.* 25th ed. Elk Grove Village, Ill: American Academy of Pediatrics; 2000.
9. Long S, Pickering LK, Prober CG, editors. Principles and practice of pediatric infectious diseases. Edinburgh: Churchill Livingstone; 1997: 1150.
10. Barron SD, Pass RF. Infectious causes of hydrops fetalis. Semin Perinatol 1995; 19:493.
11. Council of State and Territorial Epidemiologists; AIDS Program, Center for Infectious Diseases. Revision of the CDC surveillance case definition for acquired immunodeficiency syndrome. MMWR 1987; 36(suppl 1):1S-15S.
12. Centers for Disease Control and Prevention. Updated U.S. Public Health Service guidelines for the management of occupational exposures to HBV, HCV, and HIV and recommendations for postexposure prophylaxis. MMWR 2001; 50(RR-11).

16

MICROBIOLOGY AND INFECTIOUS DISEASE

NEONATOLOGY

Lisa A. Irvine, MD, PhD

I. FETAL ASSESSMENT

A. MATERNAL α-FETOPROTEIN (AFP)

1. **Elevated (>2.5 multiples of the median):** Associated with incorrect gestational dating, neural tube defects, anencephaly, multiple pregnancy, Turner's syndrome, omphalocele, cystic hygroma, epidermolysis bullosa, and renal agenesis.
2. **Low (<0.75 multiples of the median):** Associated with underestimation of gestational age, intrauterine growth retardation (IUGR), and chromosomal trisomies (13, 18, 21).

B. FETAL ANOMALY SCREENING

1. **Routine ultrasound:** Performed at 18 to 20 weeks gestation.
2. **Amniotic fluid volume (AFV) estimation**
   a. Oligohydramnios (<500 mL): Associated with Potter's syndrome, renal or urologic abnormalities, lung hypoplasia, limb deformities, premature rupture of membranes, and placental insufficiency.
   b. Polyhydramnios (>2 L): Suggestive of gastrointestinal (GI) anomalies (gastroschisis, duodenal atresia, tracheoesophageal fistula, diaphragmatic hernia), central nervous system (CNS) abnormalities (anencephaly, Werdnig-Hoffman syndrome), chromosomal trisomies, maternal diabetes, and cystic adenomatoid malformation of the lung.
3. **Fetal karyotyping**
   a. Amniocentesis: 20 to 30 mL of amniotic fluid is withdrawn under ultrasound guidance after 16 to 18 weeks gestation. Detects chromosomal abnormalities, metabolic disorders, and neural tube defects. Complications include pregnancy loss (<5/1000), chorioamnionitis (<1/1000), leakage of amniotic fluid (1/300), fetal scarring or dimpling of the skin.
   b. Chorionic villus sampling: Segment of placenta obtained either transcervically or transabdominally at 8 to 11 weeks gestation. Detects chromosomal abnormalities and metabolic disorders, but cannot detect neural tube defects or measure AFP. Complications include pregnancy loss (0.5% to 2%), maternal infection, increased risk of fetomaternal hemorrhage, and fetal limb and jaw malformation.

C. FETAL MATURITY ASSESSMENT

1. **Menstrual history:** Most accurate determination of gestational age. Nägele's rule, based on a 28-day cycle, calculates expected date of confinement (EDC) as 9 months (280 days) plus 7 days from the last menstrual period.
2. **Ultrasound:** Crown-rump length obtained between 6 and 12 weeks predicts gestational age ±3 to 4 days. After 12 weeks, the biparietal diameter is accurate within 10 days, and beyond 26 weeks accuracy diminishes to ±3 weeks.
3. **Growth:** See Table 17-1 for expected birth weight (50th percentile) by gestational age.

17

4. **Fetal lung maturity:** Lecithin (L), the active component of surfactant, is present in amniotic fluid in increasing amounts throughout gestation, compared with constant levels of sphingomyelin (S).

a. **L:S ratio:** A ratio >2:1 indicates fetal lung maturity in nondiabetic pregnancies. L/S ratio is generally 1:1 at 31 to 32 weeks gestation, and 2:1 by 35 weeks gestation.

b. **Phosphatidyl glycerol (PG):** Late-appearing surfactant component. Risk of respiratory distress syndrome (RDS) is <0.5% if PG is present in the amniotic fluid.

D. ANTEPARTUM FETAL MONITORING

1. **Nonstress test (NST):** Fetal heart rate (FHR) is monitored with the mother at rest. In a normal, reactive NST, FHR increases >15 beats per minute (bpm) for >15 seconds at least twice in 20 minutes. Reactivity can be absent in fetuses <30 weeks gestation because of CNS immaturity.

2. **Biophysical profile:** 30-minute ultrasound examination of five biophysical assessments: NST, AFV, fetal breathing, fetal movements/tone, and heart rate. Each parameter is scored as 2 (if normal) or 0 (if abnormal). Total scores of 8 to 10 are reassuring.

E. INTRAPARTUM FETAL HEART RATE MONITORING

1. **Normal baseline FHR** is 120 to 160 bpm. Mild bradycardia is 100 to 120 bpm.

2. **Normal beat-to-beat variability:** Deviation from baseline of >6 bpm. Absence of variability is <2 bpm from baseline. Abnormal beat-to-beat variability is a sign of potential fetal distress, particularly when combined with variable or late decelerations.

3. **Early decelerations:** Begin with the onset of contractions. The heart rate reaches the nadir at the peak of the contraction, and returns to baseline as the contraction ends. Occur secondary to changes in vagal tone after brief hypoxic episodes or head compression and are benign.

4. **Variable decelerations:** Represent umbilical cord compression and have no uniform temporal relationship to the onset of the contraction. They are considered severe when the heart rate drops to <60 bpm for ≥60 seconds with slow recovery to baseline.

TABLE 17-1

EXPECTED BIRTH WEIGHT BY GESTATIONAL AGE*

Gestational Age (wk)	Weight (g)
24	700
26	900
28	1100
30	1350
32	1650
34	2100
36	2600
38	3000

Data from Usher R, McLean F. J Pediatr 1969; 74:901.
*Weight is the 50th percentile for age.

5. **Late decelerations:** Occur after the peak of contraction, persist after the contraction stops, and show a slow return to baseline. Result from uteroplacental insufficiency and indicate fetal distress.

II. NEWBORN RESUSCITATION
A. NALS ALGORITHM FOR NEONATAL RESUSCITATION (Fig. 17-1)
B. ENDOTRACHEAL TUBE (ETT) SIZE (Table 17-2)

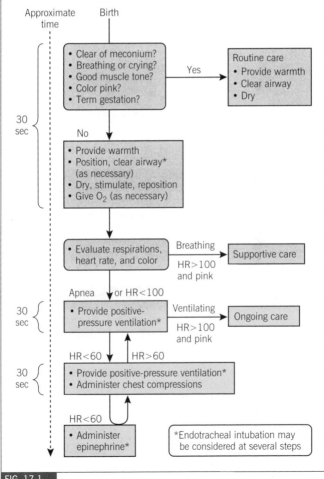

17

NEONATOLOGY

FIG. 17-1

Overview of resuscitation in the delivery room. *(From Pediatrics 2000; 106(3):e29.)*

TABLE 17-2

ENDOTRACHEAL TUBE SIZE BY WEIGHT AND GESTATIONAL AGE

Weight (g)	Gestational Age (wk)	ETT Size (mm)
<1000	<28	2.5
1000-2000	28-34	3.0
2000-3000	34-38	3.5
>3000	>38	3.5-4.0

From Pediatrics 2000; 106(3):e29.

TABLE 17-3

APGAR SCORES

Score	0	1	2
Heart rate	Absent	<100 bpm	>100 bpm
Respiratory effort	Absent, irregular	Slow, crying	Good
Muscle tone	Limp	Some flexion of extremities	Active motion
Reflex irritability (nose suction)	No response	Grimace	Cough or sneeze
Color	Blue, pale	Acrocyanosis	Completely pink

Data from Apgar V. Anesth Analg 1953; 32:260.

C. MECONIUM DELIVERY

For infants with meconium in the amniotic fluid, the mouth, pharynx, and nose should be suctioned before delivery of the thorax. Depressed infants should have residual meconium removed from the hypopharynx via suctioning under direct visualization. This should occur before drying and stimulating the infant. After intubation, a meconium aspirator attached to wall suction is connected to the endotracheal tube to suction the lower airway. Lower airway suctioning, even in the presence of thick meconium, is not routinely required for infants who are vigorous at delivery.[1]

III. NEWBORN ASSESSMENT

A. VITAL SIGNS

Average heart rate and respiratory rate are 120 to 160 bpm and 40 to 60 breaths/min, respectively. Arterial blood pressure is related to birth weight and gestational age (see Chapter 6).

B. APGAR SCORES (Table 17-3)

APGAR scores are assessed at 1 and 5 minutes and may be repeated at 5-minute intervals for infants with 5-minute scores <7.[2]

C. BALLARD GESTATIONAL AGE ESTIMATION

The Ballard score is most accurate when performed between 12 and 20 hours of age.[3] The approximate gestational age is calculated based on the sum of the neuromuscular and physical maturity ratings (Fig. 17-2).

1. Neuromuscular maturity

a. Posture: Observe infant quiet and supine. Score 0 for arms, legs extended; 1 for starting to flex hips and knees, arms extended; 2 for

Neuromuscular maturity

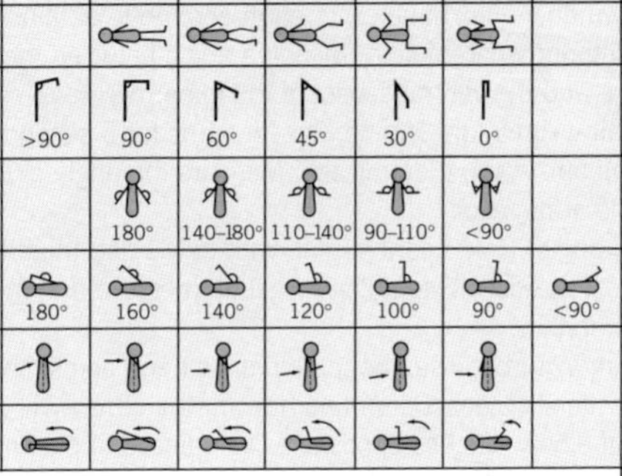

Neuromuscular maturity sign	Score							Record score here
	−1	0	1	2	3	4	5	
Posture								
Square window (wrist)	>90°	90°	60°	45°	30°	0°		
Arm recoil		180°	140–180°	110–140°	90–110°	<90°		
Popliteal angle	180°	160°	140°	120°	100°	90°	<90°	
Scarf sign								
Heel to ear								

TOTAL NEUROMUSCULAR MATURITY SCORE

Physical maturity

Physical maturity sign	Score							Record score here
	−1	0	1	2	3	4	5	
Skin	Sticky, friable, transparent	Gelatinous, red, translucent	Smooth, pink, visible veins	Superficial peeling and/or rash, few veins	Cracking, pale areas, rare veins	Parchment, deep cracking, no vessels	Leathery, cracked, wrinkled	
Lanugo	None	Sparse	Abundant	Thinning	Bald areas	Mostly bald		
Plantar surface	Heel–toe: 40–50mm: −1 <40mm: −2	>50mm: no crease	Faint red marks	Anterior transverse crease only	Creases anterior two thirds	Creases over entire sole		
Breast	Imperceptible	Barely perceptible	Flat areola, no bud	Stippled areola, 1–2mm bud	Raised areola, 3–4mm bud	Full areola, 5–10mm bud		
Eye/ear	Lids fused: loosely: −1 tightly: −2	Lids open, pinna flat, stays folded	Sl. curved pinna, soft, slow recoil	Well-curved pinna, soft but ready recoil	Formed and firm, instant recoil	Thick cartilage, ear stiff		
Genitals (male)	Scrotum flat, smooth	Scrotum empty, faint rugae	Testes in upper canal, rare rugae	Testes descending, few rugae	Testes down, good rugae	Testes pendulous, deep rugae		
Genitals (female)	Clitoris prominent and labia flat	Prominent clitoris and small labia minora	Prominent clitoris and enlarging minora	Majora and minora equally prominent	Majora large, minora small	Majora cover clitoris and minora		

TOTAL PHYSICAL MATURITY SCORE

Score		Maturity rating														Gestational age (weeks)
Neuromuscular		Score	−10	−5	0	5	10	15	20	25	30	35	40	45	50	By dates _____
Physical		Weeks	20	22	24	26	28	30	32	34	36	38	40	42	44	By ultrasound _____
Total																By exam _____

FIG. 17-2

Neuromuscular and physical maturity (New Ballard Score). *(Modified from Ballard JL et al. J Pediatr 1991; 119:417-423.)*

stronger flexion of legs, arms extended; 3 for arms slightly flexed, legs flexed and abducted; and 4 for full flexion of arms, legs.

b. Square window: Flex hand on forearm enough to obtain fullest possible flexion without wrist rotation. Measure angle between the hypothenar eminence and the ventral aspect of the forearm.

c. Arm recoil: With infant supine, flex forearms for 5 seconds, fully extend by pulling on hands, then release. Measure the angle of elbow flexion to which the arms recoil.

d. Popliteal angle: Hold infant supine with pelvis flat, thigh held in the knee-chest position. Extend leg by gentle pressure and measure the popliteal angle.

e. Scarf sign: With baby supine, pull infant's hand across the neck toward the opposite shoulder. Determine how far the elbow will go across. Score 0 if elbow reaches opposite axillary line; 1 if past midaxillary line; 2 if past midline; and 3 if elbow unable to reach midline.

f. Heel-to-ear maneuver: With baby supine, draw foot as near to the head as possible without forcing it. Observe distance between foot and head, and degree of extension at the knee.

2. **Physical maturity:** Based on the developmental stage of eyes, ears, breasts, genitalia, skin, lanugo, and plantar creases.

IV. FLUIDS, ELECTROLYTES, AND NUTRITION

A. FLUIDS

1. **Insensible water loss:** Preterm infants experience increased insensible losses through the skin because of increased surface area per unit body mass and immaturity of the skin (Table 17-4).

2. **Water requirements** (Table 17-5).

B. GLUCOSE REQUIREMENTS

Preterm neonates require approximately 5 to 6 mg/kg/min of glucose to maintain euglycemia (40 to 100 mg/dL).[4] Term neonates require about 3 to 5 mg/kg/min of glucose to maintain euglycemia. The formula to calculate rate of glucose infusion follows:

$$\text{Glucose (mg/kg/min)} = \frac{(\% \text{ Glucose in solution} \times 10) \times (\text{Rate of infusion per hour})}{60 \times \text{Weight (kg)}}$$

TABLE 17-4

ESTIMATES OF INSENSIBLE WATER LOSS AT DIFFERENT BODY WEIGHTS DURING THE FIRST FEW DAYS OF LIFE

Body Weight (g)	Insensible Water Loss (mL/kg/day)
<1000	60-70
1000-1250	60-65
1251-1500	30-45
1501-1750	15-30
1751-2000	15-20

Data from Veille JC. Clin Perinatol 1988; 15:863.

1. **Hypoglycemia:** Serum glucose <40 mg/dL in a term or preterm infant. Ensure that venous sample confirms bedside testing, assess for symptoms, and calculate glucose delivery to infant.
a. Differential diagnosis: Insufficient glucose delivery, decreased glycogen stores, increased circulating insulin (infant of diabetic mother, maternal drugs, Beckwith-Wiedemann syndrome, tumors), endocrine/metabolic disorders, sepsis, hypothermia, polycythemia, asphyxia, shock.
b. Evaluation: Serum glucose, CBC with differential, blood cultures, urine dipstick with urine cultures, and electrolytes; consider performing lumbar puncture or checking insulin level if warranted.
c. Management (Table 17-6).
d. Follow-up blood glucose should be documented every 30 to 60 minutes during therapy until normal values have been established.
2. **Hyperglycemia:** Serum blood glucose >125 mg/dL in term infants and >150 mg/dL in preterm infants. Assess glucose delivery and presence of glucosuria.

17

NEONATOLOGY

TABLE 17-5			
WATER REQUIREMENTS OF NEWBORNS			
	Water Requirements (mL/kg/24 hr) by Age		
Birthweight (g)	1-2 Days	3-7 Days	7-30 Days
<750	100-250	150-300	120-180
750-1000	80-150	100-150	120-180
1000-1500	60-100	80-150	120-180
>1500	60-80	100-150	120-180

Modified from Taeusch HW, Ballard RA, editors. Schaffer and Avery's diseases of the newborn, 7th ed. Philadelphia: WB Saunders; 1998.

TABLE 17-6		
GUIDELINES FOR THE TREATMENT OF NEONATAL HYPOGLYCEMIA		
Plasma Glucose (mg/dL) (Venous Sample)	Asymptomatic or Mildly Symptomatic	Symptomatic
35-45	Breast-feed or give formula or D_5W by nipple/gavage	IV glucose (D_5-$D_{12.5}W$) at 4-6 mg/kg/min*
25-34	IV glucose (D_5-$D_{12.5}W$) at 6-8 mg/kg/min*	IV glucose (D_5-$D_{12.5}W$) at 6-8 mg/kg/min*
<25	Minibolus of 2 mL/kg ($D_{10}W$) and continue at a rate to provide 6-8 mg/kg/min*†	

Modified from Cornblath M. In Donn SM, Fisher CW, editors. Risk management techniques in perinatal and neonatal practice. Armonk, NY: Futura; 1996.
*Changes in infusion rates should not exceed 2 mg/kg/min per change.
†If blood glucose <25 mg/dL and IV access is not available, give glucagon 0.1 mg/kg per dose (maximum 1 mg/dose) IM/SC every 30 minutes. Not as effective in small-for-gestational-age (SGA) or extremely premature infants.

a. Differential diagnosis: Excess glucose administration, sepsis, hypoxia, hyperosmolar formula, transient neonatal diabetes mellitus, medications.

b. Evaluation: Same as for hypoglycemia above.

C. ELECTROLYTES, MINERALS, AND VITAMINS

1. Electrolyte requirements: Common electrolyte abnormalities include hyponatremia, hypernatremia, hypokalemia, hyperkalemia, and hypocalcemia.

a. Sodium: None required in the first 72 hours of life unless serum sodium <135 mEq/L without evidence of volume overload. After 72 hours the sodium requirement is generally 2 to 3 mEq/kg/24 hours for term infants and 3 to 5 mEq/kg/24 hours for preterm infants.

b. Potassium: Added to fluids after adequate urinary output is established and serum level <4.5 mEq/L. Potassium requirements are generally 1 to 2.5 mEq/kg/day.

2. Mineral and vitamin requirements

a. Infants born at <34 weeks gestation have high calcium, phosphorus, sodium, iron, and vitamin D requirements and require breast-milk fortifier or special preterm formulas with iron. Fortifier should be added to breast milk only after the second week of life.

b. Iron: Enterally fed preterm infants require elemental iron supplementation of 2 mg/kg/day after 4 to 8 weeks of age.

D. NUTRITION

1. Growth rates: After approximately 10 days of life, expected weight gain in growing, stable infants is 15 to 20 g/kg/day for preterm infants and 10 g/kg/day for full-term infants in a thermoneutral environment.

2. Caloric requirements: To maintain weight, 50 to 75 kcal/kg/day are required. Adequate growth requires 100 to 120 kcal/kg/day in term, 115 to 130 kcal/kg/day for preterm, and up to 150 kcal/kg/day for very-low-birth-weight (VLBW) infants. These caloric requirements presume healthy infants in a thermoneutral environment.

3. Total parenteral nutrition (see Chapter 20).

V. CYANOSIS IN THE NEWBORN

A. DIFFERENTIAL DIAGNOSIS

1. Respiratory diseases: Persistent pulmonary hypertension (PPHN), diaphragmatic hernia, pulmonary hypoplasia, choanal atresia, pneumothorax, and lung parenchymal diseases such as respiratory distress syndrome (RDS), transient tachypnea of the newborn (TTN), pneumonia, and meconium aspiration.

2. Cardiac diseases: Severe congestive heart failure (CHF) and cyanotic heart lesions such as transposition of the great arteries (TGA), total anomalous pulmonary venous return (TAPVR), Ebstein's anomaly, tricuspid atresia, pulmonic stenosis (PS), and tetralogy of Fallot (TOF).

3. CNS diseases that can cause apnea or hypoventilation: periventricular/intraventricular hemorrhage (IVH), meningitis, seizures, and congenital myopathies.

4. Polycythemia/hyperviscosity syndrome.
5. Methemoglobinemia.
6. Hypothermia, hypoglycemia, sepsis.
7. Shock.
8. **Respiratory depression as a result of maternal medications** (magnesium sulfate, opiates).

B. EVALUATION

1. **Physical examination:** Note central versus peripheral and persistent versus intermittent cyanosis, degree of respiratory effort, single versus split S2, and presence or absence of a heart murmur. Acrocyanosis is often a normal finding in newborns.
2. **Clinical tests:** Oxygen challenge test (see p. 156), preductal and postductal arterial blood gas (ABG) levels, or pulse oximetry to assess for right-to-left shunt, transillumination of chest for possible pneumothorax.
3. **Other data:** Complete blood count (CBC) with differential, serum glucose, chest radiograph, electrocardiogram, echocardiography. Consider blood, urine, and cerebrospinal fluid (CSF) cultures if sepsis is suspected, and methemoglobin level if cyanosis does not match degree of hypoxemia.

VI. RESPIRATORY DISEASES

A. RESPIRATORY DISTRESS SYNDROME (RDS)

1. **Definition:** A deficiency of pulmonary surfactant, a phospholipid protein mixture that decreases surface tension and prevents alveolar collapse. It is produced by type II alveolar cells in increasing quantities from 32 weeks gestation. Factors that accelerate lung maturity include maternal hypertension, sickle cell disease, narcotic addiction, IUGR, prolonged rupture of membranes, fetal stress, and exogenous antenatal steroids.
2. **Incidence:** 60% in infants <30 weeks gestation without steroids, but decreases to 35% for those who have received antenatal steroids. Between 30 and 34 weeks gestation, 25% in untreated infants and 10% in those who have received antenatal steroids. For infants >34 weeks gestation, incidence is 5%.
3. **Risk factors:** Prematurity, maternal diabetes, cesarean section without antecedent labor, perinatal asphyxia, second twin, previous infant with RDS.
4. **Clinical presentation:** Respiratory distress worsens during the first few hours of life, progresses over 48 to 72 hours, and subsequently improves. Recovery is accompanied by brisk diuresis. Classically, on chest radiograph, lung fields have a "reticulogranular" pattern that may obscure the heart border.
5. **Management**
a. Support ventilation and oxygenation.
b. Surfactant therapy (see Formulary for dosing).

17

NEONATOLOGY

(1) "Rescue" therapy: Administration of surfactant to infants with diagnosed RDS.

(2) "Prophylactic" therapy: Administration of surfactant beginning immediately after delivery. May be more effective than rescue therapy in infants <26 weeks gestation.

6. **Intrauterine acceleration of fetal lung maturation:** Maternal administration of steroids antenatally has been shown to decrease neonatal morbidity and mortality. In particular, the risk of RDS is decreased in babies born >24 hours and <7 days after maternal steroid administration.

B. PERSISTENT PULMONARY HYPERTENSION OF THE NEWBORN (PPHN)

1. **Etiology:** Idiopathic or secondary to conditions leading to increased pulmonary vascular resistance. Most commonly seen in term or postterm infants, infants born via cesarean section, and infants with a history of fetal distress and low Apgar scores. Usually presents within 12 to 24 hours of birth. Accounts for up to 2% of all neonatal admissions to the intensive care unit (ICU).

a. Vasoconstriction secondary to hypoxemia and acidosis (neonatal sepsis).

b. Interstitial pulmonary disease (meconium aspiration syndrome, pneumonia).

c. Hyperviscosity syndrome (polycythemia).

d. Pulmonary hypoplasia either primary or secondary to congenital diaphragmatic hernia or renal agenesis.

2. **Diagnostic features**

a. Severe hypoxemia (Pao_2 <35 to 45 mmHg in 100% O_2) disproportionate to radiologic changes.

b. Structurally normal heart with right-to-left shunt at foramen ovale or ductus arteriosus; decreased postductal oxygen saturations compared with preductal values. (Difference of at least 7 to 15 mmHg between preductal and postductal Pao_2 is significant.)

c. Must distinguish from cyanotic heart disease. Infants with heart disease will have an abnormal cardiac examination and show little to no improvement in oxygenation with increased FiO_2 and hyperventilation. See p. 156 (Table 6-14) for interpretation of oxygen challenge test.

3. **Principles of therapy**

a. Consider transfer to a tertiary care center.

b. Minimal handling and limited invasive procedures. Sedation and occasionally paralysis of intubated babies may be necessary.

c. Maintenance of systemic blood pressure with reversal of right-to-left shunt via volume expanders and/or inotropes.

d. Optimize oxygen-carrying capacity with blood transfusions as needed.

e. Administer broad-spectrum antibiotics.

f. Mild hyperventilation to induce respiratory alkalosis (Pco_2 in low 30s) or bicarbonate infusion to induce metabolic alkalosis with pH 7.55 to 7.60. Both may improve oxygenation. Avoid severe hypocapnea (Pco_2 <25), which can be associated with myocardial ischemia and decreased cerebral blood flow. Hyperventilation may result in barotrauma, which predisposes to chronic lung disease. Consider high-frequency ventilation.

g. Nitric oxide, a selective pulmonary vasodilator, may be beneficial. Consider extracorporeal membrane oxygenation (ECMO) if infant has severe cardiovascular instability, if oxygenation index (OI) >35, or if alveolar-arterial gradient (AaO_2) is ≥610 for 8 hours (see Chapter 22 for the calculation of OI and AaO_2. PaO_2 should be measured at a postductal site.)

h. Mortality: Depends on the etiology, but overall mortality rates in North American centers approximate 30% to 40%.

VII. APNEA AND BRADYCARDIA

A. APNEA[5]

1. **Definition:** Respiratory pause >20 seconds or a shorter pause associated with cyanosis, pallor, hypotonia, or bradycardia <100 bpm. In preterm infants, apneic episodes may be central (no diaphragmatic activity), obstructive (upper airway obstruction), or mixed central and obstructive. Common causes of apnea in the newborn are listed in Fig. 17-3.

2. **Incidence:** Apnea occurs in most infants born at <28 weeks gestation, approximately 50% of infants born at 30 to 32 weeks, and <7% of infants born at 34 to 35 weeks. Apnea usually resolves by 34 to 36 weeks postconceptual age, but may persist after term in infants born at ≤25 weeks gestation.

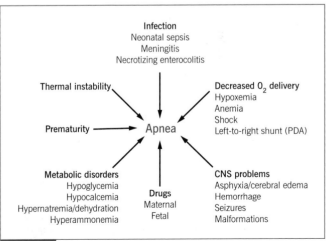

FIG. 17-3

Causes of apnea in the newborn. *(From Klaus MH, Fanaroff AA. Care of the high-risk neonate, 4th ed. Philadelphia: WB Saunders; 1993.)*

17

NEONATOLOGY

3. **Management**
a. Consider pathologic causes for apnea.
b. Pharmacotherapy with theophylline, aminophylline, caffeine, or doxapram (see Formulary for dosage information).
c. Continuous positive-airway pressure or mechanical ventilation (see Chapter 22 for details).

B. BRADYCARDIA WITHOUT CENTRAL APNEA

Obstructive apnea, mechanical airway obstruction, gastroesophageal reflux (GER), increased intracranial pressure (ICP), increased vagal tone (defecation, yawning, rectal stimulation, placement of nasogastric tube), electrolyte abnormalities, heart block.

VIII. CARDIAC DISEASES

A. PATENT DUCTUS ARTERIOSUS (PDA)

1. **Summary:** Failure of the ductus arteriosus to close in the first few days of life or reopening after functional closure. Typically results in left-to-right shunting of blood once pulmonary vascular resistance (PVR) has decreased. If the PVR remains high, blood may be shunted right to left, resulting in hypoxemia (see Persistent Pulmonary Hypertension, p. 388).

2. **Incidence:** Up to 60% in preterm infants weighing <1500 g, higher in those <1000 g. Female:male ratio is 2:1. Obligatory PDA is found in 10% of infants with congenital heart disease.

3. **Risk factors:** Most often related to hypoxia and immaturity. Term infants with PDA usually have structural defects in the walls of the ductal vessel.

4. **Diagnosis**
a. Examination: 1-4/6 continuous "machinery" murmur loudest at the left upper sternal border (LUSB) or left infraclavicular area. May have apical diastolic rumble because of increased blood flow across the mitral valve in diastole. Bounding peripheral pulses with widened pulse pressure (>60 mmHg difference between systolic and diastolic) if large shunt. Hyperactive precordium and palmar pulses may also be present.
b. Electrocardiogram (ECG): Normal or left ventricular hypertrophy in small-moderate PDA. Bilateral ventricular hypertrophy in large PDA.
c. Chest radiograph: May have cardiomegaly and increased pulmonary vascular markings depending on size of the shunt.

5. **Management**
a. Indomethacin: A prostaglandin synthetase inhibitor; 80% closure rate in preterm infants.
   (1) For dosage information and contraindications, see Formulary.
   (2) Complications: Transient decrease in glomerular filtration rate (GFR) and subsequent decreased urine output; transient GI bleeding (not associated with an increased incidence of necrotizing enterocolitis [NEC]); and prolonged bleeding time and disturbed platelet function

for 7 to 9 days independent of platelet number (not associated with increased incidence of intracranial hemorrhage).

b. Surgical ligation of the duct.

B. CYANOTIC HEART DISEASE

See Chapter 6.

IX. HEMATOLOGIC DISEASES

A. UNCONJUGATED HYPERBILIRUBINEMIA IN THE NEWBORN[6]

1. **Summary:** During the first 3 to 4 days of life, infants' serum bilirubin increases from cord bilirubin levels of 1.5 mg/dL to 6.5 ±2.5 mg/dL. The maximum rate of increase in bilirubin for otherwise normal infants with nonhemolytic hyperbilirubinemia is 5 mg/dL/24 hours or 0.2 mg/dL/hr. Visible jaundice or a total bilirubin concentration >5 mg/dL on the first day of life is outside the normal range and suggests a potentially pathologic cause. Infants <37 weeks gestation tend to have maximum serum indirect bilirubin levels 30% to 50% higher compared with term infants. Treatment guidelines for preterm infants (Table 17-7) differ from those for term infants (Table 17-8).

2. **Evaluation**

a. Maternal prenatal testing: ABO and Rh (D) typing and serum screen for isoimmune antibodies.

TABLE 17-7

GUIDELINES FOR THE USE OF PHOTOTHERAPY IN PRETERM INFANTS <1 WEEK OF AGE*

Weight (g)	Phototherapy	Consider Exchange Transfusion
500-1000	5-7	12-15
1000-1500	7-10	15-18
1500-2500	10-15	18-20
>2500	>15	>20

*Bilirubin values in milligrams per deciliter.

TABLE 17-8

MANAGEMENT OF UNCONJUGATED HYPERBILIRUBINEMIA IN THE TERM NEWBORN*

Age (hr)	Consider Phototherapy	Phototherapy	Exchange Transfusion if Intensive Phototherapy Fails	Exchange Transfusion and Intensive Phototherapy
25-48	≥12	≥15	≥20	≥25
49-72	≥15	≥18	≥25	≥30
>72	≥17	≥20	≥25	≥30

Data from American Academy of Pediatrics, Provisional Committee for Quality Improvement and Subcommittee on Hyperbilirubinemia. Pediatrics 1994; 94(4 Pt 1):558-565.
*Bilirubin values in milligrams per deciliter.

17

NEONATOLOGY

b. Infant or cord blood: Evaluation of blood smear, direct Coombs' test, blood type, and Rh typing if mother has not had prenatal blood typing or she is blood type O or Rh negative.

3. **Management**

a. Phototherapy

(1) Preterm newborn (see Table 17-7): Bilirubin levels may significantly increase in the infant who is less than 36 weeks gestation, weighs <2500 g, and who is breast-feeding. These infants may require phototherapy at lower bilirubin levels.

(2) Term newborn (see Table 17-8): Intensive phototherapy should produce a decline of the total serum bilirubin (TSB) level of 1 to 2 mg/dL within 4 to 6 hours. The TSB level should continue to fall and remain below the threshold level for exchange transfusion. If this does not occur, it is considered a failure of phototherapy.

b. Neonatal exchange transfusion: To complete double-volume exchange, transfuse 160 mL/kg for full-term infant and 160 to 200 mL/kg for preterm infant. During the exchange, blood is removed through the umbilical artery catheter and an equal volume is infused through the venous catheter. If unable to pass an arterial catheter, use a single venous catheter. Exchange in 15-mL increments in vigorous full-term infants, smaller volumes for smaller, less stable infants. Withdraw and infuse blood 2 to 3 mL/kg/min to avoid mechanical trauma to patient and donor cells. Complications include emboli, thromboses, hemodynamic instability, electrolyte disturbances, coagulopathy, and infection.

NOTE: CBC, reticulocyte count, peripheral smear, bilirubin, Ca^{2+}, glucose, total protein, infant blood type, Coombs' test, and newborn screen should be performed on a pre-exchange sample of blood because they are of no diagnostic value on postexchange blood. If indicated, save pre-exchange blood for serologic or chromosome studies.

B. POLYCYTHEMIA

1. **Definition:** Venous hematocrit >65% confirmed on two consecutive samples. May be falsely elevated when sample obtained by heel stick.

2. **Etiology:** Delayed cord clamping; twin-twin transfusion; maternal-fetal transfusion; intrauterine hypoxia; trisomy 13, 18, or 21; Beckwith-Wiedemann syndrome; maternal gestational diabetes; neonatal thyrotoxicosis; and congenital adrenal hyperplasia.

3. **Clinical findings:** Plethora, respiratory distress, cardiac failure, tachypnea, hypoglycemia, irritability, lethargy, seizures, apnea, jitteriness, poor feeding, thrombocytopenia, hyperbilirubinemia.

4. **Complications:** Hyperviscosity predisposes to venous thrombosis and CNS injury. Hypoglycemia may result from increased erythrocyte utilization of glucose.

5. **Management:** Partial exchange transfusion for symptomatic infants with isovolemic replacement of blood with isotonic fluid. Blood is exchanged in 10- to 20-mL increments to reduce hematocrit (Hct) to <55. (See p. 305 to calculate the amount of blood to be exchanged. Use birth weight (kg) × 90 for estimated blood volume [EBV].)

X. NECROTIZING ENTEROCOLITIS (NEC)

A. DEFINITION

NEC is serious intestinal inflammation and injury thought to be secondary to bowel ischemia, immaturity, and infection.

B. INCIDENCE

NEC is more common in preterm infants (3% to 4% of infants <2000 g) and African-American infants. There is no gender predominance.

C. RISK FACTORS

Prematurity, asphyxia, hypotension, polycythemia/hyperviscosity syndrome, umbilical vessel catheterization, exchange transfusion, bacterial/viral pathogens, enteral feeds, PDA, congestive heart failure, cyanotic heart disease, RDS, in utero cocaine exposure.

D. CLINICAL FINDINGS

1. **Systemic:** Temperature instability, apnea, bradycardia, metabolic acidosis, hypotension, disseminated intravascular coagulation (DIC).
2. **Intestinal:** Elevated pregavage residuals with abdominal distension, blood in stool, absent bowel sounds, and/or abdominal tenderness or mass. Elevated pregavage residuals in the absence of other clinical symptoms rarely raise suspicion of NEC.
3. **Radiologic:** Ileus, intestinal pneumatosis, portal vein gas, ascites, pneumoperitoneum.

E. MANAGEMENT

No food or water by mouth (NPO), nasogastric (NG) tube decompression, maintain adequate hydration and perfusion, antibiotics for 7 to 14 days, surgical consultation. Surgery is performed for signs of perforation or necrotic bowel.

XI. NEUROLOGIC DISEASES

A. INTRAVENTRICULAR HEMORRHAGE (IVH)

1. **Definition:** Intracranial hemorrhage usually arising in the germinal matrix and periventricular regions of the brain.
2. **Incidence:** Approximately 30% to 40% of infants weighing <1500 g; 50% to 60% of infants weighing <1000 g. Highest incidence in first 72 hours of life, 60% within 24 hours, 85% within 72 hours, <5% after 1 week postnatal age.
3. **Diagnosis and classification:** Ultrasonography is used in the diagnosis and classification of IVH. Routine screening is indicated in infants <32 weeks gestational age within the first week of life and should be repeated in the second week. The grade is based on the maximum amount of hemorrhage seen by 2 weeks of age.
   a. Grade I: Hemorrhage in germinal matrix only.
   b. Grade II: IVH without ventricular dilatation.
   c. Grade III: IVH with ventricular dilatation (30% to 45% incidence of motor/cognitive impairment).
   d. Grade IV: IVH with periventricular hemorrhagic infarct (60% to 80% incidence of motor/cognitive impairment).
4. **Prophylaxis:** Maintain acid-base balance and avoid fluctuations in blood

17

NEONATOLOGY

pressure. Pharmacologic prophylaxis includes indomethacin for prevention of severe hemorrhage (see Formulary for dosage information).

5. **Outcome:** Infants with grade III and IV hemorrhages have a higher incidence of neurodevelopmental handicap and an increased risk of posthemorrhagic hydrocephalus.

B. PERIVENTRICULAR LEUKOMALACIA (PVL)

1. **Definition and ultrasound findings:** Ischemic necrosis of periventricular white matter characterized by CNS depression within first week and ultrasound findings of cysts with or without ventricular enlargement caused by cerebral atrophy.

2. **Incidence:** More common in preterm infants, but also occurs in term infants; 3.2% in infants <1500 g.

3. **Etiology:** Primarily ischemia/reperfusion injury, hypoxia, acidosis, hypoglycemia, acute hypotension, low cerebral blood flow.

4. **Outcome:** Commonly associated with cerebral palsy with or without sensory/cognitive deficit.

C. NEONATAL SEIZURES

See pp. 427-429.

XII. RETINOPATHY OF PREMATURITY (ROP)[7]

A. DEFINITION

ROP is the interruption of the normal progression of retinal vascularization.

B. ETIOLOGY

Exposure of the immature retina to high oxygen concentrations can result in vasoconstriction and obliteration of the retinal capillary network, followed by vasoproliferation. Risk is greatest in the most immature infant.

C. DIAGNOSIS

All infants born weighing <1300 g, or at <30 weeks gestation, and any infant born weighing <1800 g, or at <35 weeks gestation, who requires oxygen should have a dilated funduscopic examination either 5 to 7 weeks after birth or before discharge home, whichever is earlier, to screen for ROP.

D. CLASSIFICATION

ROP is described by the stage of disease, the highest zone of the retina involved (Fig. 17-4), the number of clock hours or 30-degree sectors involved, and the presence or absence of plus disease.

1. **Stage 1:** Demarcation line separates avascular from vascularized retina.

2. **Stage 2:** Ridge forms along demarcation line.

3. **Stage 3:** Extraretinal fibrovascular proliferation tissue forms on ridge.

4. **Stage 4:** Retinal detachment.

5. **Plus disease:** Tortuosity and engorgement of blood vessels near the optic disc; may be present at any stage.

E. MANAGEMENT

Laser treatment is recommended when there are five contiguous or eight total 30-degree sectors of stage 3 in zone 1 or in zone 2 if accompanied by plus disease; the risk of blindness if untreated is 50%. An infant with stage 3 ROP in zone 2, stage 2 ROP with plus disease in zone 2, or any stage

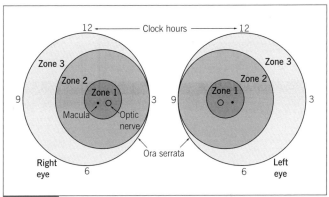

FIG. 17-4

Zones of the retina. *(From AAP: Pediatrics 1994; 94(4 Pt 1):558-565.)*

disease in zone 1 should have ophthalmologic examinations weekly to monitor progression of the ROP. All other infants should have ophthalmologic examinations every 2 weeks until the retina is fully vascularized.

XIII. CONGENITAL INFECTIONS

See Chapter 16.

REFERENCES

1. Wiswell TE et al. Delivery room management of the apparently vigorous meconium-stained neonate: results of the multicenter, international collaborative trial. Pediatrics 2000; 105:1.
2. Apgar V. A proposal for new method of evaluation of the newborn infant. Anesth Analg 1953; 32:260.
3. Ballard JL et al. New Ballard Score, expanded to include extremely premature infants. J Pediatr 1991; 119:417-423.
4. Cornblath M. Neonatal hypoglycemia. In Donn SM, Fisher CW, editors. Risk management techniques in perinatal and neonatal practice. Armonk, NY: Futura; 1996.
5. Klaus MH, Fanaroff AA. Care of the high-risk neonate, 4th ed. Philadelphia: WB Saunders, 1993.
6. American Academy of Pediatrics, Provisional Committee for Quality Improvement and Subcommittee on Hyperbilirubinemia. Practice parameter: management of hyperbilirubinemia in the healthy term newborn. Pediatrics 1994; 94(4 Pt 1):558-565.
7. Ben-Sira I et al. An international classification of retinopathy of prematurity. Pediatrics 1984; 74:127.

NEPHROLOGY

Melissa M. Sparrow, MD

I. URINALYSIS/URINE DIPSTICK

It is best if the urine specimen is evaluated within 1 hour after voiding, and ideally after the first morning void.

A. COLOR (Box 18-1)

B. TURBIDITY

Cloudy urine can be normal, and is most often the result of crystal formation at room temperature. Uric acid crystals form in acidic urine, and phosphate crystals form in alkaline urine. Cellular material and bacteria can also cause turbidity.

C. SPECIFIC GRAVITY

Specific gravity is measured in a refractometer, which requires one drop of urine, and is based on the principle that the refractive index (RI) of a solution is related to the content of dissolved solids present. The RI varies with, but is not identical to, specific gravity. The refractometer measures RI but is calibrated for specific gravity. Glucose, abundant protein, and iodine-

18

BOX 18-1

ETIOLOGIES OF ABNORMAL URINE COLOR

RED

Beets, blackberries, deferoxamine (with elevated serum iron), doxorubicin, food coloring, hemoglobin, phenazopyridine (acid urine), phenolphthalein (laxatives, alkaline urine), phenothiazines, phenytoin, porphyrins, pyrvinium pamoate, red blood cells, red diaper syndrome (nonpathogenic Serratia marcescens), urates (brick-dust phenomenon—urates reacting with chemical in diapers)

YELLOW-BROWN

Antimalarials (pamaquine, primaquine, quinacrine), B-complex vitamins, bilirubin, carotene, cascara, metronidazole, nitrofurantoin, sulfasalazine (alkaline urine), sulfonamides

BROWN-BLACK

Hemosiderin, homogentisic urine (alkaptonuria), melanin (especially in alkaline urine), myoglobin, old blood, quinine, rhubarb

BURGUNDY

Porphyrins (old urine)

DEEP YELLOW

Riboflavin

ORANGE

Phenazopyridine, rifabutin, rifampin, urates (brick-dust phenomenon), warfarin

BLUE-GREEN

Amitriptyline, biliverdin (obstructive jaundice), blue diaper syndrome (familial disorder characterized by hypercalcemia, nephrocalcinosis, indicanuria), doxorubicin, indomethacin, methylene blue, Pseudomonas, urinary tract infection (rare), riboflavin containing contrast materials can give falsely high readings. Normal specific gravity is between 1.003 and 1.030.

D. pH

pH levels are estimated using indicator paper or dipstick. To improve accuracy, use a freshly voided specimen and pH meter. Levels can be inappropriately high with hypokalemia, and they can also be used to assess various types of renal tubular acidosis (Table 18-1).

E. PROTEIN

1. Significant proteinuria, as determined by the following tests, should be confirmed by a 24-hour urine collection.

a. Dipstick is the easiest method, but it detects only albumin. Levels are significant if they are ≥1+ (30 mg/dL) on two of three random samples 1 week apart when the urine specific gravity is ≤1.015, or if ≥2+ (100 mg/dL) on similarly collected urine when the specific gravity is >1.015. False positives can occur with highly concentrated alkaline urine (pH >8), gross hematuria, pyuria, bacteriuria, and quaternary ammonium cleansers (e.g., antiseptics, chlorhexidine, or benzalkonium). False negatives can occur with very dilute or acidic urine (pH 4.5) and nonalbumin proteinuria, which can be detected by sulfosalicylic acid.

b. Protein/creatinine ratio[1]: Determine the ratio of protein (mg/dL) and creatinine (mg/dL) concentrations in randomly collected spot urine. The normal urinary protein : urinary creatinine (Upr : Ucr) is <0.2 in older children and <0.5 during the first few months of life. A Upr : Ucr ratio >1.0 is highly suspicious of nephrotic range proteinuria. All aberrant ratios should be confirmed with a 24-hour urine collection for proteinuria.

c. 24-hour urine collection. (see p. 408)
   (1) Most accurate method.[2]
   (2) Normal: ≤4 mg of protein/m^2/hr; abnormal: 4 to 40 mg/m^2/hr; nephrotic range: >40 mg/m^2/hr.[2]

2. Types of proteinuria (Fig. 18-1).

3. 24-hour urine protein excretion in children of different ages (Table 18-2).

4. Suggested evaluation of proteinuria[3] (Fig. 18-2).

NOTE: Asymptomatic patients should have dipstick/urinalysis repeated two or three times before extensive evaluation is started. Negative repeat tests indicate transient/isolated proteinuria, and only routine medical care is necessary.

F. SUGARS

Normally, urine does not contain sugars. Glucosuria is suggestive but not diagnostic of diabetes mellitus or proximal renal tubular disease (see p. 410). The presence of other reducing sugars can be confirmed by chromatography.

1. Dipstick: Easiest method but only detects glucose. False negatives occur with high levels of ascorbic acid (used as preservative in antibiotics) in urine.

TABLE 18-1
BIOCHEMICAL AND CLINICAL CHARACTERISTICS OF THE VARIOUS TYPES OF RENAL TUBULAR ACIDOSIS

	Distal Type I	Type 1 With HCO_3^- Wasting	Proximal Type II	Hyperkalemic Type IV
AT SUBNORMAL (HCO_3^-)*				
Minimal urine pH	>5.5	>5.5	<5.5	<5.5
TA and NH_4^+ excretion	↓	↓	nl or ↓	→
Urinary citrate excretion	↓	↓	↑	?
Plasma K^+ concentration	nl or ↓	nl or ↓	Usually ↓	↑
Renal K^+ clearance	>20%	>20%	>20%	<20%
Urine anion gap†	Positive	Positive	Positive or ? negative	Positive
AT NORMAL (HCO_3^-)				
TA and NH_4^+ excretion	→	→	→	→
Fractional HCO_3^- excretion	3%-5%	5%-10%	>15%	1%-15%
Urinary citrate excretion	nl	nl	↑	?
Plasma K^+ concentration	nl	nl	nl or ↓	nl or ↑
U-B P_{CO_2} (mmHg)‡	<20	<20	>20	<20
Therapeutic alkali requirement (mEq/kg/day)‡	1-3	5-10	5-20	1-5
Osteomalacia	Rare	Rare	Frequent	Absent
Nephrocalcinosis/nephrolithiasis	Common	Common	Rare	Absent

From Holliday MA et al. Pediatric nephrology. Baltimore: Williams & Wilkins; 1994.
nl, Normal; *TA*, Titratable acid.
*Plasma bicarbonate concentration.
†Urine anion gap = $[Na^+] + [K^+] - [Cl^-]$ (based on urine electrolytes).
‡Urine P_{CO_2} – blood P_{CO_2}. During bicarbonate loading, when urine pH >blood pH.

18

NEPHROLOGY

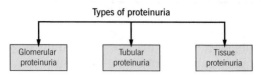

Types of proteinuria

```
                    Types of proteinuria
        ┌──────────────────┼──────────────────┐
        ▼                  ▼                  ▼
  Glomerular          Tubular            Tissue
  proteinuria         proteinuria        proteinuria
```

A. GLOMERULAR

1. Transient proteinuria: Most common in children. Associated with exercise, stress, dehydration, postural changes, cold exposure, fever, seizures, congestive heart failure, and vasoactive drugs. Serial urine tests should be negative for protein.

2. Orthostatic proteinuria: Common, not associated with renal pathology. Repeat measure of excreted urinary protein in recumbent position should be negative. Rarely exceeds 1 g/dy (see Table 18-2).

3. Proteinuria secondary to glomerulopathies

a. Primary glomerular disease: Minimal change disease, focal segmental glomerulonephritis, membranous glomerulonephritis, IgM nephropathy, IgA nephropathy.

b. Secondary glomerular disease: medications (e.g., NSAIDs, captopril, lithium), postinfectious (poststreptococcal, hepatitis B, chronic shunt infections, subacute bacterial endocarditis), infectious (bacterial, fungal, viral), neoplastic (solid tumors, leukemia), multisystem (systemic lupus erythematosus, Henoch-Schönlein purpura, sickle cell disease), reflux nephropathy, congenital nephrotic syndrome.

B. TUBULAR

1. Overload proteinuria: Occurs when excessive amount of low-molecular-weight proteins overwhelms the tubular reabsorption capacity (e.g., light chains: multiple myeloma; lysozyme: monocytic and myelocytic leukemias; myoglobin: rhabdomyolysis; hemoglobin: hemolysis).

2. Tubular dysfunction or disorders: Occurs when normal amounts of low-molecular-weight proteins (e.g., amino acids) are not adequately reabsorbed because of damaged or dysfunctional tubular cells (Fanconi's syndrome, Lowe's syndrome, reflux nephropathy, cystinosis, drugs/heavy metals [mercury, lead, cadmium, outdated tetracyclines]), ischemic tubular injury, and renal hypoplasia/dysplasia.

C. TISSUE
1. Acute inflammation of urinary tract
2. Uroepithelial tumors

FIG. 18-1

Types of proteinuria. *NSAIDs,* Nonsteroidal antiinflammatory drugs.

TABLE 18-2

24-HOUR URINE PROTEIN EXCRETION IN CHILDREN OF DIFFERENT AGES (NORMAL RANGES)

Age	Protein Concentration (mg/L)	Protein Excretion (mg/24hr)	Protein Excretion (mg/24hr/m² BSA)
Premature (5-30 days)	88-845	29 (14-60)	182 (88-377)
Full-term	94-455	32 (15-68)	145 (68-309)
2-12 mo	70-315	38 (17-85)	109 (48-244)
2-4 yr	45-217	49 (20-121)	91 (37-223)
4-10 yr	50-223	71 (26-194)	85 (31-234)
10-16 yr	45-391	83 (29-238)	63 (22-181)

From Cruz C, Spitzer A. Contemp Pediatr 1998; 15(9):89.

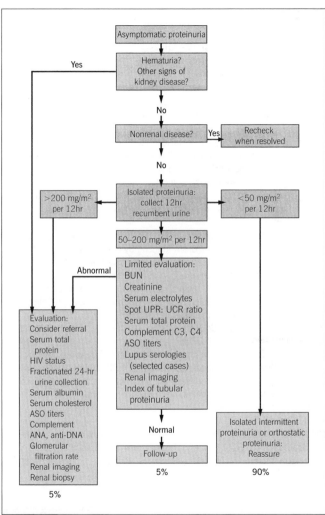

FIG. 18-2

Suggested evaluation of proteinuria in asymptomatic patients. *(From Cruz C, Spitzer A. Contemp Pediatr 1998; 15(9):89.)*

18

NEPHROLOGY

TABLE 18-3

URINALYSIS FOR BILIRUBIN/UROBILINOGEN

	Normal	Hemolytic Disease	Hepatic Disease	Biliary Obstruction
Urine urobilinogen	Normal	Increased	Increased	Decreased
Urine bilirubin	Negative	Negative	+/−	Positive

2. **Clinitest tablet (Ames Co.):** Nonspecific test; changes color if urine is positive for reducing substances, including reducing sugars (glucose, fructose, galactose, pentoses, lactose), amino acids, ascorbic acid, chloral hydrate, chloramphenicol, creatinine, cysteine, glucuronates, hippurate, homogentisic acid, isoniazid, acetoacetic acid, acetone, nitrofurantoin, oxalate, TPN, penicillin, salicylates, streptomycin, sulfonamides, tetracycline, and uric acid. Because sucrose is not a reducing sugar, it is not detected by Clinitest.

G. KETONES

Except for trace amounts, ketonuria suggests ketoacidosis, usually from either diabetes mellitus or catabolism induced by inadequate intake. Neonatal ketoacidosis may occur with a metabolic defect, such as propionic acidemia, methylmalonic aciduria, or a glycogen storage disease.

1. **Dipstick:** Detects acetoacetic acid best, acetone less well; does not detect β-hydroxybutyrate. False positives may occur after phthalein administration or with phenylketonuria.
2. **Acetest tablet (Ames Co.):** Detects only acetoacetic acid and acetone.

H. HEMOGLOBIN/MYOGLOBIN

A dipstick reads positive with intact red blood cells (RBCs), hemoglobin, and myoglobin, and can detect as few as 3 to 4 RBCs/high-power field (hpf). False positives can occur with the presence of bacterial peroxidases, high ascorbic acid concentrations, and Betadine (i.e., from fingers of medical staff).

I. BILIRUBIN/UROBILINOGEN

Dipstick measures each individually. Urine bilirubin will be positive with conjugated hyperbilirubinemia; in this form bilirubin is water soluble and excreted by the kidney. Urobilinogen will be increased in cases of hyperbilirubinemia in which there is no obstruction to enterohepatic circulation (Table 18-3).

II. URINALYSIS/MICROSCOPY

A. RBCs

Centrifuged urine usually contains fewer than 5 RBCs/hpf. Significant hematuria is 5 to 10 RBCs/hpf and corresponds to a Chemstrip reading of 50 RBCs/hpf or Labstix reading "trace hemolyzed" or "small." Microscopy is used to differentiate hemoglobinuria or myoglobinuria from hematuria (intact RBCs). In addition, examination of RBC morphology by phase contrast microscopy may help to localize the source of bleeding. Dysmorphic, small RBCs suggest a glomerular origin, whereas normal RBCs suggest lower tract bleeding.

1. **Differentiation between hemoglobinuria and myoglobinuria**

a. History: Hemoglobinuria is seen with intravascular hemolysis or in hematuric urine that has been standing for an extended period. Myoglobinuria is seen in crush injuries, vigorous exercise, major motor seizures, fever and malignant hyperthermia, electrocution, snakebites, ischemia, some muscle and metabolic disorders, and some infections such as influenza.

b. Laboratory studies: Clinical laboratories may use many techniques to measure hemoglobin or myoglobin directly. Other laboratory data may also be used to identify the source of urinary pigment indirectly. For example, in nephropathy from myoglobinuria, the blood urea nitrogen (BUN):creatinine ratio is low (creatinine is released from damaged muscles) and the creatine phosphokinase (CPK) level is high.

2. **Suggested evaluation of persistent hematuria** (Fig. 18-3)[1,2,4-6]

a. Examination of urine sediment, urine dipstick for protein, urine culture, sickle cell screen, urine calcium:creatinine ratio, family history, medication history, and audiology screen if indicated.

b. Serum electrolytes, BUN, serum creatinine, serum total protein and albumin, complete blood count (CBC) with smear, immunoglobulins, and hepatitis serologies; consider testing for human immunodeficiency virus (HIV).

c. Antistreptolysin O (ASO) titers, C3, C4, and antinuclear antibodies (ANA).

d. Renal ultrasonography and other indicated radiologic studies.

B. SEDIMENT

Using light microscopy, unstained, centrifuged urine can be examined for formed elements, including casts, cells, and crystals. Centrifuge 10 mL for 5 minutes, then decant 9 mL of supernatant. Resuspend sediment in remaining 1 mL of urine. Place drop on glass slide; use coverslip. Best results are obtained with subdued light. Focus particularly on the edge of the coverslip because formed elements collect there.

C. EPITHELIAL CELLS

Squamous epithelial cells (>10 per low power field) are useful as an index of possible contamination by vaginal secretions in females or by foreskin in uncircumcised males.

D. WHITE BLOOD CELLS (WBCs)

Greater than 5 WBCs/hpf of properly spun urine specimen is suggestive of a urinary tract infection (UTI). Sterile pyuria is rare in the pediatric population. If present, it is usually transient and accompanies systemic infection, for example, with Kawasaki disease. May also be a sign of urolithiasis.

E. BACTERIA/URINE GRAM'S STAIN

A Gram's stain is used to screen for UTIs. One organism/hpf in uncentrifuged urine represents at least 10^5 colonies/mL.

18

NEPHROLOGY

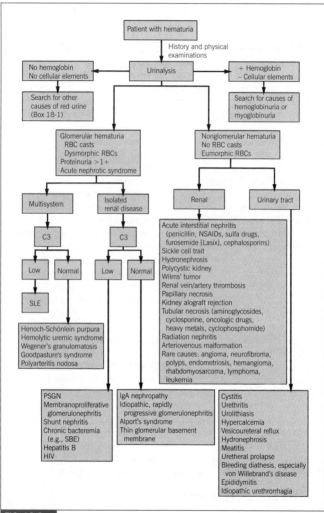

FIG. 18-3

A diagnostic strategy for hematuria. *HIV,* Human immunodeficiency virus; *NSAIDs,* nonsteroidal antiinflammatory drugs; *PSGN,* poststreptococcal glomerulonephritis; *RBC,* red blood cell; *SBE,* subacute bacterial endocarditis; *SLE,* systemic lupus erythematosus.

III. EVALUATION AND MANAGEMENT OF UTIs

NOTE: These recommendations are suggestions and vary from institution to institution and physician to physician. Use them together with the routinely practiced guidelines of your institution.

A. HISTORY

Voiding history (stool/urine) in toilet-trained children, sexual intercourse, sexual abuse, masturbation, pinworms, prolonged baths, bubble baths, evaluation of growth curve, and family history for vesicoureteral reflux/recurrent UTIs.

B. PHYSICAL EXAMINATION

Vital signs, especially blood pressure (BP); abdominal examination for flank masses, bowel distention, evidence of impaction; meatal stenosis/circumcision in males; vulvovaginitis or labial adhesions in females; neurologic examination of lower extremities; perineal sensation/reflexes; rectal/sacral examination.

C. LABORATORY STUDIES

Urinalysis with microscopic examination and urine culture (Table 18-4). NOTE: All tests must be confirmed with a urine culture. Also helpful if available are the following studies:

1. **Nitrite test:** Detects nitrites produced by the reduction of dietary nitrates by urinary gram-negative bacteria (especially *Escherichia coli* and Klebsiella and Proteus spp.). A positive test is virtually diagnostic of bacteriuria. False negatives can occur with inadequate dietary nitrates, insufficient time for bacterial proliferation, inability of bacteria to reduce nitrates to nitrites (many gram-positive organisms such as Enterococcus, Mycobacterium spp., and fungi), and large volumes of dilute urine.
2. **Leukocyte esterase test:** Detects esterases released from broken-down leukocytes, an indirect test for WBCs that may or may not be present with a UTI.
3. **BUN/Cr.**

18

NEPHROLOGY

TABLE 18-4	
URINE CULTURE: INTERPRETATION IN DIAGNOSIS OF A UTI	
Method of Collection	Quantitative Culture: UTI Present
Suprapubic aspiration	Growth of urinary pathogens in any number (the exception is up to 2×10^3 CFU/mL of coagulase-negative staphylococci)
Catheterization	Febrile infants or children usually have $>50 \times 10^3$ CFU/mL of a single urinary pathogen, but infection may be present with counts from 10×10^3 to 50×10^3 CFU/mL
Midstream clean catch, voided	Symptomatic patients usually have $>10^5$ CFU/mL of a single urinary tract pathogen
Midstream clean catch, voided	Asymptomatic patients: At least two specimens on different days with $>10^5$ CFU/mL of the same organism

From Hellerstein S. Pediatr Clin North Am 1995; 42:1142.
CFU/mL, Colony-forming units per milliliter.

D. CULTURE POSITIVE UTI

Treatment should be based on urine culture and sensitivities if possible.

1. **Cystitis:** Conventional therapy for uncomplicated lower-tract UTI is for 7 to 10 days, especially for children <5 years. Recent studies have also shown short (3 to 5 days) courses of antibiotic therapy to be effective in clearance of infection for acute uncomplicated UTIs in females >5 years and adolescents (with known normal renal function). Repeat urine culture after 48 to 72 hours of treatment for test of cure. May consider prophylactic dose antibiotics pending radiologic evaluation, if this is to be performed.

2. **Pyelonephritis**[7,8]

a. Nontoxic/clinically stable children and infants >1 to 2 months of age can be treated with oral antibiotics as outpatients as long as compliance is not an issue. It is reasonable to initiate therapy with 1 to 2 days of a long-acting, third-generation cephalosporin via the intramuscular (IM) route, or a broad spectrum oral antibiotic such as cefixime followed by 7 to 14 days of oral antibiotics and prophylaxis until urine is evaluated and urine culture/sensitivities are known.

b. Toxic children and infants <2 to 3 months old should be considered candidates for immediate hospitalization and parenteral therapy. Parenteral antibiotic therapy should be continued for 7 to 14 days in neonates, although outpatient oral antibiotic therapy to complete a full 7- to 14-day course can be substituted in patients >2 months of age when afebrile and clinically stable for 24 to 48 hours as long as compliance is ensured.[7,8]

3. **Imaging studies:**[7,8] Imaging studies of children with their first documented UTI should be pursued in all boys, in girls <5 years, and in older girls with pyelonephritis or recurrent infections. Referral to a pediatric urologist is recommended if studies reveal obstructive lesion, high-grade (grades IV or V) vesicoureteral reflux (VUR), or progressive dimercaptosuccinic acid (DMSA) or voiding cystourethrogram (VCUG) changes on follow-up studies (Fig. 18-4).

a. Abdominal radiograph: If indicated to check stool pattern and to rule out spinal dysraphism.

b. Renal sonography: A noninvasive/nonionizing evaluation for gross structural defects, lesions that are obstructive, positional abnormalities, and renal size/growth.

c. VCUG: Perform when patient is asymptomatic and cleared of bacteriuria to evaluate for vesicoureteral reflux. Indicated in all boys, girls <5 years and those >5 years with recurrent or febrile UTIs. May be substituted with radionucleotide cystography (RNC), which has 1/100th the radiation exposure of a VCUG and increased sensitivity for transient reflux. RNC does not visualize urethral anatomy, is not sensitive for low-grade reflux, and cannot grade reflux.

d. DMSA: Tc 99m DMSA is normally taken up by renal tubules; defects on DMSA image indicate tubular defects. Indicated in patients with

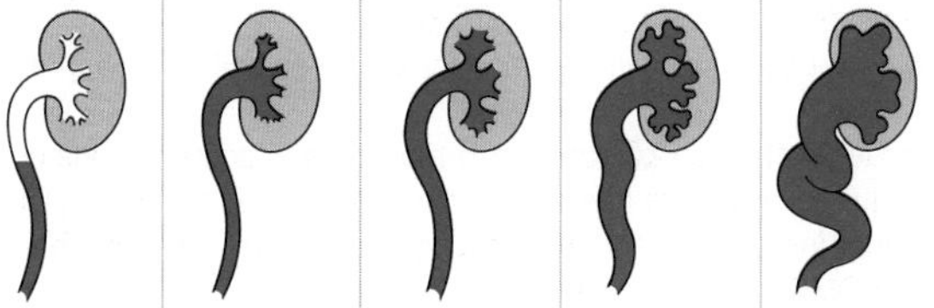

Grade I	Grade II	Grade III	Grade IV	Grade V
Ureter only	Ureter, pelvis, calyces; no dilatation, normal calyceal fornices	Mild or moderate dilatation and/or tortuosity of ureter; mild or moderate dilatation of the pelvis, but no or slight blunting of the fornices	Moderate dilatation and/or tortuosity of the ureter; mild dilatation of renal pelvis and calyces; complete obliteration of sharp angle of fornices, but maintenance of papillary impressions in majority of calyces	Gross dilatation and tortuosity of ureter; gross dilatation of renal pelvis and calyces; papillary impressions are no longer visible in majority of calyces

FIG. 18-4

International classification of vesicoureteral reflux. *(Modified from Rushton H. Pediatr Clin North Am 1997: 44:5 and International Reflux Committee. Pediatrics 1981; 67:392.)*

    an abnormal VCUG or renal sonography, in patients with history of asymptomatic bacteriuria and fever, prenatally diagnosed VUR, and in neonates/infants secondary to high incidence of hematologic spread and difficult examination. Repeat in 4 months if initial study is positive to evaluate for persistent infection and renal scarring.

e. DTPA/MAG-3: May also be used for indications given above for DMSA use. Provides quantitative assessment of renal function and drainage of dilated collecting system, as in cases of hydronephrosis in the absence of VUR.

4. **Asymptomatic bacteriuria:** Defined as bacteria in urine on microscopy/ Gram's stain in an afebrile, asymptomatic patient without pyuria. Antibiotics are not necessary if voiding habits and urinary tract are normal. Prophylaxis may be necessary in patients with bacteriuria and voiding dysfunction. DMSA may be helpful in differentiating pyelonephritis from fever and coincidental bacteriuria.

18

NEPHROLOGY

5. **Suggested indications for prophylactic antibiotics**[7,8]
a. VUR of any grade until resolution (surgically or spontaneously) (see Fig. 18-4).
b. Frequent recurrences of lower UTIs (>3 times per year), especially when associated with underlying bladder atony or abnormal voiding patterns. In conjunction with prophylactic therapy, correction of voiding disorder or constipation should also be carried out.
c. Neonates diagnosed with hydronephrosis antenatally until appropriately evaluated.[9]
d. Consider in children <2 years for 6 months after acute episode of pyelonephritis secondary to high risk of reinfection with or without VUR.[10]
e. Consider in neonates and infants <1 year who present with febrile UTI and/or DMSA changes, assuming no VUR.
f. Children with UTIs awaiting radiologic evaluations.
6. **Nonsurgical management of VUR:**[7,8] Amoxicillin recommended in first 2 months of life, otherwise TMP-SMX (trimethoprim-sulfamethoxazole) or nitrofurantoin (Macrodantin) with urine cultures every 4 months and when febrile. There is no need to discontinue antibiotics before screening urine culture. Change antibiotic therapy if patient has breakthrough UTIs while on prophylactic regimen. Repeat VCUG in 12 to 18 months to determine if VUR has resolved. Surgical correction is indicated in children >2 years with high-grade reflux (grades IV or V) and children with breakthrough pyelonephritis (especially with DMSA changes) while on prophylaxis.

IV. RENAL FUNCTION TESTS
A. TESTS OF GLOMERULAR FUNCTION
1. **Creatinine clearance (Ccr)**
a. Timed urine specimen: Standard measure of glomerular filtration rate (GFR); closely approximates insulin clearance in the normal range of GFR. When GFR is low, Ccr is greater than inulin clearance. Inaccurate in children with obstructive uropathy.
Method: Have patient empty bladder (discard specimen) before beginning the collection. Collect urine over any time period; record interval to the nearest minute. Collect all urine during that time interval, including urine voided at the end of the collection period. If the patient's renal function is stable, draw blood sample for serum creatinine once during the test period. (If function is changing rapidly, draw the blood sample at the beginning and end of the period and use the average.)

$$Ccr \ (mL/min/1.73m^2) = (U \times [V/P]) \times 1.73/BSA$$

where U (mg/dL) is urinary creatinine concentration, V (mL/min) is total urine volume (mL) divided by the duration of the collection (min) (24 hours = 1440 minutes); P (mg/dL) is serum creatinine concentration (may average two levels), and BSA (m^2) is body surface area.
b. Estimated GFR from plasma creatinine: Useful when a timed specimen cannot be collected; reasonable estimate of GFR for children with rela-

tively normal renal function and body habitus. If habitus is markedly abnormal or a precise measurement of GFR is needed, more standard methods of measuring GFR must be used.

$$\text{Estimated GFR (mL/min/1.73m}^2) = kL/Pcr$$

where k is proportionality constant, L is height (cm), Pcr is plasma creatinine (mg/dL) (Table 18-5).

2. **Glomerular function as determined by nuclear medicine scans.**
   Normal values of GFR (measured by insulin clearance) (Table 18-6).

B. TESTS OF TUBULAR FUNCTION

1. **Types of renal tubular acidosis** (see Table 18-1).
2. **Proximal tubule**
a. Proximal tubule reabsorption: The proximal tubule is responsible for the reabsorption of electrolytes, glucose, and amino acids. Studies to determine proximal tubular function compare urine and blood levels of specific compounds arriving at a percent tubular reabsorption (Tx):

$$\text{Tx} = 1 - \frac{Ux/Px}{Ucr/Pcr} \times 100\%$$

18

NEPHROLOGY

TABLE 18-5
PROPORTIONALITY CONSTANT FOR CALCULATING GFR

	k Values
Low birth weight during first year of life	0.33
Term AGA during first year of life	0.45
Children and adolescent girls	0.55
Adolescent boys	0.70

From Schwartz GJ, Brion LP, Spitzer A. Pediatr Clin North Am 1987; 34:571.
AGA, Appropriate for gestational age.

TABLE 18-6
NORMAL VALUES OF GFR

Age	GFR (Mean) (mL/min/1.73m^2)	Range (mL/min/1.73m^2)
Neonates <34 wk gestational age		
2-8 days	11	11-15
4-28 days	20	15-28
30-90 days	50	40-65
Neonates >34 wk gestational age		
2-8 days	39	17-60
4-28 days	47	26-68
30-90 days	58	30-86
1-6 mo	7	39-114
6-12 mo	103	49-157
12-19 mo	127	62-191
2 yr-adult	127	89-165

From Holliday MA et al. Pediatric nephrology. Baltimore: Williams & Wilkins; 1994.

TABLE 18-7

AGE-ADJUSTED CALCIUM/CREATININE RATIOS

Age	Ca^{2+}/Cr Ratio (mg/mg Ratio) (95th Percentile for Age)
<7 mo	0.86
7-18 mo	0.60
19 mo-6 yr	0.42
Adults	0.22

From Sargent JD et al. J Pediatr 1993; 123:393.

where Ux = concentration of compound in urine; Px = concentration of compound in plasma; Ucr = concentration of creatinine in urine; Pcr = concentration of creatinine in plasma. This formula can be used for amino acids, electrolytes, calcium, and phosphorus.

b. Glucose reabsorption: The glucose threshold is the plasma glucose concentration at which significant amounts of glucose appear in the urine. The presence of glucosuria must be interpreted in relation to simultaneously determined plasma glucose concentration. If the plasma glucose concentration is <120 mg/dL, and glucose is present in the urine, this implies incompetent tubular reabsorption of glucose and proximal renal tubular disease.

c. Bicarbonate reabsorption: The majority of bicarbonate reabsorption occurs in the proximal tubule. Abnormalities in reabsorption lead to type II renal tubular acidosis. These patients have high fractional excretion of bicarbonate in their urine at normal serum bicarbonate levels. However, they can acidify their urine when faced with metabolic acidosis (see Table 18-1).

3. **Distal tubule**

a. Urine acidification: A urine acidification defect (distal renal tubular acidosis) should be suspected when random urine pH values are >6 in the presence of moderate systemic metabolic acidosis. Acidification defects should be confirmed by simultaneous venous or arterial pH, plasma bicarbonate concentration, and pH meter (not dipstick) determination of the pH of fresh urine.

b. Urine concentration occurs in the distal tubule[11]: A random urine specific gravity of 1.023 or more indicates intact concentrating ability within the limits of clinical testing; no further tests are indicated. A first-voided specimen after an overnight fast is adequate to test concentrating ability. (For more formal testing, see water deprivation test, Chapter 9.)

c. Urine calcium: Hypercalciuria is seen usually with distal renal tubular acidosis, vitamin D intoxication, hyperparathyroidism, steroids, immobilization, excessive calcium intake, and loop diuretics. It may be idiopathic (associated with hematuria and renal calculi.) Diagnosis is as follows:
   (1) 24-hour urine: Calcium >4 mg/kg/24 hours.
   (2) Spot urine: Determine Ca:Cr ratio. It is recommended that an abnormally elevated spot urine Ca:Cr ratio be followed up with a 24-hour urine calcium determination (Table 18-7).

TABLE 18-8

LABORATORY DIFFERENTIATION OF OLIGURIA

	Prenatal Oliguria		Low Output Failure		ADH Secretion
Test	>1 Mo	Neonates	>1 Mo	Neonates	All Ages
Urine sodium	<20	<40	>40	>40	>40
Specific gravity	>1.020	>1.015	<1.010	<1.015	>1.020
Osmolality (mOsmol/L)	>500	>400	<350	<400	>500
Urine/plasma osmolality ratio	>1.3	—	<1.3	—	>2
Urea nitrogen	>20	—	<10	—	>15
Creatinine	>40	>20	<20	<15	>30
RFI*	<1	<3	>1	>3	>1
FE (Na)†	<1	<2.5	>1	>3	Close to 1

Modified from Rogers MC. Textbook of pediatric intensive care. Baltimore: Williams & Wilkins; 1992.
ADH, Antidiuretic hormone.
*RFI (renal failure index) = $(UNa \times 100)/Ucr \times Pcr$.
†FE (Na) (fractional excretion of sodium) = $(UNa/PNa)/(Ucr/Pcr) \times 100$.

V. OLIGURIA

Urine output <300 mL/m^2/24 hours, or <0.5 mL/kg/hour in children and <1.0 mL/kg/hour in infants.

A. BUN/CR RATIO (both in mg/dL)[12]

1. **Normal ratio:** 10-20; suggests intrinsic renal disease in the setting of oliguria.
2. **>20:** Suggests dehydration, prerenal azotemia, or gastrointestinal (GI) bleeding.
3. **<5:** Suggests liver disease, starvation, inborn error of metabolism.

B. LABORATORY DIFFERENTIATION OF OLIGURIA (Table 18-8)

VI. ACUTE DIALYSIS

A. INDICATIONS

1. **Acute dialysis is indicated when metabolic or fluid derangements are not controlled by aggressive medical management alone.** Generally accepted criteria include the following, although a nephrologist should always be consulted:
   a. Volume overload with evidence of pulmonary edema or hypertension that is refractory to therapy.
   b. Hyperkalemia >6.0 mEq/L if hypercatabolic or >6.5 mEq/L despite conservative measures.
   c. Metabolic acidosis with pH <7.2, or HCO_3^- <10.
   d. BUN >150; lower if rising rapidly.
   e. Neurologic symptoms secondary to uremia or electrolyte imbalance.
   f. Calcium/phosphorus imbalance (e.g., hypocalcemia with tetany or seizures in the presence of a very high serum phosphate).
2. **Dialyzable toxin or poison** (e.g., lactate, ammonia, alcohol, barbiturates, ethylene glycol, isopropanol, methanol, salicylates, theophylline).

B. TECHNIQUES[13]

1. **Peritoneal dialysis (PD):** Requires catheter to access the peritoneal cavity. May be used acutely or chronically, as in continuous ambulatory or continuous cycling peritoneal dialysis.
2. **Hemodialysis (HD):** Requires placement of special vascular access devices. May be the method of choice for certain toxins (e.g., ammonia, uric acid, or poisons) or when there are contraindications to peritoneal dialysis.
3. **Continuous arteriovenous hemofiltration/hemodialysis (CAVH/D) and continuous venovenous hemofiltration/hemodialysis (CVVH/D):** CAVH and CVVH are therapies with the primary goal of the continuous generation of a plasma ultrafiltrate. Indications include fluid management, renal failure with profound hemodynamic instability, electrolyte disturbance(s), and intoxication with substances that are freely filtered across the particular ultrafiltration membrane utilized. CAVH and CVVH can be helpful in the management of oliguric patients who are in need of better nutritional support, postoperative cardiac patients, and patients with septicemia. These therapies also require special vascular access devices.

C. PD, HD, AND CAVH/CVVH (Table 18-9)

TABLE 18-9
PD VERSUS HD VERSUS CAVH/CVVH

	PD	HD	CAVH/CVVH
BENEFITS			
Fluid removal	+	++	++
Urea and creatinine clearance	+	++	+
Potassium clearance	++	++	+
Toxin clearance	+	++	+
COMPLICATIONS			
Abdominal pain	+	−	−
Bleeding	−	+	+
Decreased cardiac output	+	+	+
Disequilibrium	−	+	−
Electrolyte imbalance	+	+	+
Need for heparinization	−	+	+
Hyperglycemia	+	−	−
Hypotension	+	++	+
Hypothermia	−	−	+
Infection (other than peritonitis)	−	+	+
Inguinal hernia	+	−	−
Lactic acidosis	Possible	−	Possible
Neutropenia	−	+	−
Pancreatitis	+	−	−
Peritonitis	+	−	−
Protein loss	++	−	−
Respiratory compromise	+	Possible	−
Thrombocytopenia	−	+	−
Vessel thrombosis	−	+	+

Modified from Rogers MC. Textbook of pediatric intensive care. Baltimore: Williams & Wilkins; 1992.

VII. CHRONIC HYPERTENSION

Note: For management of acute hypertension, see Chapter 1.

A. DEFINITION

For the definition of chronic hypertension, see Chapter 6.

1. **Normal BP:** Systolic and diastolic BP <90th percentile for age, gender, height, and weight.
2. **High normal BP:** Average systolic and/or diastolic BP between the 90th and 95th percentiles for age, gender, height, and weight.
3. **Significant hypertension:** The average of three separate systolic and/or diastolic blood pressures >95th percentile for age, gender, height, and weight.
4. **Severe hypertension:** The average of three systolic and/or diastolic blood pressures >99th percentile for age, gender, height, and weight.

B. CAUSES OF HYPERTENSION IN NEONATES, INFANTS, AND CHILDREN (Table 18-10)

C. EVALUATION OF CHRONIC HYPERTENSION[14-16]

1. **Rule out causes:** Rule out "factitious" causes of hypertension (improper cuff size—proper cuff size is two thirds of upper arm length—or measurement technique [i.e., manual versus Dynamap]), "nonpathologic" causes of hypertension (fever, pain, anxiety, muscle spasm), and iatrogenic mechanisms (medications and excessive fluid administration).
2. **History and physical examination:** Headache, blurred vision, history of UTIs, family history of renal dysfunction/hypertension, pitting edema,

18

NEPHROLOGY

TABLE 18-10		
CAUSES OF HYPERTENSION BY AGE GROUP		
	Cause	
Age	Most Common	Less Common
Neonates/ infants	Renal artery thrombosis after umbilical artery catheterization	Bronchopulmonary dysplasia
		Medications
	Coarctation of the aorta	Patent ductus arteriosus
	Renal artery stenosis	Intraventricular hemorrhage
1 to 10 yr	Renal parenchymal disease	Renal artery stenosis
	Coarctation of aorta	Hypercalcemia
		Neurofibromatosis
		Neurogenic tumors
		Pheochromocytoma
		Mineralocorticoid ↑
		Hyperthyroidism
		Transient hypertension
		Hypertension induced by immobilization
		Sleep apnea
		Essential hypertension
		Medications
11 yr to adolescence	Renal parenchymal disease Essential hypertension	All diagnoses listed above
Modified from Sinaiko A. N Engl J Med 1996; 335:26.		

dyspnea on exertion, jugular venous distention; or displaced point of maximal impulse (PMI).

3. **Laboratory studies:** Urinalysis with microscopic evaluation, urine culture, serum electrolytes, CBC, creatinine, BUN, calcium, uric acid, cholesterol, and plasma renin level.

4. **Imaging:** Renal ultrasonography, including renal artery Doppler and other imaging studies as indicated (echocardiography, renal arteriography).

5. Consider toxicology screen, hCG (human chorionic gonadotropin), thyroid function tests, urine catecholamines, plasma and urinary steroids.

6. Refer any patient with significant hypertension to a pediatric nephrologist.

D. TREATMENT OF HYPERTENSION

1. **Nonpharmacologic:** Aerobic exercise, salt restriction, smoking cessation, and weight loss. Indicated in patients with systolic BP and/or diastolic BP >90th percentile.

2. **Pharmacologic:** Indicated in patients with significant hypertension (especially diastolic hypertension.)

3. **Parenteral:** Acute hypertensive crisis.

E. ANTIHYPERTENSIVE MEDICATIONS FOR CHRONIC HYPERTENSIVE THERAPY (Box 18-2)

BOX 18-2

ANTIHYPERTENSIVE MEDICATIONS

CALCIUM CHANNEL BLOCKERS: ACT ON VASCULAR SMOOTH MUSCLES

Benefits

Renal perfusion/function minimally affected; ideal for post-renal-transplant hypertension, especially in association with cyclosporin use; ideal in low renin/volume-dependent hypertension

Nifedipine

No effect on cardiac conduction; available in short- and long-acting form; variable GI absorption and sublingual route may cause precipitous drop in BP

Verapamil

Depresses cardiac pacemaker, inhibits cyclosporin metabolism

Amlodipine

Once-daily dose, tasteless, odorless, easily made into suspension with 90% GI absorption

ACE INHIBITORS (CAPTOPRIL, ENALAPRIL): BLOCK ANGIOTENSIN I → ANGIOTENSIN II

Benefits

Decreases proteinuria while preserving renal function; ↑ potency and duration in neonatal and infantile hypertension; ↓ pulmonary vascular resistance and mean arterial pressure with little ↓ in heart rate

Side Effects

Elimination dependent on creatinine clearance; may cause hyperkalemia; contraindicated in compromised renal perfusion and in pregnancy; associated with rash, cough, angioedema, and marrow depression

cont'd

BOX 18-2—cont'd

ANTIHYPERTENSIVE MEDICATIONS

DIURETICS

Thiazides

Effective in primary hypertension; not effective when GFR <50% of normal; side effects: hypokalemia, hypercalcemia, hyperuricemia, hyperlipidemia

Furosemide/Bumetanide

Useful in renal failure; bumetanide has 40 times more diuretic activity than furosemide, but varies with patient/route; side effects: hypokalemia, hyponatremia, ototoxicity (high-dose intravenous (IV) administration)

K^+ Sparing

Spironolactone, triamterene, amiloride; modest antihypertensive medication; antiandrogenic effects

β-BLOCKERS

Benefits

↓ Heart rate, ↓ cardiac output, ↓ renin release

Side Effects

May exacerbate underlying collagen vascular disease or Raynaud's disease; may cause exaggerated hypoglycemic response in diabetes mellitus and suppress hypoglycemic symptomatology; may cause nightmares, confusion, agitation, depression; contraindicated in persons with congestive heart failure, reactive airways disease, or pulmonary insufficiency

Selective β_1 blockers: Metoprolol, atenolol

Nonselective β-blockers: Propranolol, nadolol (once-daily dosing)

α_1 BLOCKERS (PRAZOSIN): BLOCK VASOCONSTRICTION

Benefits

Effective in patients with renal failure, distorted lipid profile, Raynaud's disease/collagen vascular disease

Side Effects

Nausea, palpitations, worsening of narcolepsy, dizziness/syncope

COMBINED α AND β-BLOCKER

Labetalol (↓ peripheral resistance, ↓ heart rate) extremely potent; postural hypotension; can be used in hypertensive crisis

CENTRALLY ACTING α STIMULATORS (CLONIDINE, α-METHYLDOPA)

Stimulates brainstem α_2 receptors → peripheral adrenergic drive

Benefits

↓ Intraocular pressure, ↓ opiate withdrawal, effective in renal failure, less hyponatremia and orthostatic symptomatology

Side Effects

Dry mouth, sedation/agitation, constipation, sudden withdrawal → rebound hypertension

VASODILATORS (HYDRALAZINE, NITROPRUSSIDE, MINOXIDIL)

Direct action on vascular smooth muscle. Very potent, used in hypertensive crisis; reflex ↑ heart rate, Na^+ and H_2O retention, therefore combine with diuretics/β-blockers

Modified from Hospital for Sick Children. The HSC handbook of pediatrics. 9th ed. St Louis: Mosby; 1997; Sinaiko A. Pediatr Nephrol 1994; 8:603; and Khattak S et al. Clin Pediatr 1998; 37:31.

18

NEPHROLOGY

REFERENCES

1. Roy III S. Hematuria. Pediatr Ann 1996; 2(5):284.
2. Norman ME. An office approach to hematuria and proteinuria. Pediatr Clin North Am 1987; 34:545.
3. Cruz C, Spitzer A. When you find protein or blood in urine. Contemp Pediatr 1998; 15(9):89.
4. Feld L et al. Hematuria: an integrated medical and surgical approach. Pediatr Clin North Am 1997; 44:1191.
5. Cilento B, Stock J, Kaplan G. Hematuria in children: a practical approach. Urol Clin North Am 1995; 22:43.
6. Fitzwater D, Wyatt R. Hematuria. Pediatr Rev 1994; 15:102.
7. American Academy of Pediatrics, Committee on Quality Improvement, Subcommittee on Urinary Tract Infection. Practice parameter: the diagnosis, treatment, and evaluation of the initial urinary tract infection in febrile infants and young children. Pediatrics 1999; 103(4): 843-852.
8. Hoberman A et al. Oral versus initial intravenous therapy for urinary tract infections in young febrile children. Pediatrics 1999; 104.
9. Belman A. Vesicoureteral reflex. Pediatr Clin North Am 1997; 44:5.
10. Hellerstein S. Urinary tract infections: old and new concepts. Pediatr Clin North Am 1995; 42:6.
11. Edelmann CM Jr et al. A standardized test of renal concentrating capacity in children. Am J Dis Child 1967; 114:639.
12. Greenhill A, Gruskin AB. Laboratory evaluation of renal function. Pediatr Clin North Am 1976; 23:661.
13. Rogers MC. Textbook of pediatric intensive care. Baltimore: Williams & Wilkins; 1992.
14. Sinaiko A. Hypertension in children. N Engl J Med 1996; 335:26.
15. Rocella E et al. Update on the 1987 task force report on high blood pressure in children and adolescents: a working group report from the National High Blood Pressure Education program. Pediatrics 1996; 98(4):649-658.
16. Sadowski R, Falkner B. Hypertension in pediatric patients. Am J Kidney Dis 1996; 27:3.

NEUROLOGY

H. Scott Cameron, MD

I. WEBSITES

www.aan.com (American Academy of Neurology, patient brochures and
  information)

www.neurology.org (Neurology, on-line journal)

www.meddean.luc.edu/lumen/MedED/pedneuro/epilepsy.htm (Pediatric
  epilepsy)

www.neuro.wustl.edu/neuromuscular/index.html (neuromuscular disease)

II. NEUROLOGIC EXAMINATION[1]

A complete neurologic examination is rarely productive in the absence of
specific concerns raised by the history and must be evaluated relative to
developmental norms.

A. MENTAL STATUS

Patient should be alert and oriented to time, person, place, and current
situation. Assess attentiveness and behavior in infants.

B. CRANIAL NERVES (Table 19-1)

C. MOTOR

1. Muscle bulk.
2. Tone: High, low.
   a. Passive: Resting resistance to examiner movement.
   b. Active: Regulation of power with defined movements (e.g., posture, gait,
      pull to stand).
   c. Note anatomic distribution of abnormalities. Regional increase in tone
      (e.g., adducted thumbs, limited hand supination, equinus of feet)
      suggests cortical dysfunction. Note quality (e.g., rigid, spastic). Note
      variability with voluntary activity and sleep because tone varies with
      wakefulness and voluntary purposeful movement.
3. **Power: Observe and describe activity** (e.g., rising from the floor). Quantify (e.g., distance of broad jump, time to run 30 feet, time to climb
   stairs).

Strength rating scale

0/5: No movement
1/5: Flicker of movement or less than full range of movement in a gravity-neutral plane
2/5: Full range of movement in a gravity-neutral plane
3/5: Full range of movement against gravity but not resistance
4/5: Subnormal strength against resistance
5/5: Normal strength against resistance

D. SENSORY

Primary disorders of sensation are rare in children, but the following spinal
cord pathways and tests may be useful in anatomic localization (Fig. 19-1).

1. **Anterior cord:** Pain, fine touch, and temperature sensation.

TABLE 19-1

CRANIAL NERVES

Function/Region	Cranial Nerve	Test/Observation
Olfactory	I	Smell (e.g., coffee, vanilla, peppermint)
Vision	II	Acuity, fields, fundus
Pupils	II, III, autonomics	Shape, size, reaction to light, accommodation
Eye movements and eyelids	III, IV, VI	Range and quality of eye movements, saccades, pursuits, nystagmus, ptosis
Sensation	V	Corneal reflexes, facial sensation
Muscles of mastication	V	Clench teeth
Facial strength	VII	Observe degree of expression of emotions, eye closure strength, smile, puff out cheeks
Hearing	VIII	Localize voice, attend to finger rub
Mouth, pharynx	VII, IX, X, XII	Swallowing, speech quality (nasal deficits in labial, lingual, or palatal sound production), symmetric palatal elevation, tongue protrusion
Head control	XI	Lateral head movement, shoulder shrug

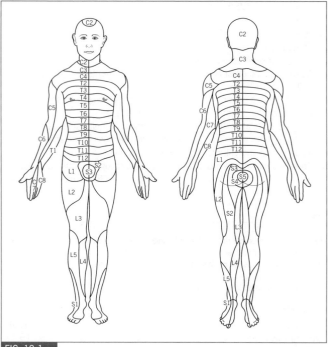

FIG. 19-1

Dermatomes. *(From Athreya BH, Silverman BK. Pediatric physical diagnosis. Norwalk, Conn; Appleton Century-Crofts; 1985.)*

418

TABLE 19-2

UPPER AND LOWER MOTOR NEURON FINDINGS

	UMN	LMN
Power	decreased	decreased
Reflexes	increased	decreased
Tone	increased	normal or decreased
Babinski	present	absent

LMN, Lower motor neuron; *UMN,* upper motor neuron.

TABLE 19-3

MUSCLE STRETCH REFLEXES

Reflex	Site
Biceps	C5, C6
Brachioradialis	C5, C6
Triceps	C7, C8
Knee	L(2,3)4
Ankle	L5-S2

19

NEUROLOGY

2. **Posterior cord:** Vibratory and joint position sense; Romberg (test of visual, proprioceptive, and cerebellar functions).

E. TENDON REFLEXES

Assessment of tendon reflexes is most helpful in localizing other abnormalities, especially in the presence of weakness or asymmetry. Isolated abnormalities of reflexes, in the setting of normal strength and coordination, have little significance. Combined with weakness, brisk reflexes indicate upper motor neuron disorder; absent reflexes reflect lower motor neuron or neuromuscular junction disorder (Table 19-2). In muscle disease, reflexes are usually diminished commensurate with power. Selective reflex dropout can help localize a spinal cord, root, or nerve lesion (Table 19-3).

Reflex rating scale

0: none

1+: Sluggish

2+: Normal

3+: Hyperactive (reflexes cross neighboring joint or cross to other side [e.g., crossed adductors in knees])

4+: Hyperactive with clonus

F. COORDINATION/MOVEMENT

Evaluate general coordination while watching activities (e.g., throwing a ball, dressing, playing video games). Tests for cerebellar function include rapid alternating and repetitive movements, finger to nose, heel to shin, orbiting, walking, and running. Note involuntary movements (e.g., tremor, dystonia, chorea, athetosis, tics, myoclonus). Note abnormal gait (e.g., waddling, wide-based, tiptoed).

III. HEADACHES[2]

A. DIFFERENTIAL DIAGNOSIS OF THE FIRST ACUTE HEADACHE

Evaluation of the first acute headache should exclude pathologic causes listed below before consideration of more common etiologies.

1. **Increased intracranial pressure (ICP):** Trauma, hemorrhage, tumor, hydrocephalus, pseudotumor cerebri, abscess, arachnoid cyst, cerebral edema.
2. **Decreased ICP:** After ventriculoperitoneal (VP) shunt, lumbar puncture (LP), cerebrospinal fluid (CSF) leak from basilar skull fracture.
3. **Meningeal inflammation:** Meningitis, leukemia, subarachnoid or sub-dural hemorrhage.
4. **Vascular:** Vasculitis, arteriovenous malformation (AVM), hypertension, cerebrovascular accident (CVA).
5. **Bone, soft tissue:** Referred pain from scalp, eyes, ears, sinuses, nose, teeth, pharynx, cervical spine, temporomandibular joint.
6. **Infection:** Systemic infection, encephalitis, etc.

B. DIFFERENTIAL DIAGNOSIS OF RECURRENT OR CHRONIC HEADACHES

1. **Migraine** (with or without aura).
2. **Cluster.**
3. **Tension.**
4. **Analgesic rebound.**
5. **Caffeine withdrawal.**
6. **Sleep deprivation** (e.g., in overweight children with sleep apnea) **or chronic hypoxia.**
7. **Tumor.**
8. **Psychogenic:** Conversion disorder, malingering.

C. EVALUATION

1. **History and physical examination:** Differentiate between acute, acute recurrent, chronic nonprogressive, and chronic progressive. Careful general, neurologic, and funduscopic examinations should be performed (Tables 19-4 and 19-5).
2. **Studies**
a. Computed tomography (CT) without contrast/magnetic resonance imaging (MRI): Obtain for focal neurologic findings, suspected increased ICP, atypical or progressive pattern, seizures, abrupt-onset severe headache (see Chapter 23 for advantages of each modality). Note that CT provides poor imaging of the posterior fossa.
b. LP: Fever, infection, papilledema, sudden severe headache (evaluate opening pressure if concern for pseudotumor). Contraindicated in increased ICP or mass effect secondary to risk of herniation.
3. **Warning signs:** Pain that awakens child from sleep, increases in morning with rising or with Valsalva's maneuver; headache associated with emesis, neurologic signs, changes in chronic pattern, and altered mental status (e.g., change in mood, personality, and school performance).
NOTE: The classic headache secondary to subarachnoid hemorrhage

TABLE 19-4

EVALUATION OF HEADACHE BY HISTORY

Questions	Comments
How many different kinds of headache do you have?	• A mixed picture implies multifactorial etiology
What has been the course of the headache?	• Try to characterize as acute, acute recurrent, chronic nonprogressive, or chronic progressive
Can you describe a typical episode?	• Is there a warning before the episode (e.g., visual aura)? • Where does it hurt? • What is the pain like? • How long do the headaches last? • How often do they occur? • How severe are they? Do they interfere with activities? • Is there abdominal pain, nausea, and/or vomiting?
Are there focal neurologic signs or symptoms?	• *Examples:* visual disturbance, paresthesia, or weakness occurring before, during, or after the headache
Does the child look sick?	• Children who have migraines look unwell during an attack
What makes the headaches worse?	• Activities that raise intracranial pressure (e.g., coughing, bending over) • Bright light or noise
What helps the headaches?	• Sleep often helps a migraine headache • Dark, quiet room? Cold cloth over forehead?
What time of day do the headaches occur?	• Headaches that waken the child may be due to increased intracranial pressure • Headaches in the late afternoon may be due to low blood glucose levels precipitating migraine
Can you identify precipitating factors?	• Are they related to the school week or term? • Certain foods, lack of sleep, stress, excitement, exercise, menstrual cycle, exertion, illness
What medications and dosages have you used?	• Was the medicine appropriate? Was the dose correct? Was the medicine used correctly?
Is there a family history of headaches?	• Many parents who have migraines attribute their headaches to other causes (e.g., sinus headaches). Ask parents to describe their headaches. Did they have headaches when they were younger?

From Forsyth R, Farrell K. Pediatr Rev 1999; 20(2):39-45.

19

NEUROLOGY

TABLE 19-5

PHYSICAL AND NEUROLOGICAL EXAMINATION OF THE CHILD WHO HAS HEADACHES

Feature	Significance
Growth parameters	• Chronic illness may affect linear growth
	• Hypothalamopituitary dysfunction may disturb growth
Head circumference	• Increased intracranial pressure before fusion of the sutures may accelerate head growth
Skin	• Evidence of trauma or a neurocutaneous disorder
Blood pressure	• Hypertension
Neurologic examination	• Signs of increased intracranial pressure
	• Focal abnormality
Cranial bruits	• May reflect an intracranial arteriovenous malformation

From Forsyth R, Farrell K. Pediatr Rev 1999; 20(2):39-45.

(SAH) is acute, severe, continuous, and generalized—the "worst headache of my life" or "thunder clap" headache. It may be associated with nausea, emesis, meningismus, focal neurologic symptoms, and loss of consciousness. If SAH is suspected, CT without contrast is the preferred method of evaluation, then LP (if CT is negative) to rule out xanthochromia (develops approximately 12 hours after event). Send tubes 1 and 4 of CSF sample for cell counts and xanthochromia. There is a persistently high red blood cell (RBC) count and xanthochromia if SAH exists. Significant decline of the RBC count between tubes 1 and 4 in the absence of xanthochromia suggests microtrauma from the LP.

D. MIGRAINE HEADACHE

1. **Characteristics:** Chronic recurrent; throbbing/pulsatile or pressure-like in children; usually bifrontal in children, unilateral in adolescents and adults; relieved by sleep; many potential triggers (e.g., stress, caffeine, diet, menses, sleep disruption); hereditary predisposition. Associated symptoms include nausea, vomiting, abdominal pain, photophobia, phonophobia, paresthesia, tinnitus, vertigo; rare associated symptoms include focal weakness, aphasia, ataxia, confusion.

2. **Classification**
a. With aura: "Classic," often frontotemporal, usually unilateral, may have associated neurologic complications. Aura is any preceding neurologic abnormality (e.g., visual aberrations, associated symptoms listed above).
b. Without aura: "Common," often bifrontal.

3. **Associated neurologic deficits (rare):** Paresthesia, visual field cuts, aphasia, hemiplegia, ophthalmoplegia, vertigo, ataxia, confusion.

4. **Treatment:** Includes reassurance and education.
a. Acute symptomatic: Dark and quiet room, sleep, nonsteroidal antiinflammatory drugs (NSAIDs) (i.e., naproxen, ketorolac), antiemetics (metoclopramide), triptans (sumatriptan), isometheptene, ergotamine, sedative/analgesic combinations (see Formulary for dosage information).

BOX 19-1

POTENTIAL DIETARY TRIGGERS FOR MIGRAINE PATIENTS*

- Ripened cheeses (cheddar, Emmentaler, Gruyère, Stilton, Brie, and Camembert)
- (Cheeses permissible: American, cottage, cream, and Velveeta)
- Herring
- Chocolate
- Vinegar (except white vinegar)
- Anything fermented, pickled, or marinated
- Sour cream, yogurt
- Nuts, peanut butter
- Hot fresh breads, raised coffeecakes and doughnuts
- Pods of broad beans (lima, navy, and pea pods)
- Any foods containing large amounts of monosodium glutamate (Chinese foods)
- Onions
- Canned figs
- Citrus foods (no more than 1 orange per day)
- Bananas (no more than ½ banana per day)
- Pizza
- Pork (no more than two or three times per week)
- Excessive tea, coffee, cola beverages (no more than 4 cups per day)
- Avocado
- Fermented sausage (bologna, salami, pepperoni, summer, and hot dogs)
- Chicken livers
- All alcoholic beverages

*Any dietary restrictions should be done in consultation with a physician.

19

NEUROLOGY

b. Prophylaxis (if frequency >3 to 4 per month or if migraines interfere with daily functioning or school)
   (1) Avoid triggers/stress, improve general health with balanced diet restrictive of certain "migraine-causing" foods (Box 19-1), aerobic exercise, regular sleep.
   (2) Explore issues of secondary gain/role of pain in family's relationships. Offer counseling when appropriate; also consider biofeedback.
   (3) Consider medications, such as β-blockers (metoprolol, nadolol), calcium channel blockers (verapamil), tricyclics (amitriptyline, nortriptyline), selective serotonin reuptake inhibitors (SSRIs) (sertraline, fluoxetine), anticonvulsants (valproic acid, gabapentin, topiramate, carbamazepine, dilantin), and cyproheptadine.

IV. PAROXYSMAL EVENTS

A. DIFFERENTIAL DIAGNOSIS OF RECURRENT EVENTS THAT MIMIC EPILEPSY IN CHILDHOOD (Table 19-6)
B. SEIZURE DISORDERS[3,4]

TABLE 19-6

DIFFERENTIAL DIAGNOSIS OF RECURRENT EVENTS THAT MIMIC EPILEPSY IN CHILDHOOD

Event	Differentiation from Epilepsy
Pseudoseizure (psychogenic seizure)	No EEG changes except movement artifact during event; movements thrashing rather than clonic; brief/absent post-ictal period; most likely to occur in patient with epilepsy
Paroxysmal vertigo (toddler)	Patient frightened and crying; no loss of awareness; staggers and falls, vomiting, dysarthria
GER in infancy, childhood	Paroxysmal dystonic posturing associated with meals (Sandifer's syndrome)
Breath-holding spells (18 mo-3 yr)	Loss of consciousness and generalized convulsion always provoked by an event that makes child cry
Syncope	Loss of consciousness with onset of dizziness and clouded or tunnel vision; slow collapse to floor; triggered by postural change, heat, emotion, etc.
Cardiogenic syncope	Abnormal ECG/Holter monitor finding (e.g., prolonged QT, atrioventricular block, other arrhythmias); exercise a possible trigger; episodic loss of consciousness without consistent convulsive movement
Cough syncope	Prolonged cough spasm during sleep in asthmatic, leading to loss of consciousness, often with urinary incontinence
Paroxysmal dyskinesias	May be precipitated by sudden movement or startle; not accompanied by change in alertness
Shuddering attacks	Brief shivering spells with continued awareness
Night terrors (4-6 yr)	Brief nocturnal episodes of terror without typical convulsive movements
Rages (6-12 yr)	Provoked and goal-directed anger
Tics/habit spasms	Involuntary, nonrhythmic, repetitive movements not associated with impaired consciousness; suppressible
Narcolepsy	Sudden loss of tone secondary to cataplexy; emotional trigger; no postictal state or loss of consciousness; EEG with recurrent REM sleep attacks
Migraine (confusional)	Headache or visual changes that may precede attack; family history of migraine; autonomic or sensory changes that can mimic focal seizure; EEG with regional area of slowing during attack

From Murphy JV, Dehkharghani F. Epilepsia 1994; 35(suppl2):S7-S17.
ECG, Electrocardiography; EEG, electroencephalography; GER, gastroesophageal reflux; REM, rapid eye movement.

1. **Seizure:** Paroxysmal synchronized discharge of cortical neurons resulting in alteration of function (motor, sensory, cognitive).
2. **Epilepsy:** Two or more seizures not precipitated by a known cause (e.g., infection, tumor).
3. **Status epilepticus:** Prolonged or recurrent seizures lasting at least 30 minutes without the patient regaining consciousness. See pp. 16-17 for treatment.
4. **Seizure etiology:** Fever, acquired cortical defect (stroke, neoplasm, in-

---

BOX 19-2

OUTLINE OF THE INTERNATIONAL CLASSIFICATION OF EPILEPTIC SEIZURES

I. Partial seizures (seizures with focal onset)
  A. Simple partial seizures (consciousness unimpaired)
    1. With motor signs
    2. With somatosensory or special sensory symptoms
    3. With autonomic symptoms or signs
    4. With psychic symptoms (higher cerebral functions)
  B. Complex partial seizures (consciousness impaired)
    1. Starting as simple partial seizures
      (a) Without automatisms
      (b) With automatisms
    2. With impairment of consciousness at onset
      (a) Without automatisms
      (b) With automatisms
  C. Partial seizures evolving into secondarily generalized seizures
II. Generalized seizures
  A. Absence seizures: Brief lapse in awareness without postictal impairment
    (Atypical absence seizures may have the following: Mild clonic, atonic, tonic, automatism, or autonomic components.)
  B. Myoclonic seizures: Brief, repetitive, symmetric muscle contractions (loss of tone)
  C. Clonic seizures: Rhythmic jerking; flexor spasm of extremities
  D. Tonic seizures: Sustained muscle contraction
  E. Tonic-clonic seizures
  F. Atonic seizures: Abrupt loss of muscle tone
III. Unclassified epileptic seizures

From Committee on Classification and Terminology of the International League Against Epilepsy, Epilepsia 1996; 38(11):1051-1059.

19

NEUROLOGY

fection, trauma), inborn error of metabolism, congenital brain malformation, neurocutaneous syndrome, neurodegenerative disease, toxins/drugs, electrolyte disturbances, idiopathic (epilepsy).

5. **Diagnosis:** Establish etiology and seizure type (e.g., primary generalized or primary partial [Box 19-2]), which generally determines treatment.

6. **Studies**

a. Depends on clinical scenario. Consider assessment of glucose, sodium, potassium, calcium, magnesium, phosphate, blood urea nitrogen (BUN), creatinine, complete blood count (CBC), toxicology screen, blood pressure (supine and upright), electroencephalography (EEG) with video monitoring, electrocardiography, head CT and/or MRI, LP, tilt table, and sleep study. If febrile, consider age-appropriate sepsis evaluation.

b. Head CT without contrast can detect mass lesions, acute hemorrhage, hydrocephalus, and calcifications secondary to congenital disease such as cytomegalovirus (CMV) infection (head ultrasound may be used in early infancy and requires open fontanelles).

c. Brain MRI with contrast should be obtained in infants with epilepsy, children with simple or complex partial seizures, focal neurologic deficits, or developmental delay. Otherwise, MRI is not routinely indicated in the evaluation of a first-time seizure.

d. EEGs should be obtained in all children with nonfebrile seizures to predict the recurrence risk and to classify the seizure type and epilepsy syndrome.[5] However, routine interictal EEGs are frequently normal; prolonged EEG monitoring with video, or studies done with sleep deprivation/photic stimulation may be more informative.

7. Treatment

a. Educate parents and patient regarding how to live with epilepsy.[6] Review seizure first aid and cardiopulmonary resuscitation (CPR). Recommend that the child participate in activities but have supervision during bath or swimming. Individualize other restrictions. Know driver's license laws in the state. Advocate teacher/school awareness.

b. Pharmacotherapy (Fig. 19-2): Weigh the risk of more seizures without therapy against the risk of treatment side effects plus residual seizures despite therapy. Treatment of single, first, afebrile seizure is not indicated routinely. Reserve pharmacotherapy for recurrent afebrile seizures. Monotherapy may reduce complications; polytherapy increases risk of complications/side effects more than efficacy.

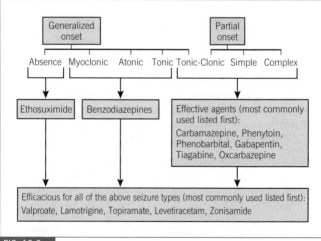

FIG. 19-2

Anticonvulsant selection by seizure type. Also consider the ketogenic diet for intractable seizure disorders. *(From Krauss G. Personal communication.)*

c. Therapeutic drug monitoring should be done at the start of therapy to screen for adverse effects when a new drug is added or stopped, if seizures are uncontrolled, if toxicity is suspected, or to assess compliance. Routine drug levels are not required with chronic therapy.

C. SPECIAL SEIZURE SYNDROMES

1. **Simple febrile seizure[7-9]:** Brief, generalized, tonic-clonic seizure associated with a febrile illness, but without any central nervous system (CNS) infection or other known neurologic cause. Genetic predisposition has been noted.

a. Incidence: 2% to 5% of children 6 months to 5 years of age.

b. Evaluation for "atypical" features: Onset more than 24 hours after onset of fever, duration >15 minutes, focality of seizure, more than one discrete seizure during illness, abnormal neurologic examination. Consider further evaluation if any one of these is present. Also include evaluation for source of fever (Fig. 19-3).

c. Treatment: Prophylactic antiepileptic drugs and antipyretics are not indicated for typical febrile seizures. Educate parents about benign nature of events and basic first aid for seizures. Rarely, rectal diazepam as needed (PRN) for seizures may be used for patients with significant parental anxiety or frequent/prolonged febrile seizures, although side effects of lethargy, drowsiness, and ataxia may mask the evolving signs of a CNS infection.

d. Outcome

(1) Risk of recurrence is 30% after first febrile seizure, 50% after second episode, declines to near zero by age 5. Recurrence risk greater with younger age (<1 year, 50%) and with family history.

(2) Risk of epilepsy: 2% versus 1% in the general population. Increased further in children with two or more of the following: atypical febrile seizures, previously abnormal development or neurologic disorder, family history of afebrile seizures.

2. **Neonatal seizure[10]:** Various paroxysmal behaviors or electrical events. May be tonic, myoclonic, clonic, or subtle (blinking, chewing, bicycling, apnea) because of immature CNS.

a. Etiologies of neonatal seizure: Almost always a symptom of acute brain disorder. Hypoxic-ischemic encephalopathy (35% to 42%); intracranial hemorrhage/infarction (15% to 20%); CNS infection (12% to 17%); CNS malformation (5%); metabolic (e.g., hypoglycemia, hypocalcemia, pyridoxine deficiency, toxins) (3% to 5%); others, including inborn errors of metabolism (5% to 20%).

b. Evaluation: Search for acute cause. Basic laboratory screens (including glucose, calcium, sodium, magnesium, and toxicology screen), sepsis workup including LP, head CT, and EEG. If basic laboratory screen is unremarkable and patient has recurrent seizures, is encephalopathic, or has signs of inborn error of metabolism, then evaluate for these disorders: plasma amino acids, urine organic acids, ammonia, lactate, pH; consider CSF amino acids, pyruvate, urine sulfites, very long chain fatty

19

NEUROLOGY

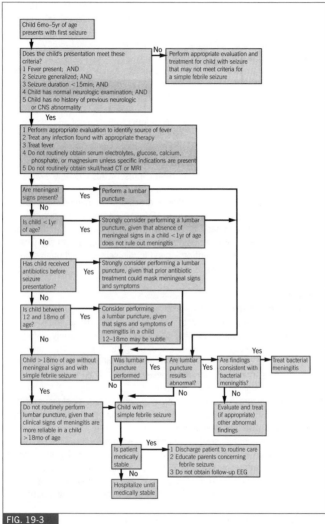

FIG. 19-3

Guidelines for febrile seizure evaluation. *(From American Academy of Pediatrics. Pediatrics 1996; 97(5):769-772.)*

> **BOX 19-3**
>
> **TREATMENT OF NEONATAL SEIZURES**
>
> 1. Establish airway, ensure oxygenation and circulation.
> 2. Treat metabolic abnormalities (see Formulary for dosage information)
>   Hypoglycemia
>   Hypocalcemia
>   Evaluate for hypomagnesemia if persistent hypocalcemia
> 3. Treat with medications (see Formulary for dosage information)
>   Phenobarbital
>   If this fails, add fosphenytoin and/or a benzodiazepine (e.g., lorazepam, diazepam)
>   Consider pyridoxine with concurrent EEG monitoring during ictal episode for intractable seizures.

Modified from Scher MS. Clin Perinatol 1997; 24(4):735-772.

19

NEUROLOGY

acids, and neurotransmitters. Prolonged or repeated EEG examinations are often needed because clinical-electrical dissociation is common.

c. Treatment: Treat underlying disorder. Prevent secondary hypoxic-ischemic or metabolic complications. Treat acute symptomatic recurring seizures quickly using combined clinical and EEG end-points. Consider trial of pyridoxine IV while EEG is recording. Maintain anticonvulsants for sufficient period of time for acute cause to subside (days to weeks); for most acute symptomatic seizures, drugs can be safely stopped before discharge from nursery (Box 19-3).

3. **Infantile spasms:** Head nodding with flexion or extension of the trunk and extremities, often in clusters during drowsiness or awakening. May be triggered by unexpected stimuli. EEG may show hypsarrhythmia. Usual onset after 2 months, peak onset 4 to 6 months. MRI examination is indicated.

a. Etiologies
   (1) Symptomatic (67%): CNS malformation, any acquired infantile brain injury, tuberous sclerosis, inborn errors of metabolism.
   (2) Cryptogenic (33%): Associated with better outcome, less mental retardation.

b. Treatment: Should be initiated as soon as possible to improve outcome. Adrenocorticotropic hormone (ACTH) (see corticotropin in Formulary for dosage information). Alternatives include valproic acid, benzo-diazepine (clonazepam), or ketogenic diet. New therapies include vigabatrin, lamotrigine, topiramate, tiagabine, zonisamide, and surgery.

c. Outcome: Often poor, correlates best with underlying brain pathology. Of cryptogenic cases, 30% to 70% may have good outcome with treatment.

V. HYDROCEPHALUS

A. DIAGNOSIS

Assess increasing head circumference, misshapen skull, frontal bossing, bulging large anterior fontanelle, separated sutures with cracked pot sign, increased ICP (sunset sign, increased tone/reflexes, vomiting, irritability, papilledema), and developmental delay. Obtain head CT if increase in head circumference crosses more than two percentile lines or if patient is symptomatic. Differentiate hydrocephalus from megalencephaly or hydrocephalus ex vacuo.

B. TREATMENT[11]

1. **Medical**
a. Emergently manage acute increase of ICP (see pp. 14-15).
b. Slowly progressive hydrocephalus: The following medications may be effective in children 2 weeks to 10 months of age with slowly progressive communicating hydrocephalus:
   (1) Acetazolamide PO or IV: 20 mg/kg/day divided Q8hr up to 100 mg/kg/day. Maximum does 2 g/24 hours.
   (2) Furosemide: 1 mg/kg/24 hours PO or IV divided Q8hr.
   (3) Polycitra: Titrate to maintain bicarbonate ≥18 mEq/L and normal Na$^+$ and K$^+$. Usual dose is 2 to 4 mEq/kg/24 hours.
2. **Surgical:** CSF shunting.
a. Shunt types: Ventriculoperitoneal (VP) shunts are used most commonly. Ventriculoatrial/pleural shunts are associated with cardiac arrhythmias, pleural effusions, and higher rates of infection.
b. Shunt complications: Shunt dysfunction may be caused by infection, obstruction (clogging or kinking), disconnection, and migration of proximal and distal tips. Patient will develop signs of increased ICP with shunt malfunction.

C. MANAGEMENT OF ACUTE SHUNT OBSTRUCTION OR INFECTION

1. **Evaluate shunt integrity:** Obtain shunt series (skull, neck, chest, and abdominal radiographs) to look for kinking or disconnection. Obtain head CT to evaluate shunt position, ventricular size, and evidence of increased ICP.
2. **Test shunt function:** Consider depressing bulb and allowing it to refill. Decreased bulb depression phase may be caused by distal shunt obstruction or a stiffened bulb. Poor refill suggests obstruction at the ventricular end, or excessive ventricular decompression. Reasons not to depress bulb include uncertainty of proximal tubing position and suspected slit ventricles.
3. **Percutaneous shunt drainage:** This procedure should be performed by a neurosurgeon; however, if a neurosurgeon is unavailable and the patient's condition is rapidly deteriorating, a percutaneous shunt drainage may be performed by any physician familiar with the procedure.
a. Cleanse the area over the shunt bulb using aseptic technique.
b. Insert a long-nose, 25G butterfly needle into the flushing device through

the bulb diaphragm into the proximal chamber. A stopcock attached to the butterfly tubing may help prevent air from entering the ventricular system. Measure the fluid pressure and remove the minimum amount of fluid needed to achieve symptomatic relief.

c. If blockage at the ventricular end is suspected and the patient's condition continues to deteriorate, insert a spinal needle (up to 18G) through the burr hole through which the shunt was placed, and direct it toward the lateral ventricles. (Aim spinal needle toward the contralateral ear.) Measure the pressure and remove the minimal amount of fluid necessary for decompression.

d. Send CSF to laboratory for culture, cell count and differential, glucose, and protein.

19

NEUROLOGY

VI. ATAXIA[12]

A. DIFFERENTIAL DIAGNOSIS OF ACUTE OR RECURRENT ATAXIA

1. **Drug ingestion** (e.g., phenytoin, carbamazepine, sedatives, hypnotics, and phencyclidine) or intoxication (e.g., alcohol, ethylene glycol, hydrocarbon fumes, lead, mercury, or thallium).
2. **Postinfectious** (cerebellitis [e.g., varicella], acute disseminated encephalomyelitis [ADEM]).
3. **Head trauma.**
4. **Basilar migraine.**
5. **Benign paroxysmal vertigo** (migraine equivalent).
6. **Brain tumor or neuroblastoma** (if accompanied by opsoclonus or myoclonus [i.e., "dancing eyes, dancing feet"]).
7. **Hydrocephalus.**
8. **Infection** (e.g., labyrinthitis, abscess).
9. **Seizure.**
10. **Vascular events** (e.g., cerebellar hemorrhage or stroke).
11. **Miller Fisher variant of Guillain-Barré syndrome** (ataxia, ophthalmoplegia, and areflexia).
12. **Inherited ataxias.**
13. **Inborn errors of metabolism** (e.g., mitochondrial disorders, amino acidopathies, urea cycle defects).
14. **Conversion reaction.**
15. **Multiple sclerosis.**

B. DIFFERENTIAL DIAGNOSIS OF CHRONIC OR PROGRESSIVE ATAXIA

1. **Hydrocephalus.**
2. **Hypothyroidism.**
3. **Tumor or paraneoplastic syndrome.**
4. **Low vitamin E levels** (e.g., cystic fibrosis).
5. **Wilson's disease.**
6. **Inborn errors of metabolism.**
7. **Inherited ataxias** (e.g., ataxia telangiectasia, Friedreich ataxia).

C. EVALUATION

Depends on clinical scenario; consider CBC, electrolytes, blood and urine toxicology screens, brain imaging, LP (if Guillain-Barré suspected), EEG, urine for vanillylmandelic acid and homovanillic acid (VMA/HVA), and imaging of the chest and abdomen if neuroblastoma is suspected.

REFERENCES

1. Athreya BH, Silverman BK. Pediatric physical diagnosis. Norwalk, Conn: Appleton Century-Crofts; 1985.
2. Forsyth R, Farrell K. Headache in childhood. Pediatr Rev 1999; 20(2):39-45.
3. Murphy JV, Dehkharghani F. Diagnosis of childhood seizure disorder. Epilepsia 1994; 35(suppl 2):S7-S17.
4. Committee on Classification and Terminology of the International League Against Epilepsy. Classification of epilepsia: its applicability and practical value of different diagnostic categories. Epilepsia 1996; 38(11):1051-1059.
5. Hirtz D et al. Practice parameter: evaluating a first nonfebrile seizure in children. Neurology 2000; 55(5):616-623.
6. Freeman J. Seizures and epilepsy in childhood: a guide to parents, 2nd ed. Baltimore: Johns Hopkins University Press; 1997.
7. American Academy of Pediatrics subcommittee. Practice parameter: the neurodiagnostic evaluation of the child with a first simple febrile seizure. Pediatrics 1996; 97(5):769-772.
8. American Academy of Pediatrics subcommittee. Practice parameter: long-term treatment of the child with simple febrile seizures. Pediatrics 1999; 103(6):1307-1309.
9. Baumann RJ, Duffner PK. Treatment of children with simple febrile seizures: the AAP practice parameter. Pediatr Neurol 2000; 23(1):11-17.
10. Scher MS. Seizures in the newborn infant: diagnosis, treatment and outcomes. Clin Perinatol 1997; 24(4):735-772.
11. Rogers M, editor. Textbook of pediatric intensive care, 3rd ed. Baltimore: Williams & Wilkins; 1996.
12. Dinolfo EA. Evaluation of ataxia. Pediatr Rev 2001; 22(5):177-178.

NUTRITION AND GROWTH

Jeanne Cox, MS, RD and Lori Chaffin Jordan, MD

I. WEBSITES

www.cdc.gov (The Centers for Disease Control and Prevention website has
   growth charts and nutrition information.)
www.eatright.org (The American Dietetic Association)
*Formula company websites for complete and up-to-date product
information:*
www.meadjohnson.com
www.nestle.com
www.rosspediatrics.com
www.Pbmproducts.com
www.hormelhealthlab.com

II. ASSESSMENT OF NUTRITIONAL STATUS

A. ELEMENTS OF NUTRITIONAL ASSESSMENT

1. **Medical history and physical examination** (medical diagnosis, clinical
   symptoms of nutritional deficiencies).
2. **Dietary evaluation** (feeding history, current intake).
3. **Laboratory findings** (comparison to age-based norms).
4. **Anthropometric measurements** (weight, length/height, head circumference, body mass index [BMI] skinfolds); data are plotted on
   growth charts according to age and compared with a reference
   population.

B. INDICATORS OF NUTRITIONAL STATUS[1]

1. **Ideally, growth should be evaluated over time, but one measurement
   can be used for screening.** Height and weight should be plotted on a
   growth chart. BMI should be determined and plotted for children over
   2 years of age. See BMI charts, pp. 447-448.

$$BMI = \frac{(Wt \ in \ kg)}{(Height \ in \ meters)^2}$$

   a. Stunting/shortness: Length or height for age <5th percentile.
   b. Underweight: BMI for age or weight for length <5th percentile.
   c. Risk of overweight: BMI for age or weight for length 85th to 95th
      percentile.
   d. Overweight: BMI for age or weight for length >95th percentile.
2. **Recommendations for management of overweight children**
   (Fig. 20-1).[2]

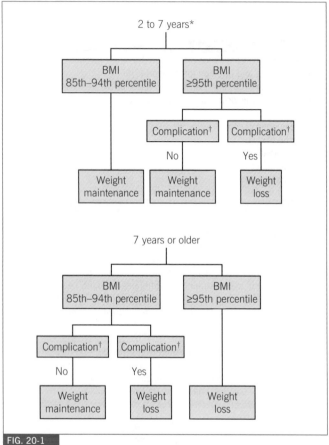

FIG. 20-1

Recommendations for obesity management. *, Indicates that children younger than 2 years should be referred to a pediatric obesity center for treatment. †, Indicates complications such as mild hypertension, dyslipidemias, and insulin resistance. Patients with acute complications, such as pseudotumor cerebri, sleep apnea, obesity hypoventilation syndrome, or orthopedic problems, should be referred to a pediatric obesity center. Weight maintenance implies no change in weight while child grows in height. *(Modified from Barlow SE, Dietz WH. Pediatrics 1998; 102(3):7.)*

III. ESTIMATING ENERGY NEEDS

A. AVERAGE ENERGY NEEDS

Several methods can be used for estimating energy needs. The most frequently used method is the average energy allowance from the Recommended Energy Intake for Age (Table 20-1).[3]

B. ADJUSTMENTS TO ENERGY NEEDS

For children who have decreased energy needs secondary to neurologic impairment, or increased needs secondary to injury, sepsis, or increased motor activity, the resting energy expenditure (REE) (see Table 20-1) can be used with the addition of factors for activity, injury, and disease.

1. Calculation of total daily energy needs using REE method:

   Total daily energy needs (kcal/kg/day) = REE (kcal/kg/day) +
   REE (kcal/kg/day) × [Maintenance + Injury + Activity factors]

2. Factors[4]

Maintenance:	0.2
Activity:	0.1-0.25
Fever:	0.13 per ° C >38°
Simple trauma:	0.2
Multiple injuries:	0.4
Burns:	0.5-1
Growth:	0.5

Example: 10-year-old boy with multiple injuries from motor vehicle accident and temperature of 39° C.

   REE + REE × (Maintenance + Activity + Fever + Injuries + Growth)
   = 40 kcal/kg/day + 40 kcal/kg/day × (0.2 + 0.1 + 0.13 + 0.4 + 0.5)
   = 40 kcal/kg/day + (40 kcal/kg/day) × (1.33)
   = 40 kcal/kg/day + 53 kcal/kg/day
   = 93 kcal/kg/day

C. CATCH-UP GROWTH REQUIREMENT FOR MALNOURISHED INFANTS AND CHILDREN

1. Calculations of energy needs for a malnourished child to catch up to expected growth parameters[5]:

Catch-up energy needs (kcal/kg/day) =

$$\frac{\text{RDA calories for age} \times \text{50th percentile weight for height (kg)}}{\text{Actual weight (kg)}}$$

a. Plot the child's height and weight on a growth chart.
b. Determine the child's recommended calories for age (RDA or DRI) or average energy needs in Table 20-1.
c. Determine the WEIGHT (50th percentile) for the child's HEIGHT. See growth charts, Figs. 20-2 to 20-25.
d. Multiply the RDA or DRI calories by the ideal body weight for height (kg).
e. Divide this value by the child's actual weight.

Text continued on p. 459

20

NUTRITION AND GROWTH

TABLE 20-1

RECOMMENDED ENERGY INTAKE FOR AGE

	Age (yr)	REE* (kcal/kg/day)	Average Energy Needs	
			(kcal/kg/day)	(kcal/day)
Infants	0.0-0.5	53	108	650
	0.5-1.0	56	98	850
Children	1-3	57	102	1300
	4-6	48	90	1800
	7-10	40	70	2000
Males	11-14	32	55	2500
	15-18	27	45	3000
Females	11-14	28	47	2200
	15-18	25	40	2200
Pregnancy	First trimester			+0
	Second and third trimesters			+300
Lactation				+500

Modifed from Food Nutrition Board, National Research Council, Recommended Dietary Allowances, 10th ed. Washington, DC: National Academy Press; 1989.

*Resting energy expenditure, based on Food and Agricultural Organization (FAO) equations.

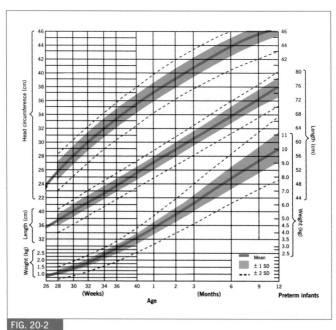

FIG. 20-2

Length, weight, and head circumference for preterm infants. *(Modified from Babson SG, Benda GI. J Pediatr 1976; 89:815.)*

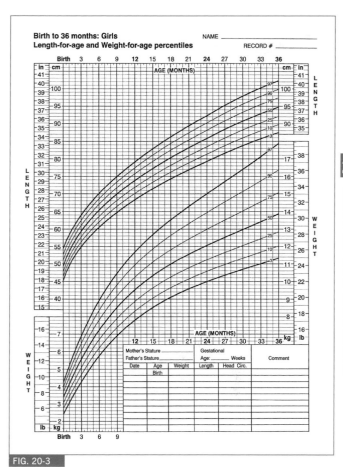

FIG. 20-3

Length and weight for girls from birth to 36 months. *(Developed by the National Center for Health Statistics in collaboration with the National Center for Chronic Disease Prevention and Health Promotion, 2000.)*

20

NUTRITION AND GROWTH

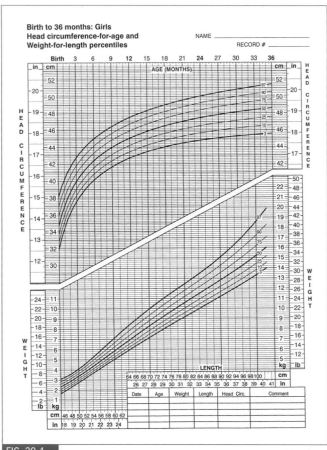

Head circumference and length:weight ratio for girls, from birth to 36 months. *(Developed by the National Center for Health Statistics in collaboration with the National Center for Chronic Disease Prevention and Health Promotion, 2000.)*

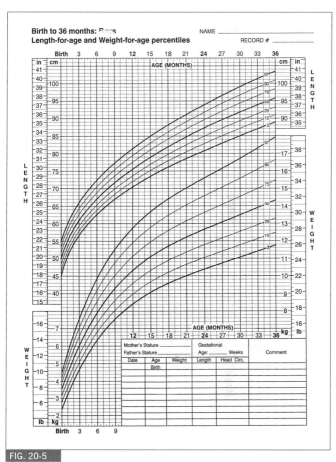

Birth to 36 months: Boys
Length-for-age and Weight-for-age percentiles

NAME _____

RECORD # _____

FIG. 20-5

Length and weight for boys from birth to 36 months. *(Developed by the National Center for Health Statistics in collaboration with the National Center for Chronic Disease Prevention and Health Promotion, 2000.)*

20

NUTRITION AND GROWTH

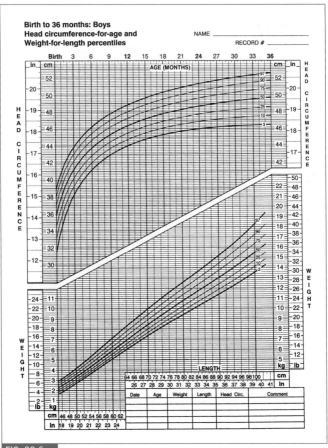

FIG. 20-6

Head circumference and length:weight ratio for boys from birth to 36 months. *(Developed by the National Center for Health Statistics in collaboration with the National Center for Chronic Disease Prevention and Health Promotion, 2000.)*

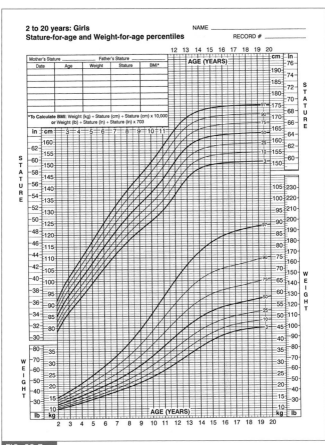

FIG. 20-7

Stature and weight for girls 2 to 20 years. *(Developed by the National Center for Health Statistics in collaboration with the National Center for Chronic Disease Prevention and Health Promotion, 2000.)*

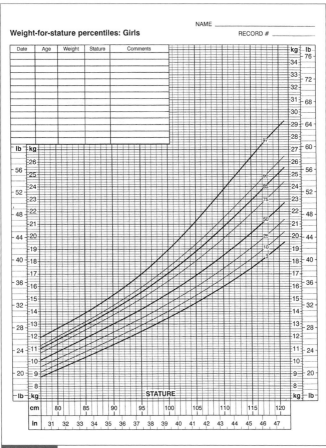

Weight-for-stature percentiles: Girls

NAME _____

RECORD # _____

Date	Age	Weight	Stature	Comments

FIG. 20-8

Stature:weight ratio for girls. *(Developed by the National Center for Health Statistics in collaboration with the National Center for Chronic Disease Prevention and Health Promotion, 2000.)*

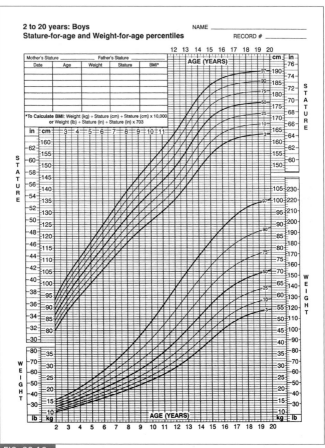

FIG. 20-10

Stature and weight for boys 2 to 20 years. *(Developed by the National Center for Health Statistics in collaboration with the National Center for Chronic Disease Prevention and Health Promotion, 2000.)*

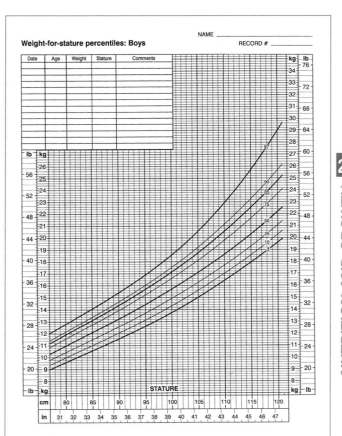

FIG. 20-11

Stature:weight ratio for boys. *(Developed by the National Center for Health Statistics in collaboration with the National Center for Chronic Disease Prevention and Health Promotion, 2000.)*

20

NUTRITION AND GROWTH

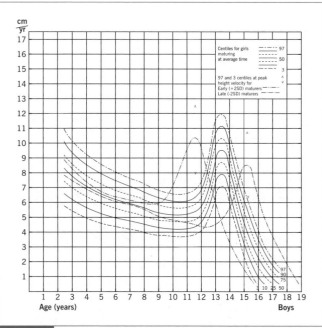

FIG. 20-12

Height velocity for boys 2 to 18 years. *(Modified from Tanner JM, Davis PS. J Pediatr 1985; 107:317-329. Courtesy Castlemead Publications, 1985. Distributed by Serono Laboratories.)*

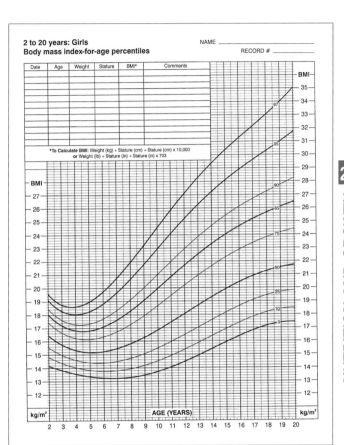

2 to 20 years: Girls
Body mass index-for-age percentiles

NAME _____

RECORD # _____

*To Calculate BMI: Weight (kg) ÷ Stature (cm) ÷ Stature (cm) x 10,000
or Weight (lb) ÷ Stature (in) ÷ Stature (in) x 703

FIG. 20-13

Body mass index for age percentiles for girls 2 to 20 years. *(Developed by the National Center for Health Statistics in collaboration with the National Center for Chronic Disease Prevention and Health Promotion, 2000.)*

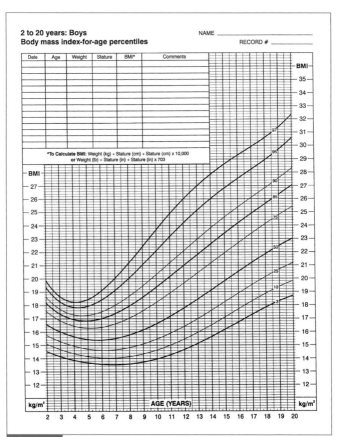

FIG. 20-14

Body mass index for age percentiles for boys 2 to 20 years. *(Developed by the National Center for Health Statistics in collaboration with the National Center for Chronic Disease Prevention and Health Promotion, 2000.)*

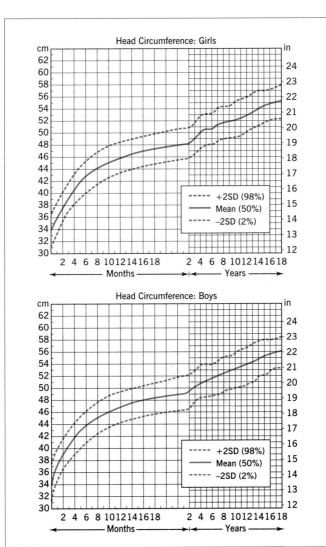

FIG. 20-15

Head circumference for girls and boys 2 to 18 years. *(Modified from Nelhaus G. J Pediatr 1968; 48:106.)*

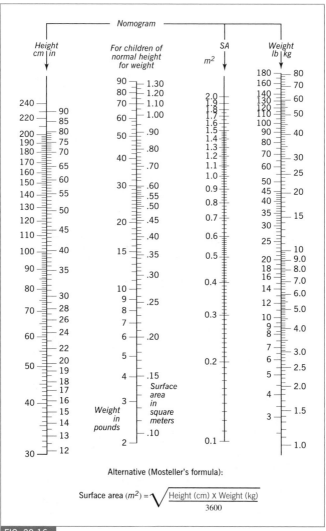

FIG. 20-16

Body surface area nomogram and equation. *(Data from Briars GL, Bailey BJ. Arch Dis Child 1994; 70:246-247.)*

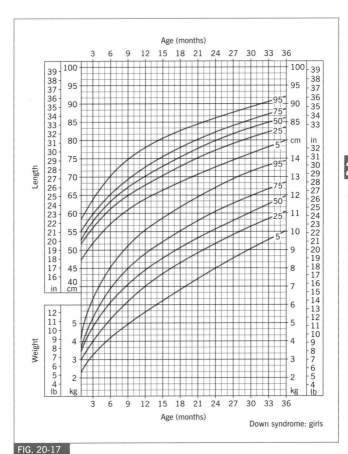

FIG. 20-17

Length and weight for girls with Down syndrome, from birth to 36 months. *(Modified from Cronk C et al. Pediatrics 1988; 81:102-110.)*

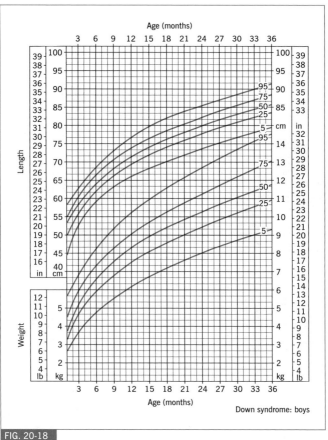

FIG. 20-18

Length and weight for boys with Down syndrome, from birth to 36 months. *(Modified from Cronk C et al. Pediatrics 1988; 81:102-110.)*

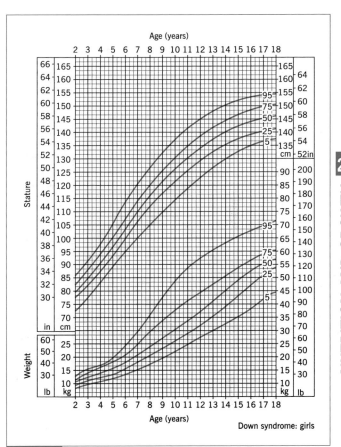

FIG. 20-19

Stature and weight for girls with Down syndrome 2 to 18 years. *(Modified from Cronk C et al. Pediatrics 1988; 81:102-110.)*

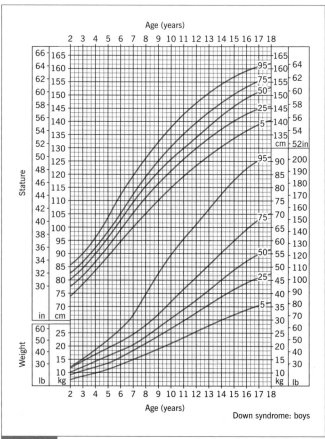

FIG. 20-20

Stature and weight for boys with Down syndrome 2 to 18 years. *(Modified from Cronk C et al. Pediatrics 1988; 81:102-110.)*

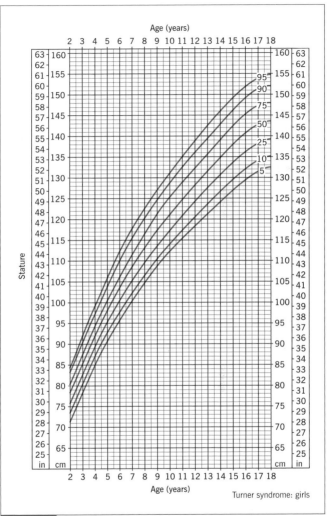

FIG. 20-21

Stature for girls with Turner's syndrome 2 to 18 years. *(From Lyon AJ, Preece MA, Grant DB. Arch Dis Child 1985; 60:932-935.)*

20

NUTRITION AND GROWTH

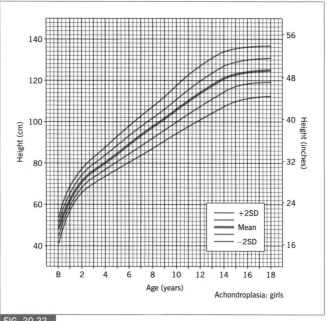

FIG. 20-22

Height for girls with achondroplasia, from birth to 18 years. *(From Horton WA et al. J Pediatr 1978; 93:435-438.)*

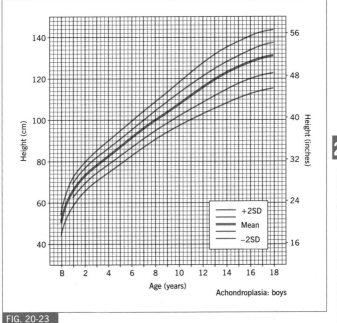

FIG. 20-23

Height for boys with achondroplasia, from birth to 18 years. *(From Horton WA et al. J Pediatr 1978; 93:435-438.)*

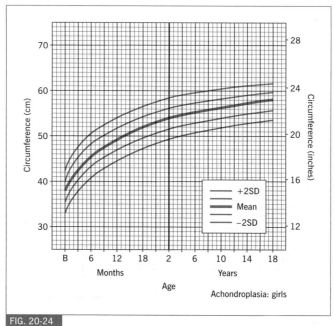

FIG. 20-24

Head circumference for girls with achondroplasia, from birth to 18 years. *(From Horton WA et al. J Pediatr 1978; 93:435-438.)*

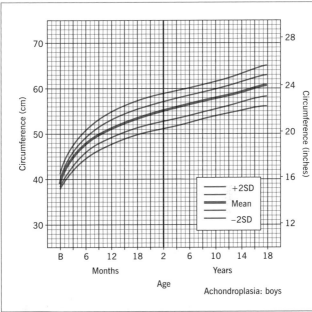

FIG. 20-25

Head circumference for boys with achondroplasia, from birth to 18 years. *(From Horton WA et al. J Pediatr 1978; 93:435-438.)*

IV. DIETARY REFERENCE INTAKES[6]
A. VITAMINS (Table 20-2)
B. MINERALS (Table 20-3)

TABLE 20-2
DIETARY REFERENCE INTAKES: RECOMMENDED INTAKES FOR INDIVIDUALS—VITAMINS

Life Stage Group	Vitamin A[a] (IU)	Vitamin C (mg/d)	Vitamin D[b,c] (IU)	Vitamin E[d] (IU)	Vitamin K (mcg/d)	Thiamin (mg/d)	Ribo-flavin (mg/d)	Niacin (mg/d)[e]	Vitamin B6 (mg/d)	Folate (mcg/d)[f]	Vitamin B12 (mcg/d)	Panto-thenic Acid (mg/d)	Biotin (mcg/d)	Choline[g] (mg/d)
Infants														
0-6 mo	1333	40*	200	4*	2.0*	0.2*	0.3*	2*	0.1*	65*	0.4*	1.7*	5*	125*
7-12 mo	1666	50*	200	5*	2.5*	0.3*	0.4*	4*	0.3*	80*	0.5*	1.8*	6*	150*
Children														
1-3 y	1000	15	200	6	30*	0.5	0.5	6	0.5	150	0.9	2*	8*	200*
4-8 y	1333	25	200	7	55*	0.6	0.6	8	0.6	200	1.2	3*	12*	250*
Males														
9-13 y	2000	45	200	11	60*	0.9	0.9	12	1.0	300	1.8	4*	20*	375*
14-18 y	3000	75	200	15	75*	1.2	1.3	16	1.3	400	2.4	5*	25*	550*
19-30 y	3000	90	200	15	120*	1.2	1.3	16	1.3	400	2.4	5*	30*	550*
Females														
9-13 y	2000	45	200	11	60*	0.9	0.9	12	1.0	300	1.8	4*	20*	375*
14-18 y	2333	65	200	15	75*	1.0	1.0	14	1.2	400	2.4	5*	25*	400*
19-30 y	2333	75	200	15	90*	1.1	1.1	14	1.3	400	2.4	5*	30*	425*

Pregnancy														
<18 y	2500	80	200	15	75*	1.4	1.4	18	1.9	600	2.6	6*	30*	450*
19-30 y	2567	85	200	15	90*	1.4	1.4	18	1.9	600	2.6	6*	30*	450*
Lactation														
<18 y	4000	115	200	19	75*	1.4	1.4	17	2.0	500	2.8	7*	35*	550*
19-30 y	4333	120	200	19	90*	1.4	1.6	17	2.0	500	2.8	7*	35*	550*

Modified from Food and Nutrition Board, the Institute of Medicine, National Academies of Science.

This table (taken from the DRI reports, see www.nap.edu) presents Recommended Dietary Allowances (RDAs) in **bold type** and Adequate Intakes (AIs) in ordinary type followed by an asterisk (*). RDAs and AIs may both be used as goals for individual intake. RDAs are set to meet the needs of almost all (97% to 98%) individuals in a group. For healthy breast-fed infants, the AI is the mean intake. The AI for other life stage and gender groups is believed to cover needs of all individuals in the group, but lack of data or uncertainty in the data prevent being able to specify with confidence the percentage of individuals covered by this intake.

ªOne IU = 0.3 mcg Retinol equivalent.

ᵇOne mcg Cholecalciferol = 40 IU Vitamin D.

ᶜIn the absence of adequate exposure to sunlight.

ᵈOne IU = 1 mg Vitamin E.

ᵉAs niacin equivalents (NE). 1 mg of niacin = 60 mg of tryptophan; 0-6 months = preformed niacin (not NE).

ᶠAs dietary folate equivalents (DFE). 1 DFE =1 mcg food folate = 0.6 mcg of folic acid from fortified food or as a supplement consumed with food = 0.5 mcg of a supplement taken on an empty stomach. In view of evidence linking folate intake with neural tube defects in the fetus, it is recommended that all women capable of becoming pregnant consume 400 mcg from supplements or fortified foods in addition to intake of food folate from a varied diet. It is assumed that women will continue consuming 400 mcg from supplements or fortified food until their pregnancy is confirmed and they enter prenatal care, which ordinarily occurs after the end of the periconceptual period—the critical time for formation of the neural tube.

ᵍAlthough AIs have been set for choline, there are few data to assess whether a dietary supply of choline is needed at all stages of the life style, and it may be that the choline requirement can be met by endogenous synthesis at some of these stages.

NUTRITION AND GROWTH

20

TABLE 20-3
DIETARY REFERENCE INTAKES: RECOMMENDED INTAKES FOR INDIVIDUALS—ELEMENTS

Life Stage Group	Calcium (mg/d)	Chromium (mcg/d)	Copper (mcg/d)	Fluoride (mg/d)	Iodine (mcg/d)	Iron (mg/d)	Magnesium (mg/d)	Manganese (mg/d)	Molybdenum (mcg/d)	Phosphorus (mg/d)	Selenium (mcg/d)	Zinc (mg/d)
Infants												
0-6 mo	210*	0.2*	200*	0.01*	110*	0.27*	30*	0.003*	2*	100*	15*	2*
7-12 mo	270*	5.5*	220*	0.5*	130*	11	75*	0.6*	3*	275*	20*	3
Children												
1-3 y	500*	11*	340	0.7*	90	7	80	1.2*	17	460	20	3
4-8 y	800*	15*	440	1.0*	90	10	130	1.5*	22	500	30	5
Males												
9-13 y	1300*	25*	700	2*	120	8	240	1.9*	34	1250	40	8
14-18 y	1300*	35*	890	3*	150	11	410	2.2*	43	1250	55	11
19-30 y	1000*	35*	900	4*	150	8	400	2.3*	45	700	55	11
Females												
9-13 y	1300*	21*	700	2*	120	8	240	1.6*	34	1250	40	8
14-18 y	1300*	24*	890	3*	150	15	360	1.6*	43	1250	55	9
19-30 y	1000*	25*	900	3*	150	18	310	1.8*	45	700	55	8
Pregnancy												
<18 y	1300*	29*	1000	3*	220	27	400	2.0*	50	1250	60	13
19-30 y	1000*	30*	1000	3*	220	27	350	2.0*	50	700	60	11
Lactation												
<18 y	1300*	44*	1300	3*	290	10	360	2.6*	50	1250	70	14
19-30 y	1000*	45*	1300	3*	290	9	310	2.6*	50	700	70	12

Modified from the Food and Nutrition Board, The Institute of Medicine, National Academies of Science.
This table presents Recommended Dietary Allowances (RDAs) in **bold type** and Adequate Intakes (AIs) in ordinary type followed by an asterisk (*). RDAs and AIs may both be used as goals for individual intake. RDAs are set to meet the needs of almost all (97 to 98%) individuals in a group. For healthy breast-fed infants, the AI is the mean intake. The AI for other life stage and gender groups is believed to cover needs of all individuals in the group, but lack of data or uncertainty in the data prevent being able to specify with confidence the percentage of individuals covered by this intake.

V. VITAMIN-MINERAL SUPPLEMENTATION FOR BREAST-FED INFANTS

A. VITAMIN D

400 IU per day is recommended for breast-fed infants, especially those who are deeply pigmented, have limited sunlight exposure, or use sunscreen. Generally an ADC multivitamin such as Tri-Vi-Sol or Vi-Daylin ADC can be used (Table 20-4). Start Vitamin D supplements by 2 months of age or sooner.[7,8]

B. FLUORIDE

Supplementation is not needed during the first 6 months of life. Thereafter 0.25 mg/day is recommended for the exclusively breast-fed infant.[8] See Formulary for complete fluoride recommendations (i.e., in areas where water is not routinely fluoridated).

C. IRON

For exclusively breast-fed infants, approximately 1 mg/kg/day is recommended after 4 to 6 months of age, preferably from iron-fortified cereal or elemental iron if sufficient cereal is not consumed.[8]

D. SELECTED MULTIVITAMINS (Table 20-5)

20

NUTRITION AND GROWTH

TABLE 20-4			
INFANT MULTIVITAMIN DROPS ANALYSIS (PER mL)*			
	Poly-Vi-Sol/ (Flor) [with iron] Vi Daylin/ F Multivitamin [with iron]	Tri-Vi-Sol/ (Flor) [with iron] Vi-Daylin/(F) ADC [with iron]	ADEK[†‡]
Vitamin A (IU)	1500	1500	1500
Vitamin D (IU)	400	400	400
Vitamin E (IU)	5	—	40
Vitamin C (mg)	35	35	45
Thiamin (mg)	0.5	—	0.5
Riboflavin (mg)	0.6	—	0.6
Niacin (mg)	8	—	6
Vitamin B6 (mg)	0.4	—	0.6
Vitamin B12 (mcg)	2[§]	—	4
Iron (mg)	[10]	[10]	—
Fluoride (mg)	(0.25)	(0.25)	—

*Standard dose = 1 mL.
[†]Also contains biotin 15 mcg; pantothenic acid 3 mg; zinc 5 mg; β-carotene 1 mg = 1666 IU vitamin A, 100 mcg vitamin K.
[‡]Recommended for use in infants with fat malabsorption such as cystic fibrosis, liver disease.
[§]Poly-Vi-Sol only.

TABLE 20-5
SELECTED MULTIVITAMIN TABLETS (ANALYSIS/TABLET)

	Multivitamins					Prenatal	
	Flintstones Original Bugs Bunny Generic Poly-Vi-Sol/(F) Vi-Daylin/(F) [with iron]	Flintstones + Extra C Sunkist + Extra C Generic + C Bugs Bunny + Extra C	Centrum Jr	Flintstones Complete Generic Complete	ADEK	Mynatal Rx Caplets Prenatal Rx Tablets	
Vitamin A (IU)*	2500	2500	5000	5000	4000	4000	
Vitamin D (IU)	400	400	400	400	400	400	
Vitamin E (IU)	15	15	30	30	150	15	
Vitamin K (mcg)	—	—	10	—	150	—	
Vitamin C (mg)	60	250	60	60	60	80	
Thiamin (mg)	1.05	1.05	1.5	1.5	1.2	1	
Riboflavin (mg)	1.2	1.2	1.7	1.7	1.3	1.6	
Niacin (mg)	13.5	13.5	20	20	10	17	
Vitamin B_6 (mg)	1.05	1	2	2	1.5	4	
Folate (mcg)	300	300	400	400	200	1000	

Vitamin B$_{12}$ (mcg)	4.5	4.5-5	6	6	12	2.5
Biotin (mcg)	—	—	45	40	50	30
Pantothenic acid (mg)	—	—	10	10	10	7
Calcium (mg)	—	—	108	100	—	200
Phosphorus (mg)	—	—	50	100	—	—
Iron (elemental) (mg)	[10-15]	—	18	18	—	60
Iodine (mcg)	—	—	150	150	—	—
Magnesium (mg)	—	—	40	20	—	—
Zinc (mg)	—	—	15	15	7.5	25
Copper (mg)	—	—	2	3	—	—
Manganese (mg)	—	—	1	—	—	—
Chromium (mcg)	—	—	20	—	—	—
Molybdenum (mcg)	—	—	20	—	—	—
β-Carotene (mg)	—	—	—	—	3	—
Fluoride	(0.25, 0.5, 1.0)	—	—	—	—	—

*Includes β-carotene.

20

NUTRITION AND GROWTH

VI. ENTERAL NUTRITION (Tables 20-6 to 20-15)

Text continued on p. 502

TABLE 20-6

PREPARATION OF INFANT FORMULAS FOR STANDARD AND SOY FORMULAS*

Formula Type	Caloric Concentration (kcal/oz)	Amount of Formula	Water (oz)
Liquid concentrates	20	13 oz	13
(40 kcal/oz)	24	13 oz	8.5
	26	13 oz	7
	28	13 oz	5.5
	30	13 oz	4.3
Small volume preparation	20	1 scoop	2
of powder (44 kcal/scoop)	24	3 scoops	5
	26	2 scoops	3
	28	7 scoops	10
	30	3 scoops	4

*Does not apply to Enfacare, Neocate, Neosure, Elecare. Enfamil AR should not be concentrated greater than 24 kcal/oz. Use a packed measure for Portagen, Nutramigen, and Pregestimil.

TABLE 20-7

COMMON CALORIC SUPPLEMENTS*

Component	Calories
PROTEIN	
Casec	3.7 kcal/g (0.9 g protein)
	17 kcal/tbsp (4 g protein)
CARBOHYDRATE	
Polycose	Powder: 3.8 kcal/g
	8 kcal/tsp
	Liquid: 2.0 kcal/mL, 10 kcal/tsp
FAT	
MCT oil[†]	7.7 kcal/mL
Vegetable oil	8.3 kcal/mL

*Use these caloric supplements when you want to increase protein or when you have reached the maximum concentration tolerated and wish to further increase caloric density.
[†]MCT oil is unnecessary unless there is fat malabsorption.

TABLE 20-8

CLASSIFICATION OF FORMULAS BY CARBOHYDRATE

	Lactose	Sucrose and Glucose Polymers	Glucose Polymers	Minimal Carbohydrate
Common ingredient names		See glucose polymers	Glucose polymers Maltodextrins Corn syrup solids Modified tapioca starch	
Comments	Requires lactase enzyme for digestion Contraindicated in galactosemia	Requires sucrase enzyme for digestion (see also glucose polymers)	Easily digested For individuals with lactose malabsorption	For severe carbohydrate intolerance
Infants	America's Store Brand Formulas (generic) Enfamil Enfamil AR Enfamil Enfacare Enfamil Premature Evaporated milk formula Neosure* Nestlé Follow-up Nestlé Good Start Similac Similac PM 60/40 Similac Special Care	Alimentum America's Store Brand Soy Isomil Isomil DF (Fiber) Nestlé Alsoy Nestlé Follow-Up Soy Portagen	Enfamil Lactofree Neocate Nutramigen Pregestimil ProSobee Similac Lactose Free	MJ3232A RCF

cont'd

20

NUTRITION AND GROWTH

TABLE 20-8
CLASSIFICATION OF FORMULAS BY CARBOHYDRATE—cont'd

	Lactose	Sucrose and Glucose Polymers	Glucose Polymers	Minimal Carbohydrate
Toddlers and young children	Cow's milk Next Step* Similac 2	Compleat Pediatric† Isomil 2 Kindercal TF (Fiber) Neocate One Plus Next Step Soy Nutren Junior PediaSure (also w/Fiber) Pediatric EO$_{28}$ Peptamen Junior‡ ProPeptide for Kids Resource Just for Kids	EleCare KetoCal Neocate Junior Pepdite One+ Vivonex Pediatric	
Older children and adolescents	Carnation Instant Breakfast Scandishake	All other formulas in Table 20-14	Criticare HN Crucial Deliver 2.0 L-Emental faa	

20

NUTRITION AND GROWTH

Glucerna
Glytrol
Isocal
Jevity (fiber)
Nestlé Modulen IBD
Nutren (all)
Osmolite
Promote
Peptamen
ProPeptide
Replete
Tolerex
Ultracal
Vivonex Plus
Vivonex TEN

*Also contains glucose polymers.
†Also contains fruit and vegetable purees.
‡Unflavored contains glucose polymers only.

TABLE 20-9

CLASSIFICATION OF FORMULAS BY PROTEIN

	Cow's Milk Protein	Soy Protein	Hydrolysate	Free Amino Acids
Common ingredient names	Cow's milk protein Nonfat milk Demineralized whey Reduced mineral whey Sodium, calcium, magnesium caseinate Casein	Soy protein Soy protein isolate	Casein hydrolysate Hydrolyzed whey, meat, and soy	—
Comments	Requires normal protein digestion and absorption	Requires normal protein digestion and absorption Not recommended for premature infants or those with cystic fibrosis	For individuals with protein allergy and/or malabsorption	For individuals with severe protein allergy and/or severe protein malabsorption
Infants	America's Store Brand formulas (generic) Enfamil Enfamil AR Enfamil Enfacare Enfamil Lactofree Enfamil Premature Evaporated milk formula Nestlé Follow-up	America's Store Brand Soy Isomil Isomil DF Nestlé Alsoy Nestlé Follow-up Soy ProSobee RCF	Alimentum MJ3232A Nutramigen Pregestimil	Neocate

	Nestlé Good Start Portagen Similac Similac Lactose Free Similac Neosure Similac PM 60/40 Similac Special Care			
Toddlers and young children	Compleat Pediatric* Cow's milk KetoCal Kindercal Next Step Nutren Junior PediaSure Resource Just for Kids Similac 2	Next Step Soy Isomil 2	Pepdite One+ Peptamen Junior Pro-Peptide for Kids	Vivonex Pediatric EleCare Neocate Junior Neocate One+ Pediatric EO$_{28}$
Older children and adolescents	All other formulas in Table 20-14	Ensure† Ensure with Nutraflora FOS† Ensure Plus† Isocal† Osmolite† Promote†	Criticare HN Crucial Peptamen ProPeptide Vital HN	L-Emental faa Tolerex Vivonex TEN Vivonex Plus

*Blenderized protein diet of meat, vegetables, and fruit.
†Also contains cow's milk.

TABLE 20-10
CLASSIFICATION OF FORMULAS BY FAT

	Long-Chain Triglycerides		Medium-Chain and Long-Chain Triglycerides

Common ingredient names	Butterfat
	Canola oil
	Coconut oil
	Corn oil
		Palm olein
		Safflower oil
		Soy oil
		Sunflower oil
			Fractioned
			  coconut oil
			Medium-chain
			  triglycerides
			  (MCT oil)

Comments	Requires normal fat digestion and absorption		For individuals
			  with fat
			  malabsorption
			Bile digestion
			  not required
			Absorbed
			  directly
			  into portal
			  circulation

Infants	America's Store
	  Brand
	  formulas
	  (generic)
	America's Store
	  Brand Soy
	Enfamil
	Enfamil AR
	Enfamil
	  Lactofree
	Evaporated milk
	  formula
	Isomil (all)
	Neocate
	Nestlé Alsoy
	Nestlé Follow-up
		Nestlé
		  Follow-up
		  Soy
		Nestlé Good
		  Start
		Nutramigen
		ProSobee
		RCF
		Similac
		Similac
		  Lactose
		  Free
		Similac PM
		  60/40
			Alimentum
			Enfamil
			  Enfacare
			Enfamil
			  Premature
			MJ3232A
			Neosure
			Portagen
			Pregestimil
			Similac
			  Special Care

cont'd

TABLE 20-10

CLASSIFICATION OF FORMULAS BY FAT—cont'd

	Long-Chain Triglycerides		Medium-Chain and Long-Chain Triglycerides	
Toddlers and young children	Compleat Pediatric Cow's milk Isomil 2 KetoCal Next Step Next Step Soy Similac 2		Elecare Kindercal Neocate Junior Neocate One+ powder Nutren Junior PediaSure Pediatric EO_{28} Peptamen Junior Pepdite One+ ProPeptide for Kids Resource Just For Kids Vivonex Pediatric	
Older children and adolescents	Carnation Instant Breakfast Criticare HN Ensure Ensure with Fiber Ensure Plus Glucerna L-Emental Tolerex Vivonex Plus Vivonex TEN	Boost Boost High-Protein Boost Plus Nepro Scandishake Suplena	Crucial Deliver 2.0 faa Isocal Jevity Glytrol Nestlé Modulen FBD Nutren 2.0 Nutren 1.0 (with Fiber)	Osmolite Peptamen Promote Propeptide Replete Subdue Traumacal Ultracal Vital HN

20

NUTRITION AND GROWTH

TABLE 20-11

INFANT FORMULA ANALYSIS (PER LITER)

Formula	kcal/mL (kcal/oz)	Protein g (% kcal)	Carbohydrate g (% kcal)	Fat g (% kcal)	Na (mEq)	K (mEq)	Ca (mg)	P (mg)	Fe (mg)	Osmolality (mOsm/kg water)	Suggested Uses
Alimentum (Ross)	0.67 (20)	19 (11) Casein hydrolysate L-Cystine, L-Tyr, L-Trp	69 (41) Sucrose 67% Modified tapioca starch	37 (48) MCT oil (33%) Safflower oil (39%) Soy oil (28%)	13	20	708	506	12	370	Infants with food allergies, protein or fat malabsorption
America's Store Brand (Wyeth Nutritionals)	0.67 (20)	14.6 (9) Nonfat milk Whey protein concentrate	71 (42) Lactose	35 (47) Oleo oil Coconut oil HO saff+ Sun oil Soy oil	6.5	14	425	284	12	—	Infants with normal GI tract
America's Store Brand for Older Infants (Wyeth Nutritionals)	0.68 (20)	22 (13) Cow's milk protein	69 (40) Lactose Corn syrup solids	37 (48) Oleo Coconut oil HO Soy	9.6	21.5	816	571	12	280	Infants 4-6 mo and older with normal GI tract

America's Store Brand Soy (Wyeth Nutritionals)	0.67 (20)	18 (11) Soy protein isolate L-Methionine	69 (41) Corn syrup solids Sucrose	35 (47) Palm olein HO saff or HO sun Coconut oil Soy oil	6.5	14	608	425	12	—	Infants with allergy to cow's milk, lactose malabsorption, galactosemia
Enfacare with iron (Mead Johnson)	0.74 (22)	21 (11) Nonfat milk Demineralized whey	79 (43) Maltodextrin Lactose Citrates	39 (46) HO sun oil Soy oil MCT oil Coconut oil	11	20	890	490	13	230	Infants with conditions such as prematurity
Enfamil AR (Mead Johnson)	0.67 (20)	16.8 (10) Nonfat milk	74 (44) Lactose (57%) Rice starch (30%) Maltodextrins (13%)	34 (46) Palm olein (45%) Soy oil (20%) Coconut oil (20%) HO sun oil (15%)	12	19	530	360	12	240	When a thickened feeding is desired (should not be concentrated >24 kcal/oz)

cont'd

20

NUTRITION AND GROWTH

TABLE 20-11
INFANT FORMULA ANALYSIS (PER LITER)—cont'd

Formula	kcal/mL (kcal/oz)	Protein g (% kcal)	Carbohydrate g (% kcal)	Fat g (% kcal)	Na (mEq)	K (mEq)	Ca (mg)	P (mg)	Fe (mg)	Osmolality (mOsm/kg water)	Suggested Uses
Enfamil with Iron [low iron] (Mead Johnson)	0.67 (20)	14 (9) Nonfat milk Demineralized whey	73 (44) Lactose	36 (48) Palm olein (45%) Soy oil (20%) Coconut oil (20%) HO Sun oil (15%)	8	19	530	360	12 [5]	300	Infants with normal GI tract
Enfamil with Iron 24 [low iron] (Mead Johnson)	0.8 (24)	17 (9) Nonfat milk Whey	88 (43) Lactose	43 (48) Palm olein (45%) Soy oil (20%) HO Sun oil (15%) Coconut oil (20%)	10	23	630	430	15 [6]	360	Infants with normal GI tract requiring additional calories
Enfamil Lactofree (Mead Johnson)	0.67 (20)	14 (9) Milk protein isolate	74 (43) Corn syrup solids	36 (48) Palm olein (45%) Soy oil (20%) Coconut oil (20%) HO Sun oil (15%)	9	19	550	370	12	200	Infants with lactose malabsorption

Product	kcal/mL (cal/oz)	Protein g (%) source	Carbohydrate g (%) source	Fat g (%) source							Indications
Enfamil Premature Formula 20 [w/Fe] (Mead Johnson)	0.67 (20)	20 (12) Demineralized whey Nonfat milk	75 (44) Corn syrup solids Lactose	35 (44) MCT oil (40%) Soy oil Coconut oil	11	18	1120	560	1.7 [12]	260	Preterm infants
Enfamil Premature Formula 24 [w/Fe] (Mead Johnson)	0.8 (24)	24 (12) Demineralized whey Nonfat milk	9 (44) Corn syrup solids Lactose	41 (44) MCT oil (40%) Soy oil Coconut oil	14	21	1340	670	2 [15]	310	Preterm infants
Evaporated milk formula*	0.67 (20)	27 (16) Cow's milk	72 (43) Lactose Corn syrup	31 (41) Butterfat	21	32	1066	832	0.8	—	Infants with normal GI tract; need vitamin C and iron supplement
Isomil (Ross)	0.67 (20)	17 (10) Soy protein isolate Methionine	70 (41) Corn syrup Sucrose	37 (49) Soy oil (30%) Coconut oil (30%) HO saff oil (40%)	13	19	709	507	12	200	Infants with allergy to cow's milk, lactose malabsorption, galactosemia

*13 oz evaporated whole milk, 19 oz water, 2 tbsp corn syrup.

cont'd

20

NUTRITION AND GROWTH

TABLE 20-11

INFANT FORMULA ANALYSIS (PER LITER)—cont'd

Formula	kcal/mL (kcal/oz)	Protein g (% kcal)	Carbohydrate g (% kcal)	Fat g (% kcal)	Na (mEq)	K (mEq)	Ca (mg)	P (mg)	Fe (mg)	Osmolality (mOsm/kg water)	Suggested Uses
Isomil DF (Ross)	0.67 (20)	18 (11) Soy protein isolate Methionine	68 (40) Corn syrup Sucrose Soy fiber	37 (49) Soy oil (60%) Coconut oil (40%)	13	19	709	507	12	240	Short-term management of diarrhea; contains fiber
MJ3232A (Mead Johnson)	0.42 (12.7)	19 (18) Casein hydrolysate L-Cystine, L-Tyr, L-Trp	28 (27) Tapioca starch CHO selected by physician	28 (55) MCT oil (85%) Corn oil (15%)	13	19	640	430	13	250	Infants with severe CHO intolerance (CHO must be added)
Neocate (SHS North America)	0.69 (21)	20 (12) Free amino acids	78 (47) Corn syrup solids	30 (41) Safflower oil Coconut oil Soy oil	11	26	837	628	12	375	Infants with severe food allergies
Nestle Carnation Alsoy (Nestlé)	0.67 (20)	21 (11) L-Methionine Soy protein isolate	68 (44) Sucrose Maltodextrin	36 (45) Palm olein (47%) Soy oil (26%) Coconut oil (21%) HO safflower oil (6%)	10	20	702	413	13	270	Infants with allergy to cow's milk, lactose malabsorption, galactosemia

Nestle Carnation Follow-up (Nestlé)	0.67 (20)	18 (10) Nonfat milk	89 (53) Corn syrup Lactose	28 (37) Palm olein (47%) Soy oil (26%) Coconut oil (21%) HO saff oil (6%)	11	23	811	603	13	326	Infants 4-12 months with normal GI tract
Nestle Carnation Follow-up Soy (Nestlé)	0.67 (20)	21 (12) Soy protein isolate Methionine	81 (48) Maltodextrin Sucrose	29 (40) Palm olein (47%) Soy oil (26%) Coconut oil (21%) HO saff oil (6%)	12	20	905	603	13	200	Infants 4-12 months with allergy to cow's milk, lactose malabsorption, galactosemia
Nestle Carnation Good Start (Nestlé)	0.67 (20)	16 (10) Partially hydrolyzed whey	74 (44) Lactose Maltodextrins	35 (46) Palm olein (47%) Soy oil (26%) Coconut oil (21%) HO saff oil (6%)	7	17	429	241	10	300	Infants with normal GI tract

cont'd

NUTRITION AND GROWTH

20

TABLE 20-11
INFANT FORMULA ANALYSIS (PER LITER)—cont'd

Formula	kcal/mL (kcal/oz)	Protein g (% kcal)	Carbohydrate g (% kcal)	Fat g (% kcal)	Na (mEq)	K (mEq)	Ca (mg)	P (mg)	Fe (mg)	Osmolality (mOsm/kg water)	Suggested Uses
Nutramigen (Mead Johnson)	0.67 (20)	19 (11) Casein hydrolysate L-Cystine, L-Tyr, L-Trp	75 (44) Corn syrup solids Modified cornstarch	34 (45) Palm olein (45%) Soy oil (20%) Coconut oil (20%) HO Sun oil (15%)	14	19	640	430	12	320	Infants with food allergies
Portagen (Mead Johnson)	0.67 (20)	24 (14) Na caseinate	78 (46) Corn syrup solids Sucrose	32 (40) MCT oil (86%) Corn oil (14%)	16	22	640	470	13	230	Infants with fat malabsorption, intestinal lymphatic obstruction, chylothorax
Pregestimil (Mead Johnson)	0.67 (20)	19 (11) Casein hydrolysate L-Cystine, L-Tyr, L-Trp	69 (41) Corn syrup solids (60%) Modified corn-starch (20%) Dextrose (20%)	38 (48) MCT oil (55%) Corn oil (10%) Soy oil (25%) HO saff oil (10%)	11	19	766	500	12	320	Infants with food allergies, protein or fat malabsorption

Product											
ProSobee (Mead Johnson)	0.67 (20)	17 (10) L-Methionine Soy protein isolate	73 (42) Corn syrup solids	37 (48) Palm olein (45%) Soy oil (20%) Coconut oil (20%) HO Sun oil (15%)	10	21	710	560	12	200	Infants with allergy to cow's milk, lactose malabsorption, galactosemia
RCF* (Ross) [w/Fe]	0.4 (12)	20 (20) Soy isolate	— Selected by physician	36 (80) Soy oil Coconut oil	13	19	709	507	12	*	Infants with severe CHO intolerance (CHO must be added) Modified for ketogenic diet
Similac with Iron [low iron] (Ross)	0.67 (20)	14 (8) Nonfat milk Whey protein	73 (43) Lactose	36 (49) Soy oil (30%) Coconut oil (30%) HO saff oil (40%)	7	18	527	284	12 [5]	300	Infants with normal GI tract
Similac with Iron 24 (Ross)	0.8 (24)	22 (11) Nonfat milk	85 (42) Lactose	42 (47) Soy oil (60%) Coconut oil (40%)	12	27	726	565	15	380	Infants with normal GI tract requiring additional calories

cont'd

20

NUTRITION AND GROWTH

TABLE 20-11

INFANT FORMULA ANALYSIS (PER LITER)—cont'd

Formula	kcal/mL (kcal/oz)	Protein g (% kcal)	Carbohydrate g (% kcal)	Fat g (% kcal)	Na (mEq)	K (mEq)	Ca (mg)	P (mg)	Fe (mg)	Osmolality (mOsm/kg water)	Suggested Uses
Similac Lactose Free (Ross)	0.67 (20)	14.5 (9) Milk protein isolate	72.3 (43) Corn syrup solids (55%) Sucrose (45%)	36.5 (49) Soy oil (60%) Coconut oil (40%)	9	18	568	378	12	200	Infants with lactose malabsorption
Similac Neosure (Ross)	0.73 (22)	19 (10) Nonfat milk Whey protein concentrate	77 (41) Lactose (50%) Maltodextrins (50%)	41 (49) MCT oil (25%) Soy oil (45%) Coconut oil (30%)	11	27	784	463	13	250	Preterm infants, after hospital discharge, until goal catch-up growth
Similac PM 60/40 (Ross)	0.67 (20)	15 (9) Whey protein concentrate Na caseinate	69 (41) Lactose	38 (50) Soy oil (12%) Coconut oil (38%) Corn oil (50%)	7	15	378	189	5	280	Infants who require lowered calcium and phosphorus levels

Similac Special Care 20 [w/Fe] (Ross)	0.67 (20)	18 (11) Nonfat milk Whey protein concentrate	72 (42) Corn syrup solids (50%) Lactose (50%)	37 (49) MCT oil (50%) Soy oil (30%) Coconut oil (20%)	13	22	1216	676	(12) 2.5	235	Preterm infants
Similac Special Care 24 [w/Fe] (Ross)	0.8 (24)	22 (11) Nonfat milk Whey protein concentrate	86 (42) Corn syrup solids (50%) Lactose (50%)	44 (49) MCT oil (50%) Soy oil (30%) Coconut oil (20%)	15	27	1452	806	(15) 3	280	Preterm infants

*Available as concentrated liquid. Nutrient values vary depending on amount of added carbohydrate (CHO) and water. A total of 12 fl oz of concentrated liquid with 15 g CHO and 12 fl oz water yields 20 kcal/fl oz formula with 68 g CHO/L.
For most current information, refer to formula websites or labels.

NUTRITION AND GROWTH

20

TABLE 20-12
HUMAN MILK AND FORTIFIERS ANALYSIS (PER LITER)

Formula	kcal/mL (kcal/oz)	Protein g (% kcal)	Carbohydrate g (% kcal)	Fat g (% kcal)	Na (mEq)	K (mEq)	Ca (mg)	P (mg)	Fe (mg)	Osmolality (mOsm/kg water)	Suggested Uses
Human milk (mature)	0.69 (20)	10 (6) Human milk protein	72 (42) Lactose	39 (54) Human milk fat	7	13	280	147	0.4	286	Infants
Human milk* (Preterm)	0.67 (20)	14 (8) Human milk protein	66 (40) Lactose	39 (52) Human milk fat	11	15	248	128	1.2	290	Preterm infants
Enfamil Human Milk Fortifier (per packet) (Mead Johnson)	3.5 (—)	0.3 (29) Whey protein isolate Na caseinate	0.26 (30) Corn syrup solids	0.16 (42) From caseinate	0.12	0.13	23	11	0.36	—	Fortifier for preterm human milk
Similac Human Milk Fortifier (Ross) per packet	3.5 kcal per packet	0.25 (29) Whey protein concentrate Nonfat milk	0.45 (51) Corn syrup solids	0.09 (23) MCT oil	0.16	0.4	29	17	0.09	—	Fortifier for preterm human milk
Similac Natural Care Human Milk Fortifier (Ross)	0.8 (24)	22 (11) Nonfat milk Whey protein concentrate	86 (42) Corn syrup solids (50%) Lactose (50%)	44 (47) MCT oil (50%) Soy oil (30%) Coconut oil (20%)	15	26.6	1694	935	3	280	Fortifier for preterm human milk

Product		Protein source	Carbohydrate source	Fat source							
Preterm Human Milk + Enfamil Human Milk Fortifier (1 pkt/25 mL)	0.79 (24)	27 (13) Human milk protein Whey protein concentrate Na caseinate	82 (41) Lactose Corn syrup solids	41 (46) Human milk fat	165	18	1140	590	15	410	Preterm infants
Preterm Human Milk + Similac Human Milk Fortifier (1 packet/25 mL)	0.79 (24)	23 (12) Nonfat milk Whey protein concentrate Human milk protein	82 (42) Lactose Corn syrup solids	41 (47) MCT oil Human milk fat	17	30	1380	776	4.6	385	Preterm infants
Preterm Human Milk + Similac Natural Care 75:25 ratio	0.7 (21)	16 (9) Human milk protein Nonfat milk Whey protein concentrate	71 (40) Lactose Corn syrup solids	40 (51) Human milk fat MCT oil Soy oil Coconut oil	12	18	610	330	1.65	288	Preterm infants
Preterm Human Milk + Similac Natural Care 50:50 ratio	0.74 (22)	18 (10) Human milk protein Nonfat milk Whey protein concentrate	71 (40) Lactose Corn syrup solids	41 (50) Human milk fat MCT oil Soy oil Coconut oil	13	21	971	531	2.1	285	Preterm infants

From Ross Products Division, Abbott Laboratories, Inc.

*Composition of human milk varies with maternal diet, stage of lactation, within feedings, diurnally, and among mothers.

20

NUTRITION AND GROWTH

TABLE 20-13

TODDLER AND YOUNG CHILD FORMULA ANALYSIS (PER LITER)

Formula	kcal/mL (kcal/oz)	Protein g (% kcal)	Carbohydrate g (% kcal)	Fat g (% kcal)	Na (mEq)	K (mEq)	Ca (mg)	P (mg)	Fe (mg)	Osmolality (mOsm/kg water)	Suggested Uses
Compleat Pediatric (Novartis)	1 (30)	38 (15) Beef Na caseinate Ca caseinate	130 (50) Vegetables Fruit Hydrolyzed cornstarch Apple juice	39 (35) HO sun oil Soy oil MCT oil	30	38	1000	1000	13	380	For those who desire a blenderized tube feeding
Cow's milk, whole	0.63 (19)	34 (22) Cow's milk	48 (31) Lactose	34 (49) Butterfat	22	40	1226	956	0.5	285	Children >1 year of age with normal GI tract
Elecare (Ross)	1 (30)	30 (15) Free L-amino acids	107 (43) Corn syrup solids	47.6 (42) HO saff oil (39%) MCT oil (33%) Soy oil (28%)	20	39	1082	808	18	596	Children with malabsorption, protein allergy
Isomil 2 (Ross)	0.67 (20)	17 (10) Soy protisolate Methionine	70 (41) Corn syrup (80%) Sucrose (20%)	37 (49) HO saff (40%) Coconut (30%) Soy oil (30%)	13	19	912	608	12	200	Milk sensitive 6-18 mo eating cereal and baby foods

Product											
KetoCal (SHS North America)	1.44 (43)	30 (8.4) Cow's milk protein	6 (1.6) Corn syrup solids	144 (90) Soybean oil	26	55	1600	1300	22	197	Children on ketogenic diet
Kindercal TF (contains fiber) (Mead Johnson)	1.06 (32)	30 (11) Milk protein concentrate	135 (52) Maltodextrins Sucrose	44 (37) Canola oil (40%) HO sun oil (28%) Corn oil (12%) MCT oil (20%)	16	34	1010	850	11	345 institutional and retail 440 vanilla 520 chocolate	Tube feeding and oral supplement for children with normal GI tract
Neocate Junior (SHS North America)	1 (30)	30 (12) Free amino acids	104 (42) Corn syrup solids	50 (46) Canola oil MCT oil (25%) Saff oil	18	35	1130	940	14	602	Children with malabsorption, protein allergy
Neocate One+ Powder (SHS North America)	1 (30)	25 (10) Free amino acids	146 (58) Corn syrup solids	35 (22) MCT oil (35%) Canola oil Saff oil	9	24	620	620	8	610	Children with malabsorption, protein allergy

20

NUTRITION AND GROWTH

TABLE 20-13
TODDLER AND YOUNG CHILD FORMULA ANALYSIS (PER LITER)—cont'd

Formula	kcal/mL (kcal/oz)	Protein g (% kcal)	Carbohydrate g (% kcal)	Fat g (% kcal)	Na (mEq)	K (mEq)	Ca (mg)	P (mg)	Fe (mg)	Osmolality (mOsm/kg water)	Suggested Uses
Next Step (Mead Johnson)	0.67 (20)	18 (10) Nonfat milk protein	75 (45) Lactose Corn syrup solids	34 (45) Palm olein (45%) Soy oil (20%) Coconut oil (20%) HO sun oil (15%)	12	23	810	570	12	270	Toddlers with normal GI tract
Next Step Soy (Mead Johnson)	0.67 (20)	22 (13) Soy protein isolate	80 (47) Corn syrup solids Sucrose	30 (40) Palm olein (45%) Soy oil (20%) Coconut oil (20%) HO sun oil (15%)	13	26	780	610	12	260	Toddlers with cow's milk allergy, galactosemia
Nutren Junior (also with fiber) (Nestlé)	1 (30)	30 (12) Casein (50%) Whey (50%)	128 (51) Maltodextrins Sucrose (Soy polysaccharides)	42 (37) Soy oil MCT oil (25%) Canola oil Soy lecithin	20	34	1000	800	14	350	Tube feeding and oral supplement for children with normal GI tract

Product											
PediaSure (also with fiber) (Ross)	1 (30)	30 (12) Na caseinate Whey protein concentrate	110 (44) Maltodextrins Sucrose (Soy fiber)	50 (44) HO saff oil (50%) Soy oil (30%) MCT oil (20%)	17	34	970	800	14	335 (institutional) 430 (retail/oral)	Tube feeding and oral supplement for children with normal GI tract
Pediatric EO$_{28}$ (SHS North America)	1 (30)	25 (10) Free amino acids	146 (58) Maltodextrins Sucrose	35 (32) MCT oil Canola oil HO saff oil	9	24	620	620	8	820	Children with malabsorption, protein allergy
Pepdite One+ (SHS North America)	1 (30)	31 (12) Hydrolyzed meat and soy protein Free amino acids	106 (42) Corn syrup solids	50 (46) MCT oil Canola oil Saff oil	18	35	1130	940	14	432-440	Children with malabsorption
Peptamen Junior (Nestlé) (also with fiber)	1 (30)	30 (12) Enzymatically hydrolyzed whey protein	138 (55) Maltodextrin Sucrose (flavored) Cornstarch	38.5 (33) MCT oil (60%) Soy oil Canola oil Lecithin	20	33	1000	800	14	260 (unflavored) 360 (flavored)	Children with malabsorption
Propeptide for Kids (Hormel Health Labs)	1 (30)	30 (12) Enzymatically hydrolyzed whey protein	137.5 (55) Maltodextrin Sucrose Cornstarch	38.5 (33) MCT oil (18.5%) Soy oil (22%) Canola oil (60%) Lecithin	20	34	1000	800	14	360	Children with malabsorption

cont'd

20

NUTRITION AND GROWTH

TABLE 20-13

TODDLER AND YOUNG CHILD FORMULA ANALYSIS (PER LITER)—cont'd

Formula	kcal/mL (kcal/oz)	Protein g (% kcal)	Carbohydrate g (% kcal)	Fat g (% kcal)	Na (mEq)	K (mEq)	Ca (mg)	P (mg)	Fe (mg)	Osmolality (mOsm/kg water)	Suggested Uses
Resource Just for Kids (Novartis)	1 (30)	30 (12) Na caseinate Ca caseinate Whey protein concentrates	110 (44) Hydrolyzed cornstarch Sucrose	50 (44) HO Sun oil Soy oil MCT oil	17	33	1140	800	14	390	Tube feeding and oral supplement for children with normal GI tract
Similac 2	0.67 (20)	14 (8) Nonfat milk Whey protein concentrate	72 (43) Lactose	37 (49) HO saff (40%) Coconut oil (30%) Soy oil (30%)	7	18	797	432	12	300	6-18 months eating cereal and baby foods
Vivonex Pediatric (Novartis)	0.8 (24)	24 (12) Free amino acids	130 (63) Maltodextrins Modified starch	24 (25) MCT oil (68%) Soy oil (32%)	17	31	970	800	10	360	Children with malabsorption, protein allergy

TABLE 20-14
OLDER CHILD AND ADULT FORMULA ANALYSIS (PER LITER)

Formula	kcal/mL (kcal/oz)	Protein g (% kcal)	Carbohydrate g (% kcal)	Fat g (% kcal)	Na (mEq)	K (mEq)	Ca (mg)	P (mg)	Fe (mg)	Osmolality (mOsm/kg water)	Suggested Uses
Boost (Mead Johnson)	1 (30)	42 (17) Milk protein concentrate	171 (67) Corn syrup solids Sucrose	17 (16) Canola oil HO sun oil Corn oil	24	43	1248	1040	15	610	Oral supplement
Boost High Protein (Mead Johnson)	1 (30)	61 (24) Na caseinate Ca caseinate Milk protein concentrate	139 (55) Corn syrup solids Sucrose	23 (21) Canola oil HO sun oil Corn oil	31	41	1390	1310	19	540	Oral supplement or tube feeding for patients with increased protein needs
Boost Plus (Mead Johnson)	1.5 (45)	59 (16) Na caseinate Ca caseinate Milk protein concentrate	200 (50) Corn syrup solids Sucrose	58 (34) Canola oil HO sun oil Corn oil	31	41	1390	1310	19	720	Oral supplement or tube feeding for patients with high calorie needs, normal GI tract, volume fluid restriction

cont'd

TABLE 20-14

OLDER CHILD AND ADULT FORMULA ANALYSIS (PER LITER)—cont'd

Formula	kcal/mL (kcal/oz)	Protein g (% kcal)	Carbohydrate g (% kcal)	Fat g (% kcal)	Na (mEq)	K (mEq)	Ca (mg)	P (mg)	Fe (mg)	Osmolality (mOsm/kg water)	Suggested Uses
Carnation Instant Breakfast w/whole milk (Nestlé)	1.2 (36)	53 (18) Cow's milk	161 (54) Lactose Maltodextrin Sucrose	34 (26) Butterfat	42	67	1632	1400	17	590	High-calorie supplement for patients with normal GI tract
Criticare HN (Mead Johnson)	1.06 (32)	38 (14) Hydrolyzed casein Amino acids	220 (81.5) Maltodextrin Modified cornstarch	5 (4.5) Safflower oil	27	34	530	530	9.7	650	Patients with malabsorption IBD, short bowel
Crucial (Nestlé)	1.5 (45)	94 (25) Enzymatically hydrolyzed casein arginine glutamine	135 (36) Maltodextrin Corn starch	68 (39) Marine oil MCT oil (50%) Soybean oil	51	48	1000	1000	18	490	Volume-restricted critically ill patients

Product	kcal/mL (mOsm)	Protein g (% cal)	Carbohydrate g (% cal)	Fat g (% cal)						mOsm	Indications
Deliver 2.0 (Mead Johnson)	2 (60)	75 (15) Ca caseinate Na caseinate	200 (40) Corn syrup	101 (45) Soy oil (70%) MCT oil (30%)	35	43	1010	1010	18	640	Oral supplement or tube feeding for patients with fluid restriction or liver disease increased calorie needs
Ensure (Ross)	1.06 (32)	37 (14) Na caseinate Ca caseinate Soy protein isolate Whey protein concentrate	167 (64) Corn syrup Maltodextrin Sucrose	25 (22) HO saff oil (40%) Canola oil (40%) Corn oil (20%)	36	40	1250	1250	18.7	590	Oral supplement or tube feeding for patients with normal GI tract
Ensure Fiber with FOS (Ross)	1.06 (32)	37 (14) Na caseinate Ca caseinate Soy protein isolate	175 (64) Maltodextrin (65%) Sucrose (29%) Soy fiber (2%) Oat fiber (2%) Fructooligosaccharides (2%)	25 (22) Corn oil (20%) HO saff oil (40%) Canola oil (40%)	37	40	1458	1250	19	500	Oral supplement or tube feeding with fiber, normal GI tract

cont'd

NUTRITION AND GROWTH

20

TABLE 20-14
OLDER CHILD AND ADULT FORMULA ANALYSIS (PER LITER)—cont'd

Formula	kcal/mL (kcal/oz)	Protein g (% kcal)	Carbohydrate g (% kcal)	Fat g (% kcal)	Na (mEq)	K (mEq)	Ca (mg)	P (mg)	Fe (mg)	Osmolality (mOsm/kg water)	Suggested Uses
Ensure Plus (Ross)	1.5 (45)	54 (15) Na caseinate Ca caseinate Soy protein isolate	208 (56) Corn syrup Sucrose Maltodextrin	48 (29) Corn oil (25%) Canola oil (50%) HO saff (25%)	43	47	833	833	19	680	Oral supplement or tube feeding for patients with higher calorie needs, normal GI tract
faa (Nestlé)	1.0 (30)	50 (20) Free amino acids	176 (70) Maltodextrin	11 (10) Soy oil MCT oil	24	38	800	700	18	700	Tube feeding or oral supplement for malabsorption, not for protein allergy
Glucerna (Ross)	1 (30)	42 (17) Na caseinate Ca caseinate	96 (34) Soy fiber Fructose Maltodextrin	54 (49) HO saff oil (85%) Canola oil (10%) Lecithin (5%)	40	40	705	705	13	355	Patients with impaired glucose tolerance, also contains fiber

Glytrol (Nestlé)	1.0 (30)	45 (18) Ca Potassium caseinates	100 (40) Maltodextrin Modified corn starch Fructose Gum arabic Soy polysaccharide Pectin	48 (42) Canola oil HO saff MCT oil Soy lecithin	32	36	720	720	13	380	Tube feeding or oral supplement for patients with impaired glucose tolerance
Isocal (Mead Johnson)	1.06 (32)	34 (13) Na caseinate Ca caseinate Soy protein	135 (50) Maltodextrin	44 (37) MCT oil (20%) Soy oil (80%)	23	34	630	530	10	270	Tube feeding for patients with normal GI tract
Jevity (Ross)	1.06 (32)	44 (17) Na caseinate Ca caseinate	155 (54) Corn syrup Maltodextrin Soy fiber	35 (29) HO saff oil (48%) Canola oil (29%) MCT oil (20%) Lecithin (3%)	40	40	910	760	14	300	Tube feeding with fiber, normal GI tract

cont'd

TABLE 20-14

OLDER CHILD AND ADULT FORMULA ANALYSIS (PER LITER)—cont'd

Formula	kcal/mL (kcal/oz)	Protein g (% kcal)	Carbohydrate g (% kcal)	Fat g (% kcal)	Na (mEq)	K (mEq)	Ca (mg)	P (mg)	Fe (mg)	Osmolality (mOsm/kg water)	Suggested Uses
L-Emental (Hormel Health Labs)	1 (30)	38 (15) Free amino acids	210 (82) Maltodextrins	2.85 (3) Safflower oil	20	20	500	500	9	630	Patients with malabsorption, protein allergy
Nepro (Ross)	2 (60)	70 (14) Ca caseinate Mg caseinate Na caseinate Milk protein isolate	222 (43) Corn syrup Sucrose Fructo oligo-saccharides	96 (43) HO saff oil (67%) Canola oil (29%) Lecithin (4%)	36	27	1370	685	19	665	Patients with renal failure undergoing dialysis
Nestlé Modulen IBD (Nestlé)	1 (30)	36 (14) Acid casein with TGF-β₂	108 (44) Corn syrup Sucrose	46 (42) Milk fat MCT oil Corn oil Soy oil Lecithin	15	31	888	600	12	370	Patients with Crohn's disease
Nutren 1.0 with fiber (Nestlé)	1 (30)	40 (16) K caseinate Ca caseinate	127 (51) Maltodextrin Corn syrup solids (Soy polysacch)	38 (33) Canola oil MCT oil (25%) Corn oil	38	32	668	668	12	315-370	Standard tube feeding with fiber

Product										
Nutren 2.0 (Nestlé)	2 (60)	80 (16) K caseinate Ca caseinate	196 (39) Corn syrup solids Maltodextrin Sucrose	106 (45) MCT oil (75%) Canola oil Corn oil Soy lecithin	57	49	1340	1340	24	745	Oral supplement or tube feedings for patients with fluid restriction or increased calorie needs
Osmolite (Ross)	1.06 (32)	37 (14) Na caseinate Ca caseinate Soy protein isolate	151 (57) Maltodextrin	35 (29) HO saff oil (48%) Canola oil (29%) MCT oil (20%) Lecithin (3%)	28	26	535	535	9.6	300	Tube feeding for patients with normal GI tract
Peptamen (Nestlé)	1 (30)	40 (16) Enzymatically hydrolyzed whey protein	127 (51) Maltodextrin Corn starch	39 (33) MCT oil (70%) Soybean oil (30%)	24	39	800	700	18	270-380	Patients with malabsorption
Promote (Ross)	1 (30)	63 (25) Na caseinate Ca caseinate Soy protein isolate	130 (52) Maltodextrin Sucrose	26 (23) HO saff oil (47%) Canola oil (28%) MCT oil (19%) Lecithin (6%)	43	50	1200	1200	18	340	Tube feeding or oral supplement for patients with increased protein needs

cont'd

20

NUTRITION AND GROWTH

TABLE 20-14

OLDER CHILD AND ADULT FORMULA ANALYSIS (PER LITER)—cont'd

Formula	kcal/mL (kcal/oz)	Protein g (% kcal)	Carbohydrate g (% kcal)	Fat g (% kcal)	Na (mEq)	K (mEq)	Ca (mg)	P (mg)	Fe (mg)	Osmolality (mOsm/kg water)	Suggested Uses
ProPeptide (unflavored) (Hormel Health Labs)	1 (30)	40 (16) Hydrolyzed whey	127 (51) Maltodextrins Starch	39 (33) Sunflower oil (30%) MCT oil (70%)	22	32	800	700	14	270	Patients with malabsorption
Replete (with fiber) (Nestlé)	1 (30)	62 (25) Ca Potassium Caseinate	113 (40) Maltodextrin Corn syrup solids	34 (30) Canola oil MCT oil Soy lecithin	38	39	1000	1000	18	300-398	Tube feeding or oral supplement for patients with increased protein needs
Scandishake w/ whole milk (Scandipharm)	2.5 (75)	50 (8) Cow's milk	292 (47) Lactose Maltodextrin Soy oil	125 (45) Coconut oil Safflower oil Palm oil	240	103	391	478	trace	1094	High-calorie supplement and for fat malabsorption
Subdue (Mead Johnson)	1 (30)	50 (20) Hydrolyzed whey protein concentrate	127 (50) Maltodextrin Corn starch Sucrose	34 (30) Canola oil HO sun Corn oil MCT oil	48	41	1081	1040	15	330	Patients with malabsorption, IBD

Product										
Suplena (Ross)	2 (60)	30 (6) Na caseinate Ca caseinate	255 (51) Maltodextrin Sucrose (10%)	96 (43) HO saff oil (86%) Soy oil (10%) Lecithin (4%)	34	29	1430	730	19	600	Patients with renal failure not undergoing dialysis
Tolerex (Novartis)	1 (30)	21 (8) Free amino acids	230 (91) Maltodextrin	1.5 (1) Safflower oil	20	30	560	560	10	550	Patients with chylothorax, malabsorption, or severe food allergy
Traumacal (Mead Johnson)	1.5 (45)	82 (22) Na caseinate Ca caseinate	144 (38) Corn syrup Sucrose	68 (40) Soy oil (70%) MCT oil (30%)	51	36	750	750	9	560	Patients with increased protein and calorie needs
Ultracal (Mead Johnson)	1.06 (32)	45 (17) Na caseinate Ca caseinate Milk protein concentrate	132 (50) Maltodextrin Soy fiber Microcrystalline cellulose Acacia	39 (33) MCT oil (30%) Canola oil (35%) HO sun oil (25%) Corn oil (10%)	59	47	1000	1000	18	360	Oral supplement or tube feeding with fiber, normal GI tract

cont'd

NUTRITION AND GROWTH

20

TABLE 20-14
OLDER CHILD AND ADULT FORMULA ANALYSIS (PER LITER)—cont'd

Formula	kcal/mL (kcal/oz)	Protein g (% kcal)	Carbohydrate g (% kcal)	Fat g (% kcal)	Na (mEq)	K (mEq)	Ca (mg)	P (mg)	Fe (mg)	Osmolality (mOsm/kg water)	Suggested Uses
Vital HN (Ross)	1 (30)	42 (17) Hydrolyzed whey, meat, and soy protein (87%) Free amino acids (13%)	185 (74) Maltodextrin Sucrose Lactose (<0.5%)	11 (9) Safflower oil (55%) MCT oil (45%)	25	36	667	667	12	500	Patients with malabsorption, IBD
Vivonex Plus (Novartis)	1 (30)	45 (18) Free amino acids	190 (76) Maltodextrin Modified cornstarch	6.7 (6) Soybean oil	27	27	560	560	10	650	Patients with malabsorption or severe food allergy
Vivonex TEN (Novartis)	1 (30)	38 (15) Free amino acids	210 (82) Maltodextrin Modified cornstarch	2.8 (3) Safflower oil	26	24	500	500	9	630	Patients with malabsorption or severe food allergy

TABLE 20-15
ORAL REHYDRATION SOLUTIONS

Solution	Kcal/mL (kcal/oz)	Carbohydrate (g/L)	Na (mEq/L)	K (mEq/L)	Osmolality (mOsm/kg H_2O)
CeraLyte-70 (Cera)	0.16 (4.9)	Rice digest 40	70	20	232
CeraLyte-50 (Cera)	0.16 (4.9)	Rice digest, Glucose 40	50	20	200
Enfalyte (Mead Johnson)	0.12 (3.7)	Rice syrup solids 30	50	25	200
Oral Rehydration Salts (WHO) (Jianas)	0.06 (2)	Dextrose 20	90	20	330
Pedialyte Unflavored (Ross)	0.1 (3)	Dextrose 25	45	20	250
Rehydralyte (Ross)	0.1 (3)	Dextrose 25	75	20	305

20

NUTRITION AND GROWTH

VII. PARENTERAL NUTRITION (Tables 20-16 to 20-18)

TABLE 20-16
INITIATION AND ADVANCEMENT OF PARENTERAL NUTRITION*

Nutrient	Initial Dose	Advancement	Maximum
Glucose	5% to 10%	2.5% to 5%/day	12.5% peripheral
			18 mg/kg/min (maximum rate of infusion)
Protein	1 g/kg/day	0.5-1 g/kg/day	3 g/kg/day
			10%-16% of calories
Fat	0.5-1 g/kg/day	1 g/kg/day	4 g/kg/day
			0.17 g/kg/hr (maximum rate of infusion)

Modified from Baker RD, Baker SS, Davis AM. Pediatric parenteral nutrition. New York: Chapman and Hall; 1997 and Cox JH, Cooning SW. Parenteral nutrition. In Samour PQ, Helm KK, Lang CE, editors. Handbook of pediatric nutrition. Gaithersburg, Md; Aspen; 1999.
*Acceptable osmolarity of parenteral nutrition through a peripheral line varies between 900-1050 osm/L by institution. An estimate of the osmolarity of parenteral nutrition can be obtained with the following formula: Estimated osmolarity = (dextrose concentration × 50) + (amino acid concentration × 100) + (mEq of electrolytes × 2). Consult individual pharmacy for hospital limitations.

TABLE 20-17
DAILY PARENTERAL NUTRIENT RECOMMENDATIONS

Component	0-1 yr	1-7 yr	>7 yr
Energy (kcal/kg)	80-120	55-90	55-75
Protein (g/kg)	2-3	1.5-2.5	1.5-2.5
Sodium (mEq/kg)	3-4	2-4	2-4
Potassium (mEq/kg)	2-3	2-3	2-3
Magnesium (mEq/kg)	0.25-1	0.25-1	0.25-1
Calcium (mg/kg)	40-60	10-50	10-50
Phosphorus (mg/kg)	20-45	15-40	15-40
Zinc (mcg/kg)	400 (preterm) 100	100	100 (maximum 4 mg/day)
Copper (mcg/kg)	20	20	20 (maximum 1.5 mg/day)
Chromium (mcg/kg)	0.2	0.2	0.2 (maximum 15 mcg/day)
Manganese (mcg/kg)	2-10	2-10	2-10 (maximum 0.8 mg/day)
Selenium (mcg/kg)	3	3	3 (maximum 40 mcg/day)

Modified from Baker RD, Baker SS, Davis AM. Pediatric parenteral nutrition. New York: Chapman and Hall; 1997 and Cox JH, Cooning SW. Parenteral nutrition. In Samour PQ, Helm KK, Lang CE, editors. Handbook of pediatric nutrition. Gaithersburg, Md; Aspen; 1999.

TABLE 20-18		
MONITORING SCHEDULE FOR PATIENTS RECEIVING PARENTERAL NUTRITION*		
Variable	Initial Period[†]	Later Period[‡]
GROWTH		
Weight	Daily	2 times/wk
Height	Weekly (infants) Monthly	Monthly
Head circumference (infants)	Weekly	Monthly[§]
Arm circumference	Monthly	Monthly
Skinfold thickness	Monthly	Monthly
LABORATORY STUDIES		
Electrolytes and glucose	Daily until stable	Weekly
BUN/creatinine	2 times/wk	Weekly
Albumin or prealbumin	Weekly	Weekly
Ca^{2+}, Mg^{2+}, P	2 times/wk	Weekly
ALT, AST, Alk P	Weekly	Weekly
Total and direct bilirubin	Weekly	Weekly
CBC	Weekly	Weekly
Triglycerides	With each increase	Weekly
Vitamins	—	As indicated
Trace minerals	—	As indicated

Alk P, Alkaline phosphatase; *ALT,* alanine transaminase; *AST,* aspartate transaminase; *BUN,* blood urea nitrogen; *CBC,* complete blood count.

*For patients on long-term parenteral nutrition, monitoring every 2 to 4 weeks is adequate in most cases.

[†]The period before nutritional goals are reached or during any period of instability.

[‡]When stability is reached, no changes in nutrient composition.

[§]Weekly in preterm infants.

REFERENCES

1. CDC website. www.cdc.gov/growth.
2. Barlow SE, Dietz WH. Obesity evaluation and treatment: expert committee recommendations. Pediatrics 1998; 102(3):7.
3. Food Nutrition Board, National Research Council, Recommended Dietary Allowances, 10th ed. Washington, DC: National Academy Press; 1989.
4. Seashore JH. Nutritional support of children in the intensive care unit. Yale J Biol Med 1984; 57:111-132.
5. Corrales KM, Utter SL. Failure to thrive. In Samour PQ, Helm KK, Lang CE, editors. Handbook of pediatric nutrition, 2nd ed. Gaithersburg, Md: Aspen, 1999.
6. Food and Nutrition Board, National Research Council. Dietary Reference Intakes, Washington, DC: National Academy Press, 2001.
7. Kreiter SR et al. Nutritional rickets in African American breast-fed infants. J Pediatr 2000; 137: 153-157.
8. Kleinman RE, editor. Committee on Nutrition of the AAP. Pediatric nutrition handbook, 4th ed. Elk Grove Village, Ill: 1998.

20

NUTRITION AND GROWTH

ONCOLOGY

Michelle Hudspeth, MD and Heather Symons, MD

I. WEBSITES

http://www.cancer.gov/cancer_information/
http://www.hopkinscancercenter.org

II. PRESENTING SIGNS AND SYMPTOMS OF PEDIATRIC MALIGNANCIES (Table 21-1)

NOTE: Common presenting signs and symptoms of many malignancies include weight loss, failure to thrive, anorexia, malaise, fever, pallor, and lymphadenopathy.

21

III. FEVER AND NEUTROPENIA[1,2]

A. DEFINITION

Absolute neutrophil count (ANC ≤500) or falling toward this level, and fever >38.3° C (orally), or >38.0° C when measured twice ≥4 hours apart in a 24-hour period. Patients who develop low-grade fever while on steroids

---

TABLE 21-1

COMMON SIGNS AND SYMPTOMS OF PEDIATRIC MALIGNANCIES

Type of Malignancy	Signs/Symptoms
Leukemia	Limp, hepatomegaly, splenomegaly, petechiae/bruising, bone pain, anemia, thrombocytopenia
Lymphoma	Night sweats; pruritus; stridor; persistent respiratory symptoms; GI bleeding; back pain; hepatomegaly; splenomegaly; abdominal, head, neck, or chest mass
Wilms tumor	Emesis, hypertension, abdominal mass, abdominal distension, hepatomegaly
Neuroblastoma	Emesis; diarrhea; hypertension; opsoclonus-myoclonus; periorbital ecchymoses; Horner's syndrome; stridor; persistent respiratory symptoms; abdominal, head, neck or chest mass; limp; blue subcutaneous nodules
CNS tumors	Irritability, clumsiness, headache, emesis, seizure, cranial nerve palsies, visual changes, proptosis, ataxia
Testicular tumors	Abdominal pain or tenderness, scrotal swelling or mass
Bone tumors	Limp, back pain, persistent limb pain, fracture
Histiocytic disease	Polyuria, polydipsia, otorrhea, hepatomegaly, splenomegaly, cutaneous lesions, osteolytic lesions, pulmonary infiltrates, anemia, thrombocytopenia
Retinoblastoma	Leukocoria, asymmetric red reflex, orbital inflammation, hyphema, pupil irregularity

Modified from Crist WM. Principles of diagnosis. In Behrman RE, Kliegman RM, Jenson NB, editors. Nelson's text book of pediatrics, 16th ed. Philadelphia: WB Saunders; 2000 and Hogarty MD et al. Oncologic emergencies. Fleisher G, Ludwig S, editors. Text book of pediatric emerging medicine. Philadelphia: Lippincott, Williams and Wilkins; 2000.

or who appear ill, even in the absence of fever, also require similar evaluation.

B. MANAGEMENT

1. Detailed history and physical examination, including line sites, incisions, and perianal area (avoid rectal examination).
2. Begin laboratory evaluation: Complete blood count (CBC) with differential, blood cultures from all central line lumens, urinalysis and urine culture (do not catheterize), with blood type and screen, electrolytes, and PT/aPTT if clinically indicated. Mucosal surveillance cultures are controversial. Obtain chest radiographs if clinically indicated.
3. Antibiotic therapy
a. If patient is not ill-appearing and has no apparent focus of infection, start antibiotics with gram-negative (including *Pseudomonas*) and gram-positive coverage (e.g., cefepime or piperacillin/tazobactam). Take into account local bacterial sensitivities. Select an antibiotic that covers previous blood culture isolates.
b. If patient appears ill, provide double coverage for *Pseudomonas* (e.g., cefepime or piperacillin/tazobactam with an aminoglycoside).
c. If blood culture remains negative and patient is afebrile, continue broad-spectrum coverage until early evidence of marrow recovery (e.g., rising ANC).
d. If patient is persistently febrile after 3 days, consider adding a semisynthetic penicillin such as oxacillin or vancomycin (for better coverage of gram-positive organisms), especially if central line infection is suspected. Also consider broader gram-negative coverage.
e. If patient is persistently febrile, or has a new fever 4 to 7 days into therapy, consider intravenous (IV) amphotericin B (0.5 mg/kg/day) for empiric antifungal coverage after appropriate cultures are taken. May increase dose to 1 mg/kg/day if fever persists for 2 days beyond initiation of amphotericin therapy.

C. FURTHER EVALUATION

For further evaluation and modifications based on focus of infections, see Table 21-2.

IV. ONCOLOGIC EMERGENCIES[1,3]

A. TUMOR LYSIS SYNDROME

1. **Etiology:** Lysis of tumor cells before or during early stages of chemotherapy (especially Burkitt's lymphoma/leukemia, T-cell acute lymphocytic leukemia [ALL]).
2. **Presentation:** Hyperuricemia, hypocalcemia, hyperkalemia, hyperphosphatemia, acidosis. Can lead to acute renal failure.
3. Prevention/management
a. Hydration and alkalinization: D_5 0.2 normal saline (NS) + 25 to 50 mEq $NaHCO_3$ (without K^+) at two times maintenance rate. Keeping urine specific gravity <1.010 and pH 7.0 to 7.5 reduces risk of urate crystal formation. Reduce $NaHCO_3$ if pH >7.5 to avoid calcium phosphate precipitation.

TABLE 21-2

FURTHER EVALUATION AND MODIFICATIONS BASED ON FOCUS OF INFECTIONS

Site	Presentation	Diagnostic Evaluation	Treatment Modification
Central line	Erythema, warmth, discharge (may not be present in neutropenic patient)	Blood cultures from all lumens	Additional gram-positive coverage (i.e., vancomycin, oxacillin) Rotation of antibiotics through all lumens Removal of line for tunnel infection, fungal, or prolonged infection
HEENT	Gingivitis Vesicles or ulcerative lesions Sinus tenderness	HSV cultures, PCR, Tzanck test CT scan	Add anaerobic coverage Add acyclovir Consider antifungal coverage
Respiratory	Increased work of breathing, cough, tachypnea, hypoxia	Chest radiographs with or without CT, sputum culture Consider early BAL HSV, CMV serology CMV culture, early antigen Sputum for PCP, fungal stain	Consider fungal, PCP coverage Consider *Mycoplasma* coverage Consider CMV, HSV coverage Consider early steroids for suspected PCP (contraindicated in fungal infection)
Gastrointestinal	Retrosternal pain Acute abdominal pain	Consider endoscopy or upper GI Abdominal radiographs with or without CT, MRI, or ultrasound	Add fungal and/or HSV coverage, H_2 blocker If suspect typhlitis*, add anaerobic and gram-negative coverage; in addition, monitor closely, provide aggressive fluid replacement, keep patient NPO, seek surgical consult (reserved for severe bleeding, shock, peritonitis)
	Diarrhea	Stool cultures, *Clostridium difficile* toxin	Consider treatment for *C. difficile*
	Perianal tenderness		Add anaerobic coverage

From Hogarty MD, Lange B. Oncologic emergencies. In Fleisher G, Ludwig S, editors. Textbook of pediatric emergency medicine. Philadelphia: Lippincott, Williams and Wilkins; 2000.
*Typhlitis: Inflammation of the bowel wall, usually localized to the cecum. Most common in patients treated for leukemia or lymphoma, especially when Ara-C is used. Presentation includes right-lower-quadrant abdominal pain, nausea, fever, and diarrhea. Abdominal radiograph may show pneumatosis, paucity of air, and/or bowel-wall edema. Consider CT/MRI to confirm diagnosis.

BAL, Bronchoalveolar lavage; *CMV,* cytomegalovirus; *HEENT,* head, eyes, ears, nose, throat; *HSV,* herpes simplex virus; *PCP, Pneumocystis carinii* pneumonia; *PCR,* polymerase chain reaction.

21

ONCOLOGY

b. Allopurinol (100 mg/m^2 per dose) Q8hr by mouth (PO).

c. Check K$^+$, Ca^{2+}, phosphate, and uric acid frequently.

d. Manage abnormal electrolytes as described in Chapter 10. See p. 411 for dialysis indications.

e. Consider stopping alkalinization soon after starting chemotherapy (if uric acid is normal).

B. SPINAL CORD COMPRESSION

1. **Etiology:** Extension of tumor into spinal cord.

2. **Presentation:** Back pain (localized/radicular), weakness, sensory loss, change in bowel/bladder function. Prognosis for recovery based on duration and level of disability at presentation.

3. **Management**

a. With back pain and no neurologic abnormalities, may start dexamethasone 0.25 to 0.5 mg/kg/day PO divided Q6hr and perform magnetic resonance imaging (MRI) of the spine within 24 hours. Be aware that steroids may prevent diagnosis of lymphoma; therefore plan diagnostic procedure as soon as possible.

b. In the presence of neurologic abnormalities, immediately start dexamethasone 1 to 2 mg/kg/day IV and obtain an emergent MRI of the spine.

c. If the cause of the tumor is known, emergent radiotherapy or chemotherapy is indicated for sensitive tumors; otherwise, emergent neurosurgery consultation is warranted.

d. If cause of tumor is unknown, surgery is indicated to decompress the spine.

C. INCREASED INTRACRANIAL PRESSURE

1. **Etiology:** Ventricular obstruction, obstruction of cerebrospinal fluid (CSF) flow.

2. **Diagnosis:** Obtain computed tomography (CT) scan or MRI of the head. MRI is more sensitive for diagnosis of posterior fossa tumors.

3. **Management**

a. See pp. 14-15 for basic management.

b. If tumor is identified, add dexamethasone 2 mg/kg/day IV divided Q6hr.

c. Obtain emergent neurosurgical consultation.

D. CEREBROVASCULAR ACCIDENT

1. **Etiology:** Hyperleukocytosis, coagulopathy, thrombocytopenia, chemotherapy-related (e.g., L-asparaginase–induced hemorrhage or thrombosis).

2. **Diagnosis and management**

a. Platelet transfusions, fresh frozen plasma (FFP) as needed to replace factors (e.g., if depleted by L-asparaginase).

b. Brain CT scan with contrast, MRI, or magnetic resonance angiography/venography (MRA/MRV) if venous thrombosis is suspected.

c. Administer heparin acutely, followed by warfarin, for thromboses (if no venous hemorrhage is observed on MRI).

d. Avoid L-asparaginase.

E. RESPIRATORY DISTRESS/SUPERIOR VENA CAVA SYNDROME

1. **Etiology:** Hodgkin's disease, non-Hodgkin's lymphoma (e.g., lympho-blastic lymphoma), ALL (T-lineage), germ cell tumors.
2. **Presentation:** Orthopnea, headaches, facial swelling, dizziness, plethora.
3. **Diagnosis:** Chest radiograph. Consider CT or MRI scan to assess airway. Attempt diagnosis of malignancy (if not known) by the least invasive method possible.
4. **Management**
   a. Control airway.
   b. Biopsy (e.g., bone marrow, pleurocentesis, lymph-node biopsy) before therapy if patient can tolerate sedation or general anesthesia.
   c. Empiric therapy: Radiotherapy, steroids, cyclophosphamide.

F. HYPERLEUKOCYTOSIS

1. **Etiology:** In acute myeloid leukemia (AML) (especially M4 and M5), hyperleukocytosis occurs with a white blood cell (WBC) count as low as $100,000/mm^3$. It occurs in ALL with a WBC count above $300,000/mm^3$.
2. **Presentation:** Hypoxia/dyspnea from pulmonary leukostasis, mental status changes, headaches, seizures, papilledema from leukostasis in cerebral vessels; occasionally, gastrointestinal (GI) bleeding, abdominal pain, renal failure, priapism, and tumor lysis syndrome.
3. **Management**
   a. Transfuse platelets as needed to keep count above $20,000/mm^3$ (reduce risk of intracranial hemorrhage).
   b. Avoid red blood cell (RBC) transfusions because they will raise viscosity (keep hemoglobin ≤ 10 g/dL). If RBCs are required, consider partial exchange transfusion.
   c. Hydration, alkalinization, and allopurinol should be initiated (as discussed under tumor lysis syndrome).
   d. Administer FFP and vitamin K if patient is coagulopathic.
   e. Before cytotoxic therapy, consider leukopheresis to lower WBC count.

21

ONCOLOGY

V. HEMATOLOGIC CARE AND COMPLICATIONS[1]

NOTE: Transfuse only irradiated packed RBC (pRBC)/platelets, cytomegalo-virus (CMV)-negative or leuko-filtered pRBC/platelets for CMV-negative patients. Use leuko-filtered pRBC/platelets for those who may receive a bone marrow transplant (BMT) in the future to prevent alloimmunization, or for those who have had nonhemolytic febrile transfusion reactions.

A. ANEMIA

1. **Etiology:** Blood loss, chemotherapy, marrow infiltration, hemolysis
2. **Management**
   a. See pp. 303-304 for specific details on pRBC transfusions.
   b. Generally, pRBC transfusions in cancer patients are not recommended until hematocrit falls below 20% to 22%, or if the patient is symptomatic.

B. THROMBOCYTOPENIA

1. **Etiology:** Chemotherapy, marrow infiltration, consumptive coagulopathy, medications.

2. Management

a. See pp. 304-305 for specific details on platelet transfusions.

b. Generally, maintain platelet count above 10,000/mm^3 unless patient is clinically bleeding or febrile, or before procedure (e.g., lumbar puncture or intramuscular [IM] injection requires >50,000/mm^3). Consider maintaining platelet counts at higher levels for patients who have brain tumors or those who have had brain surgery.

VI. NAUSEA TREATMENT IN CANCER PATIENTS[1]

1. **Etiology:** The usual cause of nausea is chemotherapy treatment. Also suspect opiate therapy, GI/central nervous system (CNS) radiotherapy, abdominal process, and CNS mass.

2. **Therapy:** Hydration plus one or more antinausea medications (see Formulary for dosing):

a. Ondansetron or granisetron: Usually a first-line therapy. Patients may respond preferentially to one of these agents.

b. Diphenhydramine.

c. Dexamethasone: Especially helpful in patients with brain tumor.

d. Lorazepam: Used as an adjunct antiemetic agent.

e. Metoclopramide: Especially helpful in patients with brain tumor. Use diphenhydramine to reduce extrapyramidal symptoms (EPS).

f. Phenothiazines (promethazine, chlorpromazine). Use diphenhydramine to reduce EPS.

g. Droperidol can be used as continuous infusion.

h. Cannabinoids (e.g., dronabinol) can be helpful in resistant cases, especially in patients with large tumor burden. May also be used as an appetite stimulant in malnourished patients.

VII. ANTIMICROBIAL PROPHYLAXIS IN ONCOLOGY PATIENTS
(Table 21-3)

NOTE: Treatment length and dosage may vary per protocol.

TABLE 21-3

ANTIMICROBIAL PROPHYLAXIS IN ONCOLOGY PATIENTS

Organism	Medication	Indication
Pneumocystis carinii	TMP-SMX, dapsone, or pentamidine	Chemotherapy and BMT per protocol (usually at least 6 mo after chemotherapy, 12 mo after BMT)
HSV	Acyclovir (dosing is different for zoster, varicella, and mucocutaneous HSV)	After BMT if patient or donor is HSV or CMV positive; recurrent zoster
Candida albicans	Fluconazole	After BMT (usual minimum 28 days)
Gram-positive organisms	Penicillin	After BMT (usually at least 1 mo)

REFERENCES

1. Poplack D, Pizzo P. Principles and practice of pediatric oncology, 3rd ed. Philadelphia: Lippincott-Raven; 1997.
2. Chanock SJ, Pizzo PA. Fever in the neutropenic host. Infect Dis Clin North Am. 1996; 10(4): 777-796.
3. Kelly KM, Lange B. Oncologic emergencies. Pediatr Clin North Am. 1997; 44(4):809-30.

21

ONCOLOGY

PULMONOLOGY

Melissa M. Greenfield, MD

I. WEBSITES

www.lungusa.org (American Lung Association)
www.cff.org (Cystic Fibrosis Foundation)
cfcenter.stanford.edu (Stanford University CF Center)
www.aaaai.org (American Academy of Allergy, Asthma & Immunology)

II. NORMAL RESPIRATORY RATES (Table 22-1)

III. ASTHMA GUIDELINES

22

A. ACUTE ASTHMA

For management of acute asthma exacerbation and status asthmaticus, please refer to pp. 9-10.

B. CLASSIFICATION OF CHRONIC ASTHMA SEVERITY AND MANAGEMENT IN CHILDREN (Table 22-2)

1. In addition to long-term medications, all patients should receive short-acting bronchodilator agents for quick relief of symptoms.
2. Attempt to gain control quickly by starting with the most aggressive options in a step, or even at the next highest step.
3. Step down gradually to the least medication needed to maintain control.
4. Step up to a more aggressive therapy if control is not maintained.[1]
5. Systemic corticosteroids and other therapy may be needed at times of acute exacerbation.
6. Provide written asthma action plan for all children with persistent asthma.
7. Identify and control environmental asthma triggers (e.g., dust mites, cigarette smoke, pet dander, cockroaches, pollens).

TABLE 22-1

NORMAL RESPIRATORY RATES IN CHILDREN

Age (yr)	Respiratory Rate (per minute)
0-1*	24-38
1-3	22-30
4-6	20-24
7-9	18-24
10-14	16-22
14-18	14-20

Modified from Bardella IJ. Am Fam Phys 1999; 60(6):1743-1750.
*Slightly higher respiratory rates in the neonatal period (i.e., 40-50) may be normal in the absence of other signs and symptoms.

TABLE 22-2

CLASSIFICATION OF CHRONIC ASTHMA SEVERITY AND MANAGEMENT IN CHILDREN

	Clinical Features	Long-term Medication	Quick Relief
Mild intermittent	• Daytime symptoms ≤2 times per week • Nocturnal symptoms ≤2 times per month • FEV_1 or PEF ≥80% predicted • PEF variability <20%	No antiinflammatory agents needed	• Short-acting BD* as needed for symptoms • Intensity of acute treatment will depend on severity of exacerbation • Use of short-acting BD >2 times per week may indicate the need for long-term control therapy
Mild persistent	• Daytime symptoms >2 times per week but <1 time per day • Nocturnal symptoms >2 times per month • FEV_1 or PEF ≥80% predicted • PEF variability 20% to 30%	*One daily medication:* • Cromolyn or nedocromil or • ICS low dose or • Leukotriene modifiers (≥2 years old) or • Theophylline (not preferred)	• Short-acting BD* as needed for symptoms • Intensity of acute treatment will depend on severity of exacerbation • Daily or increasing use of short-acting BD indicates the need for additional long-term control therapy

Moderate persistent	• Daily symptoms • Nocturnal symptoms >1 time per week • FEV_1 or PEF >60% and <80% predicted • PEF variability >30%	*Daily medication:* • ICS medium dose or • ICS low-medium dose + long-acting BD[†] *If needed:* • ICS medium-high dose + long-acting BD or • ICS medium-high dose + leukotriene modifier and • Consider referral to asthma specialist[‡]	• Short-acting BD* as needed for symptoms • Intensity of acute treatment will depend on severity of exacerbation • Daily or increasing use of short-acting BD indicates the need for additional long-term control therapy
Severe persistent	• Continuous symptoms • Frequent nighttime symptoms • FEV_1 or PEF ≤60% predicted • PEF variability >30%	*Daily medication:* • ICS high dose + long-acting BD[†] + systemic corticosteroids long-term if needed and • Referral to asthma specialist[‡]	• Short-acting BD* as needed for symptoms • Intensity of acute treatment will depend on severity of exacerbation • Daily or increasing use of short-acting BD indicates the need for additional long-term control therapy

Modified from NIH. Guidelines for the diagnosis and management of asthma, Expert Panel Report 2. NIH Publication No. 97-4051, April 1997.

BD, Bronchodilators; FEV_1, forced expiratory volume in one second; *ICS*, inhaled corticosteroid; *PEF*, peak expiratory flow.

*Short-acting BD = short-acting inhaled β_2-agonist.

[†]Long-acting BD include long-acting inhaled β_2-agonist, sustained-release theophylline, or long-acting β_2-agonist tablets.

[‡]Consider comorbid conditions (e.g., allergic rhinitis, sinusitis, gastroesophageal reflux).

PULMONOLOGY 22

IV. PULMONARY FUNCTION TESTS

Pulmonary function tests (PFTs) provide objective and reproducible measurements of airway function and lung volumes. PFTs are used to characterize disease, assess severity, and follow response to therapy.

A. PEAK EXPIRATORY FLOW RATE

The peak expiratory flow rate (PEFR) is the maximum flow rate generated during a forced expiratory maneuver. It is effort dependent and insensitive to small airway function. It is useful in following the course of asthma and response to therapy. Compare a patient's PEFR to the previous "personal best" and the normal predicted value (Table 22-3).

B. SPIROMETRY

Spirometry is the plot of airflow versus time. Measurements are made from a rapid, forceful, and complete expiration from total lung capacity (TLC) to residual volume (forced vital capacity maneuver). Spirometry is often done before and after use of bronchodilators to assess response to therapy, or after bronchial challenge to assess airway hyperreactivity. It can be performed reliably by most children 6 years and older.

1. **Forced vital capacity (FVC):** FVC is the maximum volume of air exhaled from the lungs after a maximum inspiration. Bedside measurement of vital capacity with a hand-held spirometer can be useful in confirming or predicting hypoventilation. FVC <15 mL/kg may be an indication for ventilatory support.

2. **Forced expiratory volume in one second (FEV$_1$):** Volume exhaled during the first second of an FVC maneuver. It is the single best measure of airway function.

TABLE 22-3

PREDICTED AVERAGE PEAK EXPIRATORY FLOW RATES FOR NORMAL CHILDREN

Height (in)	PEFR (L/min)	Height (in)	PEFR (L/min)
43	147	56	320
44	160	57	334
45	173	58	347
46	187	59	360
47	200	60	373
48	214	61	387
49	227	62	400
50	240	63	413
51	254	64	427
52	267	65	440
53	280	66	454
54	293	67	467
55	307		

From Voter KZ. Pediatr Rev 1996; 17(2):53-63.

3. **Forced expiratory flow (FEF$_{25-75}$):** Mean rate of airflow over the middle half of the FVC between 25% and 75% of FVC. Sensitive to small airway obstruction.

C. FLOW-VOLUME CURVES

Flow-volume curves are the plot of airflow versus lung volume. They are useful in characterizing different patterns of airway obstruction (Fig. 22-1).

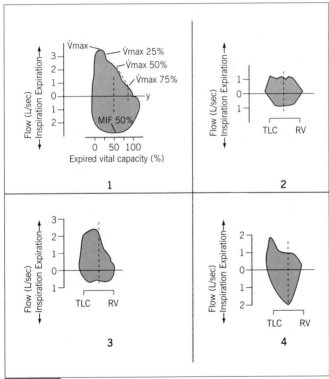

FIG. 22-1

1. Normal flow–volume curve. 2. Fixed upper airway obstruction (tracheal stenosis): Flattening of both inspiratory and expiratory phases. 3. Variable extrathoracic obstruction (tracheomalacia, paralyzed vocal cords): Flattened inspiratory phase as negative inspiratory pressure favors extrathoracic airway collapse. 4. Variable intrathoracic obstruction (tumor): Flattened expiratory phase as positive pleural pressure compresses trachea and increases resistance.

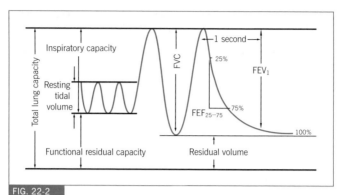

Lung volumes. See text for abbreviations.

D. LUNG VOLUMES
Total lung capacity, functional residual capacity (FRC), and residual volume (RV) cannot be determined by spirometry and require determination by helium dilution, nitrogen washout, or body plethysmography (Fig. 22-2).

E. MAXIMAL INSPIRATORY AND EXPIRATORY PRESSURES
Obtained by asking patient to inhale and exhale against a fixed obstruction. Low pressures suggest a neuromuscular problem or submaximal effort. An inspiratory pressure <20-25 cmH$_2$O (negative inspiratory force [NIF]) may be an indication for ventilatory support.

F. INTERPRETATION OF PFTs (Table 22-4)

V. SWEAT CHLORIDE TEST[2]
Normal (1 week to adult) <40 mmol/L
Patients with cystic fibrosis (CF) >60 mmol/L
(mmol/L = mEq/L)
1. Sweat is obtained through quantitative pilocarpine iontophoresis.
2. Results between 40 to 60 mmol/L require repeat testing or other tests for CF.
3. Normal levels (false negatives) may be found in patients with CF in the presence of edema and hypoproteinemia or inadequate sweat rate.
4. Elevated chloride levels may be from CF, untreated adrenal insufficiency, glycogen storage disease type I, fucosidosis, hypothyroidism, nephrogenic diabetes insipidus, ectodermal dysplasia, malnutrition, mucopolysaccharidosis, panhypopituitarism, or poor testing technique.

TABLE 22-4

INTERPRETATION OF SPIROMETRY AND LUNG VOLUME READINGS

	Obstructive Disease (Asthma, Cystic Fibrosis)	Restrictive Disease (Interstitial Fibrosis, Scoliosis, Neuromuscular Disease)
SPIROMETRY		
FVC[a]	Normal or reduced	Reduced
FEV$_1$[a]	Reduced	Reduced[d]
FEV$_1$/FVC[b]	Reduced	Normal
FEF$_{25-75}$	Reduced	Normal or reduced[d]
PEFR[a]	Normal or reduced	Normal or reduced[d]
LUNG VOLUMES		
TLC[a]	Normal or increased	Reduced
RV[a]	Increased	Reduced
RV/TLC[c]	Increased	Unchanged
FRC	Increased	Reduced

[a]Normal range: ±20% of predicted.
[b]Normal range: >85%.
[c]Normal range: 20 ± 10%.
[d]Reduced proportional to FVC.

VI. PULMONARY GAS EXCHANGE

A. ARTERIAL BLOOD GAS

Measurement of arterial blood gas (ABG) is used to assess oxygenation (Pao$_2$), ventilation (V), Paco$_2$, and acid-base status (pH and HCO$_3^-$). See Chapter 24 for normal mean ABG values.

B. VENOUS BLOOD GAS

Measurement of venous blood gas (VBG) through peripheral venous samples is strongly affected by the local circulatory and metabolic environment. It can be used to assess acid-base status. Pvco$_2$ averages 6 to 8 mmHg higher than Paco$_2$, and pH is slightly lower.

C. CAPILLARY BLOOD GAS

Correlation of capillary blood gas (CBG) with arterial sampling is generally best for pH, moderate for Pco$_2$, and worst for Po$_2$.

D. ANALYSIS OF ACID-BASE DISTURBANCES[3,4]

1. **Pure respiratory acidosis (or alkalosis):** 10 mmHg rise (fall) in Paco$_2$ results in an average 0.08 fall (rise) in pH.
2. **Pure metabolic acidosis (or alkalosis):** 10 mEq/L fall (rise) in HCO$_3^-$ results in an average 0.15 fall (rise) in pH.
3. **Determine primary disturbance and then assess for mixed disorder by calculating expected compensatory response** (Table 22-5).

E. PULSE OXIMETRY[5,6]

1. **Arterial oxygen saturation:** Noninvasive method of indirectly measuring arterial oxygen saturation (Sao$_2$). Uses light absorption characteristics of oxygenated and deoxygenated hemoglobin to estimate O$_2$ saturation.
2. **The oxyhemoglobin dissociation curve** (Fig. 22-3): This relates O$_2$

TABLE 22-5

CALCULATION OF EXPECTED COMPENSATORY RESPONSE

Disturbance	Primary Change	pH	Expected Compensatory Response
Acute respiratory acidosis	↑ $Paco_2$	↓ pH	↑HCO_3^- by 1 mEq/L for each 10 mmHg rise in $Paco_2$
Acute respiratory alkalosis	↓ $Paco_2$	↑ pH	↓ HCO_3^- by 1-3 mEq/L for each 10 mmHg fall in $Paco_2$
Chronic respiratory acidosis	↑ $Paco_2$	↓ pH	↑ HCO_3^- by 4 mEq/L for each 10 mmHg rise in $Paco_2$
Chronic respiratory alkalosis	↓ $Paco_2$	↑ pH	↓ HCO_3^- by 2-5 mEq/L for each 10 mmHg fall in $Paco_2$
Metabolic acidosis	↓ HCO_3^-	↓ pH	↓ $Paco_2$ by 1 to 1.5 × fall in HCO_3^-
Metabolic alkalosis	↑ HCO_3^-	↑ pH	↑ $Paco_2$ by 0.25-1 × rise in HCO_3^-

Modified from Schrier RW. Renal and electrolyte disorders, 3rd ed. Boston: Little, Brown; 1986.

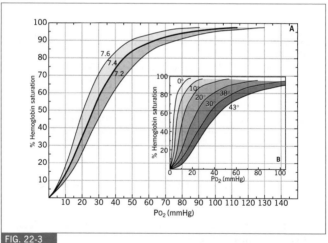

FIG. 22-3

Oxyhemoglobin dissociation curve. **A,** Curve shifts to the left as pH increases. **B,** Curve shifts to the left as temperature decreases. *(Modified from Lanbertsten CJ. Transport of oxygen, CO_2, and inert gases by the blood. In Mountcastle VB, editor. Medical physiology, 14th ed. St Louis: Mosby; 1980.)*

saturation to Pao_2. Increased hemoglobin affinity for oxygen (shift to the left) occurs with alkalemia, hypothermia, hypocapnia, decreased 2,3-diphosphoglycerate (2,3-DPG), increased fetal hemoglobin, and anemia. Decreased hemoglobin affinity for oxygen (shift to the right) occurs with acidemia, hyperthermia, hypercapnia, and increased 2,3-DPG.

3. **Important uses of pulse oximetry**

a. Rapid and continuous assessment of oxygenation in acutely ill patients.

b. Monitoring of patients requiring oxygen therapy.

c. Assessment of oxygen requirements during feeding, sleep, and exercise.

d. Home monitoring of physiologic effects of apnea/bradycardia.

4. **Limitations of pulse oximetry**

a. Measures saturation (Sao_2) and not O_2 delivery to tissues. A marginally low saturation may be clinically significant in an anemic patient because a normal O_2 saturation does not ensure a normal O_2-carrying capacity (see oxygen content calculation on p. 526).

b. Unreliable when detection of pulse signal is poor as a result of physiologic conditions (hypothermia, hypovolemia, shock) or movement artifact. The oximeter's pulse rate should match the patient's heart rate to ensure an accurate measurement.

c. Insensitive to hyperoxia because of the sigmoid shape of the oxyhemoglobin curve.

d. Sao_2 is artificially increased by carboxyhemoglobin levels >1% to 2% (e.g., in chronic smokers, or with smoke inhalation).

e. Sao_2 is artificially decreased by patient motion, intravenous dyes, such as methylene blue and indocyanine green, and opaque nail polish.

f. Sao_2 is artificially increased or decreased by methemoglobin levels >1% to 2%, electrosurgical interference, or xenon arc surgical lamps.

g. An Sao_2 reading often does not correlate with Pao_2 in sickle cell disease.[7]

F. CAPNOGRAPHY

Capnography measures CO_2 concentration of expired gas by infrared spectroscopy or mass spectroscopy. End-tidal CO_2 ($ETCO_2$) correlates with $Paco_2$ (usually within 5 mmHg of $Paco_2$ in healthy subjects). Capnography can be used for demonstrating proper placement of an endotracheal tube, continuous monitoring of CO_2 trends in ventilated patients, and monitoring ventilation during polysomnography.

VII. OXYGEN DELIVERY SYSTEMS (Table 22-6)

22

PULMONOLOGY

TABLE 22-6
OXYGEN DELIVERY SYSTEMS

	O_2 Concentration Delivered (%)	Flow Rate (L/min)	Important Information
Nasal cannula	22-40	0.25-4	High flow rates may cause dry mucous membranes, gastric distension, headaches
Simple mask	35-50	6-10	Insufficient flow rates may cause CO_2 retention
Partial rebreather	60-95	>6	Collapsed reservoir bag indicates air leak or inadequate flow of oxygen
Nonrebreather	Approaches 100	10-15	Requires tight seal and high flow rate to deliver maximum oxygen concentration
Venturi mask	24-50 (mask specific)	Variable	Useful in COPD. If back pressure develops on jet, less room air enters and FiO_2 can elevate unpredictably
Tracheostomy mask	Unpredictable unless attached to Venturi circuit	Variable	Provides humidity and controlled O_2; FiO_2 should be analyzed for each individual patient
Oxygen hoods/ head boxes	Approaches 100	>10	Insufficient flow rates may cause CO_2 retention *Disadvantages:* O_2 gradient may develop within the hood/box; patients must be taken out for feeding/care
Oxygen tents	Up to 50	>10	Insufficient flow rates may cause CO_2 retention; can be used to provide humidified air *Disadvantages:* Development of O_2 gradient; sparks in or near tent may be hazardous; claustrophobia in older children; requires close monitoring of patient and apparatus

VIII. CRITICAL CARE
A. MECHANICAL VENTILATION
1. Types of ventilatory support
a. Volume limited
   (1) Delivers a preset tidal volume to a patient regardless of pressure required.
   (2) Risk of barotrauma reduced by pressure alarms and pressure pop-off valves that limit peak inspiratory pressure (PIP).
b. Pressure limited
   (1) Gas flow is delivered to the patient until a preset pressure is reached and then held for the set inspiratory time (reduces the risk of barotrauma).
   (2) Useful for neonatal and infant ventilatory support (<10 kg) in which the volume of gas being delivered is small in relation to the volume of compressible air in the ventilator circuit, which makes reliable delivery of a set tidal volume difficult.
c. High-frequency ventilation[8]
   (1) High-frequency oscillatory ventilation (HFOV)
      (a) High-amplitude and high-frequency pressure waveform generated in the ventilator circuit. Tidal volumes are less than dead space. Bias gas flow provides fresh gas at ventilator and maintains airway pressure.
      (b) Minimizes barotrauma and oxygen toxicities.
   (2) High-frequency jet ventilation
      (a) Used simultaneously with a conventional ventilator.
      (b) A jet injector port delivers short bursts of inspiratory gas.
      (c) Adequate gas exchange can be achieved at low airway pressures providing maintenance of lung volume and minimal risk of barotrauma.

2. Ventilator parameters
a. PIP: Peak inspiratory pressure attained during the respiratory cycle.
b. Positive end-expiratory pressure (PEEP): Airway pressure maintained between inspiratory and expiratory phases (prevents alveolar collapse during expiration, decreasing work of reinflation and improving gas exchange).
c. Rate (intermittent mandatory ventilation) or frequency (Hz): Number of mechanical breaths delivered per minute, or rate of oscillations in HFOV.
d. Inspired oxygen concentration (Fio_2): Fraction of oxygen present in inspired gas.
e. Inspiratory time (ti): Length of time spent in the inspiratory phase of the respiratory cycle.
f. Tidal volume (TV): Volume of gas delivered during inspiration.
g. Power (ΔP): Amplitude of the pressure waveform in HFOV.
h. Mean airway pressure (MAP): Average pressure over entire respiratory cycle.

3. Modes of operation

22

PULMONOLOGY

a. Intermittent mandatory ventilation (IMV): A preset number of breaths is delivered each minute. The patient can take breaths on his or her own, but the ventilator may cycle on during a patient breath.

b. Synchronized IMV (SIMV): Similar to IMV, but the ventilator synchronizes delivered breaths with inspiratory effort, and allows the patient to finish expiration before cycling on.

c. Assist control (AC or AMV): Every inspiratory effort by the patient triggers a ventilator-delivered breath at the set tidal volume. Ventilator-initiated breaths are delivered when the spontaneous rate falls below the backup rate.

d. Pressure support ventilation (PSV): Inspiratory effort opens a valve allowing airflow at a preset positive pressure. Patient determines rate and inspiratory time. May be used in combination with other modes of operation.

e. Noninvasive positive-pressure ventilation (NIPPV): Respiratory support provided through face mask.

    (1) Continuous positive airway pressure (CPAP): Delivers airflow (with set Fio_2) to maintain a set airway pressure.

    (2) Bilevel positive airway pressure (BiPAP): Delivers airflow to maintain set pressures for inspiration and expiration.

4. **Initial ventilator settings**

a. Volume limited

    (1) Rate: Approximately normal range for age (see Table 22-1).

    (2) Tidal volume: Approximately 10 to 15 mL/kg.

    (3) Inspiratory time: Generally use inspiration:expiration (I:E) ratio of 1:2. More prolonged expiratory phases are required for obstructive diseases to avoid air trapping.

    (4) Fio_2: Selected to maintain targeted oxygen saturation and Pao_2.

b. Pressure limited

    (1) Rate: Approximately normal range for age (see Table 22-1).

    (2) PEEP: Start with 3 to 4 cmH_2O and increase as clinically indicated. (Monitor for decreases in cardiac output with increasing PEEP.)

    (3) PIP: Set at pressure required to produce adequate chest-wall movement (approximate this using hand bagging and manometer).

    (4) Fio_2: Selected to maintain targeted oxygen saturation and Pao_2.

c. High-frequency oscillatory ventilator

    (1) Frequency: 10 to 15 Hz for neonates.

    (2) Power: Select to achieve adequate chest-wall movement.

    (3) MAP: 1 to 4 cmH_2O higher than settings on a conventional ventilator.

    (4) Fio_2: Selected to maintain targeted oxygen saturation and Pao_2.

d. High frequency jet ventilator

    (1) PIP: Increase 2 cmH_2O over conventional ventilator setting.

    (2) Inspiratory time: Set at 0.02 seconds.

    (3) Frequency: In neonates, set at 420 cycles per second.

5. **Further ventilator management**

TABLE 22-7

EFFECTS OF VENTILATOR SETTING CHANGES

Ventilator Setting Changes	Typical Effects on Blood Gases	
	$Paco_2$	Pao_2
↑ PIP	↓	↑
↑ PEEP	↑	↑
↑ Rate (IMV)	↓	Minimal ↑
↑ I:E ratio	No change	↑
↑ Fio2	No change	↑
↑ Flow	Minimal ↓	Minimal ↑
↑ Power (in HFOV)	↓	No change
↑ MAP (in HFOV)	Minimal ↓	↑

Modified from Carlo WA, Chatburn RL. Neonatal respiratory care, 2nd ed. St Louis: Mosby; 1988.

22

PULMONOLOGY

a. Follow patient closely with serial blood gas measurements and clinical assessment. Adjust ventilator parameters as indicated (Table 22-7).
b. Parameters for initiating high-frequency ventilation[7]
   (1) Oxygenation Index (OI) >40 (see p. 526 for calculation of OI).
   (2) Inability to provide adequate oxygenation or ventilation with conventional ventilator.
c. Parameters predictive of successful extubation
   (1) $Paco_2$ appropriate for patient.
   (2) PIP generally 14 to 16 cmH_2O.
   (3) PEEP 2 to 3 cmH_2O (infants) or 5 cmH_2O (children).
   (4) IMV 2 to 4 breaths per minute (infants); children may wean to CPAP or pressure support.
   (5) Fio_2 <40% (maintaining Pao_2 >70).
   (6) Adequate air leak around endotracheal tube in cases of airway edema or stenosis.
   (7) Maximum negative inspiratory pressure (NIF) >20-25 cmH_2O.

B. CRITICAL CARE REFERENCE DATA

1. Minute ventilation (V_E)

$$V_E = \text{Respiratory rate} \times \text{Tidal volume (TV)}$$

a. $V_E \times Paco_2 = $ Constant (for volume-limited ventilation)
b. Normal TV = 10 to 15 mL/kg

2. Alveolar gas equation

$$PAo_2 = Pio_2 - (Paco_2/R)$$
$$Pio_2 = Fio_2 \times (P_B - 47 \text{ mmHg})$$

a. $PiO_2 = $ Partial pressure of inspired $O_2 \cong 150$ mmHg at sea level on room air.
b. R = Respiratory exchange quotient (CO_2 produced/O_2 consumed) = 0.8.
c. $PAco_2 = $ Partial pressure of alveolar $CO_2 \cong $ Partial pressure of arterial CO_2 ($Paco_2$).

d. P_B = Atmospheric pressure = 760 mmHg at sea level. Adjust for high altitude environment.
e. Water vapor pressure = 47 mmHg.
f. P_{AO_2} = Partial pressure of O_2 in the alveoli.
3. **Alveolar-arterial oxygen gradient (A-a gradient)**

$$\text{A-a gradient} = P_{AO_2} - Pa_{O_2}$$

a. Obtain ABG measuring P_{AO_2} and Pa_{CO_2} with patient on 100% Fio_2 for at least 15 minutes.
b. Calculate the P_{AO_2} (see above) and then the A-a gradient.
c. The larger the gradient, the more serious the respiratory compromise. A normal gradient is 20 to 65 mmHg on 100% O_2, or 5 to 20 mmHg on room air.
4. **Oxygen content (CAO_2)**

O_2 content of sample (mL/dL) =
$$(O_2 \text{ capacity} \times O_2 \text{ saturation [as decimal]}) + \text{Dissolved } O_2$$

a. O_2 capacity = Hemoglobin (g/dL) × 1.34.
b. Dissolved O_2 = Po_2 (of sample) × 0.003.
c. Hemoglobin carries more than 99% of O_2 in blood under standard conditions.
5. **Arteriovenous O_2 difference ($AVDo_2$)**

$$AVDo_2 = Cao_2 - Cvo_2 = \text{Arterial } O_2 \text{ content} - \text{Mixed venous } O_2 \text{ content}$$

a. Usually done after placing patient on 100% Fio_2 for 15 minutes.
b. Obtain ABG and mixed venous blood sample (best obtained from pulmonary artery catheter), and measure O_2 saturation in each sample.
c. Calculate arterial and mixed venous oxygen contents (see section 4 above) and then $AVDo_2$ (normal: 5 mL/100 dL).
d. Used in the calculation of O_2 extraction ratio.
6. **O_2 extraction ratio**

$$O_2 \text{ extraction} = (AVDo_2/Cao_2) \times 100$$

Normal range 28% to 33%.
a. Calculate $AVDO_2$ and O_2 contents (see sections 4 and 5 above).
b. Extraction ratios are indicative of the adequacy of O_2 delivery to tissues, with increasing extraction ratios suggesting that metabolic needs may be outpacing the oxygen content being delivered.[9]
7. **Oxygenation Index (OI)**

$$OI = \frac{\text{Mean airway pressure (cmH}_2\text{O)} \times FiO_2 \times 100}{PaO_2}$$

OI >35 for 5 to 6 hours is one criterion for ECMO (extracorporeal membrane oxygen) support.

8. Intrapulmonary shunt fraction (Qs/Qt)

$$\frac{Qs}{Qt} = \frac{(\text{A-a gradient}) \times 0.003}{(AVDO_2) + (\text{A-a gradient} \times 0.003)}$$

where Qt is cardiac output and Qs is flow across right-to-left shunt.
a. Formula assumes blood gases obtained on 100% Fio_2.
b. Represents the mismatch of ventilation and perfusion and is normally <5%.
c. A rising shunt fraction (usually >15% to 20%) is indicative of progressive respiratory failure.

REFERENCES

1. Kwong KYC, Jones CA. Chronic asthma therapy. Pediatr Rev 1999; 20(10):329.
2. Soldin SJ, Brugnara C, Hicks JM. Pediatric reference ranges. Washington, DC: AACC Press; 1995.
3. Schrier RW. Renal and electrolyte disorders, 3rd ed. Boston: Little, Brown; 1986.
4. Brenner BM, Floyd CR Jr, editors. The kidney, vol. 1. Philadelphia: WB Saunders; 1991.
5. Murray CB, Loughlin GM. Making the most of pulse oximetry. Contemp Pediatr 1995; 12(7):45-52, 55-57, 61-62.
6. Lanbertsten CJ. Transport of oxygen, CO_2, and inert gases by the blood. In Mountcastle VB, editor. Medical physiology, 14th ed. St Louis: Mosby; 1980.
7. Comber JT, Lopez BL. Examination of pulse oximetry in sickle cell anemia patients presenting to the emergency department in acute vasoocclusive crisis. Am J Emerg Med 1996; 14(1):16.
8. Charney J. Pediatric ventilation outside the operating room. Anesthesiol Clin North Am 2001; 19(2):399.
9. Rogers M. Textbook of pediatric intensive care, 2nd ed. Baltimore: Williams & Wilkins; 1992.

22

PULMONOLOGY

RADIOLOGY

Chicky Dadlani, MD and Shalloo Sachdev, MD

I. PLAIN FILMS[1]

A. CHEST

1. **Anatomy** (Figs. 23-1 and 23-2).
2. **Pneumonia:** Lobar or segmental consolidation and atelectasis are more typical of bacterial infections, whereas hyperinflation, bilateral patchy or streaky densities, and peribronchial thickening are more typical of nonbacterial disease.
3. **Atelectasis versus infiltrate**
a. Atelectasis: When air is removed from the lung, the tissue collapses, resulting in volume loss on chest radiographs. Air may still remain in the larger bronchi, creating air bronchograms on the radiograph. Collapse and re-expansion can happen very quickly, unlike infiltrates.
b. Infiltrate: A fluid (blood, pus, edema) that invades one of the compartments of the lung (bronchoalveolar air space or peribronchial interstitial space) shows as a density on a radiograph. When alveolar air is displaced by fluid, but air remains in the bronchi, the classic pneumonic infiltrate with air bronchograms is seen. When the infiltrate is interstitial, its borders are more vague, and bronchial walls may be thickened. Typically, infiltrates resolve in 2 to 6 weeks.
4. **Central line placement:** Central venous catheters are ideally placed with the catheter tip at the junction of the superior vena cava and right atrium. Some extension into the right atrium is acceptable, but if the catheter is noted to curve to the patient's left on the posteroanterior (PA) film, the catheter may be positioned in the right ventricle.
5. **Endotracheal tube (ETT) placement:** The end of the ETT should rest approximately 2 to 3 cm above the carina, at the level of T3-T4. (This may vary somewhat depending on the size of the patient.) The lung fields should show symmetric aeration.

B. ABDOMEN

Plain films of the abdomen are useful in evaluating for obstruction, pneumoperitoneum, and mass effect. In the radiologic evaluation of the acute abdomen, at least two of the following films should be obtained.
1. **Supine:** Useful for evaluating bowel distention.
2. **Either a left lateral decubitus of the abdomen, a supine cross-table lateral film or an upright abdomen:** For free air, air-fluid levels, necrotizing enterocolitis, or intussusception.
3. **Chest radiographs:** Chest radiographs should always be considered so that pulmonary pathology, which can mimic an abdominal process, can be excluded.

C. CERVICAL SPINE

After immobilization in a collar, lateral/anteroposterior (lateral/AP) radiologic examinations of the cervical spine (C-spine) (Figs. 23-3 and 23-4) should be performed in all children who have sustained significant head trauma or

23

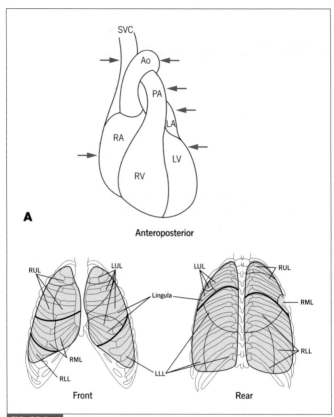

A, Lung and cardiac anatomy on an AP chest radiograph. Divisions within lobes indicate segments matched with X-rays. Arrows indicate contours seen on anteroposterior chest x-ray films. *Ao,* Aorta; *LA,* left atrium; *LLL,* left lower lobe; *LUL,* left upper lobe; *LV,* left ventricle; *PA,* pulmonary artery; *RA,* right atrium; *RLL,* right lower lobe; *RML,* right middle lobe; *RUL,* right upper lobe; *RV,* right ventricle; *SVC,* superior vena cava. *(Heart diagram modified from Kirks DR et al. Practical pediatric imaging: diagnostic radiology of infants and children. 3rd ed. Lippincott-Raven, Philadelphia, 1998.)*

deceleration injury, or who have undergone unwitnessed trauma for which no history can be obtained. The seventh cervical vertebrae and the C7-T1 junction must be visualized. Flexion/extension films may be helpful, especially in patients with Down syndrome who are at risk for atlantoaxial subluxation. Odontoid views may be helpful in older children with suspected occipitocervical injury (e.g., whiplash) (Fig. 23-5). C-spine

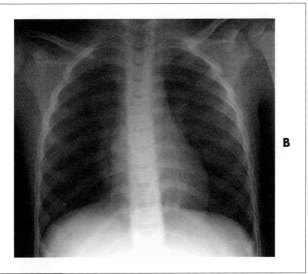

B

FIG. 23-1—cont'd

B, AP chest radiograph.

injuries are most common from the occiput to C3 in children (especially subluxation of the atlantooccipital joint or atlantoaxial joint in infants and toddlers) and in the lower C-spine in older children and adults.

1. **Reading C-spine films:** The following **ABCDs** mnemonic is useful:
a. **A**lignment: The anterior vertebral body line, posterior vertebral body line, facet line, and spinous process line should each form a straight line with smooth contour and no step-offs.
b. **B**ones: Assess each bone looking for chips or fractures.
c. **C**ount: Must see C7 body in its entirety.
d. **D**ens: Examine for chips or fractures.
e. **D**isc spaces: Should see consistent distance between each vertebral body.
f. **S**oft tissue: Assess for swelling, especially in the prevertebral area (see below).
2. **SCIWORA: S**pinal **C**ord **I**njury **W**ith **O**ut **R**adiographic **A**bnormality (SCIWORA) is a functional C-spine injury that cannot be excluded by abnormality on a radiograph; it is thought to be attributable to the increased mobility of a child's spine. SCIWORA should be suspected in the setting of normal C-spine images when clinical signs or symptoms (e.g., point tenderness or focal neurologic symptoms) suggest C-spine injury. If neurologic symptoms persist despite normal C-spine and flexion/extension views, magnetic resonance imaging (MRI) is indicated to rule out swelling or intramedullary hemorrhage of the spinal cord.

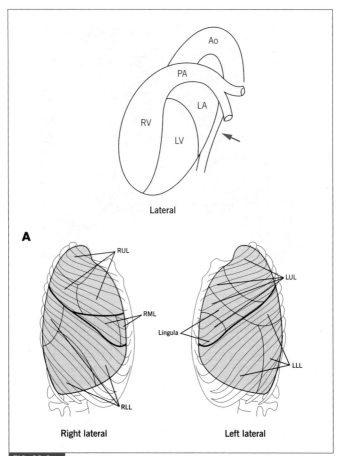

A

Lateral

Right lateral   Left lateral

FIG. 23-2

A, Lung and cardiac anatomy on lateral chest radiograph. Divisions within lobes indicate segments matched with X-rays. Arrows indicate contours seen on lateral chest x-ray films. *Ao,* Aorta; *LA,* left atrium; *LLL,* left lower lobe; *LUL,* left upper lobe; *LV,* left ventricle; *PA,* pulmonary artery; *RLL,* right lower lobe; *RML,* right middle lobe; *RUL,* right upper lobe. *RV,* right ventricle. *(Heart diagram modified from Kirks DR et al. Practical pediatric imaging: diagnostic radiology of infants and children. 3rd ed. Lippincott-Raven, Philadelphia, 1998.)*

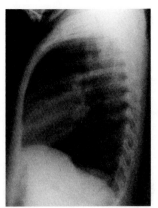

FIG. 23-2—cont'd
B, Lateral chest radiograph.

D. AIRWAY FILMS

The lateral view of the upper airway is the single most useful film for evaluating a child with stridor. If possible, this view should be obtained on inspiration. A radiologic workup should always include AP and lateral views of the chest, with inclusion of the upper airway on the AP chest film.

1. **Diagnosis of diseases based on airway radiologic examination** (Table 23-1; see also Figs. 23-3 and 23-4).

2. **Foreign bodies**

a. Lower airway foreign bodies: In the absence of a radiopaque foreign body, radiologic findings include air trapping, hyperinflation, atelectasis, consolidation, pneumothorax, and pneumomediastinum. If suspected clinically or on the basis of an initially abnormal chest radiograph, further studies should include expiratory films (cooperative patient), bilateral decubitus chest films (uncooperative patient), or airway fluoroscopy.

b. Esophageal foreign bodies: Esophageal foreign bodies usually lodge at one of three locations: at the thoracic inlet, at the level of the aortic arch-left mainstem bronchus, or at the gastroesophageal junction. Evaluation should include the following:

   (1) Lateral airway film.

   (2) AP film of the chest and abdomen (including the supraclavicular region).

   (3) If these films are normal and an esophageal foreign body is still suspected, a contrast study of the esophagus may reveal it. If perforation is suspected, use nonionic, water-soluble contrast.

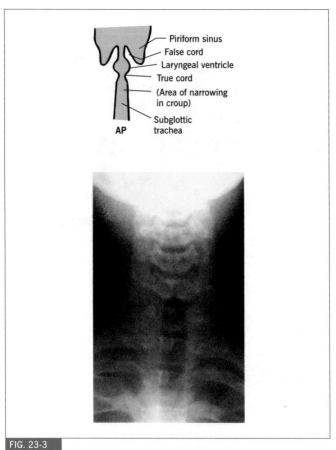

FIG. 23-3
AP neck film with normal anatomy on AP airway view.

E. EXTREMITY STUDIES

In suspected trauma, an adequate evaluation requires at least two views, usually an AP and a lateral. Restricting the film to include only the area of interest improves the resolution (e.g., for a thumb injury, ask for an image of the thumb, not the hand). In general, comparison films of the uninvolved extremity are not necessary, but they may be helpful in several instances, such as the evaluation of joint effusions (particularly the hip), suspected osteomyelitis, or pyarthrosis and/or the evaluation of subtle fractures, especially in areas of multiple ossification centers such as the elbow. Bone age determinations traditionally use a PA view of the left hand and wrist. See Chapter 4 for the Salter-Harris classification of growth-plate injury.

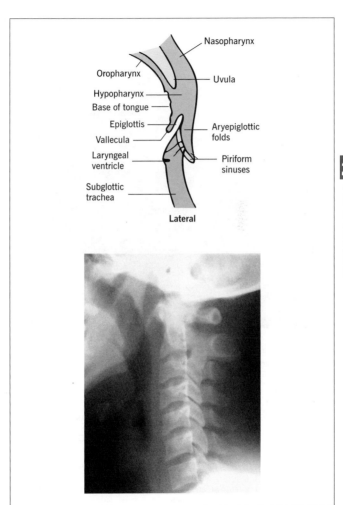

Nasopharynx

Oropharynx

Uvula

Hypopharynx

Base of tongue

Epiglottis

Aryepiglottic folds

Vallecula

Laryngeal ventricle

Piriform sinuses

Subglottic trachea

Lateral

23

RADIOLOGY

FIG. 23-4

Lateral neck film with normal anatomy on lateral airway view.

F. SKELETAL SURVEY

The skeletal survey is the appropriate radiologic series to order in cases of suspected child abuse or metastatic oncologic disease. This survey should include a lateral skull film with a C-spine film, an AP chest film (bone technique), an oblique view of the ribs, an AP view of the pelvis, an abdominal film (bone technique) with the lateral thoracic and lumbar spine,

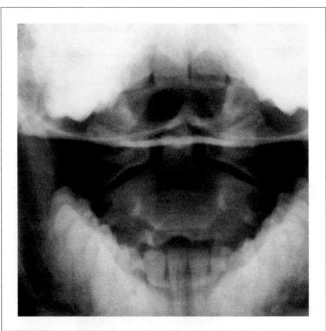

FIG. 23-5

Open-mouth odontoid C-spine view.

TABLE 23-1

DIAGNOSIS OF DISEASES BASED ON AIRWAY RADIOLOGIC EXAMINATION

Diagnosis	Findings on Airway Films
Croup	AP and lateral films with subglottic narrowing ("steeple sign")
Epiglottitis	Enlarged, indistinct epiglottis on lateral film ("thumb sign")
Vascular ring	AP and lateral films with narrowing; double or right aortic arch
Retropharyngeal abscess or pharyngeal mass	Soft tissue air or persistent enlargement of prevertebral soft tissues; more than half of a vertebral body above C3 and one vertebral body below C3
Immunodeficiency	Absence of adenoidal and tonsillar tissue after age 6 mo

and AP long bone films. Classic findings are multiple epiphyseal and metaphyseal injuries of various ages (especially "bucket handle fractures"). In addition, suspicion should be raised by fracture at unusual sites, such as posterior rib fractures or solitary spiral and transverse fractures of the long bones with an inconsistent history of trauma, or by multiple fractures of varying ages.

G. SPINE FILMS
Scoliosis is evaluated by an erect AP spine radiograph. PA views can be used in postpubertal girls to decrease breast radiation dose. For evaluation and management, see Chapter 5. For spondylolysis and spondylolisthesis, oblique lumbar spine films should also be obtained.

II. ULTRASONOGRAPHY[2]

23

RADIOLOGY

A. APPLICATIONS
Common uses for ultrasonography include pyloric stenosis, abdominal masses in young children, intussusception, tuboovarian abscess, acute intracranial hemorrhage in newborns, definition of renal pathology, congenital hip dislocation in children <4 months of age, evaluation for spinal dysraphism in young infants, fluid collections (e.g., hip effusions, pleural effusions, ascites), biliary tree and gallbladder evaluation, and pregnancy evaluation.

B. ADVANTAGES
There is no radiation exposure, the procedures is painless, no sedation is required, and the machine is portable.

C. DISADVANTAGES
Gas and fat may degrade the image. The procedure is operator dependent.

D. PREPARATION
Obtain ultrasound examinations before barium studies. The patient should have a full bladder for pelvic and lower abdomen studies, with no voiding for the previous 1 to 3 hours.

E. COLOR DOPPLER FLOW IMAGING
Moving blood is detected by ultrasonographic frequency shifts. Color Doppler flow imaging can be used to evaluate deep-vein thrombosis, vascular patency, intracranial blood flow (including transcranial Doppler to screen for ischemic brain injury risk in sickle cell disease), cardiac shunt flow, transplant vascularity, and testicular perfusion in acute scrotum. Power Doppler, available in some centers, is particularly sensitive in detecting slow flow in small vessels (e.g., infant testes).

III. COMPUTED TOMOGRAPHY AND MAGNETIC RESONANCE IMAGING[2]

A. INDICATIONS FOR COMPUTED TOMOGRAPHY (CT) VERSUS MRI
(Table 23-2)

B. ULTRAFAST CT
Ultrafast CT permits cine imaging of a dynamic process such as trachea shape with breathing, uses reduced radiation dosing, and takes only 50 to

TABLE 23-2

INDICATIONS FOR CT VS. MRI

	CT	MRI
Applications		
CNS	Acute intracranial trauma, hemorrhage, hydrocephalus, acute child abuse evaluation (shaken baby syndrome), 3-D CT reconstruction for craniofacial injuries and complex skeletal deformities.	Posterior fossa, brainstem, spinal cord (including meningomyelocele), demyelination disorders, evaluation for structural lesions in focal seizure disorders, detects diffuse axonal injury, determines ages of multiple extraaxial hemorrhages (i.e., useful for suspected intentional injury).
Chest	Chest trauma, pulmonary parenchymal disease, evaluation of tracheal, bronchial, pleural or chest wall lesions.	Mediastinal lymphadenopathy, mediastinal vasculature, congenital anomalies of the heart and great vessels.
Abdomen	Blunt abdominal trauma, complicated inflammatory bowel disease, appendicitis, intraabdominal solid masses, abscesses, many hepatobiliary abnormalities, retroperitoneal masses.	Delineating hepatic tumors before resection.
Skeletal	Calcifying processes, delineation of extent of bony lesions, stress fractures.	Osteomyelitis, avascular necrosis of the femoral head, extension of bone tumors, marrow replacement by leukemic infiltrates.
Advantages	Faster and less costly than MRI, sensitive to calcium, operator-independent interpretation, wide field of view; spiral scanning also decreases the need for sedation.	No ionizing radiation, multiple imaging planes, sensitive to the presence of abnormal tissues.

Disadvantages	Ionizing radiation exposure, not sensitive to diffuse white matter or cutaneous abnormalities, limited scanning planes, and risks of IV contrast exposure.	Difficult to accommodate critical care equipment. Patients with implanted ferromagnetic devices (e.g., pacemakers, implanted heart valves, osteotomy hardware) cannot be scanned. Sensitive to motion degradation. Frequently requires sedation. Poor signal from calcium and gas.
Indications for contrast	For abdominal study, use both oral and IV contrast. For a chest study, use only IV contrast. Avoid oral contrast in the child with intractable vomiting. Avoid IV contrast if there is renal compromise or allergy to IV contrast. Use water-soluble contrast if perforation is suspected or there is risk of aspiration. Rectal contrast for appendicitis evaluation may be used.	Contrast is not used routinely; consult a radiologist.
Preparation	No solid foods 3 hr before study. No liquids 30 min before. Sedation protocols require longer periods without solids or liquids.	Depends on sedation protocol considerations; consider a mild anxiolytic for older children.

TABLE 23-3

T1- AND T2-WEIGHTED IMAGING

	T1-Weighted Images*	T2-Weighted Images*
Fat	Increased	Intermediate
Flowing blood	No signal	No signal
Acute hematoma	Intermediate	Decreased
Subacute hematoma	Increased	Increased
Chronic blood (hemosiderin)	Decreased	Decreased
Muscle	Intermediate	Intermediate

Courtesy Laureen Sena, MD.

*Increased means brighter; decreased means darker.

100 msec to complete. A disadvantage is a somewhat decreased image quality compared with conventional CT.

C. HIGH-RESOLUTION CT
High-resolution CT permits edge enhancement and is good for imaging lung parenchyma.

D. COMPARISON OF T1 VERSUS T2 IMAGING ON MRI (Table 23-3)

IV. SPECIAL TESTS[2]

A. GASTROINTESTINAL
Barium is usually the contrast of choice. Water-soluble contrast medium should be used if perforation or leak is suspected. Gas-producing agents may be used for providing double contrast.

1. **Upper gastrointestinal study:** Contrast is ingested; esophagus, stomach, and duodenum are visualized by fluoroscopy and plain films. Test can be expanded to include small intestine if small bowel follow-through is requested.
a. Indications: Esophageal webs and rings, masses, gastric volvulus, gastroesophageal reflux evaluation (to exclude anatomic causes of reflux symptoms; reflux visualized during study is neither sensitive nor specific in quantifying reflux disease); motility problems, ulcerations, strictures/obstruction, hiatal hernias, varices, and gastric outlet obstruction (e.g., pyloric stenosis). Limited sensitivity in detecting mucosal disease.
b. Preparation: <18 months: Nothing by mouth (NPO) for 3 hours before study. >18 months: NPO for 4 hours before study. Clear liquids only after midnight. Consider bisacodyl pills or suppositories and magnesium citrate for older children.

2. **Barium enema**
a. Indications: Polyps, strictures/Hirschsprung's disease, colitis, volvulus, meconium ileus, intussusception.
b. Preparation: <18 months: Liquid diet starting the evening before the study. >18 months: Liquid diet for 24 hours before study. Consider bisacodyl suppositories and enemas, and magnesium citrate for older children. Colon preparation is not advised for evaluation of Hirschsprung's disease because it may stretch the transition zone.

B. GENITOURINARY

1. **Voiding cystourethrogram:** Water-soluble contrast fills the bladder through a urinary catheter; the catheter is then removed. Plain films are taken during filling and voiding.

a. Indications: Vesicoureteral reflux, abnormalities of bladder or urethral function and anatomy.

b. Preparation: No urination just before examination. (Some urine needs to be in the bladder.) Can be uncomfortable and requires urinary catheterization.

2. **Intravenous pyelogram:** Intravenous contrast is given, and timed plain films are taken as contrast is excreted in the kidneys.

a. Indications: Collecting system abnormalities, duplex kidneys. An IV pyelogram is rarely the first examination of the urinary tract (ultrasound is preferred).

b. Preparation: No food or fluid 2 to 3 hours before. Invasive, requires IV contrast, which may aggravate renal failure.

V. COMMONLY USED NUCLEAR MEDICINE PROCEDURES[2]
(Table 23-4)

23

RADIOLOGY

TABLE 23-4

COMMONLY USED NUCLEAR MEDICINE PROCEDURES

Study/Agent	Indication	Patient Preparation/Technique	Physiology/Mechanism
MUSCULOSKELETAL			
Bone scan ^{99m}Tc-MDP	Benign or metastatic bone disorders Unexplained bone pain Child abuse	No preparation IV injection Delayed imaging at 3-4 hr	Localizes at sites of osteoblastic or osteoclastic activity
Three-phase bone scan (^{99m}Tc-MDP)	Infection or inflammation (osteomyelitis, septic arthritis), AVN, fracture	No preparation Immediate blood flow, extracellular phases Delayed imaging at 3-4 hr	Blood flow and extracellular information helpful in infection or inflammation
Gallium scan (^{67}Ga citrate)	Infections Some tumors (Hodgkin's lymphoma)	Bowel preparation Imaging times dependent on indication or interference from bowel activity (24, 48, 72, 96 hr)	Ga^{2+} is an Fe^{2+} analog, binds to serum proteins Partial excretion in colon Sometimes better for chronic infection
White blood cell scan (^{111}In-labeled WBCs)	Infections	Blood withdrawal WBC labeling, reinjection Imaging at 24 and/or 48 hr	Localizes active inflammation or infection No bowel excretion
NEUROLOGIC			
Brain blood flow scan (^{99m}Tc-DTPA)	Adjunct in assessment of brain death	No preparation	Absent perfusion is compatible with brain death

Brain scan (^{99m}Tc-ECD or ^{99m}Tc-HMPAO)	Localization of epileptic foci Cerebral vascular disease	No preparation	Ictal foci show increased flow Tracer follows blood flow
Cisternography (^{111}In-DTPA)	Hydrocephalus CSF leak	No preparation Tracer injected into subarachnoid space	Tracer follows CSF flow
CSF shunt patency (^{111}In-DTPA)	Assess patency of VP, LP, VA shunts	No preparation Injection into reservoir/shunt	Tracer follows CSF flow
RESPIRATORY			
V/Q scan (^{99m}Tc-MAA perfusion, ^{133}Xe ventilation)	Assess congenital pulmonary or vascular anomalies Pulmonary embolus	No preparation	IV-injected MAA trapped in the pulmonary capillary bed ^{133}Xe gas inhaled
GASTROINTESTINAL			
Gastric emptying or reflux study (^{99m}Tc-sulfur colloid)	Quantitative assessment of solid or liquid emptying Gastric reflux	NPO the evening before study	Tracer is not absorbed in the gastrointestinal tract Assess for GER or pulmonary aspiration
Hepatobiliary (^{99m}Tc-mebrofenin)	Neonatal hepatitis versus biliary atresia Biliary leak after trauma or transplant	Phenobarbital 2.5 mg/kg Q12hr 3-5 days before imaging No preparation	Phenobarbital increases bile secretion; in hepatitis, helps in tracer transit In leaks, tracer extravasates into peritoneal cavity

AVN, Avascular necrosis; *CSF,* cerebrospinal fluid; *DTPA,* diethylenetriaminepentaacetic acid; *GER,* gastroesophageal reflux; *GFR,* glomerular filtration rate; *LP,* lumbar peritoneal; *MAA,* macroaggregated albumin; *MDP,* methylene diphosphonate; *NPO,* nothing by mouth; *PE,* pulmonary embolism; *RAS,* renal artery stenosis; *RES,* reticuloendothelial system; *VA,* ventriculoatrial; *VP,* ventriculoperitoneal; *V/Q,* ventilation/perfusion; *VUR,* vesicoureteral reflux; *WBC,* white blood cell.

23

RADIOLOGY

TABLE 23-4

COMMONLY USED NUCLEAR MEDICINE PROCEDURES—cont'd

Study/Agent	Indication	Patient Preparation/Technique	Physiology/Mechanism
GASTROINTESTINAL—cont'd			
Liver-spleen scan (⁹⁹ᵐTc-sulfur colloid)	Defining organs in congenital anomalies (splenosis, asplenia) Assess splenic function	No preparation	Tracer taken up by RES in liver (Kupffer's cells), spleen, bone marrow
Meckel's scan (⁹⁹ᵐTc-pertechnetate)	Gastrointestinal bleeding	(Optional) pentagastrin, cimetidine, glucagon	Tracer localizes to mucinous cells in Meckel's diverticula
GENITOURINARY			
Radionuclide cystogram (⁹⁹ᵐTc-pertechnetate)	Vesicoureteral reflux Functional bladder capacity	Bladder catheterization Direct infusion of tracer via bladder catheter	Dynamic imaging of bladder filling and voiding Sensitive in detection of VUR
Renal scan			
⁹⁹ᵐTc-DTPA or ⁹⁹ᵐTc-MAG₃	Renal function Renovascular hypertension (RAS) Ureteral obstruction	Bladder catheterization (optional if no obstruction) Initial 30-min imaging Lasix washout 30 min (optional)	⁹⁹ᵐTc-DTPA is excreted by filtration (GFR) Captopril challenge for RAS Lasix washout slower in obstruction
⁹⁹ᵐTc-DMSA or ⁹⁹ᵐTc-glucoheptonate	Renal cortical scarring Pyelonephritis	⁹⁹ᵐTc-DMSA: Imaging at 4 hr *Glucoheptonate:* Initial 2-hr delayed imaging	Tracers localize in the renal tubules, providing an indicator of function
Testicular scan (⁹⁹ᵐTc-pertechnetate)	Suspected testicular torsion versus epididymitis	No preparation	Absent flow in torsion; increased in epididymitis

REFERENCES

1. Kirks DR et al. Practical pediatric imaging: diagnostic radiology of infants and children. 3rd ed. Philadelphia: Lippincott-Raven; 1998.
2. Blickman H. Pediatric radiology: the requisites. 2nd ed, St. Louis: Mosby; 1998.

PART III

Reference

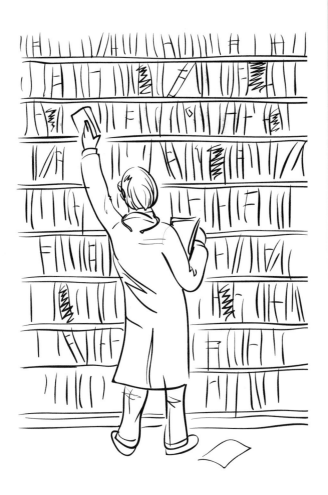

BLOOD CHEMISTRIES AND BODY FLUIDS

Christian Nechyba, MD

These values are compiled from the published literature[1-6] and from the Johns Hopkins Hospital Department of Laboratory Medicine. Normal values vary with the analytic method used. Consult your laboratory for its analytic method and range of normal values and for less commonly used parameters, which are beyond the scope of this text. Additional normal laboratory values may be found in the Chapters 9, 13, and 14.

24

I. REFERENCE VALUES (Table 24-1)

Text continued on p. 556

TABLE 24-1

REFERENCE VALUES[1-6]

	Conventional Units	SI Units
ACID PHOSPHATASE		
(Major sources: prostate and erythrocytes)		
Newborn	7.4-19.4 U/L	7.4-19.4 U/L
2-13 yr	6.4-15.2 U/L	6.4-15.2 U/L
Adult male	0.5-11.0 U/L	0.5-11.0 U/L
Adult female	0.2-9.5 U/L	0.2-9.5 U/L
ALANINE AMINOTRANSFERASE (ALT)		
(Major sources: liver, skeletal muscle, and myocardium)		
Neonate/infant	13-45 U/L	13-45 U/L
Adult male	10-40 U/L	10-40 U/L
Adult female	7-35 U/L	7-35 U/L
ALBUMIN		
(See Proteins)		
ALDOLASE		
(Major sources: skeletal muscle and myocardium)		
10-24 mo	3.4-11.8 U/L	3.4-11.8 U/L
2-16 yr	1.2-8.8 U/L	1.2-8.8 U/L
Adult	1.7-4.9 U/L	1.7-4.9 U/L
ALKALINE PHOSPHATASE		
(Major sources: liver, bone, intestinal mucosa, placenta, and kidney)		
Infant	150-420 U/L	150-420 U/L
2-10 yr	100-320 U/L	100-320 U/L
Adolescent males	100-390 U/L	100-390 U/L
Adolescent females	100-320 U/L	100-320 U/L
Adult	30-120 U/L	30-120 U/L
AMMONIA		
(Heparinized venous specimen on ice analyzed within 30 min)		
Newborn	90-150 mcg/dL	64-107 mcmol/L
0-2 wk	79-129 mcg/dL	56-92 mcmol/L
>1 mo	29-70 mcg/dL	21-50 mcmol/L
Adult	0-50 mcg/dL	0-35.7 mcmol/L

cont'd

REFERENCE VALUES[1-6]—cont'd

	Conventional Units	SI Units
AMYLASE		
(Major sources: pancreas, salivary glands, and ovaries)		
Newborn	5-65 U/L	5-65 U/L
Adult	27-131 U/L	27-131 U/L
ANTINUCLEAR ANTIBODY (ANA)		
Not significant	<1:80	
Likely significant	>1:320	
Patterns with clinical correlation:		
Centromere—CREST		
Nucleolar—Scleroderma		
Homogeneous—SLE		
ANTISTREPTOLYSIN O TITER		
(4-fold rise in paired serial specimens is significant)		
Preschool	<1:85	
School age	<1:170	
Older adult	<1:85	
NOTE: Alternatively, values up to 200 Todd units are normal.		
ASPARTATE AMINOTRANSFERASE (AST)		
(Major sources: liver, skeletal muscle, kidney, myocardium, and erythrocytes)		
Newborn	25-75 U/L	25-75 U/L
Infant	15-60 U/L	15-60 U/L
1-3 yr	20-60 U/L	20-60 U/L
4-6 yr	15-50 U/L	15-50 U/L
7-9 yr	15-40 U/L	15-40 U/L
10-11 yr	10-60 U/L	10-60 U/L
12-19 yr	15-45 U/L	15-45 U/L
BICARBONATE		
Newborn	17-24 mEq/L	17-24 mmol/L
2 mo-2 yr	16-24 mEq/L	16-24 mmol/L
>2 yr	22-26 mEq/L	22-26 mmol/L
BILIRUBIN (TOTAL)		
Cord		
Preterm	<2 mg/dL	<34 mcmol/L
Term	<2 mg/dL	<34 mcmol/L
0-1 days		
Preterm	<8 mg/dL	<137 mcmol/L
Term	<8.7mg/dL	<149 mcmol/L
1-2 days		
Preterm	<12 mg/dL	<205 mcmol/L
Term	<11.5 mg/dL	<197 mcmol/L
3-5 days		
Preterm	<16 mg/dL	<274 mcmol/L
Term	<12 mg/dL	<205 mcmol/L
Older infant		
Preterm	<2 mg/dL	<34 mcmol/L
Term	<1.2 mg/dL	<21 mcmol/L
Adult	0.3-1.2 mg/dL	5-21 mcmol/L

TABLE 24-1
REFERENCE VALUES[1-6]—cont'd

	Conventional Units	SI Units	
BILIRUBIN (CONJUGATED)			
Neonate	<0.6 mg/dL	<10 mcmol/L	
Infants/children	<0.2 mg/dL	<3.4 mcmol/L	

BLOOD GAS, ARTERIAL[7]

	PH	Pao_2 (mmHg)	$Paco_2$ (mmHg)	HCO_3^- (mEq/L)
Newborn (birth)	7.26-7.29	60	55	19
Newborn (>24 hr)	7.37	70	33	20
Infant (1-24 mo)	7.40	90	34	20
Child (7-19 yr)	7.39	96	37	22
Adult (>19 yr)	7.35-7.45	90-110	35-45	22-26

NOTE: Venous blood gases can be used to assess acid-base status, not oxygenation. Pco_2 averages 6-8 mmHg higher than $Paco_2$, and pH is slightly lower. Peripheral venous samples are strongly affected by the local circulatory and metabolic environment. Capillary blood gases correlate best with arterial pH and moderately well with $Paco_2$.

	Conventional Units	SI Units
CALCIUM (TOTAL)		
Preterm	6.2-11 mg/dL	1.6-2.8 mmol/L
Full term <10 days	7.6-10.4 mg/dL	1.9-2.6 mmol/L
10 days-24 mo	9.0-11.0 mg/dL	2.3-2.8 mmol/L
2-12 yr	8.8-10.8 mg/dL	2.2-2.7 mmol/L
Adult	8.6-10 mg/dL	2.2-2.5 mmol/L
CALCIUM (IONIZED)		
Newborn <36 hr	4.20-5.48 mg/dL	1.05-1.37 mmol/L
Newborn 36-84 hr	4.40-5.68 mg/dL	1.10-1.42 mmol/L
1-18 yr	4.80-5.52 mg/dL	1.20-1.38 mmol/L
Adult	4.64-5.28 mg/dL	1.16-1.32 mmol/L
CARBON DIOXIDE (CO_2 CONTENT)		
Cord blood	14-22 mEq/L	14-22 mmol/L
Newborn	13-22 mEq/L	13-22 mmol/L
Premature, 1 wk	14-27 mEq/L	14-27 mmol/L
Infant/child	20-28 mEq/L	20-28 mmol/L
Adult	22-28 mEq/L	22-28 mmol/L
CARBON MONOXIDE (CARBOXYHEMOGLOBIN)		
Nonsmoker	0.5-1.5% of total hemoglobin	
Smoker	4%-9% of total hemoglobin	
Toxic	20%-50% of total hemoglobin	
Lethal	>50% of total hemoglobin	
CHLORIDE (SERUM)		
Newborn	98-113 mEq/L	98-113 mmol/L
Child/Adult	98-107 mEq/L	98-107 mmol/L
CHOLESTEROL		
(See Lipids)		
C-REACTIVE PROTEIN		
(Other laboratories may have different reference values)	0-0.5 mg/dL	

cont'd

24

BLOOD CHEMISTRIES AND BODY FLUIDS

TABLE 24-1

REFERENCE VALUES[1-6]—cont'd

	Conventional Units	SI Units
CREATINE KINASE (CREATINE PHOSPHOKINASE)		
(Major sources: myocardium, skeletal muscle, smooth muscle, and brain)		
Newborn	10-200 U/L	10-200 U/L
Man	15-105 U/L	15-105 U/L
Woman	10-80 U/L	10-80 U/L
CREATININE (SERUM)		
Cord	0.6-1.2 mg/dL	53-106 mcmol/L
Newborn	0.3-1.0 mg/dL	27-88 mcmol/L
Infant	0.2-0.4 mg/dL	18-35 mcmol/L
Child	0.3-0.7 mg/dL	27-62 mcmol/L
Adolescent	0.5-1.0 mg/dL	44-88 mcmol/L
Man	0.7-1.3 mg/dL	62-115 mcmol/L
Woman	0.6-1.1 mg/dL	53-97 mcmol/L
ERYTHROCYTE SEDIMENTATION RATE (ESR)		
Term neonate	0-4 mm/hr	
Child	4-20 mm/hr	
Adult (male)	1-15 mm/hr	
Adult (female)	4-25 mm/hr	
FERRITIN		
Newborn	25-200 ng/mL	20-200 ng/mL
1 mo	200-600 ng/mL	200-600 ng/mL
2-5 mo	50-200 ng/mL	50-200 ng/mL
6 mo-15 yr	7-140 ng/mL	7-140 ng/mL
Adult male	20-250 ng/mL	20-250 ng/mL
Adult female	10-120 ng/mL	10-120 ng/mL
FIBRINOGEN		
(See Table 13-5, p. 296)		
FOLATE (SERUM)		
Newborn	5-65 ng/mL	11-147 nmol/L
Infant	15-55 ng/mL	34-125 nmol/L
2-16 yr	5-21 ng/mL	11-48 nmol/L
>16 yr	3-20 ng/mL	7-45 nmol/L
FOLATE (RBC)		
Newborn	150-200 ng/mL	340-453 nmol/L
Infant	75-1000 ng/mL	170-2265 nmol/L
2-16 yr	>160 ng/mL	>362 nmol/L
>16 yr	140-628 ng/mL	317-1422 nmol/L
GALACTOSE		
Newborn	0-20 mg/dL	0-1.11 mmol/L
Thereafter	<5 mg/dL	<0.28 mmol/L

TABLE 24-1°
REFERENCE VALUES[1-6]—cont'd

	Conventional Units	SI Units
γ-GLUTAMYL TRANSFERASE (GGT)		
(Major sources: liver [biliary tree] and kidney)		
Cord	19-270 U/L	19-270 U/L
Preterm	56-233 U/L	56-233 U/L
0-3 wk	0-130 U/L	0-130 U/L
3 wk-3 mo	4-120 U/L	4-120 U/L
3-12 mo boy	5-65 U/L	5-65 U/L
3-12 mo girl	5-35 U/L	5-35 U/L
1-15 yr	0-23 U/L	0-23 U/L
Adult male	11-50 U/L	11-50 U/L
Adult female	7-32 U/L	7-32 U/L
GLUCOSE (SERUM)		
Preterm	20-60 mg/dL	1.1-3.3 mmol/L
Newborn, <1 day	40-60 mg/dL	2.2-3.3 mmol/L
Newborn, >1 day	50-80 mg/dL	2.8-4.5 mmol/L
Child	60-100 mg/dL	3.3-5.6.mmol/L
>16 yr	74-106 mg/dL	4.1-5.9 mmol/L
HAPTOGLOBIN		
Newborn	5-48 mg/dL	50-480 mg/L
>30 days	26-185 mg/dL	260-1850 mg/L
HEMOGLOBIN A₁C	5.0-7.5% total Hgb	
HEMOGLOBIN F [MEAN (SD) % TOTAL Hgb]		
1 day	77.0 (7.3)	
5 days	76.8 (5.8)	
3 wk	70.0 (7.3)	
6-9 wk	52.9 (11)	
3-4 mo	23.2 (16)	
6 mo	4.7 (2.2)	
8-11 mo	1.6 (1.0)	
Adult	<2.0	
IRON		
Newborn	100-250 mcg/dL	17.9-44.8 mcmol/L
Infant	40-100 mcg/dL	7.2-17.9 mcmol/L
Child	50-120 mcg/dL	9.0-21.5 mcmol/L
Adult male	65-175 mcg/dL	11.6-31.3 mcmol/L
Adult female	50-170 mcg/dL	9.0-30.4 mcmol/L
KETONES (SERUM)		
Quantitative	0.5-3.0 mg/dL	5-30 mg/L
LACTATE		
Capillary blood		
Newborn	<27 mg/dL	0.0-3.0 mmol/L
Child	5-20 mg/dL	0.56-2.25 mmol/L
Venous	5-20 mg/dL	0.5-2.2 mmol/L
Arterial	5-14 mg/dL	0.5-1.6 mmol/L

cont'd

	Conventional Units	SI Units
LACTATE DEHYDROGENASE (AT 37° C)		
(Major sources: myocardium, liver, skeletal muscle, erythrocytes, platelets, and lymph nodes)		
0-4 days	290-775 U/L	290-775 U/L
4-10 days	545-2000 U/L	545-2000 U/L
10 days-24 mo	180-430 U/L	180-430 U/L
24 mo-12 yr	110-295 U/L	110-295 U/L
>12 yr	100-190 U/L	100-190 U/L
LEAD		
(See pp. 35-38)		
Child	<10 mcg/dL	<0.48 mcmol/L
LIPASE		
0-90 days	10-85 U/L	
3-12 mo	9-128 U/L	
1-11 yr	10-150 U/L	
>11 yr	10-220 U/L	
LIPIDS[8]		

	Cholesterol (mg/dL)			LDL (mg/dL)			HDL (mg/dL)
	Desirable	Borderline	High	Desirable	Borderline	High	Desirable
Child/adolescent	<170	170-199	>200	<110	110-129	>130	45
Adult	<200	200-239	>240	<130	130-159	>160	45

	Conventional Units	SI Units
MAGNESIUM	1.3-2.0 mEq/L	0.65-1.0 mmol/L
METHEMOGLOBIN	<1.5% total Hgb	
OSMOLALITY	275-295 mOsm/kg	275-295 mmol/kg
PHENYLALANINE		
Preterm	2.0-7.5 mg/dL	121-454 mcmol/L
Newborn	1.2-3.4 mg/dL	73-206 mcmol/L
Adult	0.8-1.8 mg/dL	48-109 mcmol/L
PHOSPHORUS		
Newborn	4.5-9.0 mg/dL	1.45-2.91 mmol/L
10 days-24 mo	4.5-6.7 mg/dL	1.45-2.16 mmol/L
24 mo-12 yr	4.5-5.5 mg/dL	1.45-1.78 mmol/L
>12 yr	2.7-4.5 mg/dL	0.87-1.45 mmol/L
PORCELAIN[9]	7.24-8.19 mg/dL	8.32-9.93 mmol/L
POTASSIUM		
Newborn	3.7-5.9 mEq/L	3.7-5.9 mmol/L
Infant	4.1-5.3 mEq/L	4.1-5.3 mmol/L
Child	3.4-4.7 mEq/L	3.4-4.7 mmol/L
Adult	3.5-5.1 mEq/L	3.5-5.1 mmol/L
PREALBUMIN		
Newborn	7-39 mg/dL	
1-6 mo	8-34 mg/dL	
6 mo-4 yr	2-36 mg/dL	
4-6 yr	12-30 mg/dL	
6-19 yr	12-42 mg/dL	

TABLE 24-1

REFERENCE VALUES[1-6]—cont'd

PROTEINS

Protein Electrophoresis (g/dL)

Age	TP	Albumin	α-1	α-2	β	γ
Cord	4.8-8.0	2.2-4.0	0.3-0.7	0.4-0.9	0.4-1.6	0.8-1.6
Newborn	4.4-7.6	3.2-4.8	0.1-0.3	0.2-0.3	0.3-0.6	0.6-1.2
1 day-1 mo	4.4-7.6	2.5-5.5	0.1-0.3	0.3-1.0	0.2-1.1	0.4-1.3
1-3 mo	3.6-7.4	2.1-4.8	0.1-0.4	0.3-1.1	0.3-1.1	0.2-1.1
4-6 mo	4.2-7.4	2.8-5.0	0.1-0.4	0.3-0.8	0.3-0.8	0.1-0.9
7-12 mo	5.1-7.5	3.2-5.7	0.1-0.6	0.3-1.5	0.4-1.0	0.2-1.2
13-24 mo	3.7-7.5	1.9-5.0	0.1-0.6	0.4-1.4	0.4-1.4	0.4-1.6
25-36 mo	5.3-8.1	3.3-5.8	0.1-0.3	0.4-1.1	0.3-1.2	0.4-1.5
3-5 yr	4.9-8.1	2.9-5.8	0.1-0.4	0.4-1.0	0.5-1.0	0.4-1.7
6-8 yr	6.0-7.9	3.3-5.0	0.1-0.5	0.5-0.8	0.5-0.9	0.7-2.0
9-11 yr	6.0-7.9	3.2-5.0	0.1-0.4	0.7-0.9	0.6-1.0	0.8-2.0
12-16 yr	6.0-7.9	3.2-5.1	0.1-0.4	0.5-1.1	0.5-1.1	0.6-2.0
Adult	6.0-8.0	3.1-5.4	0.1-0.4	0.4-1.1	0.5-1.2	0.7-1.7

		Conventional Units	SI Units
PYRUVATE		0.3-0.9 mg/dL	0.03-0.10 mmol/L
RHEUMATOID FACTOR		<30 U/mL	
SODIUM			
Preterm		130-140 mEq/L	130-140 mmol/L
Older		133-146 mEq/L	133-146 mmol/L
TOTAL IRON-BINDING CAPACITY (TIBC)			
Infant		100-400 mcg/dL	17.9-71.6 mcmol/L
Adult		250-425 mcg/dL	44.8-76.1 mcmol/L
TOTAL PROTEIN			
(See Proteins)			
TRANSAMINASE (SGOT)			
(See Aspartate aminotransferase [AST])			
TRANSAMINASE (SGPT)			
(See Alanine aminotransferase [ALT])			
TRANSFERRIN			
Newborn		130-275 mg/dL	1.30-2.75 g/L
3 mo-10 yr		203-360 mg/dL	2.03-3.6 g/L
Adult		215-380 mg/dL	2.15-3.8 g/L

TRIGLYCERIDES (FASTING)[10]

	Male (mg/dL)	Female (mg/dL)	Male (g/L)	Female (g/L)
Cord blood	10-98	10-98	0.10-0.98	0.10-0.98
0-5 yr	30-86	32-99	0.30-0.86	0.32-0.99
6-11 yr	31-108	35-114	0.31-1.08	0.35-1.14
12-15 yr	36-138	41-138	0.36-1.38	0.41-1.38
16-19 yr	40-163	40-128	0.40-1.63	0.40-1.28
20-29 yr	44-185	40-128	0.44-1.85	0.40-1.28
Adults	40-160	35-135	0.40-1.60	0.35-1.35

cont'd

24

BLOOD CHEMISTRIES AND BODY FLUIDS

REFERENCE VALUES[1-6]—cont'd

	Conventional Units	SI Units
TROPONIN-I	0-0.1 mcg/L	
UREA NITROGEN		
Premature (<1 week)	3-25 mg/dL	1.1-8.9 mmol/L
Newborn	4-12 mg/dL	1.4-4.3 mmol/L
Infant/child	5-18 mg/dL	1.8-6.4 mmol/L
Adult	6-20 mg/dL	2.1-7.1 mmol/L
URIC ACID		
0-2 yr	2.4-6.4 mg/dL	0.14-0.38 mmol/L
2-12 yr	2.4-5.9 mg/dL	0.14-0.35 mmol/L
12-14 yr	2.4-6.4 mg/dL	0.14-0.38 mmol/L
Adult male	3.5-7.2 mg/dL	0.20-0.43 mmol/L
Adult female	2.4-6.4 mg/dL	0.14-0.38 mmol/L
VITAMIN A		
(Retinol)		
Preterm	13-46 mcg/dL	0.46-1.61 mcmol/L
Full term	18-50 mcg/dL	0.63-1.75 mcmol/L
1-6 yr	20-43 mcg/dL	0.7-1.5 mcmol/L
7-12 yr	20-49 mcg/dL	0.9-1.7 mcmol/L
13-19 yr	26-72 mcg/dL	0.9-2.5 mcmol/L
VITAMIN B_1		
(Thiamine)	5.3-7.9 mcg/dL	0.16-0.23 mcmol/L
VITAMIN B_2		
(Riboflavin)	4-24 mcg/dL	106-638 nmol/L
VITAMIN B_{12}		
(Cobalamin)		
Newborn	160-1300 pg/mL	118-959 pmol/L
Child/adult	200-835 pg/mL	148-616 pmol/L
VITAMIN C		
(Ascorbic acid)	0.4-1.5 mg/dL	23-85 mcmol/L
VITAMIN D_3		
(1,25-dihydroxy-vitamin D)	16-65 pg/mL	42-169 pmol/L
VITAMIN E		
<11 yr	3-15 mg/L	7.0-35 mcmol/L
>11 yr	5-20 mg/L	11.6-46.4 mcmol/L
ZINC	70-120 mcg/dL	10.7-18.4 mcmol/L

II. EVALUATION OF BODY FLUIDS

A. EVALUATION OF TRANSUDATE VERSUS EXUDATE (Table 24-2)

B. EVALUATION OF CEREBROSPINAL FLUID (Table 24-3)

C. EVALUATION OF SYNOVIAL FLUID (Table 24-4)

TABLE 24-2

EVALUATION OF TRANSUDATE vs. EXUDATE (PLEURAL, PERICARDIAL, OR PERITONEAL FLUID)

Measurement[a]	Transudate	Exudate[b]
Specific gravity	<1.016	>1.016
Protein (g/dL)	<3.0	>3.0
Fluid:serum ratio	<0.5	>0.5
LDH (IU)	<200	>200
Fluid:serum ratio (isoenzymes not useful)	<0.6	>0.6
WBCs[c]	<1000/mm^3	>1000/mm^3
RBCs	<10,000	Variable
Glucose	Same as serum	Less than serum
pH[d]	7.4-7.5	<7.4

LDH, Lactate dehydrogenase; *RBCs,* red blood cells; *WBCs,* white blood cells.
[a]Always obtain serum for glucose, LDH, protein, amylase, etc.
[b]Not required to meet all of the following criteria to be considered an exudate.
[c]In peritoneal fluid, WBC >800/mm^3 suggests peritonitis.
[d]Collect anaerobically in a heparinized syringe.
NOTE: Amylase >5000 U/mL or pleural fluid:serum ratio >1 suggests pancreatitis.

TABLE 24-3

EVALUATION OF CEREBROSPINAL FLUID

	WBC Count	Mean % PMNs
Preterm	0-25 WBCs/mm^3	57%
Term	0-22 WBCs/mm^3	61%
Child	0-7 WBCs/mm^3	5%
GLUCOSE		
Preterm	24-63 mg/dL	1.3-3.5 mmol/L
Term	34-119 mg/dL	1.9-6.6 mmol/L
Child	40-80 mg/dL	2.2-4.4 mmol/L
CSF GLUCOSE/BLOOD GLUCOSE		
Preterm	55%-105%	
Term	44%-128%	
Child	50%	
LACTIC ACID DEHYDROGENASE		
Normal range	5-30 U/L (or about 10% of serum value)	
MYELIN BASIC PROTEIN	<4 ng/mL	
OPENING PRESSURE		
(Lateral recumbent)		
Newborn	80-110 mmH$_2$O	
Infant/child	<200 mmH$_2$O	
Respiratory variations	5-10 mmH$_2$O	
PROTEIN		
Preterm	65-150 mg/dL	0.65-1.5 g/L
Term	20-170 mg/dL	0.20-1.7 g/L
Child	5-40 mg/dL	0.05-0.40 g/L

Modified from Oski FA. Principles and practice of pediatrics, 3rd ed. Philadelphia: JB Lippincott; 1999.
CSF, Cerebrospinal fluid; *PMNs,* polymorphonuclear lymphocytes; *WBC,* white blood cell.

TABLE 24-4

EVALUATION OF SYNOVIAL FLUID

Group	Condition	Color/Clarity	Viscosity	Mucin clot	WBC Count	PMNs (%)	Miscellaneous Findings
Noninflammatory	Normal	Yellow/clear	VH	G	<200	<25	—
	Traumatic arthritis	Xanthochromic/ turbid	H	F-G	<2000	<25	Debris
Inflammatory	Osteoarthritis	Yellow/clear	H	F-G	1000	<25	—
	SLE	Yellow/clear	M	M	5000	10	LE cells
	Rheumatic fever	Yellow/cloudy	D	F	5000	10-50	—
	Juvenile rheumatoid arthritis	Yellow/cloudy	D	Poor	15,000-20,000	75	—
	Reiter's syndrome and Lyme disease	Yellow/opaque	D	Poor	20,000	80	Reiter's cells in Reiter's syndrome
Pyogenic	Tuberculous arthritis	Yellow-white/cloudy	D	Poor	25,000	50-60	Acid-fast bacilli
	Septic arthritis	Serosanguineous/ turbid	D	Poor	50,000-300,000	>75	Low glucose, bacteria

From Cassidy JT, Petty RE. Textbook of pediatric rheumatology, 3rd ed. Philadelphia: WB Saunders; 1995.

D, Decreased; *F,* fair; *G,* good; *H,* high; *M,* moderate; *PMNs,* polymorphonuclear neutrophils (leukocytes); *SLE,* systemic lupus erythematosus; *VH,* very high.

III. CONVERSION FORMULAS

A. TEMPERATURE

1. **To convert degrees Celsius to degrees Fahrenheit:** ([9/5] × Temperature) + 32.
2. **To convert degrees Fahrenheit to degrees Celsius:** (Temperature − 32) × (5/9).

B. LENGTH AND WEIGHT

1. **Length:** To convert inches to centimeters, multiply by 2.54.
2. **Weight:** To convert pounds to kilograms, divide by 2.2.

REFERENCES

1. Meites S, editor. Pediatric clinical chemistry, 2nd and 3rd eds. Washington, DC: American Association for Clinical Chemistry; 1981.
2. Burtis CA, Ashwood ER. Tietz textbook of clinical chemistry, 3rd ed. Philadelphia: WB Saunders; 1999.
3. Soldin SJ et al. Pediatric reference ranges, 3rd ed. Washington: AACC Press; 1999.
4. Lundberg GD. SI unit implementation: the next step. JAMA 1988; 260:73.
5. Wallach J. Interpretation of diagnostic tests. Boston: Little, Brown & Co; 1992.
6. Berkow R. The Merck manual of diagnosis and therapy. Rahway, NJ: Merck Research Laboratories; 1992.
7. Rogers M. Textbook of pediatric intensive care, 2nd ed. Baltimore: Williams & Wilkins, 1992.
8. Summary of the NCEP adult treatment panel II report: highlights of the report of the expert panel on blood and cholesterol levels in children and adolescents, 1991, U.S. Department of Health and Human Services. JAMA 1993; 269.
9. Nechyba LD, Nechyba AS, Gunn P. Surviving pediatric chief residency at Hopkins: patience and virtue. 2001-2002, Baltimore.
10. Behrman RE et al. Nelson textbook of pediatrics, 15th ed. Philadelphia: WB Saunders; 1996.

24

BLOOD CHEMISTRIES AND BODY FLUIDS

BIOSTATISTICS AND EVIDENCE-BASED MEDICINE

Veronica L. Gunn, MD, MPH

I. BIOSTATISTICS FOR MEDICAL LITERATURE

A. STUDY DESIGN COMPARISON (Table 25-1)

B. MEASUREMENTS IN CLINICAL STUDIES (Table 25-2)

1. Prevalence

a. Proportion of study population who have a disease (at one point or period in time).

b. Number of old cases and new cases divided by total population.

c. In cross-sectional studies (use Table 25-2): $(A + B)/(A + B + C + D)$.

2. Incidence

a. Number of people in study population who newly develop an outcome (disease) per total study population per given time period.

b. Number of new cases divided by the total population over a given time period (use Table 25-2).

c. For cohort studies and clinical trials: $(A + B)/(A + B + C + D)$.

3. Relative risk (RR)

a. Ratio of incidence of disease among people with risk factor to incidence of disease among people without risk factor.

b. For cohort studies or clinical trials (use Table 25-2): $[A/(A + C)]/[B/(B + D)]$.

c. RR = 1 means no effect of exposure (or treatment) on outcome (or disease). RR <1 indicates exposure or treatment protective against disease. RR >1 indicates exposure/treatment increases probability of outcome/disease.

4. Odds ratio (OR)

a. For case-control studies, ratio of odds of having risk factor in people with disease (A/B) to odds of having risk factor in people without disease (C/D), or $(A/B)/(C/D) = (A \times D)/(B \times C)$. (Use Table 25-2.)

b. Good estimate of RR if disease is rare. OR = 1 means no risk factor-disease association. OR >1 suggests risk factor associated with increased disease, and OR <1 suggests risk factor protective against disease.

5. α (Significance level of statistical test)

a. Probability of finding a statistical association by chance alone when there truly is no association (type I error).

b. Often set at 0.05; low α especially important when interpreting a finding of an association.

6. Power (of a statistical test)

a. β = Probability of finding no statistical association when there truly is one (type II error).

b. Power = 1-β = Probability of finding a statistical association when there truly is one.

TABLE 25-1
STUDY DESIGN COMPARISON

Design Type	Definition	Advantages	Disadvantages
Case-control (often called *retrospective*)	Define diseased subjects (cases) and nondiseased subjects (controls); compare proportion of cases with exposure (risk factor) with proportion of controls with exposure (risk factor).	Good for rare diseases Smaller sample size Faster (not followed over time) Less expensive	Highest potential for biases (recall, selection and others) Weak evidence for causality No prevalence, PPV, NPV
Cohort (usually prospective; occasionally retrospective)	In study population, define exposed group (with risk factor) and nonexposed group (without risk factor). Over time, compare proportion of exposed group with outcome (disease), with proportion of nonexposed group with outcome (disease).	Defines incidence Stronger evidence for causality Decreases biases (sampling, measurement, reporting)	Expensive Long study times May not be feasible for rare diseases/ outcomes Factors related to exposure and outcome may falsely alter effect of exposure on outcome (confounding)
Cross-sectional	In study population, concurrently measure outcome (disease) and risk factor. Compare proportion of diseased group with risk factor, with proportion of nondiseased group with risk factor.	Defines prevalence Short time to complete	Selection bias Weak evidence for causality
Clinical trial (experiment)	In study population, assign (randomly) subjects to receive treatment or receive no treatment. Compare rate of outcome (e.g., disease cure) between treatment and nontreatment groups.	Randomized blinded trial is gold standard Randomization reduces confounding Best evidence for causality	Expensive Risks of experimental treatments in humans Longer time Bad for rare outcomes/ diseases

NPV, Negative predictive value; *PPV*, positive predictive value.

TABLE 25-2

GRID FOR CALCULATIONS IN CLINICAL STUDIES

Disease or Outcome	Exposure or Risk Factor or Treatment	
	Positive	Negative
Positive	A	B
Negative	C	D

TABLE 25-3

GRID FOR EVALUATING A CLINICAL TEST

Test Result	Disease Status	
	Positive	Negative
Positive	A (true positive)	B (false positive)
Negative	C (false negative)	D (true negative)

c. Power often set at 0.80; high power especially important when interpreting a finding of no association.

7. **Sample size**

Number of subjects required in a clinical study to achieve a sufficiently high power and sufficiently low α to obtain a clinically relevant result.

8. ***p* value**

a. Probability of a finding by chance alone.

b. If *p* value is < preset α level (often 0.05), then finding is interpreted as unlikely to be due to chance simply from sampling.

9. **Confidence interval (95%)**

95% probability that the reported interval contains the true value.

C. MEASUREMENTS FOR EVALUATING A CLINICAL TEST (Table 25-3)

1. **Sensitivity (Sens)**

a. Proportion of all diseased who have positive test (use Table 25-3): $A/(A + C)$.

b. Use highly sensitive test to help exclude a disease. (Low false-negative rate. High likelihood ratio [LR] negative. This is good for screening.)

2. **Specificity (Spec)**

a. Proportion of all nondiseased who have a negative test (use Table 25-3): $D/(B + D)$.

b. Use highly specific test to help confirm a disease. (Low false-positive rate. High LR positive.)

3. **Positive predictive value (PPV)**

a. Proportion of all those with positive tests who truly have disease (use Table 25-3): $A/(A + B)$.

b. Increased PPV with higher disease prevalence and higher specificity (and, to a lesser degree, higher sensitivity).

4. **Negative predictive value (NPV)**

a. Proportion of all those with negative tests who truly do not have disease (use Table 25-3): $D/(C + D)$.

b. Increased NPV with lower prevalence (rarer disease) and higher sensitivity.

5. Likelihood ratio (LR)

a. LR positive: Ability of positive test result to confirm diseased status: LR positive = (Sens)/(1 − Spec).

b. LR negative: Ability of negative test result to confirm nondiseased status: LR negative = (Spec)/(1 − Sens). [Alternative LR negative = (1- Sens)/ Spec.]

c. Good tests have LR ≥10. (Good tests ≤0.1 if using alternative LR negative formula.) Physical examination findings often have LR of about 2.

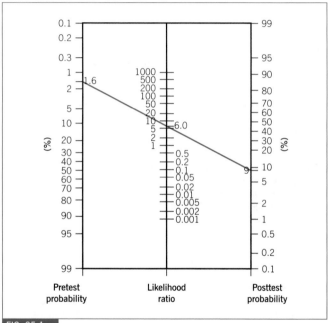

FIG. 25-1

Nomogram for calculating the change in probability by applying tests with known LRs. For example, the prevalence (i.e., pretest probability) of occult bacteremia in a well-appearing 3- to 36-month-old with temperature ≥39° C without source is 1.6%. LR positive for WBC >20 × 10^9/L is 6.0. For such infants, then, with a WBC >20 × 10^9/L, you can use the nomogram to determine the increased probability from the positive test. Anchor a straight edge at 1.6% on the left pretest probability column and direct the straight edge through the central column at the LR of 6.0. The straight edge will intersect the right column with your answer to give a posttest probability of approximately 9%. It is then up to you to decide the clinical importance of a 9% probability of bacteremia. *(From Fagan TJ. N Engl J Med 1975; 293:257 and Lee GM, Harper MB. Arch Pediatr Adolesc Med 1998; 152:624-628.)*

d. LR should not be affected by disease prevalence. LR can be used to calculate increase in probability of disease from baseline prevalence with positive test (LR positive) and decrease in probability of disease from baseline prevalence with negative test (using alternative LR negative) for any level of disease prevalence (Fig. 25-1).

II. EVIDENCE-BASED MEDICINE

A. DEFINITION

Evidence-Based Medicine (EBM) is a method of using critically analyzed or peer-reviewed information to guide clinical decision making.

B. SAMPLE LIKELIHOOD RATIOS

NOTE: These sample likelihood ratios are derived from a variety of recent studies. These are not meant to be exhaustive nor reflective of all available areas in which LRs would be helpful. Rather, these are used as examples of how to utilize available clinical tests to make educated decisions regarding patient care. Table 25-4 can be used as an example of how to use an LR. Positive nitrites on urinalysis are 26.5 times more likely to be found in a person with urinary tract infection (UTI), than in a person without UTI. Conversely, a patient with neither positive leukocyte esterase, nitrites, nor microscopy on urinalysis is *very unlikely* to have a UTI. In calculating LRs, if the specificity or sensitivity is 100%, the LR+ or LR– respectively, is an infinitely large number, ∞. One should interpret the LRs in such instances as an indication of a strongly positive (or negative) LR.

1. Components of the urinalysis (Table 25-4).
2. Denver Developmental Screening Test as a predictor of outcome (Table 25-5).
3. Using ligase chain reaction (LCR) for detection of chlamydia and gonorrhea in urine (Table 25-6).
4. Capillary blood lead levels as screening tool for plumbism (Table 25-7).

TABLE 25-4

SENSITIVITY, SPECIFICITY, AND LIKELIHOOD RATIOS FOR COMPONENTS OF THE URINALYSIS

Test	Sensitivity (%)	Specificity (%)	LR+	LR–
Leukocyte esterase	83	78	3.8	4.6
Nitrite	53	98	**26.5**	2.1
Leukocyte esterase *or* nitrite positive	93	72	3.3	**10.3**
Microscopy: WBCs	73	81	3.8	3.0
Microscopy: Bacteria	81	83	4.8	4.4
Leukocyte esterase *or* nitrite *or* microscopy positive	99.8	70	3.3	**350**

From: The AAP policy statement on urinary tract infections in febrile infants and young children. American Academy of Pediatrics. Available online at: http://www.aap.org/policy/ac9830.htm.

TABLE 25-5

SENSITIVITY, SPECIFICITY, AND LIKELIHOOD RATIOS FOR ASPECTS OF THE DENVER DEVELOPMENTAL SCREENING TEST (DDST)[a]

Study	Assessment	Sensitivity (%)	Specificity (%)	LR+	LR−
Pooled DDST data from five studies[b,c]	School performance	20	94	3.3	1.2
Comparison of DDST and speech-language screening[d]	Speech-language skills	46.2	100	∞[e]	1.8

[a]One should note that the DDST was not designed to predict developmental outcomes; however, this is often the manner in which this tool is used by providers.
[b]Data from Greer S, Bauchner H, Zuckerman B. Dev Med Child Neurol 1989; 31:774-781.
[c]Data from Meisels SJ. Pediatrics 1989; 83:578-585.
[d]Data from Borowitz KC, Glascoe FP. Pediatrics 1986; 78:1075-1078.
[e]N = 71 patients.

TABLE 25-6

SENSITIVITY, SPECIFICITY, AND LIKELIHOOD RATIOS FOR DETECTION OF *CHLAMYDIA TRACHOMATIS* AND *NEISSERIA GONORRHEA* IN URINE USING LIGASE CHAIN REACTION VERSUS CERVICAL CULTURE

Infection	Test	Sensitivity (%)	Specificity (%)	LR+	LR−
Chlamydia[a]					
HIV positive	LCR	86.2	95.6	**19.6**	6.9
HIV negative	LCR	100	100	∞[b]	∞[b]
N. gonorrhea[a]					
HIV positive	LCR	91.6	99.4	**1527**	11.8
HIV negative	LCR	100	100	∞[c]	∞[c]
N. gonorrhea[d]	LCR	88.2	100	∞[e]	8.5
	Culture	82.3	98.9	**74.8**	5.6

For both *Chlamydia trachomatis* and *N. gonorrhea,* a positive urine LCR test is strongly indicative of infection.
[a]Data from Perlalta L et al. J Adol Health 2001; 29S:87-92.
[b]Note that N = 82 for this study population subgroup, with only 10 testing positive for *Chlamydia trachomatis.*
[c]Note that N = 82 for this study population subgroup with only 2 testing positive for *N. gonorrhea.*
[d]Data from Xu K et al. Sex Trans Dis 1998; 25:533-538.
[e]N = 330 patients

TABLE 25-7

SENSITIVITY, SPECIFICITY, AND LIKELIHOOD RATIOS FOR CAPILLARY PEDIATRIC BLOOD LEAD SCREENING

Sample	Cutoff (mcg/dL)	Sensitivity (%)	Specificity (%)	LR+	LR−
Capillary[a]	≥20	88	100	∞[b]	8.3
Capillary[c]	≥10	94	99	94	16.5
	≥20	78	100	∞[d]	4.5

These values were obtained using comparable sampling methods, and the correlation coefficient of capillary samples with venous samples was 0.96 in both studies. Patients with a capillary lead level of ≥10 mcg/dL are more likely to truly have plumbism than patients without similar capillary lead results.

[a]Data from Schlenker TL et al. JAMA 1994; 271:1346-1348.
[b]N = 39 patients
[c]Data from Holtrop TG et al. Arch Pediatr Adolesc Med 1998; 152:455-458.
[d]N = 120 patients

C. WEBSITES

1. www.welch.jhu.edu/internet/ebr.html
2. www.pedsccm.wustl.edu/EBJ/EB_Resources.html
3. www.tripdatabase.com
4. www.cochranelibrary.com
5. www.guideline.gov/body_home_nf.asp?view=home
6. www.ncbi.nlm.nih.gov/entrez/query/stastic/clinical.html

25

BIOSTATISTICS AND EVIDENCE-BASED MEDICINE

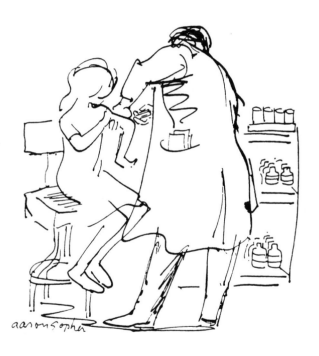

DRUG DOSES

Carlton Lee, PharmD, MPH; Christian Nechyba, MD;
and Veronica L. Gunn, MD, MPH

I. NOTE TO THE READER

The authors have made every attempt to check dosages and medical content for accuracy. Because of the incomplete data on pediatric dosing, many drug dosages will be modified after the publication of this text. We recommended that the reader check product information and published literature for changes in dosing, especially for newer medicines.

26

II. SAMPLE ENTRY

Pregnancy: Refer to explanation of pregnancy categories (on facing page).

Breast: Refer to explanation of breast-feeding categories (on facing page).

Kidney: Indicates need for caution or need for dose adjustment in renal failure (see also Chapter 29).

How supplied

ACETAZOLAMIDE ← Generic name
Diamox ← Trade name and other names
Carbonic anhydrase inhibitor, diuretic ← Drug category

Yes 1 C

Tabs: 125, 250 mg
Suspension: 25, 30, 50 mg/mL 🗹 ← Mortar and pestle: Indicates need for extemporaneous compounding by a pharmacist
Caps (sustained release): 500 mg
Inj (sodium): 500 mg/5 mL
Contains 2.05 mEq Na/500 mg drug

Diuretic (PO, IV)
Child: 5 mg/kg/dose QD-QOD
Adult: 250–375 mg/dose QD-QOD
Glaucoma
Child: 20–40 mg/kg/24 hr ÷ Q6 hr IM/IV; 8–30 mg/kg/24 hr ÷ Q6–8 hr PO
Adult: 1000 mg/24 hr ÷ Q6 hr PO; for rapid decrease in intraocular pressure, administer 500 mg/dose IV
Seizures: 8–30 mg/kg/24 hr ÷ Q6–12 hr PO
Max. dose: 1 g/24 hr
Urine alkalinization: 5 mg/kg/dose PO repeated BID-TID
Management of hydrocephalus: Start with 20 mg/kg/24 hr ÷ Q8 hr PO/IV; may increase to 100 mg/kg/24 hr up to a **max. dose** of 2 g/24 hr

Drug dosing

Contraindicated in hepatic failure, severe renal failure (GFR <10 mL/min), and hypersensitivity to sulfonamides.

$T_{1/2}$: 2–6 hr; **do not use** sustained-release capsules in seizures; IM injection may be painful; bicarbonate replacement therapy may be required during long-term use (see *Citrate* or *Sodium Bicarbonate*).

Possible side effects (more likely with long-term therapy) include GI irritation, paresthesias, sedation, hypokalemia, acidosis, reduced urate secretion, aplastic anemia, polyuria, and development of renal calculi.

May increase toxicity of cyclosporine. May decrease the effects of salicylates and phenobarbital. False-positive urinary protein may occur with several assays. **Adjust dose in renal failure (see p. 947).**

Brief remarks about side effects, drug interactions, precautions, therapeutic monitoring, and other relevant information

III. EXPLANATION OF BREAST-FEEDING CATEGORIES

See sample entry.

1 Compatible
2 Use with caution
3 Unknown with concerns
X Contraindicated
? Safety not established

IV. EXPLANATION OF PREGNANCY CATEGORIES

A Adequate studies in pregnant women have not demonstrated a risk to the fetus in the first trimester of pregnancy, and there is no evidence of risk in later trimesters.
B Animal studies have not demonstrated a risk to the fetus, but there are no adequate studies in pregnant women; or animal studies have shown an adverse effect, but adequate studies in pregnant women have not demonstrated a risk to the fetus during the first trimester of pregnancy, and there is no evidence of risk in later trimesters.
C Animal studies have shown an adverse effect on the fetus, but there are no adequate studies in humans; or there are no animal reproduction studies and no adequate studies in humans.
D There is evidence of human fetal risk, but the potential benefits from the use of the drug in pregnant women may be acceptable despite its potential risks.
X Studies in animals or humans demonstrate fetal abnormalities or adverse reaction; reports indicate evidence of fetal risk. The risk of use in pregnant woman clearly outweighs any possible benefit.

26

DRUG DOSES

ABACAVIR SULFATE

Ziagen, 1592
*Antiviral agent, nucleoside analogue reverse transcriptase
inhibitor*

No   3   C

Tabs: 300 mg
Oral solution: 20 mg/mL (240 mL)
In combination with zidovudine (AZT) and lamivudine (3TC) as Trizivir:
 Tabs: 300 mg abacavir + 300 mg zidovudine + 150 mg lamivudine

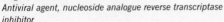

 1–3 mo (investigational dose): 8 mg/kg/dose PO BID
 3 mo–16 yr: 8 mg/kg/dose PO BID; **max. dose:** 300 mg BID
 Adult: 300 mg/dose PO BID
Trizivir:
 Adolescents and adults (≥40 kg): 1 tablet PO BID

 Fatal hypersensitivity reactions (5%) have been associated with signs or symptoms of fever, skin rash, fatigue, GI symptoms (nausea, vomiting, diarrhea, or
 abdominal pain), and respiratory symptoms (cough, dyspnea, and pharyngitis).
If signs or symptoms are present, discontinue drug immediately and monitor closely.
Do not restart medication following hypersensitivity reaction because more severe
life-threatening symptoms will recur. Adverse reactions not related to hypersensitivity
include nausea, vomiting, diarrhea, decreased appetite, and insomnia. Lactic acidosis
and severe hepatomegaly with steatosis have also been reported.

 Adolescent dosing: Patients in early puberty (Tanner I-II) should be dosed with
pediatric regimens and those in late puberty (Tanner V) should be dosed with adult
regimens. Adolescents who are at the midst of their growth spurt (Tanner III females
and Tanner IV males) can be dosed by either pediatric or adult regimen with close
monitoring of efficacy and toxicity.

 Use in combination with other antiretrovirals. Drug is primarily metabolized by
alcohol dehydrogenase and glucuronyl transferase. Ethanol decreases the elimination
of abacavir. Pharmacokinetic properties in renal or hepatic impairment are
incompletely understood. Doses may be administered with food or on an empty
stomach.

ACETAMINOPHEN

Tylenol, Tempra, Panadol, Feverall, Anacin-3, and others
Analgesic, antipyretic

Yes   1   B

Tabs: 160, 325, 500, 650 mg
Extended-release tabs: 650 mg
Chewable tabs: 80 mg

Continued

ACETAMINOPHEN *continued*

Infant drops, solution/suspension: 80 mg/0.8 mL
Child solution/suspension: 160, 166.7 mg/5 mL
Elixir: 80, 120, 160, 325 mg/5 mL
Caplet: 160, 500, 650 mg
Gelcap: 500 mg
Caps: 325, 500 mg
Sprinkle caps: 80, 160 mg
Suppositories: 80, 120, 125, 300, 325, 650 mg
(Combination product with Codeine, see *Codeine and Acetaminophen*)

See remarks for additional information on higher rectal dosing.
Neonates: 10–15 mg/kg/dose PO/PR Q6–8 hr
Pediatric: 10–15 mg/kg/dose PO/PR Q4–6 hr
Dosing by age:
   0–3 mo: 40 mg/dose
   4–11 mo: 80 mg/dose
   12–24 mo: 120 mg/dose
   2–3 yr: 160 mg/dose
   4–5 yr: 240 mg/dose
   6–8 yr: 320 mg/dose
   9–10 yr: 400 mg/dose
   11–12 yr: 480 mg/dose
Adult: 325–650 mg/dose
Max. dose: 4 g/24 hr, 5 doses/24 hr

Does not possess antiinflammatory activity. Use with **caution** in patients with known G6PD deficiency.
   For rectal dosing, some may advocate the use of a 40–45 mg/kg/dose loading dose.
   $T_{1/2}$: 1–3 hr, 2–5 hr in neonates; metabolized in the liver; see p. 24 for management of overdosage.
   Some preparations contain alcohol (7%–10%) and/or phenylalanine; all suspensions should be shaken before use.
   May decrease the activity of lamotrigine and increase the activity of zidovudine. Rifampin and anticholinergic agents (e.g., scopolamine) may decrease the effect of acetaminophen. Increased risk for hepatotoxicity may occur with barbiturates, carbamazepine, phenytoin, carmustine (with high acetaminophen doses), and chronic alcohol use.
   Adjust dose in renal failure (see p. 947).

ACETAZOLAMIDE

Diamox
Carbonic anhydrase inhibitor, diuretic

Yes   1   C

Tabs: 125, 250 mg
Suspension: 25, 30, 50 mg/mL

Continued

ACETAZOLAMIDE *continued*

Caps (sustained release): 500 mg
Inj (sodium): 500 mg/5 mL
Contains 2.05 mEq Na/500 mg drug

Diuretic (PO, IV)
  Child: 5 mg/kg/dose QD-QOD
  Adult: 250–375 mg/dose QD-QOD
Glaucoma
  Child: 20–40 mg/kg/24 hr ÷ Q6 hr IM/IV; 8–30 mg/kg/24 hr ÷ Q6–8 hr PO
  Adult: 1000 mg/24 hr ÷ Q6 hr PO; for rapid decrease in intraocular pressure, administer 500 mg/dose IV
Seizures: 8–30 mg/kg/24 hr ÷ Q6–12 hr PO
Max. dose: 1 g/24 hr
Urine alkalinization: 5 mg/kg/dose PO repeated BID-TID
Management of hydrocephalus: Start with 20 mg/kg/24 hr ÷ Q8 hr PO/IV; may increase to 100 mg/kg/24 hr up to a **max. dose** of 2 g/24 hr

Contraindicated in hepatic failure, severe renal failure (GFR <10 mL/min), and hypersensitivity to sulfonamides.

$T_{1/2}$: 2–6 hr; **do not use** sustained-release capsules in seizures; IM injection may be painful; bicarbonate replacement therapy may be required during long-term use (see *Citrate* or *Sodium Bicarbonate*).

Possible side effects (more likely with long-term therapy) include GI irritation, paresthesias, sedation, hypokalemia, acidosis, reduced urate secretion, aplastic anemia, polyuria, and development of renal calculi.

May increase toxicity of cyclosporine. May decrease the effects of salicylates and phenobarbital. False-positive urinary protein may occur with several assays. **Adjust dose in renal failure (see p. 947).**

ACETYLCYSTEINE
Mucomyst, Mucomyst 10 IV
Mucolytic, antidote for acetaminophen toxicity

No   ?   B

Solution: 100 mg/mL (10%) or 200 mg/mL (20%) (4, 10, 30 mL)

For acetaminophen poisoning, see Chapter 2, p. 24.
  Meconium ileus: 5–10 mL/kg of 10% solution PR by soft rubber catheter. This may be given up to Q6 hr.
Nebulizer:
  Children: 3–5 mL of 20% solution (diluted with equal volume of H_2O, or sterile saline to equal 10%), or 6–10 mL of 10% solution; administer TID-QID.
  Adolescents: 5–10 mL of 10% or 20% solution; administer TID-QID.

Continued

For nebulized use, give inhaled bronchodilator 10–15 min before use and follow with postural drainage and/or suctioning after acetylcysteine administration. Prior hydration is essential for meconium ileus treatment.

May induce bronchospasm, stomatitis, drowsiness, rhinorrhea, nausea, vomiting, and hemoptysis.

ACTH
See Corticotropin

ACYCLOVIR
Zovirax
Antiviral   Yes   1   C

Caps: 200 mg
Tabs: 400, 800 mg
Suspension: 200 mg/5 mL
Ointment: 5% (15 g)
Inj. (with sodium): 500 mg/10 mL, 1000 mg/20 mL
Contains 4.2 mEq Na/1 g drug

IMMUNOCOMPETENT:
Neonatal HSV and HSV encephalitis:
   <35 weeks postconceptional age: 40 mg/kg/24 hr ÷ Q12 hr IV × 14–21 days
   ≥35 weeks postconceptional age: 60 mg/kg/24 hr ÷ Q8 hr IV × 14–21 days
Mucocutaneous HSV (including genital):
   Initial infection:
      IV: 15 mg/kg/24 hr or 750 mg/m^2/24 hr ÷ Q8 hr × 5–7 days
      PO: 1200 mg/24 hr ÷ Q8 hr × 7–10 days with a **max. dose** in children at 80 mg/kg/24 hr ÷ Q6–8 hr
   Recurrence:
      PO: 1200 mg/24 hr ÷ Q8 hr or 1600 mg/24 hr ÷ Q12 hr × 5 days with a **max. dose** in children at 80 mg/kg/24 hr ÷ Q6–8 hr
   Chronic suppressive therapy:
      PO: 800–1000 mg/24 hr ÷ 2–5 × day for up to 1 year with a **max. dose** in children at 80 mg/kg/24 hr ÷ Q6–8 hr
Zoster:
   IV: 30 mg/kg/24 hr or 1500 mg/m^2/24 hr ÷ Q8 hr × 7–10 days
   PO: 4000 mg/24 hr ÷ 5 times/24 hr × 5–7 days for patients ≥12 yr
Varicella:
   IV: 30 mg/kg/24 hr or 1500 mg/m^2/24 hr ÷ Q8 hr × 7–10 days
   PO: 80 mg/kg/24 hr ÷ QID × 5 days (begin treatment at earliest signs/symptoms); **max. dose:** 3200 mg/24 hr

Continued

ACYCLOVIR *continued*

Max. dose of oral acyclovir in children = 80 mg/kg/24 hr
IMMUNOCOMPROMISED:
HSV:
   IV: 750–1500 mg/m^2/24 hr ÷ Q8 hr × 7–14 days
   PO: 1000 mg/24 hr ÷ 3–5 times/24 hr × 7–14 days
HSV prophylaxis:
   IV: 750 mg/m^2/24 hr ÷ Q8 hr during risk period
   PO: 600–1000 mg/24 hr ÷ 3–5 times/24 hr during risk period
Varicella or zoster:
   IV: Same as immunocompetent dosing × 7–10 days
   PO: 250–600 mg/m^2/dose 4–5 times/24 hr
CMV prophylaxis:
   IV: 1500 mg/m^2/24 hr ÷ Q8 hr during risk period
   PO: 800–3200 mg/24 hr ÷ Q6–24 hr during risk period
Max. dose of oral acyclovir in children = 80 mg/kg/24 hr
TOPICAL:
   Apply 0.5-inch ribbon of 5% ointment for 4-inch square surface area 6 times per
   day × 7 days.

See most recent edition of the AAP *Red Book* for further details. Oral absorption is unpredictable (15%–30%). Use ideal body weight for obese patients when calculating dosages. Resistant strains of HSV and VZV have been reported in immunocompromised patients (e.g., advanced HIV infection).

Adequate hydration and slow (1 hr) IV administration are essential to prevent crystallization in renal tubules; **dose alteration necessary in patients with impaired renal function (see p. 938).**

Can cause renal impairment; has been infrequently associated with headache, vertigo, insomnia, encephalopathy, GI tract irritation, rash, urticaria, arthralgia, fever, and adverse hematologic effects. Probenecid decreases acyclovir renal clearance.

ADENOSINE

Adenocard
Antiarrhythmic

No ? C

Inj: 3 mg/mL (2, 5 mL)

Supraventricular tachycardia:
  Children: 0.1–0.2 mg/kg rapid IV push over 1–2 seconds; may increase dose by
  0.05-mg/kg increments every 2 min to **max.** of 0.25 mg/kg (up to 12 mg), or
until termination of SVT. **Max. single dose:** 12 mg
Adolescents and adults ≥ 50 kg: 6 mg rapid IV push over 1-2 seconds; if no
response after 1–2 min, give 12 mg rapid IV push. May repeat a second 12-mg
dose after 1–2 minutes if required. **Maximum single dose:** 12 mg

Continued

ADENOSINE *continued*

Alternate dosing for children <50 kg: 0.05–0.1 mg/kg rapid IV bolus given centrally or peripherally followed by saline flush. If conversion of SVT does not occur within 1 to 2 min, give additional bolus injections at incrementally higher doses, increasing the amount given by 0.05 to 0.1 mg/kg (follow each bolus with a saline flush). Continue until sinus rhythm is established or a **max. single dose** of 0.3 mg/kg is used.

Contraindicated in second- and third-degree AV block or sick-sinus syndrome unless pacemaker placed.

Follow each dose with NS flush. $T_{1/2}$: <10 sec.

May precipitate bronchoconstriction, especially in asthmatics. Side effects include transient asystole, facial flushing, headache, shortness of breath, dyspnea, nausea, chest pain, and lightheadedness.

Carbamazepine and dipyridamole may increase the effects/toxicity of adenosine. Methylxanthines (e.g., caffeine and theophylline) may decrease the effects of adenosine.

ALBUMIN, HUMAN

Albuminar, Albutein, Buminate, Plasbumin, Normal Serum
Albumin (Human), and others

Blood product derivative, plasma volume expander

No ? C

Inj: 5% (50 mg/mL) (5, 10, 20, 50, 250, 500, 1000 mL) ; 25% (250 mg/mL) (20, 50, 100 mL); both concentrations contain 130–160 mEq Na/L

Hypoproteinemia:
  Children: 0.5–1 g/kg/dose IV over 30–120 min; repeat Q1–2 days PRN
  Adult: 25 g/dose IV over 30–120 min; repeat Q1–2 days PRN
Hypovolemia:
  Children: 0.5–1 g/kg/dose IV rapid infusion
  Adult: 25 g/dose IV rapid infusion; may repeat PRN
Max. dose: 6 g/kg/24 hr or 250 g/48 hr

Contraindicated in cases of CHF or severe anemia; rapid infusion may cause fluid overload; hypersensitivity reactions may occur; may cause rapid increase in serum sodium levels.

Caution: 25% concentration contraindicated in preterm infants because of risk of IVH. For infusion, use 5 micron filter or larger. Both 5% and 25% products are isotonic but differ in oncotic effects. Dilutions of the 25% product should be made with D_5W or NS.

ALBUTEROL

Proventil, Ventolin, Ventolin HFA (aerosol inhaler), AccuNeb
(prediluted nebulized solution)

No   2   C

Beta-2-adrenergic agonist

Tabs: 2, 4 mg
Sustained release tabs: 4, 8 mg
Oral solution: 2 mg/5 mL (473 mL)
Aerosol inhaler: 90 mcg/actuation (200 actuations/inhaler) (17 g)
Rotacaps for inhalation: 200 mcg/capsule
Nebulization solution: 0.5% (5 mg/mL) (20 mL)
Prediluted nebulized solution: 0.63 mg in 3 mL NS, 1.25 mg in 3 mL NS, and
2.5 mg in 3 mL NS (0.083%)

Inhalations:
  Aerosol (MDI): 1–2 puffs (90–180 mcg) Q4–6 hr PRN
    Rotacaps: 200–400 mcg Q4–6 hr
Nebulization:
    <1 yr: 0.05–0.15 mg/kg/dose Q4–6 hr
    1–5 yr: 1.25–2.5 mg/dose Q4–6 hr
    5–12 yr: 2.5 mg/dose Q4–6 hr
    >12 yr: 2.5–5 mg/dose Q6 hr
For use in acute exacerbations, more aggressive dosing may be employed.
Oral:
  Children <6 yr: 0.3 mg/kg/24 hr PO ÷ TID; **max. dose:** 12 mg/24 hr
  6–11 yr: 6 mg/24 hr PO ÷ TID; **max. dose:** 24 mg/24 hr
  >12 yr and adults: 2–4 mg/dose PO TID-QID; **max. dose:** 32 mg/24 hr

Nebulization may be given more frequently than indicated. In such cases,
consider cardiac monitoring and monitoring of serum potassium. Systemic
effects are dose related. Please verify the concentration of the nebulization
solution used.

Use of oral dosage form is discouraged due to increased side effects and decreased
efficacy compared to inhaled formulations.

Possible side effects include tachycardia, palpitations, tremor, insomnia,
nervousness, nausea, and headache.

The use of tube spacers or chambers may enhance efficacy of the metered dose
inhalers. Proventil HFA is a CFC-free metered dose inhaler.

For explanation of icons, see p. 572.

ALLOPURINOL

Zyloprim, Alloprim, and others
Uric acid lowering agent, xanthine oxidase inhibitor

Yes   1   C

Tabs: 100, 300 mg
Suspension: 10, 20 mg/mL
Inj (Alloprim): 500 mg

Child:
  Oral: 10 mg/kg/24 hr PO ÷ BID-QID; **max. dose:** 800 mg/24 hr
  Inj: 200 mg/m^2/24 hr IV ÷ Q 6–12 hr; **max. dose:** 600 mg/24 hr
Adult:
  Oral: 200–800 mg/24 hr PO ÷ BID-TID
  Inj: 200–400 mg/m^2/24 hr IV ÷ Q 6–12 hr; **max. dose:** 600 mg/24 hr
For use in tumor lysis syndrome, see Chapter 21, p. 508.

Adjust dose in renal insufficiency (see p. 947). Must maintain adequate urine output and alkaline urine.
  Drug interactions: Increases serum theophylline level; may increase the incidence of rash with ampicillin and amoxicillin; and increases risk of hypersensitivity reactions with ACE inhibitors and thiazide diuretics.
  Side effects include rash, neuritis, hepatotoxicity, GI disturbance, bone marrow suppression, and drowsiness.
  IV dosage form is very alkaline and must be **diluted to a minimum concentration of** 6 mg/mL and infused over 30 min.

ALPROSTADIL

Prostin VR, Prostaglandin E$_1$, PGE$_1$
Prostaglandin E$_1$, vasodilator

No   ?   X

Inj: 500 mcg/mL (contains dehydrated alcohol)

Neonates:
  Initial: 0.05–0.1 mcg/kg/min. Advance to 0.2 mcg/kg/min if necessary.
  Maintenance: When increase in PaO$_2$ is noted, decrease immediately to lowest effective dose. *Usual dosage range:* 0.01–0.4 mcg/kg/min; doses above 0.4 mcg/kg/min not likely to produce additional benefit.
To prepare infusion: See inside front cover.

  For palliation only. Continuous vital sign monitoring essential. May cause apnea, fever, seizures, flushing, bradycardia, hypotension, diarrhea, gastric outlet obstruction, and reversible cortical proliferation of long bones (with prolonged use). Decreases platelet aggregation.

ALTEPLASE

Activase, tPA
Thrombolytic agent, tissue plasminogen activator

No ? C

Inj: 50 mg (29 million unit), 100 mg (58 million unit)
Contains L-arginine and polysorbate 80.

Occluded IV catheter:
Aspiration method: Use 1 mg/1 mL concentration as follows:

Age/Weight	Single-Lumen CVL	Double-Lumen CVL
Neonate	0.5 mg	0.5 mg each lumen
<10 kg	1 mg	1 mg each lumen
≥10 kg	1-2 mg	1-2 mg each lumen

Instill into catheter over 1-2 min and leave in place for 2-4 hr before attempting
blood withdrawal. Dose may be repeated once in 24 hr using a longer catheter dwell
time. **DO NOT** infuse into patient.
Systemic thrombolytic therapy (**use in consultation with a hematologist**): 0.1–0.6
mg/kg/hr × 6 hr has been recommended (*Chest* 2001; 119:344-370S). The length of
continuous infusion is variable because patients may respond to longer or shorter
courses of therapy.

Current use in the pediatric population is limited. May cause bleeding, rash, and
increased prothrombin time.
   THROMBOLYTIC USE: History of stroke, transient ischemic attacks, other
neurologic disease, and hypertension are **contraindicated** for adults but considered
relative contraindications for children. Monitor fibrinogen, thrombin clotting time, PT,
and APTT when used as a thrombolytic.
   Newborns have reduced plasminogen levels (~50% of adult values), which decrease
the thrombolytic effects of alteplase. Plasminogen supplementation may be necessary.

ALUMINUM HYDROXIDE

Amphojel, Dialume, Alu-Cap, Alu-Tab, AlternaGEL, and others
Antacid, phosphate binder

Yes ? C

Tabs: 300, 500, 600 mg
Caps: 400, 500 mg
Suspension: 320, 450, 600, 675 mg/5 mL (180, 360, 480 mL)
Each tablet, capsule, and 5-mL suspension contains <0.13 mEq Na.

Continued

ALUMINUM HYDROXIDE *continued*

 (mL volume dosages are based on the 320 mg/5 mL suspension concentration):
 Peptic ulcer:
 Child: 5–15 mL PO Q3–6 hr or 1–3 hr PC and HS
 Adult: 15–45 mL PO Q3–6 hr or 1–3 hr PC and HS
Prophylaxis against GI bleeding:
 Neonates: 1 mL/kg/dose PO Q4 hr PRN
 Infant: 2–5 mL PO Q1–2 hr
 Child: 5–15 mL PO Q1–2 hr
 Adults: 30–60 mL PO Q1–2 hr
Hyperphosphatemia:
 Child: 50–150 mg/kg/24 hr ÷ Q4–6 hr PO
 Adult: 30–40 mL TID-QID PO between meals and QHS

Use with caution in patients with renal failure and upper GI hemorrhage. Interferes with the absorption of several orally administered medications, including digoxin, indomethacin, isoniazid, tetracyclines, and iron. Do not take oral medications within 1-2 hr of taking aluminum dose unless specified by your physician.

May cause constipation, decreased bowel motility, encephalopathy, and phosphorus depletion.

ALUMINUM HYDROXIDE WITH MAGNESIUM HYDROXIDE

No   ?   C

Maalox, Mylanta, Mylanta Double Strength, Mintox, Rulox, and others
Antacid

Chewable tabs: (Al (OH)$_3$: Mg (OH)$_2$)
 200 mg: 200 mg (Mintox, Rulox)
 400 mg: 400 mg (Mintox, Rulox)
 200 mg: 200 mg + simethicone 20 mg (Mylanta)
 400 mg: 400 mg + simethicone 40 mg (Mylanta Double Strength)
 Each tablet contains 0.03–0.06 mEq Na
Suspension:
 Mylanta: Each 5 mL contains 200 mg AlOH, 200 mg MgOH, and 20 mg simethicone
 Mylanta Double Strength: Each 5 mL contains 400 mg AlOH, 400 mg MgOH, and 40 mg simethicone
 Maalox: Each 5 mL contains 225 mg AlOH, 200 mg MgOH
 Extra Strength Maalox Plus: Each 5 mL contains 500 mg AlOH, 450 mg MgOH, and 40 mg simethicone
 Many other combinations exist
 Contains 0.03–0.06 mEq Na/5 mL

Continued

FORMULARY

ALUMINUM HYDROXIDE WITH MAGNESIUM HYDROXIDE *continued*

Same as for aluminum hydroxide preparations. **Do not use** combination product for hyperphosphatemia.

May have laxative effect. May cause hypokalemia. Use with **caution** in patients with renal insufficiency (magnesium), gastric outlet obstruction.

Interferes with the absorption of the benzodiazepines, chloroquine, ciprofloxacin, digoxin, phenytoin, tetracyclines, and iron. Do not take oral medications within 1-2 hr of taking antacid dose unless specified by your physician.

AMANTADINE HYDROCHLORIDE
Symmetrel, and others
Antiviral agent

         Yes   2   C

Caps: 100 mg
Syrup: 50 mg/5 mL (480 mL)

Influenza A prophylaxis and treatment:
  1–9 yr: 5 mg/kg/24 hr PO ÷ QD-BID; **max. dose:** 150 mg/24 hr
  >9 yr:
    <40 kg: 5 mg/kg/24 hr PO ÷ QD-BID; **max. dose:** 200 mg/24 hr
    ≥40 kg: 200 mg/24 hr ÷ QD-BID
Alternative dosing for influenza A prophylaxis:
  Children >20 kg and adults: 100 mg/24 hr PO ÷ QD-BID
Prophylaxis (duration of therapy):
  Single exposure: At least 10 days
  Repeated/uncontrolled exposure: Up to 90 days
  Use with influenza A vaccine when possible
Symptomatic treatment (duration of therapy):
  Continue for 24–48 hr after disappearance of symptoms

Use with **caution** in patients with liver disease, seizures, renal disease, CHF, peripheral edema, orthostatic hypotension, history of recurrent eczematoid rash, and in those receiving CNS stimulants. **Dose must be adjusted in patients with renal insufficiency (see p. 938).**

May cause dizziness, anxiety, depression, mental status change, rash (livedo reticularis), nausea, orthostatic hypotension, edema, CHF, and urinary retention.

For treatment of influenza A, it is best to initiate therapy immediately after the onset of symptoms (within 2 days).

For explanation of icons, see p. 572.

AMIKACIN SULFATE

Amikin
Antibiotic, aminoglycoside

Yes   ?   C

Inj: 50, 250 mg/mL

Neonates: See table below.
Infants and children:
    15–22.5 mg/kg/24 hr ÷ Q8 hr IV/IM
Adults:
    15 mg/kg/24 hr ÷ Q8–12 hr IV/IM
Initial **max. dose:** 1.5 g/24 hr, then monitor levels

Adjust dose in renal failure (see p. 938). Rapidly eliminated in patients with cystic fibrosis, burns, and in febrile neutropenic patients. CNS penetration is poor beyond early infancy.

Therapeutic levels: Peak, 20–30 mg/L; trough 5–10 mg/L. Recommended serum sampling time at steady-state: Trough within 30 min before the third consecutive dose and peak 30–60 min after the administration of the third consecutive dose. Peak levels of 25–30 mg/L have been recommended for pulmonary, bone, and life-threatening infections and in febrile neutropenic patients.

May cause ototoxicity, nephrotoxicity, neuromuscular blockade, and rash. Loop diuretics may potentiate the ototoxicity of all aminoglycoside antibiotics.

NEONATES: IV/IM

Postconceptional Age (weeks)	Postnatal Age (days)	Dose (mg/kg/dose)	Interval (hr)
≤29*	0–28	7.5	24
	>28	10	24
30–36	0–14	10	24
	>14	7.5	12
≥37	0–7	7.5	12
	>7	7.5	8

*Or significant asphyxia.

AMINOCAPROIC ACID

Amicar and others
Hemostatic agent

Yes   ?   C

Tabs: 500 mg
Syrup: 250 mg/mL (480 mL) (may contain 0.2% methylparaben and 0.05% propylparaben)
Inj: 250 mg/mL (contains 0.9% benzyl alcohol)

Continued

AMINOCAPROIC ACID *continued*

Children:
Loading dose: 100–200 mg/kg IV/PO
Maintenance: 100 mg/kg/dose Q4–6 hr; **max. dose:** 30 g/24 hr

Contraindications: DIC, hematuria. Use with **caution** in patients with cardiac, renal, or hepatic disease. Dose should be reduced by 75% in oliguria or end-stage renal disease. Hypercoagulation may be produced when given in conjunction with oral contraceptives.

May cause nausea, diarrhea, malaise, weakness, headache, decreased platelet function, hypotension, and false increase in urine amino acids. Elevation of serum potassium may occur, especially in patients with renal impairment.

AMINOPHYLLINE

Aminophyllin, Phylocontin, and others
Bronchodilator, methylxanthine

No   1   C

Tabs: 100, 200 mg (79% theophylline)
Liquid (oral): 105 mg/5 mL (240 mL) (86% theophylline)
Inj: 25 mg/mL (79% theophylline)
Suppository: 250, 500 mg (79% theophylline)
Tabs (sustained release): 225 mg (79% theophylline)
Note: Pharmacy may dilute IV and oral dosage forms to enhance accuracy of neonatal dosing.

PO:
Infants: (see *Theophylline* and convert to mg of aminophylline)
1–9 yr: 27 mg/kg/24 hr ÷ Q4–6 hr
9–12 yr: 20 mg/kg/24 hr ÷ Q6 hr
12–16 yr: 16 mg/kg/24 hr ÷ Q6 hr
Adults: 12.5 mg/kg/24 hr ÷ Q6 hr
Neonatal apnea:
Loading dose: 5–6 mg/kg IV or PO
Maintenance dose: 1–2 mg/kg/dose Q6–8 hr, IV or PO
IV loading: 6 mg/kg IV over 20 min (each 1.2 mg/kg dose raises the serum theophylline concentration 2 mg/L)
IV maintenance: Continuous IV drip:
Neonates: 0.2 mg/kg/hr
6 wk–6 mo: 0.5 mg/kg/hr
6 mo–1 yr: 0.6–0.7 mg/kg/hr
1–9 yr: 1–1.2 mg/kg/hr
9–12 yr and young adult smokers: 0.9 mg/kg/hr
>12 yr healthy nonsmokers: 0.7 mg/kg/hr
The above total daily doses may also be administered IV ÷ Q4–6 hr.

Continued

For explanation of icons, see p. 572.

AMINOPHYLLINE *continued*

Consider mg of theophylline available when dosing aminophylline.
Monitoring serum levels is essential, especially in infants and young children.

Intermittent dosing for infants and children 1–5 yr may require Q4 hr dosing regimen due to enhanced metabolism. Side effects: Restlessness, GI upset, headache, tachycardia, and seizures (may occur in absence of other side effects with toxic levels).

Therapeutic level (theophylline): For asthma, 10–20 mg/L; for neonatal apnea, 6–13 mg/L.

Recommended guidelines for obtaining levels:

IV bolus: 30 min after infusion

IV continuous: 12–24 hr after initiation of infusion

PO liquid, immediate-release tab:

Peak: 1 hr post dose

Trough: Just before dose

PO sustained-release:

Peak: 4 hr post dose

Trough: Just before dose

Ideally, obtain levels after steady state has been achieved (after at least 1 day of therapy). See *Theophylline* for drug interactions.

Use in breastfeeding may cause irritability in infant.

AMIODARONE HCl

Cordarone
Antiarrhythmic, Class III

No 3 D

Tabs: 200 mg
Suspension: 5 mg/mL
Inj: 50 mg/mL (3 mL) (contains 20.2 mg/mL benzyl alcohol and 100 mg/mL polysorbate 80 or Tween 80)
Inj (without benzyl alcohol and polysorbate 80): 15 mg/mL (10 mL)
Contains 37% iodine by weight.

See algorithms in back of book for arrest dosing.
Children PO:

<1 yr: 600–800 mg/1.73 m^2/24 hr ÷ Q12–24 hr × 4–14 days and/or until adequate control achieved, then reduce to 200–400 mg/1.73 m^2/24 hr

≥1 yr: 10–15 mg/kg/24 hr ÷ Q12–24 hr × 4–14 days and/or until adequate control achieved, then reduce to 5 mg/kg/24 hr ÷ Q12–24 hr if effective

Children IV (limited data):

5 mg/kg over 30 min followed by a continuous infusion starting at 5 micrograms (mcg)/kg/min; infusion may be increased up to a **maximum** of 10 mcg/kg/min or 20 mg/kg/24 hr.

Adults PO:

Loading dose: 800–1600 mg QD for 1–3 wk

Maintenance: 600–800 mg QD × 1 mo, then 200–400 mg QD

Use lowest effective dose to minimize adverse reactions.

Continued

AMIODARONE HCl *continued*

Adults IV:

Loading dose: 150 mg over 10 min (15 mg/min) followed by 360 mg over 6 hrs (1 mg/min); followed by a maintenance dose of 0.5 mg/min. Supplemental boluses of 150 mg over 10 min may be given for breakthrough VF or hemodynamically unstable VT and the maintenance infusion may be increased to suppress the arrhythmia.

Amiodarone replaces bretyllium in the resuscitation algorithm for ventricular fibrillation/pulseless ventricular tachycardia **(see front cover for arrest dosing and back cover for PALS algorithm).**

Contraindicated in severe sinus node dysfunction, marked sinus bradycardia, and second- and third-degree AV block.

Long elimination half-life (40–55 days). Major metabolite is active.

Increases cyclosporine, digoxin, phenytoin, tacrolimus, warfarin, calcium channel blockers, theophylline, and quinidine levels. Amiodarone is a substrate for CYP 450 and inhibits CYP P450 3A3/4, 2C9, and 2D6.

Proposed therapeutic level with chronic oral use: 1–2.5 mg/L.

Asymptomatic corneal microdeposits should appear in all patients. Alters liver enzymes, thyroid function. Pulmonary fibrosis reported in adults. May cause worsening of preexisting arrhythmias with bradycardia and AV block. May also cause anorexia, nausea, vomiting, dizziness, paresthesias, ataxia, tremor, and hypothyroidism or hyperthyroidism.

Intravenous continuous infusion concentration for peripheral administration **should not exceed** 2 mg/mL and **must be** diluted with D_5W. The intravenous dosage form can leach out plasticizers such as DEHP. It is recommended to reduce the potential exposure to plasticizers in pregnant women and children at the toddler stages of development and younger by using alternative methods of IV drug administration. The preservative-free intravenous product is available as an orphan drug from Academic Pharmaceuticals, Inc. at (847) 735-1170.

AMITRIPTYLINE

Elavil and others
Antidepressant, tricyclic

No   3   D

Tabs: 10, 25, 50, 75, 100, 150 mg
Inj: 10 mg/mL (10 mL)

Antidepressant:

Children (PO): Start with 1 mg/kg/24 hr ÷ TID for 3 days; then increase to 1.5 mg/kg/24 hr. Dose may be gradually increased to a **maximum** of 5 mg/kg/24 hr if needed. Monitor ECG, BP, and heart rate for doses >3 mg/kg/24 hr.

Adolescents (PO): 10 mg TID with 20 mg QHS; dose may be gradually increased to a **maximum** of 200 mg/24 hr if needed.

Continued

For explanation of icons, see p. 572.

AMITRIPTYLINE *continued*

Adults:

PO: 40–100 mg/24 hr ÷ QHS-BID; dose may be gradually increased to 300 mg/24 hr if needed; gradually decrease dose to lowest effective dose when symptoms are controlled.

IM: 20–30 mg QID (convert to oral therapy as soon as possible)

Augment analgesia for chronic pain:

Initial: 0.1 mg/kg/dose QHS PO; increase as needed and tolerated over 2–3 weeks to 0.5–2 mg/kg/dose QHS

Migraine prophylaxis:

Adults: 25–50 mg/dose QHS PO

Contraindicated in narrow-angle glaucoma, seizures, severe cardiac disorders, and patients who received MAO inhibitors within 14 days. See p. 44 for management of toxic ingestion.

$T_{1/2}$ = 9–25 hr in adults. Maximum antidepressant effects may not occur for 2 or more weeks after initiation of therapy. **Do not abruptly discontinue therapy in patients receiving high doses for prolonged periods.**

Therapeutic levels (sum of amitriptyline and nortriptyline): 100–250 ng/mL. Recommended serum sampling time: Obtain a single level 8 or more hr after an oral dose (following 4–5 days of continuous dosing).

Side effects include sedation, urinary retention, constipation, dry mouth, dizziness, drowsiness, and arrhythmia. May discolor urine (blue/green). QHS dosing during first weeks of therapy will reduce sedation. Monitor ECG, BP, CBC at start of therapy and with dose changes. Decrease dose if PR interval reaches 0.22 sec, QRS reaches 130% of baseline, HR rises above 140/min, or if BP is more than 140/90. Tricyclics may cause mania.

AMLODIPINE

Norvasc
Calcium channel blocker, antihypertensive

No ? C

Tabs: 2.5, 5, 10 mg
Suspension: 1 mg/mL

Hypertension:

Child: Start with 0.1 mg/kg/dose PO QD-BID; dosage may be gradually increased to a **maximum** of 0.6 mg/kg/24 hr up to 20 mg/24 hrs.

Adult: 5–10 mg/dose QD PO; use 2.5 mg/dose QD PO in patients with hepatic insufficiency. **Max. dose:** 10 mg/24 hr

Continued

FORMULARY

AMLODIPINE *continued*

Use with **caution** in combination with other antihypertensive agents. Younger children may require higher mg/kg doses than older children and adults. A BID dosing regimen may provide better efficacy in children.

Reduce dose in hepatic insufficiency. Allow 5-7 days of continuous initial dose therapy before making dosage adjustments because of the drug's gradual onset of action and lengthy elimination half-life.

Dose-related side effects include edema, dizziness, flushing, fatigue, and palpitations. Other side effects include headache, nausea, abdominal pain, and somnolence.

AMMONIUM CHLORIDE
Diuretic, urinary acidifying agent

Yes ? B

Tabs: 500 mg
Enteric coated tabs: 486 mg
Inj: 5 mEq/mL (26.75%) (20 mL);
1 mEq = 53 mg

Urinary acidification:
Child: 75 mg/kg/24 hr ÷ Q6 hr PO or IV; **max. dose:** 6 g/24 hr
Adult:
Intravenous: 1.5 g/dose IV Q6 hr; **max. IV dose:** 6 g/24 hr
Oral: 2–3 g/dose PO Q6 hr; **max. PO dose:** 12 g/24 hr
Inj: Dilute to concentration not >0.4 mEq/mL.
Infusion **not to exceed** 50 mg/kg/hr or 1 mEq/kg/hr.

Contraindicated in hepatic or renal insufficiency; use with **caution** in infants. May produce acidosis, hyperammonemia, and GI irritation. Monitor serum chloride level, acid/base status, and ammonia.
Administer oral doses after meals.

AMOXICILLIN
Amoxil, Trimox, Wymox, Polymox, and others
Antibiotic, aminopenicillin

Yes 1 B

Drops: 50 mg/mL (15, 30 mL)
Suspension: 125, 250 mg/5 mL (80, 100, 150, 200 mL); and 200, 400 mg/5 mL (50, 75, 100 mL)
Caps: 250, 500 mg
Tabs: 500, 875 mg
Chewable tabs: 125, 200, 250, 400 mg

Continued

For explanation of icons, see p. 572.

AMOXICILLIN *continued*

Child:
  Standard dose: 25–50 mg/kg/24 hr ÷ TID PO
    High dose: 80–90 mg/kg/24 hr ÷ BID PO
Adult: 250–500 mg/dose TID PO
Max. dose: 2–3 g/24 hr
Reccurent otitis media prophylaxis: 20 mg/kg/dose QHS PO
SBE prophylaxis: See pp. 158–160

Renal elimination. **Adjust dose in renal failure (see p. 938).** Serum levels about twice those achieved with equal dose of ampicillin. Less GI effects, but otherwise similar to ampicillin. Side effects: Rash and diarrhea.

High-dose regimen increasingly useful in respiratory infections, especially acute otitis media and sinusitis, due to increasing incidence of penicillin-resistant pneumococci.

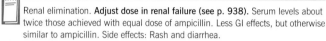

AMOXICILLIN-CLAVULANIC ACID
Augmentin, Augmentin ES-600
Antibiotic, aminopenicillin with beta lactamase inhibitor   Yes   1   B

Tabs:
  For TID dosing: 250, 500 (with 125 mg clavulanate)
  For BID dosing: 875 mg amoxicillin (with 125 mg clavulanate)
Chewable tabs:
  For TID dosing: 125, 250 mg amoxicillin (31.25 and 62.5 mg clavulanate, respectively)
  For BID dosing: 200, 400 mg amoxicillin (28.5 and 57 mg clavulanate, respectively)
Suspension:
  For TID dosing: 125, 250 mg amoxicillin/5 mL (31.25 and 62.5 mg clavulanate/ 5 mL, respectively) (75, 100, 150 mL)
  For BID dosing: 200, 400 mg amoxicillin/5 mL (28.5 and 57 mg clavulanate/ 5 mL, respectively) (50, 75, 100 mL)
  Augmentin ES-600: 600 mg amoxicillin/5 mL (42.9 mg clavulanate/5 mL) (50, 75, 100, 150 mL)
  Contains 0.63 mEq K^+ per 125 mg clavulanate (Augmentin ES-600 contains 0.23 mEq K^+ per 42.9 mg clavulanate)

Dosage based on amoxicillin component.
  Children <3 mo: 30 mg/kg/24 hr ÷BID PO (recommended dosage form is 125 mg/5 mL suspension)
Children ≥3 mo:
  TID dosing (see remarks):
    20–40 mg/kg/24 hr ÷ TID PO
  BID dosing (see remarks):
    25–45 mg/kg/24 hr ÷ BID PO

Continued

AMOXICILLIN-CLAVULANIC ACID *continued*

Augmentin ES-600:
  ≥3 mo and <40 kg: 90 mg/kg/24 hr ÷ BID PO × 10 days
Adult: 250–500 mg/dose TID PO or 875 mg/dose BID PO for more severe and respiratory infections
Max. dose: 2 g/24 hr

Clavulanic acid extends the activity of amoxicillin to include beta-lactamase–producing strains of *H. influenzae, M. catarrhalis, N.gonorrhoeae,* and some *S. aureus.* **Adjust dose in renal failure (see p. 938).**

The BID dosing schedule is associated with less diarrhea. For BID dosing, the 875-mg tablet, the 200 mg, 400 mg chewable tablets or the 200 mg/5 mL, 400 mg/5 mL, 600 mg/5 mL suspensions should be used. These BID dosage forms contain phenylalanine and **should not be used** by phenylketonurics. For TID dosing, the 250 mg, 500 mg tabs, the 125 mg, 250 mg chewable tabs, or the 125 mg/5 mL, 250 mg/5 mL suspensions should be used.

Higher doses of 80–90 mg/kg/24 hr (amoxicillin component) have been recommended for resistant strains of *S. pneumoniae* in acute otitis media (use BID formulations containing 7:1 ratio of amoxicillin to clavulanic acid or Augmentin ES-600).

AMPHOTERICIN B

Fungizone, Amphocin
Antifungal

Yes   ?   B

Inj: 50-mg vials
Cream: 3% (20 g)
Lotion: 3% (30 mL)
Ointment, topical: 3% (20 g)

Topical: Apply BID-QID
IV: Mix with D_5W to concentration 0.1 mg/mL (peripheral administration) or 0.25 mg/mL (central line only). pH >4.2. Infuse over 2–6 hr.
Test dose: 0.1 mg/kg/dose IV up to **maximum** of 1 mg (followed by remaining initial dose)
Initial dose: 0.25–0.5 mg/kg/24 hr
Increment: Increase as tolerated by 0.25–0.5 mg/kg/24 hr QD or QOD
Maintenance:
  QD dosing: 0.25–1 mg/kg/24 hr QD
  QOD dosing: 1.5 mg/kg/dose QOD
Max. dose: 1.5 mg/kg/24 hr
Intrathecal: 25–100 mcg Q48–72 hr. Increase to 500 mcg as tolerated.

Monitor renal, hepatic, electrolyte, and hematologic status closely. Hypercalciuria, hypokalemia, hypomagnesemia, RTA, renal failure, acute hepatic failure, hypotension, and phlebitis may occur. **For dosing information in renal failure, see p. 938.**

Continued

AMPHOTERICIN B *continued*

Common infusion-related reactions include fever, chills, headache, hypotension, nausea, and vomiting; may premedicate with acetaminophen and diphenhydramine 30 min before and 4 hr after infusion. Meperidine useful for chills. Hydrocortisone, 1 mg/mg amphotericin (**max.** 25 mg) added to bottle may help prevent immediate adverse reactions.

Salt loading with 10-15 mL/kg of NS infused prior to each dose may minimize the risk of nephrotoxicity.

AMPHOTERICIN B CHOLESTERYL SULFATE

Amphotec
Antifungal

No   ?   B

Inj: 50, 100 mg (vials)
(formulated as a 1:1 molar ratio of amphotericin B complexed to cholesteryl sulfate)

IV: Start at 3–4 mg/kg/24 hr QD, dose may be increased to 6 mg/kg/24 hr if necessary.

Mix with D_5W to concentration 0.16–0.83 mg/mL.
Test dose: 10 mL of the diluted solution administered over 15–30 min has been recommended.
Infusion rate: Give first dose at 1 mg/kg/hr; if well tolerated, infusion time can be gradually shortened to a minimum of 2 hr.

Monitor renal, hepatic, electrolyte, and hematologic status closely. Thrombocytopenia, tachycardia, hypokalemia, hypomagnesemia, hypocalcemia, hyperglycemia, diarrhea, dyspnea, back pain, and increases in aminotransferases and bilirubin may occur.

Common infusion-related reactions include fever, chills, rigors, nausea, vomiting, hypotension, and headache; may premedicate with acetaminophen, diphenhydramine and meperidine (see *Amphotericin B* remarks).

Doses as high as 7.5 mg/kg/24 hr have been used to treat invasive fungal infections in BMT patients.

AMPHOTERICIN B LIPID COMPLEX

Abelcet
Antifungal

No   ?   B

Inj: 5 mg/mL (10, 20 mL)
(formulated as a 1:1 molar ratio of amphotericin B to lipid complex comprised of dimyristoylphosphatidylcholine and dimyristoylphosphatidylglycerol)

Continued

AMPHOTERICIN B LIPID COMPLEX *continued*

IV: 2.5–5 mg/kg/24 hr QD
Mix with D₅W to concentration 1 mg/mL or 2 mg/mL for fluid-restricted patients.
Infusion rate: 2.5 mg/kg/hr; shake the infusion bag every 2 hr if total infusion time exceeds 2 hr.

Monitor renal, hepatic, electrolyte, and hematologic status closely. Thrombocytopenia, anemia, leukopenia, hypokalemia, hypomagnesemia, diarrhea, respiratory failure, skin rash, and increases in liver enzymes and bilirubin may occur.
Common infusion-related reactions include fever, chills, rigors, nausea, vomiting, hypotension, and headache; may premedicate with acetaminophen, diphenhydramine, and meperidine (see *Amphotericin B* remarks).

AMPHOTERICIN B, LIPOSOMAL

AmBisome
Antifungal

No   ?   B

Inj: 50 mg (vials)
(formulated in liposomes composed of hydrogenated soy phosphatidylcholine, cholesterol, distearoylphosphatidylglycerol, and alpha-tocopherol)

IV: 3–5 mg/kg/24 hr QD
Mix with D₅W to concentration 1–2 mg/mL (0.2–0.5 mg/mL may be used for infants and small children).
Infusion rate: Administer dose over 2 hr; infusion may be reduced to 1 hr if well tolerated.

Monitor renal, hepatic, electrolyte, and hematologic status closely. Thrombocytopenia, tachycardia, hypokalemia, hypomagnesemia, hypocalcemia, hyperglycemia, diarrhea, dyspnea, skin rash, low back pain, and increases in liver enzymes and bilirubin may occur.
Common infusion-related reactions include fever, chills, rigors, nausea, vomiting, hypotension, and headache; may premedicate with acetaminophen, diphenhydramine, and meperidine (see *Amphotericin B* remarks).
Doses as high as 6 mg/kg/24 hr have been used in patients with aspergillus.

AMPICILLIN

Omnipen, Principen, Totacillin, and others
Antibiotic, aminopenicillin

Yes   2   B

Suspension: 125, 250 mg/5 mL (80, 100, 150, 200 mL); 500 mg/5 mL (100 mL)
Caps: 250, 500 mg

Continued

AMPICILLIN *continued*

Inj: 125, 250, 500 mg; 1, 2, 10 g
Contains 3 mEq Na/1 g IV drug

Neonate IM/IV:
    <7 days:
        <2 kg: 50–100 mg/kg/24 hr IM/IV ÷ Q12 hr
        >2 kg: 75–150 mg/kg/24 hr IM/IV ÷ Q8 hr
≥7 days:
    <1.2 kg: 50–100 mg/kg/24 hr ÷ Q12 hr IM/IV
    1.2–2 kg: 75–150 mg/kg/24 hr ÷ Q8 hr IM/IV
    >2 kg: 100–200 mg/kg/24 hr ÷ Q6 hr IM/IV
Child:
    Mild-moderate infections:
        IM/IV: 100–200 mg/kg/24 hr ÷ Q6 hr
        PO: 50–100 mg/kg/24 hr ÷ Q6 hr; **max. PO dose:** 2–3 g/24 hr
    Severe infections: 200–400 mg/kg/24 hr ÷ Q4–6 hr IM/IV
Adult:
    IM/IV: 500–3000 mg Q4–6 hr
    PO: 250–500 mg Q6 hr
Max. IV/IM dose: 12 g/24 hr
SBE prophylaxis: See Chapter 6, pp. 159–160

Use higher doses to treat CNS disease. CSF penetration occurs only with inflammed meninges. **Adjust dose in renal failure (see p. 939).**

Produces the same side effects as penicillin, with cross-reactivity. Rash commonly seen at 5–10 days, and rash may occur with concurrent EBV infection. May cause interstitial nephritis, diarrhea, and pseudomembranous enterocolitis.

AMPICILLIN/SULBACTAM

Unasyn
Antibiotic, aminopenicillin with beta-lactamase inhibitor

Yes   ?   B

Inj:
1.5 g = ampicillin 1 g + sulbactam 0.5 g
3 g = ampicillin 2 g + sulbactam 1 g
Contains 5 mEq Na per 1.5 g drug combination

Dosage based on ampicillin component:
    Infant ≥1 month:
        Mild/moderate infections: 100–150 mg/kg/24 hr ÷ Q6 hr IM/IV
    Meningitis/severe infections: 200–300 mg/kg/24 hr ÷ Q6 hr IM/IV
Children:
    Mild/moderate infections: 100–200 mg/kg/24 hr ÷ Q6 hr IM/IV
    Meningitis/severe infections: 200–400 mg/kg/24 hr ÷ Q4–6 hr IM/IV

Continued

AMPICILLIN/SULBACTAM *continued*

Adult: 1–2 g Q6–8 hr IM/IV
Max. dose: 8 g ampicillin/24 hr

Similar spectrum of antibacterial activity to ampicillin with the added coverage of beta-lactamase–producing organisms. Total sulbactam dose **should not exceed 4 g/24 hr.**

Adjust dose in renal failure (see p. 939). Similar CSF distribution and side effects to ampicillin.

AMPRENAVIR

Agenerase, APV
Antiviral, protease inhibitor   Yes   3   C

Caps: 50, 150 mg
Each 150-mg capsule contains 109 IU Vitamin E (*d*-alpha-tocopherol)
Oral solution: 15 mg/mL (240 mL)
Each 1 mL contains 46 IU Vitamin E (*d*-alpha-tocopherol) and 1100 mg propylene glycol

Children 4-12 yr and adolescents <50 kg (Tanner I-II):
Oral solution: 22.5 mg/kg/dose PO BID or 17 mg/kg/dose PO TID up to a **max. dose** of 2800 mg/24 hr
Capsules: 20 mg/kg/dose PO BID or 15 mg/kg/dose PO TID up to a **max. dose** of 2400 mg/24 hr
Adolescents ≥50 kg (Tanner V) and adults: 1200 mg PO BID

Drug contains significant amounts of vitamin E and propylene glycol (oral solution only); oral solution is **contraindicated** in children <4 yr, pregnant women, patients with hepatic or renal failure, and patients receiving metronidazole or disulfiram. Therapeutic dosages of the oral solution will provide 1650 mg/kg/24 hr of propylene glycol and 138 IU/kg/24 hr of vitamin E.

May cause nausea, vomiting, diarrhea, perioral paresthesias, and rash (including severe life-threatening rashes in 1% of patients). Amprenavir is a substrate and inhibitor of CYP 450 3A4. **Do not** coadminister the following drugs: astemizole, terfenadine, cisapride, midazolam, triazolam, ergot derivatives, lipid-lowering agents (e.g., atorvastatin and cervistatin), and rifampin. Efavirenz and St. John's Wort can lower amprenavir levels. **Always check the potential for other drug interactions when either initiating therapy or adding a new drug onto an existing regimen.**

Adolescent dosing: Patients in early puberty (Tanner I-II) should be dosed with pediatric regimens and those in late puberty (Tanner V) should be dosed with adult regimens. Adolescents who are at the midst of their growth spurt (Tanner III females and Tanner IV males) can be dosed by either pediatric or adult regimen with close monitoring of efficacy and toxicity.

Continued

AMPRENAVIR *continued*

Oral liquid and capsules are not interchangeable on a mg per mg basis; oral solution is 14% less bioavailable. Drug may be taken with or without food; avoid administering with high-fat meals. Administer drug 1 hr before or after antacid or didanosine use. **Noncompliance can quickly promote resistant HIV strains.**

ANTIPYRINE AND BENZOCAINE

Auralgan and others
Otic analgesic, cerumenolytic

No   ?   C

Otic solution: Antipyrine 5.4%, benzocaine 1.4% (10, 15 mL)

Otic analgesia: Fill external ear canal (2–4 drops) Q1–2 hr PRN. After instillation of the solution, a cotton pledget should be moistened with the solution and inserted into the meatus.
Cerumenolytic: Fill external ear canal (2–4 drops) TID–QID for 2–3 days

Benzocaine sensitivity may develop. **Contraindicated** if tympanic membrane perforated or PE tubes in place.

ASCORBIC ACID

Vitamin C, others
Water-soluble vitamin

No   1   A/C

Tabs (OTC): 25, 50, 100, 200, 250, 500 mg, 1 g
Chewable tabs (OTC): 60, 100, 250, 500, 1000 mg
Tabs (timed release) (OTC): 0.5, 1, 1.5 g
Caps (timed release) (OTC): 500 mg
Inj: 500 mg/mL
Liquid (OTC): 35 mg/0.6 mL (50 mL)
Solution (OTC): 100 mg/mL (50 mL)
Syrup (OTC): 500 mg/5 mL (120, 480 mL)
Lozenges (OTC): 25, 60 mg
Some products may contain approximately 5 mEq Na/1 g drug and/or calcium

Scurvy PO/IM/IV/SC:
  Children: 100–300 mg/24 hr ÷ QD-BID for at least 2 weeks
  Adults: 100–250 mg QD-BID for at least 2 weeks
U.S. Recommended Daily Allowance (RDA):
  See pp. 460–461.

Continued

ASCORBIC ACID *continued*

Adverse reactions: Nausea, vomiting, heartburn, flushing, headache, faintness, dizziness, and hyperoxaluria. Use high doses with **caution** in G6PD patients.

Oral dosing is preferred with or without food. IM route is the preferred parenteral route. Protect the injectable dosage form from light.

Pregancy category changes to "C" if used in doses above the RDA.

ASPIRIN

ASA, Anacin, Bufferin, and various trade names
Nonsteroidal antiinflammatory agent, antiplatelet agent, analgesic

Yes   2   C/D

Tabs: 325, 500 mg
Tabs, enteric-coated: 81, 165, 325, 500, 650 mg
Tabs, time-release: 81, 650, 800 mg
Tabs, buffered: 81, 325, 500 mg
Tabs, caffeinated: 400 mg ASA + 32 mg caffeine, 500 mg ASA + 32 mg caffeine
Tabs, chewable: 81 mg
Suppository: 60, 120, 125, 130, 195, 200, 300, 325, 600, 650 mg, and 1.2 g

Analgesic/antipyretic: 10–15 mg/kg/dose PO/PR Q4–6 hr up to total 60–80 mg/kg/24 hr
Max. dose: 4 g/24 hr
Antiinflammatory: 60–100 mg/kg/24 hr PO ÷ Q6–8 hr
Kawasaki disease: 80–100 mg/kg/24 hr PO ÷ QID during febrile phase until defervesces, then decrease to 3–5 mg/kg/24 hr PO QAM. Continue for at least 8 weeks or until both platelet count and ESR are normal.

Do not use in children <16 yr for treatment of varicella or flu-like symptoms (risk of Reye's syndrome), in combination with other nonsteroidal antiinflammatory drugs, or in severe renal failure. Use with **caution** in bleeding disorders, renal dysfunction, gastritis, and gout. May cause GI upset, allergic reactions, liver toxicity, and decreased platelet aggregation. See p. 41 for management of overdose.

Drug interactions: May increase effects of methotrexate, valproic acid, and warfarin, which may lead to toxicity (protein displacement). Buffered dosage forms may decrease absorption of ketoconazole, and tetracycline.

Therapeutic levels: Antipyretic/analgesic: 30–50 mg/L, antiinflammatory: 150–300 mg/L. Tinnitus may occur at levels of 200–400 mg/L. Recommended serum sampling time at steady state: Obtain trough level just prior to dose following 1–2 days of continuous dosing. Peak levels obtained 2 hr (for nonsustained release dosage forms) after a dose may be useful for monitoring toxicity.

Pregnancy category changes to "D" if full-dose aspirin is used during the third trimester. **Adjust dose in renal failure (see p. 947).**

ATENOLOL

Tenormin
Beta-1 selective adrenergic blocker

Yes 2 C

Inj: 0.5 mg/mL (10 mL)
Tab: 25, 50, 100 mg
Suspension: 2 mg/mL

Children: 1–1.2 mg/kg/dose PO QD; **max. dose:** 2 mg/kg/24 hr
Adults:

PO: 25–100 mg/dose PO QD; **max. dose:** 200 mg/24 hr
Post myocardial infarction: 5 mg IV × 1 over 5 min and then repeat in 10 min if initial dose tolerated. Then start 50 mg/dose PO Q 12 hr × 2 doses 10 min after last IV dose followed by 100 mg/24 hr PO ÷ QD–BID × 6-9 days. Discontinue atenolol if bradycardia or hypotension requiring treatment or any other untoward effects occur.

Contraindicated in pulmonary edema, and cardiogenic shock. May cause bradycardia, hypotension, second- or third-degree AV block, dizziness, fatigue, lethargy, and headache. Use with **caution** in diabetes and asthma. Wheezing and dyspnea have occurred when daily dosage exceeds 100 mg/24 hr. Postmarketing evaluation reports a temporal relationship for causing elevated LFTs and/or bilirubin, hallucinations, psoriatic rash, thrombocytopenia, visual disturbances, and dry mouth. **Avoid** abrupt withdrawal of the drug. Does not cross the blood-brain barrier; lower incidence of CNS side effects compared to propranolol. **Adjust dose in renal impairment (see p. 947).** IV administration rate **not to exceed** 1 mg/min.

ATROPINE SULFATE

Anticholinergic agent

No 1 C

Tabs: 0.4 mg
Inj: 0.05, 0.1, 0.3, 0.4, 0.5, 0.8, 1 mg/mL
Ointment (ophthalmic): 1% (1, 3.5 g)
Solution (ophthalmic): 0.5%, 1%, 2% (1, 2, 5, 15 mL)

Preanesthesia dose (30-60 min pre op):
Child: 0.01 mg/kg/dose SC/IV/IM, **max. dose:** 0.4 mg/dose; **min. dose:** 0.1 mg/dose; may repeat Q4–6 hr
Adult: 0.5 mg/dose SC/IV/IM
Cardiopulmonary resuscitation:
Child: 0.02 mg/kg/dose IV Q5 min × 2–3 doses PRN; **min. dose:** 0.1 mg; **max. single dose:** 0.5 mg in children, 1 mg in adolescents; **max. total dose:** 1 mg children, 2 mg adolescents

Continued

FORMULARY

ATROPINE SULFATE *continued*

Adult: 0.5–1 mg/dose IV Q5 min; **max. total dose:** 2 mg
Bronchospasm: 0.025–0.05 mg/kg/dose in 2.5 mL NS; **max. dose:** 2.5 mg/dose
Q6–8 hr via nebulizer
Ophthalmic:
    Child: (0.5% solution) 1–2 drops in each eye QD-TID
    Adult: (1% solution) 1–2 drops in each eye QD-QID

Contraindicated in glaucoma, obstructive uropathy, tachycardia, and thyrotoxicosis. **Caution** in patients sensitive to sulfites.

Doses <0.1 mg have been associated with paradoxical bradycardia. Side effects include dry mouth, blurred vision, fever, tachycardia, constipation, urinary retention, CNS signs (dizziness, hallucinations, restlessness, fatigue, headache).

In case of bradycardia, may give via endotracheal tube (dilute with NS to volume of 1–2 mL). Use injectable solution for nebulized use; can be mixed with albuterol for simultaneous administration.

ATTAPULGITE

Children's Kaopectate, Diasorb, Donnagel, Kaopectate Advanced Formula, Kaopectate Maximum Strength, K-Pek, Parepectolin, Rheaban Maximum Strength
Antidiarrheal

No   ?   B

Liquid: 600 mg/15 mL (120, 180, 240 mL); 750 mg/15 mL (120, 237, 354 mL)
Chewable tabs: 300, 600 mg
Tabs: 750 mg
Caplets: 750 mg
Some preparations may contain alcohol and/or saccharin

PO (administer dose after each loose stool):
3–6 yrs: 300–750 mg/dose PRN up to a **max.** of 7 doses/24 hr or 2250 mg/24 hr
6–12 yrs: 600–1500 mg/dose PRN up to a **max.** of 7 doses/24 hr or 4500 mg/24 hr
>12 yrs and adults: 1200–3000 mg/dose PRN up to a **max.** of 8 doses/24 hr or 9000 mg/24 hr

Plain Kaopectate's active ingredients are kaolin and pectin. Different versions of Kaopectate may contain different active ingredients.

Do not use in children <3 yr, diarrhea caused by *C. difficile* or other toxigenic bacterias. Allow a 2–3 hr interval between the administration of attapulgite and other medications (concurrent administration may lead to reduced absorption). Prolonged use or excessive doses may cause constipation.

For explanation of icons, see p. 572.

AZATHIOPRINE

Imuran and others
Immunosuppressant

Yes   ?   D

Suspension: 50 mg/mL
Tabs: 50 mg
Inj: 100 mg (20 mL)

Immunosuppression:
Initial: 3–5 mg/kg/24 hr IV/PO QD
Maintenance: 1–3 mg/kg/24 hr IV/PO QD

Toxicity: Bone marrow suppression, rash, stomatitis, hepatotoxicity, alopecia, arthralgias, and GI disturbances. Use ¼–⅓ dose when given with allopurinol.
Severe anemia has been reported when used in combination with captopril or enalapril. Monitor CBC, platelets, total bilirubin, alkaline phosphatase, BUN, and creatinine. **Adjust dose in renal failure (see p. 947).**
Administer oral doses with food to minimize GI discomfort.

AZELASTINE

Astelin, Opitvar
Antihistamine

Yes   ?   C

Nasal spray (Astelin): 1% (137 mcg/spray), 100 actuations (17 mL)
Ophthalmic drops (Opitvar): 0.05% (0.5 mg/mL) (6 mL)

Seasonal allergic rhinitis:
Children 5–11 yrs: 1 spray each nostril BID
≥12 yrs and adults: 2 sprays each nostril BID
Ophthalmic:
≥3 yrs and adults: Instill 1 drop into each affected eye BID

Use with **caution** in asthmatics. Reduced dosages have been recommended in patients with renal and hepatic dysfunction.
Drowsiness may occur despite the nasal route of administration (avoid concurrent use of alcohol or CNS depressants). Bitter taste, nasal burning, epistaxis may also occur with nasal route. Eye burning and stinging have been reported in about 30% of patients receiving the ophthalmic dosage form.

AZITHROMYCIN

Zithromax
Antibiotic, macrolide

No ? B

Tabs: 250, 600 mg
Suspension: 100 mg/5 mL (15 mL), 200 mg/5 mL (15, 22.5, 30 mL)
Oral powder (sachet): 1 g
Inj: 500 mg (10 mL)

Children:
Otitis media or community-acquired pneumonia (≥6 mo): 10 mg/kg PO
day 1 (**not to exceed** 500 mg), followed by 5 mg/kg/24 hr PO QD (**not to
exceed** 250 mg/24 hr) on days 2–5
Pharyngitis/tonsillitis (≥2 yrs): 12 mg/kg/24 hr PO QD × 5 days (**not to exceed**
500 mg/24 hr)
M. avium complex prophylaxis: 20 mg/kg/dose PO Q 7 days (**not to exceed**
1200 mg/dose)
Adolescents and adults:
Respiratory tract, skin, and soft tissue infection: 500 mg PO day 1, then 250
mg/24 hr PO on days 2–5
Uncomplicated chlamydial urethritis or cervicitis: Single 1-g dose PO
M. avium complex prophylaxis: 1200 mg PO Q 7 days
M. avium complex treatment: 600 mg PO QD with ethambutol 800–1200 mg
PO QD
Acute PID (chlamydia): 500 mg IV QD × 1–2 days followed by 250 mg PO QD to
complete a 7–10 day regimen.

Contraindicated in hypersensitivity to macrolides. Can cause increase in hepatic
enzymes, cholestatic jaundice, GI discomfort, and pain at injection site (IV use).
Compared to other macrolides, less risk for drug interactions. CNS penetration
is poor.
Aluminum- and magnesium-containing antacids decrease absorption. Capsules and
oral suspension should be administered on an empty stomach, at least 1 hr before or
2 hr after meals. Tablets and oral powder (sachet) may be administered with food.
Intravenous administration is over 1–3 hours; do not give as a bolus or IM injection.
Single 2-g oral dose may be indicated for *N. gonorrhoeae* urethritis or cervicitis.

AZTREONAM

Azactam
Antibiotic, monobactam

Yes 1 B

Inj: 0.5, 1, 2 g
Each 1-g drug contains approximately 780 mg L-Arginine

Continued

AZTREONAM *continued*

Neonate:
30 mg/kg/dose:
   <1.2 kg and 0–4 wk age: Q12 hr IV/IM
   1.2–2 kg and 0–7 days: Q12 hr IV/IM
   1.2–2 kg and >7 days: Q8 hr IV/IM
   >2 kg and 0–7 days: Q8 hr IV/IM
   >2 kg and >7 days: Q6 hr IV/IM
Children:
  90–120 mg/kg/24 hr ÷ Q6–8 hr IV/IM
Cystic fibrosis:
  150–200 mg/kg/24 hr ÷ Q6–8 hr IV/IM
Max. dose: 8 g/24 hr

Typically indicated in multidrug-resistant aerobic gram-negative infections when beta-lactam therapy is contraindicated. Well-absorbed IM. Low cross-allergenicity between aztreonam and other beta-lactams. *Adverse reactions:* Thrombophlebitis, eosinophilia, leukopenia, neutropenia, thrombocytopenia, elevation of liver enzymes, hypotension, seizures, and confusion. Good CNS penetration. **Adjust dose in renal failure (see p. 939).**

BACITRACIN ± POLYMYXIN B

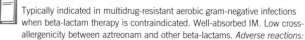

AK-Tracin Ophthalmic, Baciguent Topical, and others; in combination with polymyxin b: AK-Poly-Bac Ophthalmic, Polysporin Ophthalmic, Polysporin Topical, and others
Antibiotic, topical

No ? C

Ophthalmic ointment: 500 U/g (3.5, 3.75 g)
Topical ointment: 500 U/g (1, 15, 30, 120, 454 g)
In combination with polymyxin B:
Ophthalmic ointment: 500 Units bacitracin + 10,000 Units polymyxin B/g (3.5, 3.75 g)
Topical ointment: 500 Units bacitracin + 10,000 Units polymyxin B/g (15, 30 g)
Topical powder: 500 Units bacitracin + 10,000 Units polymyxin B/g (10 g)

BACITRACIN
Children and adults:
  Topical: Apply to affected area 1–5 times/24 hrs.
  Ophthalmic: Apply 0.25–0.5-inch ribbon into the conjunctival sac of the infected eye(s) Q 3–12 hr; frequency depends on severity of infection.
BACITRACIN + POLYMYXIN B
Children and adults:
  Topical: Apply ointment or powder to affected area QD–TID
  Ophthalmic: Apply 0.25–0.5-inch ribbon into the conjunctival sac of the infected eye(s) Q 3–12 hr; frequency depends on severity of infection

Continued

B

FORMULARY

BACITRACIN ± POLYMYXIN B *continued*

 Hypersensitivity reactions to bacitracin and/or polymyxin B can occur. **Do not use** topical ointment for the eyes. Side effects may include rash, itching, burning, and edema. Ophthalmic dosage form may cause temporary blurred vision and retard corneal healing.

BACLOFEN

Lioresal
Centrally acting skeletal muscle relaxant

Yes 1 C

Tabs: 10, 20 mg
Suspension: 5, 10 mg/mL
Intrathecal inj: 0.5, 2 mg/mL

Dosage increments are made at 3-day intervals until desired effect or max. dose is achieved.
Children; PO:
≥2 yr: 10–15 mg/24 hr ÷ Q8 hr
Max. dose, <8 yr: 40 mg/24 hr
Max. dose, ≥ 8 yr: 60 mg/24 hr
Adults; PO:
5 mg TID; **max. dose:** 80 mg/24 hr

Avoid abrupt withdrawal of drug. Use with **caution** in patients with seizure disorder, impaired renal function. Approximately 70%-80% of the drug is excreted in the urine unchanged. Administer oral doses with food or milk.
Adverse effects: Drowsiness, fatigue, nausea, vertigo, psychiatric disturbances, rash, urinary frequency, and hypotonia. Intrathecal dosing in children is not well established.

BECLOMETHASONE DIPROPIONATE

Beconase, Beconase AQ, Vanceril, Vanceril Double Strength,
Vancenase, Vancenase Pockethaler, Vancenase AQ, Vancenase
AQ 84, QVAR
Corticosteroid

No ? C

Inhalation, oral:
QVAR: 40 mcg/inhalation (100 inhalations, 7.3 g), 80 mcg/inhalation
(100 inhalations, 7.3 g)
Vanceril: 42 mcg/inhalation (80 inhalations, 6.7 g; 200 inhalations, 16.8 g)
Vanceril Double Strength: 84 mcg/inhalation (40 inhalations, 5.4 g;
120 inhalations, 12.2 g)

Continued

BECLOMETHASONE DIPROPIONATE *continued*

Inhalation, nasal:
  Beconase or Vancenase: 42 mcg/inhalation (80 inhalations, 6.7 g; 200 inhalations, 16.8 g)
  Vancenase Pockethaler: 42 mcg/inhalation (200 metered doses, 7 g)
Spray, aqueous nasal:
  Beconase AQ or Vancenase AQ: 42 mcg/inhalation (200 metered doses, 25 g)
  Vancenase AQ 84: 84 mcg/inhalation (120 metered doses, 19 g)

Oral inhalation (1 inhalation = 40 or 42 mcg):
  6–12 yr: 1–2 inhalations TID-QID or 2–4 inhalations BID; **max.** 10 inhalations/24 hr
  >12 yr: 2 inhalations TID-QID; **max.** 20 inhalations/24 hr
Oral Inhalation, Double Strength (1 inhalation = 84 mcg):
  6–12 yr: 2 inhalations BID; **max.** 5 inhalations/24 hr
  >12 yr: 2 inhalations BID; **max.** 10 inhalations/24 hr
Oral inhalation (NIH-National Heart Lung and Blood Institute recommendations):
see, pp. 514–515
Nasal inhalation:
  6–12 yr: 1 spray each nostril TID
  >12 yr: 1 spray each nostril BID-QID or 2 sprays each nostril BID
Aqueous nasal spray:
  >6 yr and adults: 1–2 sprays each nostril BID

Not recommended for children <6 yr. Dose should be titrated to lowest effective dose. **Avoid** using higher than recommended doses.
  Monitor for hypothalamic, pituitary, or adrenal suppression, and hypercortism. Rinse mouth and gargle with water after oral inhalation; may cause thrush. Consider using with tube spacers for oral inhalation.

BENZOYL PEROXIDE

Benzac AC Wash 2½, Benzac 5, Benzac 10, Brevoxyl-4
Creamy Wash, Desquam-E 5, Desquam-E 10, Oxy-5,
Oxy-10 and various other names
Topical acne product

No   ?   C

Liquid wash: 2.5% (240 mL), 5%* (120, 150, 240 mL), 10%* (120, 150, 240 mL)
Liquid cream wash: 4% (170 g), 8% (170 g)
Bar: 5%* (113 g), 10%* (106, 113 g)
Lotion: 4%* (297 g), 5%* (25, 30, 50, 60 mL), 5.5%* (25 mL), 8%* (297 g), 10%* (12, 30, 60 mL)
Mask: 5%* (60 g)
Cream: 5%* (18 g), 10%* (18, 28 g)
Gel: 2.5%* (30, 45, 60, 90, 113 g), 4% (42.5, 90 g), 5%* (45, 60, 90, 113.4 g), 6% (42.5 g), 8% (42.5, 90 g), 10%* (45, 60, 85, 90, 113.4 g), 20%* (30, 60 g)

Continued

BENZOYL PEROXIDE *continued*

Cleanser: 10% (85.1 g)
Combination product with erythromycin:
  Gel: 30 mg erythromycin and 50 mg benzoyl peroxide per g (23.3 g)
* = Available OTC without a prescription

Children and adults:
  Cleanser, liquid wash, or bar: Wet affected area prior to application. Apply and
    wash QD–BID; rinse thoroughly and pat dry. Modify dose frequency or
  concentration to control the amount of drying or peeling.
  Lotion, cream, or gel: Cleanse skin and apply small amounts over affected areas QD
  initially; increase frequency to BID–TID if needed. Modify dose frequency or
  concentration to control drying or peeling.

Avoid contact with mucous membranes, and eyes. May cause skin irritation,
stinging, dryness, peeling, erythema, edema, and contact dermatitis. Concurrent
use with tretinoin (Retin-A) will increase risk of skin irritation. Any single
application resulting in excessive stinging or burning may be removed with mild soap
and water. Lotion, cream, and gel dosage forms should be applied to dry skin.

BERACTANT

See Surfactant, pulmonary

BETHANECHOL CHLORIDE

Urecholine and other brand names
Cholinergic agent

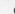

No   ?   C

Tabs: 5, 10, 25, 50 mg
Suspension: 1 mg/mL
Inj: 5 mg/mL

Children:
  Abdominal distention/urinary retention
    PO: 0.6 mg/kg/24 hr ÷ Q6–8 hr
    SC: 0.12–0.2 mg/kg/24 hr ÷ Q6–8 hr
  Gastroesophageal reflux:
    0.1–0.2 mg/kg/dose 30 min.–1 hr AC and HS
      Max.: 4 doses/24 hr
Adults:
  PO: 10–50 mg Q6–12 hr
  SC: 2.5–5 mg TID-QID, up to 7.5–10 mg Q4 hr for neurogenic bladder

Continued

BETHANECHOL CHLORIDE *continued*

 Contraindicated in asthma, mechanical GI or GU obstruction, peptic ulcer disease, hyperthyroidism, cardiac disease, seizure disorder. May cause hypotension, nausea, bronchospasm, salivation, flushing, and abdominal cramps. **Warning:** Severe hypotension may occur when given with ganglionic blockers (trimethaphan). Do not give IV or IM. Atropine is the antidote.

BICITRA
See Citrate Mixtures

BISACODYL
Dulcolax, Fleet Laxative, Fleet Bisacodyl, and various others
Laxative, stimulant

No   ?   B

Tabs (enteric-coated): 5 mg
Suppository: 10 mg
Enema: 10 mg/30 mL (37.5 mL)

 Oral:
  Child: 0.3 mg/kg/24 hr or 5–10 mg to be given 6 hr before desired effect; **max. dose:** 30 mg/24 hr
  Adult (>12 yr): 5–15 mg to be given 6 hr before desired effect; **max. dose:** 30 mg/24 hr
Rectal (as a single dose):
  <2 yr: 5 mg
  2–11 yr: 5–10 mg
  >11 yr: 10 mg

 Do not chew or crush tablets; do not give within 1 hr of antacids or milk. **Do not use** in newborn period. May cause abdominal cramps, nausea, vomiting, rectal irritation. Oral usually effective within 6–10 hr; rectal usually effective within 15–60 min.

BISMUTH SUBSALICYLATE
Pepto-Bismol and others
Antidiarrheal, gastrointestinal ulcer agent

Yes   2   C/D

Liquid: 130 mg/15 mL (240 mL), 262 mg/15 mL (120, 240, 360, 480 mL), 524 mg/15mL (120, 240, 360 mL)

Continued

BISMUTH SUBSALICYLATE *continued*

Caplet: 262 mg
Chewable tabs: 262 mg
Contains 102 mg salicylate per 262 mg tablet; or 129 mg salicylate per 15 mL of the 262 mg/15 mL suspension.

Diarrhea:
  Children: 100 mg/kg/24 hr ÷ 5 equal doses for 5 days; **max. dose:** 4.19 g/24 hr
    *Dosage by age; give following dose Q30 min to 1 hr PRN up to a **maximum** 8 doses/24 hrs:*
    3–6 yrs: 87.3 mg (⅓ tablet or 5 mL of 262 mg/15 mL)
    6–9 yrs: 174.7 mg (⅔ tablet or 10 mL of 262 mg/15 mL)
    9–12 yrs: 262 mg (1 tablet or 15 mL of 262 mg/15 mL)
    Adults: 524 mg (2 tablets or 30 mL of 262 mg/15 mL)
H. pylori gastric infection (in combination with ampicillin and metronidazole or with tetracycline and metronidazole for adults; doses not well established for children):
  <10 yr: 262 mg PO QID × 6 weeks
  ≥10 yr–adults: 524 mg PO QID × 6 weeks

Generally not recommended in children <16 yr with chickenpox or flu-like symptoms (risk of Reye's syndrome), in combination with other nonsteroidal antiinflammatory drugs, or in severe renal failure. Use with **caution** in bleeding disorders, renal dysfunction, gastritis, and gout. May cause darkening of tongue and/or black stools, GI upset, impaction, and decreased platelet aggregation.

Drug combination appears to have antisecretory and antimicrobial effects with some antiinflammatory effects. Absorption of bismuth is negligible, whereas approximately 80% of the salicylate is absorbed.

Pregnancy category changes to "D" during the third trimester.

BRETYLIUM TOSYLATE
Bretylol
Antiarrhythmic, class III

Yes ? C

Inj: 50 mg/mL (10, 20 mL)
Premixed inj: 1, 2, 4 mg/mL in D_5W (250, 500 mL)

IV: 5–10 mg/kg/dose; may repeat Q10–20 min for total dose of 30 mg/kg.
IM: 2–5 mg/kg × 1
Maintenance dose (IM, IV): 5 mg/kg/dose Q6–8 hr

Contraindicated in arrhythmias induced by digoxin toxicity. May cause initial hypertension followed by hypotension. May cause PVCs and increased sensitivity to digitalis and catecholamines. **Reduce dose in renal failure (see p. 948).**

BROMPHENIRAMINE ± PSEUDOEPHEDRINE

Yes   1   C

Bromphen Elixir, Dimetane Extentabs, and various other names; in combination with pseudoephedrine: Bromfed, Dimetapp, Rondec Chewable, and various other names

Antihistamine ± decongestant

Elixir: 2 mg/5 mL (120, 480 mL) (contains 3% alcohol)
Tab: 4 mg
Extended release tabs: 12 mg
Inj: 10 mg/mL (10 mL)
In combination with pseudoephedrine:
Elixir: Brompheniramine 1 mg + pseudoephedrine 15 mg/5 mL (120, 240, 360, 480 mL), brompheniramine 2 mg + pseudoephedrine 30 mg/5 mL (120, 473 mL), brompheniramine 4 mg + pseudoephedrine 30 mg/5 mL (473 mL), brompheniramine 4 mg + pseudoephedrine 60 mg/5 mL (473 mL)
Chewable tabs (Rondec Chewable): Brompheniramine 4 mg + pseudoephedrine 60 mg (contains aspartame)
Tabs: Brompheniramine 4 mg + pseudoephedrine 60 mg
Extended-released capsules: Brompheniramine 6 mg + pseudoephedrine 60 mg, brompheniramine 12 mg + pseudoephedrine 120 mg

BROMPHENIRAMINE:
Oral:
　<6 yr: 0.5 mg/kg/24 hr ÷ Q6–8 hr; **max. dose:** 6–8 mg/24 hr
　6–12 yr: 2–4 mg/dose Q6–8 hr; **max. dose:** 12–16 mg/24 hr
　>12 yr: 4–8 mg/dose Q6–8 hr or 8–12 mg of the sustained-release dosage form Q8–12 hr; **max. dose:** 24 mg/24 hr
IV/IM/SC:
　<12 yr: 0.5 mg/kg/24 hr ÷ Q6–8 hr
　≥12 yr: 5–20 mg Q6–12 hr; **max. dose:** 40 mg/24 hr
BROMPHENIRAMINE + PSEUDOEPHEDRINE
Oral, elixir (based on brompheniramine component):
　Children 6–11 yr: 2 mg Q4 hr up to a **max.** of 4 doses in 24 hr
　≥12 yr and adult: 4 mg Q4 hr up to a **max.** of 4 doses in 24 hr
Oral, chewable tablet, and tablet:
　Children 6–11 yr: ½ tab QID; **max.** 8 mg/24 hr of brompheniramine
　≥12 yr and adult: 1 tab QID; **max.** 16 mg/24 hr of brompheniramine
Extended-released caps:
　Children 6–11 yr:
　　Product containing 6 mg brompheniramine: 1 cap BID
　≥12 yr and adult:
　　Product containing 6 mg brompheniramine: 2 caps BID
　　Product containing 12 mg brompheniramine: 1 cap BID

Continued

BROMPHENIRAMINE ± PSEUDOEPHEDRINE *continued*

 Generally **not recommended** for treating URIs for infants. No proven benefit for infants and young children with URIs. **Contraindicated** in narow-angle glaucoma, bladder neck obstruction, asthma, and with concurrent use of MAO inhibitors. In addition, pseudoephedrine product is **contraindicated** in severe hypertension, coronary artery disease, diabetes mellitus, and thyroid disease. Discontinue use 48 hours prior to allergy skin testing.

Both products may cause drowsiness, fatigue, CNS excitation, xerostomia, blurred vision, and wheezing. The combination products have been reformulated without phenylpropanolamine (PPA) as the decongestant. PPA has been associated with an increased risk for hemorrhagic strokes.

Dosage adjustment may be necessary in renal failure for patients receiving the combination product because pseudoephedrine and its metabolite are significantly excreted in the urine.

BUDESONIDE
Pulmicort Respules, Pulmicort Turbuhaler, Rhinocort,
Rhinocort Aqua
Corticosteroid

No   ?   C

Nasal aerosol (Rhinocort): 32 mcg/actuation (7 g, delivers approx. 200 sprays)
Nasal spray (Rinocort Aqua): 32 mcg/actuation (10 mL, delivers approx. 120 sprays)
Nebulized inhalation suspension: 0.25 mg/2 mL, 0.5 mg/2 mL (30s)
Oral inhaler: 200 mcg/metered dose (1 inhaler delivers approx. 200 doses)

Nebulized inhalation suspension:
  Children 1–8 yr:
    No prior steroid use: 0.5 mg/24 hr ÷ QD–BID; **max. dose:** 0.5 mg/24 hr
    Prior inhaled steroid use: 0.5 mg/24 hr ÷ QD–BID; **max. dose:** 1 mg/24 hr
    Prior oral steroid use: 1 mg/24 hr ÷ QD–BID; **max. dose:** 1 mg/24 hr
Oral inhalation:
  Children ≥6 yr: Start at 1 inhalation (200 mcg) BID and increase, as needed, up to a **maximum** of 4 inhalations/24 hr
  Adult:
    No prior steroid use: 1–2 inhalations BID; **max. dose:** 4 inhalations/24 hr
    Prior inhaled steriod use: Start at 1–2 inhalations BID and increase, as needed, up to a **maximum** of 8 inhalations/24 hr
    Prior oral steroid use: Start at 2–4 inhalations BID; **max. dose:** 8 inhalations/ 24 hr
Oral inhalation (NIH-National Heart Lung and Blood Institute recommendations): see pp. 514–515.
Nasal inhalation (aerosol and spray):
  >6 yr: Initial: 2 sprays in each nostril QAM and QHS or, 4 sprays in each nostril QAM. Reduce dose gradually to the lowest effective dose after resolution of symptoms.
  Max. total dose 256 mcg/24 hr (8 sprays/24 hr)

Continued

BUDESONIDE *continued*

Reduce maintenance dose to as low as possible to control symptoms. May cause pharyngitis, cough, epistaxis, nasal irritation, and HPA-axis suppression. Rinse mouth after each use via the oral inhalation route. Nebulized budesonide has been shown effective in mild to moderate croup at doses of 2 mg × 1. Ref: N Engl J Med 331(5):285.

Onset of action for oral inhalation and nebulized suspension is within 1 day and 2–8 days, respectively, with peak effects at 1–2 weeks and 4–6 weeks, respectively.

For nasal use, onset of action is seen after 1 day, with peak effects after 3–7 days of therapy. Discontinue therapy if no improvement in nasal symptoms after 3 weeks of continuous therapy.

BUMETANIDE

Bumex
Loop diuretic

No ? C

Tabs: 0.5, 1, 2 mg
Inj: 0.25 mg/mL (some preparations may contain 1% benzyl alcohol)

Children: PO, IM, IV
≥6 *mo:* 0.015–0.1 mg/kg/dose QD-QOD; **max. dose:** 10 mg/24 hr
Adults:
PO: 0.5–2 mg/dose QD-BID
IM/IV: 0.5–1 mg over 1–2 min. May give additional doses Q2–3 hr PRN
Usual **max. dose** (PO/IM/IV): 10 mg/24 hr

Cross-allergenicity may occur in patients allergic to sulfonamides. Dosage reduction may be necessary in patients with hepatic dysfunction. Administer oral doses with food.

Side effects include cramps, dizziness, hypotension, headache, electrolyte losses (hypokalemia, hypocalcemia, hyponatremia, hypochloremia), and encephalopathy. May also lead to metabolic alkalosis.

Drug elimination has been reported to be slower in neonates with respiratory disorders compared to neonates without. May displace bilirubin in critically ill neonates.

BUPIVICAINE

Marcaine, Sensorcaine, Sensorcaine-MPF Spinal, and others
Local anesthetic

No ? C

Inj (preservative-free): 0.25%, 0.5%, 0.75% (2.5, 5, 7.5 mg/mL, respectively)
Inj: 0.25%, 0.5% (some preparations may contain 1 mg/mL methylparabens)

Continued

BUPIVICAINE *continued*

Inj with 1:200,000 epinephrine (preservative-free): 0.25%, 0.5%, 0.75%
Inj with 1:200,000 epinephrine: 0.25%, 0.5%
Spinal injection (preservative-free): 0.75% in dextrose 8.25%

Caudal block: 1–3.7 mg/kg; with or without epinephrine
Epidural block: 1.25 mg/kg
Local anesthesia: See Chapter 27.

Contraindicated in patients allergic to other amide-type anesthetics, regional intravenous anesthesia (Bier block), obstetrical paracervical block. May cause hypotension, asystole, seizures, and respiratory arrest. Prolonged use, particularly in neonates and infants, may lead to toxicity. Use with **caution** in severe liver disease.

Solutions containing epinephrine contain metabisulfate, which can induce allergic reactions, including anaphylaxis. See p. 911 for additional information.

CAFFEINE CITRATE
Cafcit
Methylxanthine, respiratory stimulant

No   1   B

Inj: 20 mg/mL (3 mL)
Oral liquid: 20 mg/mL (3 mL), (also available as powder for compounding)
20 mg/mL caffeine citrate salt = 10 mg/mL caffeine base

Doses expressed in mg of caffeine citrate.
Neonatal apnea:
Loading dose: 10–20 mg/kg IV/PO × 1
Maintenance dose: 5–10 mg/kg/dose PO/IV QD, to begin 24 hr after loading dose

Avoid use in symptomatic cardiac arrhythmias. **Do not use** caffeine benzoate formulation because it has been associated with kernicterus in neonates.
Therapeutic levels: 5–25 mg/L. Cardiovascular, neurologic, or GI toxicity reported at serum levels >50 mg/L. *Recommended serum sampling time:* Obtain trough level within 30 min prior to a dose. Steady-state is typically achieved 3 weeks after the initiation of therapy. Levels obtained prior to steady-state are useful for preventing toxicity.

For explanation of icons, see p. 572.

CALCITONIN

Cibacalcin, Miacalcin, Miacalcin Nasal Spray, Salmonine
Hypercalcemia antidote, antiosteoporotic

No   ?   B

Inj:
  Salmon: 200 U/mL (2 mL); contains phenol
  Human (Cibacalcin): 0.5 mg (1 mL)
Nasal spray:
  Salmon: 200 U/metered dose (2 mL, provides 14 doses)

Osteogenesis imperfecta:
  6 mo.–15 yrs: (Salmon calcitonin) 2 U/kg/dose IM/SC 3 times per week with oral calcium supplements.
Hypercalcemia (adult doses):
  Salmon calcitonin: Start with 4 U/kg/dose IM/SC Q12 hr; if response is unsatisfactory after 1 or 2 days, increase dose to 8 U/kg/dose Q12 hr. If response remains unsatisfactory after 2 more days, increase to a **maximum** of 8 U/kg/dose Q6 hr.
Paget's disease (adult doses):
  Salmon calcitonin:
    IM/SC: Start with 100 U QD initially, followed by a usual maintenance dose of 50 U QD OR 50–100 U Q 1–3 days
    Intranasal: 1–2 sprays (200–400 U) QD
  Human calcitonin: Start with 0.5 mg SC QD initially, followed by a usual maintenance dose of 0.5 mg SC 2–3 times per week **OR** 0.25 mg SC QD

Contraindicated in patients sensitive to salmon protein or gelatin. If using salmon calcitonin product, prepare a 10 U/mL dilution with normal saline and administer 0.1 mL intradermally as a skin test (observe for 15 min). Nausea, abdominal pain, flushing, and inflammation at the injection site have been reported with IM/SC route of administration. Nasal irritation, rhinitis, epistaxis may occur with use of the nasal spray. If the injection volume exceeds 2 mL, use IM route and multiple sites of injection.

CALCITRIOL

1,25-dihydroxycholecalciferol, Rocaltrol, Calcijex
Active form vitamin D, fat soluble

No   ?   A/D

Caps: 0.25, 0.5 mcg
Oral solution: 1 mcg/mL (15 mL)
Inj: (Calcijex) 1, 2 mcg/mL (1 mL)

Renal failure:
Children:
  Oral: Suggested dose range 0.01–0.05 mcg/kg/24 hr. Titrate in 0.005–0.01 mcg/kg/24 hr increments Q4–8 wk based on clinical response.

Continued

CALCITRIOL *continued*

IV: 0.01–0.05 mcg/kg/dose given 3 times per week
Adults:
Oral initial: 0.25 mcg/dose PO QD–QOD
Oral increment: 0.25 mcg/dose PO Q4–8 wk. Usual dose is 0.5–1 mcg/24 hr.
IV: 0.5 mcg/24 hr given 3 times per week. Usual dose is 0.5–3 mcg/24 hr given 3 times per week

Hypoparathyroidism:

For children >1 yr and adults, initial dose is 0.25 mcg/dose PO QD. May increase daily dosage by 0.25 mcg at 2–4 week intervals. Usual maintenance dosage as follows:

<1 yr: 0.04–0.08 mcg/kg/dose PO QD
1–5 yr: 0.25–0.75 mcg/dose PO QD
>6 yr and adults: 0.5–2 mcg/dose PO QD

Most potent vitamin D metabolite available. Monitor serum calcium and phosphorus. Avoid concomitant use of Mg^{++}-containing antacids. IV dosing applies if patient undergoing hemodialysis.

Contraindicated in patients with hypercalcemia, and vitamin D toxicity. Side effects include weakness, headache, vomiting, constipation, hypotonia, polydipsia, polyuria, myalgia, metastatic calcification, etc.

Pregnancy category changes to "D" if used in doses above the recommended daily allowance.

CALCIUM CARBONATE

Tums, Os-Cal, and others; 40% Elemental Ca
Calcium supplement, antacid

No   ?   C

Chewable tab: 350, 420, 500, 600, 750, 850, 1000, 1250 mg
Tabs: 250, 364, 500, 600, 650, 667, 1000, 1250, 1500 mg
Susp: 1250 mg/5 mL
Caps: 125, 364, 1250 mg
Powder: 6500 mg/packet
Each 1000 mg of salt contains 20 mEq elemental Ca (400 mg elemental Ca)

Doses expressed in mg of elemental calcium. To convert to mg of salt, divide elemental dose by 0.4.

Hypocalcemia:
Neonates: 50–150 mg/kg/24 hr ÷ Q4–6 hr PO
   Max. dose: 1 g/24 hr
Children: 45–65 mg/kg/24 hr PO ÷ QID
Adults: 1–2 g/24 hr PO ÷ TID-QID

Continued

CALCIUM CARBONATE *continued*

Side effects: Constipation, hypercalcemia, hypophosphatemia, hypomagnesemia, nausea, vomiting, headache, and confusion. May reduce absorption of
tetracycline, iron, and effectiveness of polystyrene sulfonate. May potentiate
effects of digoxin. Some products may contain trace amounts of Na. Administer each
dose with meals or with lots of fluid.

CALCIUM CHLORIDE

27% Elemental Ca
Calcium supplement

No   ?   C

Inj: 100 mg/mL (10%) (1.36 mEq Ca/mL); 1g of salt contains 13.6 mEq (273 mg)
elemental Ca

Doses expressed in mg of CaCl
Cardiac arrest:
  Infant/child: 20 mg/kg/dose IV Q10 min
Adults: 250–500 mg/dose IV Q10 min or 2–4 mg/kg/dose Q10 min
MAXIMUM IV ADMINISTRATION RATES:
  IV push: **Do not exceed** 100 mg/min
  IV infusion: **Do not exceed** 45–90 mg/kg/hr with a **maximum** concentration of
  20 mg/mL.

Use IV with **extreme caution.** Extravasation may lead to necrosis. Hyaluronidase
may be helpful for extravasation. Central-line administration is preferred IV route
of administration. **Do not use** scalp veins. **Do not administer** IM or SC route.
Rapid IV infusion associated with bradycardia, hypotension, and peripheral vasodilation. May cause hyperchloremic acidosis.

CALCIUM GLUBIONATE

Neo-Calglucon; 6.4% Elemental Ca
Calcium supplement

No   ?   C

Syrup: 1.8 g/5 mL (480 mL) (1.2 mEq Ca/mL); 1 g of salt contains 3.2 mEq (64 mg)
elemental Ca

Doses expressed in mg calcium glubionate
Neonatal hypocalcemia: 1200 mg/kg/24 hr PO ÷ Q4–6 hr
  Maintenance:
Infant/child: 600–2000 mg/kg/24 hr PO ÷ QID; **max. dose:** 9 g/24 hr
Adult: 6–18 g/24 hr PO ÷ QID

Continued

CALCIUM GLUBIONATE *continued*

Side effects include GI irritation, dizziness, and headache. Best absorbed when given before meals. Absorption inhibited by high phosphate load. High osmotic load of syrup (20% sucrose) may cause diarrhea.

CALCIUM GLUCEPTATE

8.2% Elemental Ca
Calcium supplement

No ? C

Inj: 220 mg/mL (22%) (0.9 mEq Ca/mL); 1 g of salt contains 4.1 mEq (82 mg) elemental Ca

Doses expressed in mg of calcium gluceptate
Hypocalcemia:
   Children: 200–500 mg/kg/24 hr IV ÷ Q6 hr
  Adult: 500–1100 mg/dose IV as needed
Cardiac arrest:
  Children: 110 mg/kg/dose IV Q10 min
MAXIMUM IV ADMINISTRATION RATES:
  IV push: **Do not exceed** 100 mg/min
  IV infusion: **Do not exceed** 150–300 mg/kg/hr with a **maximum** concentration of 55 mg/mL

See *Calcium gluconate.*

CALCIUM GLUCONATE

9% Elemental Ca
Calcium supplement

No ? C

Tabs: 500, 650, 975, 1000 mg
Inj: 100 mg/mL (10%) (0.45 mEq Ca++/mL)
1 g of salt contains 4.5 mEq (90 mg) elemental Ca

Doses expressed in mg calcium gluconate
Maintenance/hypocalcemia:
  Neonates: IV: 200–800 mg/kg/24 hr ÷ Q6 hr
Infants:
  IV: 200–500 mg/kg/24 hr ÷ Q6 hr
  PO: 400–800 mg/kg/24 hr ÷ Q6 hr
Child: 200–500 mg/kg/24 hr IV or PO ÷ Q6 hr
Adult: 5–15 g/24 hr IV or PO ÷ Q6 hr

Continued

CALCIUM GLUCONATE *continued*

For cardiac arrest:
　Infants and children: 100 mg/kg/dose IV Q10 min
　Adults: 500–800 mg/dose IV Q10 min
　Max. dose: 3 g/dose
MAXIMUM IV ADMINISTRATION RATES:
　IV push: **Do not exceed** 100 mg/min
　IV infusion: **Do not exceed** 120–240 mg/kg/hr with a **maximum** concentration of 50 mg/mL

Avoid peripheral infusion because extravasation may cause tissue necrosis. IV infusion associated with hypotension and bradycardia. Also associated with arrythmias in digitalized patients. May precipatate when used with bicarbonate. **Do not use** scalp veins. **Do not administer** IM or SC.

CALCIUM LACTATE
13% Elemental Ca
Calcium supplement

No　?　C

Tabs: 325, 650 mg
Caps: 500 mg
1 g of salt contains 6.5 mEq (130 mg) elemental Ca

Doses expressed in mg of calcium lactate
　Infants: 400–500 mg/kg/24 hr PO ÷ Q4–6 hr
　Children: 500 mg/kg/24 hr PO ÷ Q6–8 hr
Adult: 1.5–3 g PO Q8 hr
Max. dose: 9 g/24 hr

Give with meals. Do not dissolve tablets in milk.

CALFACTANT
See Surfactant, pulmonary

CAPTOPRIL

Capoten
Angiotensin converting enzyme inhibitor, antihypertensive

Yes   1   C/D

Tabs: 12.5, 25, 50, 100 mg
Suspension: 0.75, 1 mg/mL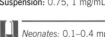

Neonates: 0.1–0.4 mg/kg/24 hr PO ÷ Q6–8 hr
Infants: Initially 0.15–0.3 mg/kg/dose; titrate upward if needed; **max. dose:**
6 mg/kg/24 hr ÷ QD-QID
Children: Initially 0.3–0.5 mg/kg/dose Q8 hr; titrate upward if needed; **max. dose:**
6 mg/kg/24 hr ÷ BID-QID
Adolescents and adults: Initially 12.5–25 mg/dose PO BID–TID; increase weekly if
necessary by 25 mg/dose to **max. dose:** 450 mg/24 hr

Onset within 15–30 min of administration. Peak effect within 1–2 hr. **Adjust
dose with renal failure (see p. 948).** Should be administered on an empty
stomach 1 hr before or 2 hr after meals. Titrate to minimal effective dose.
Use with **caution** in collagen vascular disease and concomitant potassium-sparing
diuretics. **Avoid use** with dialysis with high-flux membranes because anaphylactoid
reactions have been reported. May cause rash, proteinuria, neutropenia, cough,
angioedema, hyperkalemia, hypotension, or diminution of taste perception (with long-
term use). Known to decrease aldosterone and increase renin production.
Pregnancy category is a "C" during the first trimester but changes to a "D" for the
second and third trimester (fetal injury and death have been reported).

CARBAMAZEPINE

Atretol, Epitol, Tegretol, Tegretol-XR, Carbatrol
Anticonvulsant

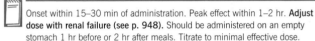

Yes   1   D

Tabs: 200 mg
Chewable tabs: 100 mg
Extended-release tabs: 100, 200, 400 mg
Extended-release caps: 200, 300 mg
Suspension: 100 mg/5 mL (450 mL)

<6 yr:
Initial: 10–20 mg/kg/24 hr PO ÷ BID-TID (QID for suspension)
Increment: Q5–7 days up to 35 mg/kg/24 hr PO
6–12 yr:
Initial: 10 mg/kg/24 hr PO ÷ BID up to **max. dose:** 100 mg/dose BID
Increment: 100 mg/24 hr at 1-wk intervals (÷ TID-QID) until desired response is
obtained

Continued

CARBAMAZEPINE *continued*

Maintenance: 20–30 mg/kg/24 hr PO ÷ BID-QID; usual maintenance dose is 400–800 mg/24 hr; **max. dose:** 1000 mg/24 hr
>12 yr:
  Initial: 200 mg PO BID
  Increment: 200 mg/24 hr at 1-wk intervals (÷ BID-QID) until desired response is obtained
  Maintenance: 800–1200 mg/24 hr PO ÷ BID-QID
Max. dose:
  Children 12–15 yr: 1000 mg/24 hr
  Children >15 yr: 1200 mg/24 hr
  Adult: 1.6–2.4 g/24 hr

Contraindicated for patients taking MAO inhibitors or who are sensitive to tricyclic antidepressants. Should **not** be used in combination with clozapine because of increased risk for bone marrow suppression and agranulocytosis. Erythromycin, verapamil, cimetidine, and INH may increase serum levels. Carbamazepine may decrease activity of warfarin, doxycycline, oral contraceptives, cyclosporin, theophylline, phenytoin, benzodiazepines, ethosuximide, and valproic acid. Carbamazepine is a substrate and inducer of CYP 450 3A3/4.

Suggested dosing intervals for specific dosage forms: Extended-release tabs or caps (BID); chewable and immediate-release tablets (BID–TID); suspension (QID). Doses may be administered with food. Do not crush or chew extended-release dosage forms. Shake bottle well prior to dispensing oral suspension dosage form, and do not administer simultaneously with other liquid medicines or diluents.

Drug metabolism typically increases after the first month of therapy due to hepatic autoinduction. $T_{1/2}$ = 25–65 hrs, initially. $T_{1/2}$ for children = 8–14 hrs. $T_{1/2}$ for adults = 12–17 hrs.

Therapeutic blood levels: 4–12 mg/L. *Recommended serum sampling time:* Obtain trough level within 30 minutes prior to an oral dose. Steady-state is typically achieved 1 mo after the initiation of therapy (following enzymatic autoinduction). Levels obtained prior to steady-state are useful for preventing toxicity.

Side effects include sedation, dizziness, diplopia, aplastic anemia, neutropenia, urinary retention, nausea, SIADH, and Stevens-Johnson syndrome. Pretreatment CBC and LFT are suggested. Patient should be monitored for hematologic and hepatic toxicity. **Adjust dose in renal impairment (see p. 948).**

See p. 26 for management of ingestions.

CARBENICILLIN
Geocillin, Geopen, Pyopen
Antibiotic, penicillin (extended spectrum)

Yes ? B

Tabs (as Indanyl sodium): 382 mg; each 382-mg tab contains 1 mEq Na

Continued

CARBENICILLIN continued

Mild infection:
Children: 30–50 mg/kg/24 hr PO ÷ Q6 hr; **max. dose:** 2–3 g/24 hr
Adults (UTI): 382–764 mg PO Q6 hr

Use with **caution** in penicillin-allergic patients. Most frequent side effects are nausea, vomiting, diarrhea, abdominal cramps, and flatulence. May cause hepatotoxicity. Furry tongue is a reported side effect. **Adjust dose in renal failure** (see p. 939).

CARNITINE

Levocarnitine, Carnitor, VitaCarn
L-Carnitine

No　?　B

Tabs: 330 mg
Caps: 250 mg
Solution: 100 mg/mL (118 mL)
Inj: 200 mg/mL (5 mL) (preservative free)

Oral:
Children: 50–100 mg/kg/24 hr PO ÷ Q8–12 hr; increase slowly as needed and tolerated to **max. dose** of 3 g/24 hr
Adults: 330 mg to 1 g/dose BID-TID PO
IV:
Children and adults: 50 mg/kg as loading dose; may follow with 50 mg/kg/24 hr IV infusion; maintenance: 50 mg/kg/24 hr ÷ Q4–6 hr. Increase to **maximum** of 300 mg/kg/24 hr if needed.

May cause nausea, vomiting, abdominal cramps, diarrhea, and body odor. Seizures have been reported in patients with or without a history of seizures. Give bolus IV infusion over 2–3 min.

CEFACLOR

Ceclor, Ceclor CD
Antibiotic, cephalosporin (second generation)

Yes　1　B

Caps: 250, 500 mg
Extended-release tabs: 375, 500 mg
Suspension: 125, 187, 250, 375 mg/5 mL (75, 150 mL)

Continued

CEFACLOR *continued*

 Infant and child: 20–40 mg/kg/24 hr PO ÷ Q8 hr; **max. dose:** 2 g/24 hr
(Q12 hr dosage interval optional in otitis media or pharyngitis)
 Adult: 250–500 mg/dose PO Q8 hr; **max. dose:** 4 g/24 hr
Extended-release tabs: 375–500 mg/dose PO Q12 hr

Use with **caution** in patients with penicillin allergy or renal impairment. May
cause positive Coomb's test or false-positive test for urinary glucose. Serum
sickness reactions have been reported in patients receiving multiple courses of
cefaclor.
 Do not crush, cut, or chew extended-release tabs. Extended-release tabs not
recommended for children. **Adjust dose in renal failure (see p. 939).**

CEFADROXIL
Duricef, Ultracef
Antibiotic, cephalosporin (first generation)   Yes   1   B

Suspension: 125, 250, 500 mg/5 mL (50, 75, 100 mL)
Tabs: 1 g
Caps: 500 mg

Infant and child: 30 mg/kg/24 hr PO ÷ Q12 hr (daily dose may be administered
QD for group A beta-hemolytic streptococci pharyngitis/tonsillitis)
Adolescents and adult: 1–2 g/24 hr PO ÷ Q12 hr; **max. dose:** 2 g/24 hr

See *Cephalexin.* Side effects include nausea, vomiting, pseudomembranous
colitis, pruritus, neutropenia, vaginitis, and candidiasis. **Adjust dose in renal
failure (see p. 939).**

CEFAMANDOLE
Mandol
Antibiotic, cephalosporin (second generation)   Yes   1   B

Inj: 1, 2 g (3.3 mEq Na/g)

Child: 50–150 mg/kg/24 hr IM/IV ÷ Q4–6 hr
Adult: 1.5–12 g/24 hr IM/IV ÷ Q4–8 hr; **max. dose:** 12 g/24 hr, 2 g/dose

See *Cefaclor.* May cause elevated liver enzymes, coagulopathy, transient
neutropenia, and disulfiram-like reaction with ethanol. Does not penetrate well
into CSF. **Adjust dose in renal failure (see p. 939).**

CEFAZOLIN

Ancef, Kefzol, Zolicef, and others
Antibiotic, cephalosporin (first generation)   Yes   1   B

Inj: 0.5, 1, 5, 10, 20 g
Frozen Inj: 500 mg/50 mL 5% dextrose, 1 g/50 mL 5% dextrose (iso-osmotic solutions)
Contains 2.1 mEq Na/g drug

Neonate IM, IV:
Postnatal age ≤7 days: 40 mg/kg/24 hr ÷ Q12 hr
   Postnatal age >7 days:
   ≤2000 g: 40 mg/kg/24 hr ÷ Q12 hr
   >2000 g: 60 mg/kg/24 hr ÷ Q8 hr
Infant >1 mo/children: 50–100 mg/kg/24 hr ÷ Q8 hr IV/IM; **max. dose:** 6 g/24 hr
Adult: 2–6 g/24 hr ÷ Q6–8 hr IV/IM; **max. dose:** 12 g/24 hr

See *Cephalexin.* Use with **caution** in renal impairment or in penicillin-allergic patients. Does not penetrate well into CSF. May cause phlebitis, leukopenia, thrombocytopenia, transient liver enzyme elevation, false-positive urine reducing substance (Clinitest) and Coombs' test. **Adjust dose in renal failure (see p. 939).**

CEFDINIR

Omnicef
Antibiotic, cephalosporin (third generation)   Yes   1   B

Caps: 300 mg
Suspension: 125 mg/5 mL (60, 100 mL)

6 mo-12 yr:
   Otitis media, sinusitis, pharyngitis/tonsillitis: 14 mg/kg/24 hr PO ÷ Q12–24 hr;
   max. dose: 600 mg/24 hr
   Uncomplicated skin infections: 14 mg/kg/24 hr PO ÷ Q12 hr; **max. dose:**
   600 mg/24 hr
≥13 yr and adults:
   Bronchitis, sinusitis, pharyngitis/tonsillitis: 600 mg/24 hr PO ÷ Q12–24 hr
   Community-acquired pneumonia, uncomplicated skin infections: 600 mg/24 hr
   PO ÷ Q12 hr

Use with **caution** in penicillin-allergic patients or in presence of renal impairment. Good gram-positive cocci activity. May cause diarrhea and false-positive urine reducing substance (Clinitest) and Coombs' test. Eosinophilia and abnormal LFTs have been reported with higher than usual doses.

Continued

CEFDINIR *continued*

Once daily dosing has not been evaluated in pneumonia and skin infections. Avoid concomitant administration with iron and iron-containing vitamins (space by 2 hrs apart) to reduce the risk for decreasing antibiotic absorption. Doses may be taken without regard to food. **Adjust dose in renal failure (see p. 939).**

CEFEPIME

Maxipime
Antibiotic, cephalosporin (fourth generation)

Yes   1   B

Inj: 0.5, 1, 2 g
Each 1 g drug contains 725 mg L-Arginine

Children ≥2 mo: 100 mg/kg/24 hr ÷ Q12 hr IV/IM
Meningitis, fever, and neutropenia, or serious infections: 150 mg/kg/24 hr ÷ Q8 hr IV/IM
Max. dose: 6 g/24 hr
Cystic fibrosis: 150 mg/kg/24 hr ÷ Q8 hr IV/IM, up to a **maximum** of 6 g/24 hr.
Adult: 1–4 g/24 hr ÷ Q12 hr IV/IM
Severe infections: 6 g/24 hr ÷ Q8 hr IV/IM
Max. dose: 6 g/24 hr

Use with **caution** in patients with penicillin allergy or renal impairment. Good activity against *P. aeruginosa* and other gram-negative bacteria plus most gram-positive bacteria *(S. aureus).* May cause thrombophlebitis, GI discomfort, transient increases in liver enzymes, and false-positive urine reducing substance (Clinitest) and Coombs' test. **Adjust dose in renal failure (see p. 940).**

CEFIXIME

Suprax
Antibiotic, cephalosporin (third generation)

Yes   1   B

Tabs: 200, 400 mg
Suspension: 100 mg/5 mL (50, 75, 100 mL)

Infant and child: 8 mg/kg/24 hr ÷ Q12–24 hr PO; **max. dose:** 400 mg/24 hr
Adolescent/adult: 400 mg/24 hr ÷ Q12–24 hr PO
Uncomplicated cervical, urethral, or rectal infections caused by N. gonorrhoeae:
400 mg × 1 PO

Continued

CEFIXIME *continued*

Use with **caution** in patients with penicillin allergy or renal failure. Adverse reactions include diarrhea, abdominal pain, nausea, and headaches. **Do not use** tablets for the treatment of otitis media because of reduced bioavailability. May cause false-positive urine reducing substance (Clinitest), Coombs' test, and nitroprusside test for ketones. **Adjust dose in renal failure (see p. 940).**

CEFOPERAZONE

Cefobid
Antibiotic, cephalosporin (third generation)

No 1 B

Inj: 1, 2, 10 g (1.5 mEq Na/g)

Infant and child: 100–150 mg/kg/24 hr ÷ Q8–12 hr IV/IM
Adult: 2–4 g/24 hr ÷ Q12 hr IV/IM; **max. dose:** 12 g/24 hr

Use with **caution** in penicillin-allergic patients or in patients with hepatic failure or biliary obstruction. Drug is extensively excreted in bile. May cause disulfiram-like reaction with ethanol, and false-positive urine reducing substance (Clinitest) and Coombs' test. Bleeding and bruising may occur, especially in patients with vitamin-K deficiency. Does not penetrate well into CSF.

CEFOTAXIME

Claforan
Antibiotic, cephalosporin (third generation)

Yes 1 B

Inj: 0.5, 1, 2, 10 g
Frozen inj: 1 g/50 mL 3.4% dextrose, 2 g/50 mL 1.4% dextrose (iso-osmotic solutions)
Contains 2.2 mEq Na/g drug

Neonates: IV/IM:
Postnatal age ≤7 days:
  <2000 g: 100 mg/kg/24 hr ÷ Q12 hr
  ≥2000 g: 100–150 mg/kg/24 hr ÷ Q8–12 hr
Postnatal age >7 days:
  <1200 g: 100 mg/kg/24 hr ÷ Q12 hr
  ≥1200 g: 150 mg/kg/24 hr ÷ Q8 hr
Infant and child: (<50 kg): 100–200 mg/kg/24 hr ÷ Q6–8 hr IV/IM (see remarks)
  Meningitis: 200 mg/kg/24 hr ÷ Q6 hr IV/IM (see remarks)
Max. dose: 12 g/24 hr

Continued

CEFOTAXIME *continued*

Adult: (≥50 kg): 1–2 g/dose Q6–8 hr IV/IM
  Severe infection: 2 g/dose Q4–6 hr IV/IM
  Max. dose: 12 g/24 hr
  Uncomplicated gonorrhea: 1 g × 1 IM

Use with **caution** in penicillin-allergic patients or in presence of renal impairment (reduce dosage). Toxicities are similar to other cephalosporins and include allergy, neutropenia, thrombocytopenia, eosinophilia, false-positive urine reducing substance (Clinitest) and Coombs' test, and elevated BUN, creatinine, and liver enzymes.

Good CNS penetration. Doses of 225–300 mg/kg/24 hr ÷ Q6–8 hr, in combination with vancomycin (60 mg/kg/24 hr), have been recommended for meningitis caused by penicillin-resistant pneumococci. Doses of 150–225 mg/kg/24 hr ÷ Q6–8 hr have been recommended for infections outside the CSF caused by penicillin-resistant pneumococci. Pediatrics 99(2);1997:293.

Adjust dose in renal failure (see p. 940).

CEFOTETAN
Cefotan
Antibiotic, cephalosporin (second generation)

Yes 1 B

Inj: 1, 2, 10 g
Frozen inj: 1 g/50 mL 3.8% dextrose, 2 g/50 mL 2.2% dextrose (iso-osmotic solutions)
Contains 3.5 mEq Na/g drug

Infant and child: 40–80 mg/kg/24 hr ÷ Q12 hr IV/IM
Adult: 2–6 g/24 hr ÷ Q12 hr IV/IM
Max. dose: 6 g/24 hr

Use with **caution** in penicillin-allergic patients or in presence of renal impairment. Has good anaerobic activity. May cause disulfiram-like reaction with ethanol, false-positive urine reducing substance (Clinitest), and false elevations of serum and urine creatinine (Jaffe method). CSF penetration is poor. **Adjust dose in renal failure (see p. 940).**

CEFOXITIN
Mefoxin
Antibiotic, cephalosporin (second generation)

Yes 1 B

Inj: 1, 2, 10 g
Frozen inj: 1 g/50 mL 4% dextrose, 2 g/50 mL 2.2% dextrose (iso-osmotic solutions)
Contains 2.3 mEq Na/g drug

Continued

CEFOXITIN *continued*

Infant and child: 80–160 mg/kg/24 hr ÷ Q4–8 hr IM/IV
Adult: 4–12 g/24 hr ÷ Q6–8 hr IM/IV
Max. dose: 12 g/24 hr

Use with **caution** in penicillin-allergic patients or in presence of renal impairment. Has good anaerobic activity. May cause false-positive urine reducing substance (Clinitest and other copper reduction method tests) and false elevations of serum and urine creatinine (Jaffe and KDA methods). CSF penetration is poor.
Adjust dose in renal failure (see p. 940).

CEFPODOXIME PROXETIL

Vantin
Antibiotic, cephalosporin (second generation)   Yes   1   B

Tabs: 100, 200 mg
Suspension: 50, 100 mg/5 mL (50, 75, 100 mL)

2 mo–12 yr: 10 mg/kg/24 hr PO ÷ Q12–24 hr
Max. dose: 400 mg/24 hr
≥13 yr–adult: 200–800 mg/24 hr PO ÷ Q12 hr
Uncomplicated gonorrhea: 200 mg PO × 1

Use with **caution** in penicillin-allergic patients or in presence of renal impairment. May cause diarrhea, nausea, vomiting, vaginal candidiasis, and false-positive Coombs' test.
Tabs should be administered with food to enhance absorption. Suspension may be administered without regard to food. High doses of antacids or H_2 blockers may reduce absorption.
Adjust dose in renal failure (see p. 941).

CEFPROZIL

Cefzil
Antibiotic, cephalosporin (second generation)   Yes   1   B

Tabs: 250, 500 mg
Suspension: 125, 250 mg/5 mL (50, 75, 100 mL) (contains aspartame and phenylalanine)

Continued

CEFPROZIL *continued*

Otitis media:
  6 mo–12 yr: 30 mg/kg/24 hr PO ÷ Q12 hr
    Pharyngitis/tonsillitis:
  2–12 yrs: 15 mg/kg/24 hr PO ÷ Q12 hr
Acute sinusitis:
  6 mo–12 yr: 15–30 mg/kg/24 hr PO ÷ Q12–24 hr
Uncomplicated skin infections:
  2–12 yr: 20 mg/kg/24 hr PO ÷ Q24 hr
Other:
  ≥12 yr and adults: 500–1000 mg/24 hr PO ÷ Q12–24 hr
Max. dose: 1 g/24 hr

Use with **caution** in penicillin-allergic patients or in presence of renal impairment. Oral suspension contains aspartame and phenylalanine and should not be used by phenylketonurics. May cause false-positive urine reducing substance (Clinitest and other copper reduction method tests) and Coombs' test. Absorption is not affected by food. **Adjust dose in renal failure (see p. 941).**

CEFTAZIDIME

Fortaz, Tazidime, Tazicef, Ceptaz (arginine salt)
Antibiotic, cephalosporin (third generation)

Yes   1   B

Inj: 0.5, 1, 2, 6, 10 g
Frozen inj: 1 g/50 mL 4.4% dextrose, 2 g/50 mL
3.2% dextrose (iso-osmotic solutions)
(Fortaz, Tazicef, Tazidime contains 2.3 mEq Na/g drug)
(Ceptaz contains 349 mg L-arginine/g drug)

Neonates: IV/IM:
  Postnatal age ≤7 days: 100 mg/kg/24 hr ÷ Q12 hr
    Postnatal age >7 days:
  <1200 g: 100 mg/kg/24 hr ÷ Q12 hr
  ≥1200 g: 150 mg/kg/24 hr ÷ Q8 hr
Infant and child: 90–150 mg/kg/24 hr ÷ Q8 hr IV/IM
Meningitis: 150 mg/kg/24 hr ÷ Q8 hr IV/IM
Cystic fibrosis: 150 mg/kg/24 hr ÷ Q8 hr IV/IM
Adult: 2–6 g/24 hr ÷ Q8–12 hr IV/IM
Max. dose: 6 g/24 hr

Use with **caution** in penicillin-allergic patients or in presence of renal impairment. Good *Pseudomonas* coverage and CSF penetration. May cause false-positive urine reducing substance (Clinitest and other copper reduction method tests) and Coombs' test. **Adjust dose in renal failure (see p. 941).**

CEFTIBUTEN
Cedax
Antibiotic, cephalosporin (third generation)

Yes   1   B

Suspension: 90 mg/5 mL (30, 60, 90, 120 mL); 180 mg/5 mL (30, 60, 120 mL)
Caps: 400 mg

Children: 9 mg/kg/24 hr PO QD
≥*12 yr:* 400 mg PO QD
Max. dose: 400 mg/24 hr

Use with **caution** in penicillin-allergic patients or in presence of renal impairment. Suspension should be administered 2 hours before or 1 hour after a meal. **Adjust dose in renal failure (see p. 941).**

CEFTIZOXIME
Cefizox
Antibiotic, cephalosporin (third generation)

Yes   1   B

Inj: 0.5, 1, 2, 10 g
Frozen inj: 1 g/50 mL 3.8% dextrose, 2 g/50 mL 1.9% dextrose (iso-osmotic solutions)
Contains 2.6 mEq Na/g drug

>1 mo and <6 mo: 100–200 mg/kg/24 hr ÷ Q6–8 hr IV/IM
≥*6 mo and children:* 150–200 mg/kg/24 hr ÷ Q6–8 hr IV/IM
Adult: 2–12 g/24 hr ÷ Q8–12 hr IV/IM
Uncomplicated gonorrhea: 1 g IM × 1
Max. dose: 12 g/24 hr

Use with **caution** in penicillin-allergic patients or in presence of renal impairment. May cause false-positive urine reducing substances (Clinitest). Good CNS penetration. **Adjust dose in renal failure (see p. 941).**

CEFTRIAXONE
Rocephin
Antibiotic, cephalosporin (third generation)

No   1   B

Inj: 0.25, 0.5, 1, 2, 10 g
Frozen inj: 1 g/50 mL 3.8% dextrose, 2 g/50 mL 2.4% dextrose (iso-osmotic solutions)
Contains 3.6 mEq Na/g drug

Neonate:
  Gonococcal ophthalmia or prophylaxis: 25–50 mg/kg/dose IM/IV × 1;
    max. dose: 125 mg/dose
Infant and child: 50–75 mg/kg/24 hr ÷ Q12–24 hr IM/IV (see remarks)
  Meningitis (including penicillin-resistant pneumococci): 100 mg/kg/24 hr IM/IV ÷
    Q12 hr; **max. dose:** 4 g/24 hr
  Acute otitis media: 50 mg/kg IM × 1; **max. dose:** 1 g
Adult: 1–4 g/24 hr ÷ Q12–24 hr IV/IM; **max. dose:** 4 g/24 hr
  Uncomplicated gonorrhea or chancroid: 250 mg IM × 1

Use with **caution** in penicillin-allergic patients or in presence of renal impairment. May cause reversible cholelithiasis, sludging in gallbladder, and jaundice.

Use with **caution** in neonates and continuous dosing because of risk for hyperbilirubinemia. Consider using an alternative third-generation cephalosporin with similar activity.

80–100 mg/kg/24 hr ÷ Q12–24 hr has been recommended for infections outside the CSF caused by penicillin-resistant pneumococci. Pediatrics 99(2);1997:293.

CEFUROXIME (IV, IM)/
CEFUROXIME AXETIL (PO)
IV: Zinacef, Kefurox; PO: Ceftin
Antibiotic, cephalosporin (second generation)

Yes   1   B

Inj: 0.75, 1.5, 7.5 g
Frozen inj: 750 mg/50 mL 2.8% dextrose, 1.5 g/50 mL water (iso-osmotic solutions)
Injectable dosage forms contain 2.4 mEq Na/g drug
Tabs: 125, 250, 500 mg
Suspension: 125, 250 mg/5 mL (50, 100 mL)

IM/IV:
  Neonates: 20–60 mg/kg/24 hr ÷ Q12 hr
    Infant/Child: 75–150 mg/kg/24 hr ÷ Q8 hr
  Max. dose: 6 g/24 hr
  Adults: 750–1500 mg/dose Q8 hr
  Max. dose: 9 g/24 hr

Continued

CEFUROXIME (IV, IM)/CEFUROXIME AXETIL (PO) *continued*

PO:
  Children:
    Pharyngitis:
      Suspension: 20 mg/kg/24 hr ÷ Q12 hr; **max. dose:** 500 mg/24 hr
      Tab: 125 mg Q12 hr
    Otitis media/impetigo:
      Suspension: 30 mg/kg/24 hr ÷ Q12 hr; **max. dose:** 1 g/24 hr
      Tab: 250 mg Q12 hr
  Adults: 250–500 mg BID
  Max. dose: 1 g/24 hr

Use with **caution** in penicillin-allergic patients or in presence of renal impairment. May cause thrombophlebitis at the infusion site; false-positive urine reducing substance (Clinitest and other copper reduction method tests) and Coombs' test; may interfere with serum and urine creatinine determinations by the alkaline picrate method. Not recommended for meningitis.

Tablets and suspension are **NOT** bioequivalent and are **NOT** substitutable on a mg/mg basis. Administer suspension with food. Concurrent use of antacids, H₂ blockers, and proton pump inhibitors may decrease oral absorption. **Adjust dose in renal failure (see p. 941).**

CEFALEXIN

Keflex, Biocef, and others
Antibiotic, cephalosporin (first generation)   Yes   1   B

Tabs: 250, 500 mg, 1 g
Caps: 250, 500 mg
Suspension: 125, 250 mg/5 mL (100, 200 mL)

Infant and child: 25–100 mg/kg/24 hr PO ÷ Q6 hr
Adult: 1–4 g/24 hr PO ÷ Q6 hr
Max. dose: 4 g/24 hr

Some cross-reactivity with penicillins. Use with **caution** in renal insufficiency. May cause false-positive urine reducing substance (Clinitest and other copper reduction method tests) and Coombs' test; false elevation of serum theophylline levels (HPLC method); and false urinary protein test.

Administer doses on an empty stomach; 2 hr before or 1 hr after meals. Less frequent dosing (Q8-12 hr) can be used for uncomplicated infections. **Adjust dose in renal failure (see p. 941).**

CEPHALOTHIN

Keflin
Antibiotic, cephalosporin (first generation)

Yes   1   B

Inj: 1, 2 g
Frozen inj: 1 g/50 mL 3.5% dextrose, 2 g/50 mL 1.1% dextrose (iso-osmotic solutions)
Contains 2.8 mEq Na/g drug

Neonates:
  IV: <2 kg:
    0–7 days: 40 mg/kg/24 hr ÷ Q12 hr
    >7 days: 40–60 mg/kg/24 hr ÷ Q8–12 hr
  ≥2 kg:
    0–7 days: 60 mg/kg/24 hr ÷ Q8 hr
    >7 days: 80 mg/kg/24 hr ÷ Q6 hr
Infant and child: 80–160 mg/kg/24 hr ÷ Q4–6 hr IV or deep IM
Adults: 2–12 g/24 hr ÷ Q4–6 hr IV/IM
Max. dose: 12 g/24 hr

Use with **caution** in penicillin-allergic patients and in renal insufficiency. May cause phlebitis. Similar spectrum to cefazolin but with a shorter $T_{1/2}$. CSF penetration is poor. **Adjust dose in renal failure (see p. 941).**

CEPHRADINE

Velosef and others
Antibiotic, cephalosporin (first generation)

Yes   1   B

Suspension: 125, 250 mg/5 mL (100, 200 mL)
Caps: 250, 500 mg
Inj: 0.25, 0.5, 1, 2 g (6 mEq Na/1g)

Child: PO: 25–50 mg/kg/24 hr ÷ Q6–12 hr
Adult: PO: 1–4 g/24 hr ÷ Q6–12 hr
Max. dose: 4 g/24 hr

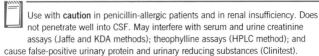

Use with **caution** in penicillin-allergic patients and in renal insufficiency. Does not penetrate well into CSF. May interfere with serum and urine creatinine assays (Jaffe and KDA methods); theophylline assays (HPLC method); and cause false-positive urinary protein and urinary reducing substances (Clinitest).
Adjust dose in renal failure (see p. 941).

CETIRIZINE

Zyrtec, Zyrtec-D 12 Hour
Antihistamine, less-sedating

Yes   ?   B

Syrup: 5 mg/5 mL (120 mL)
Tabs: 5, 10 mg
Extended-release tabs in combination with pseudoephedrine (PE):
  Zyrtec-D 12 Hour: 5 mg cetirizine + 120 mg PE

Cetirizine:
  Children 2–5 yr: Initial dose: 2.5 mg PO QD; if needed, may increase dose to a
    maximum of 5 mg/24hr.
  ≥*6 yr–adult:* 5–10 mg PO QD
Extended-release tabs of cetirizine and pseudoephedrine:
  ≥*12 yr and adult:*
    Zyrtec-D 12 Hour: 1 tablet PO BID

May cause headache, pharyngitis, GI symptoms, dry mouth, and sedation. Has
NOT been implicated in causing cardiac arrhythmias when used with other
drugs that are metabolized by hepatic microsomal enzymes (e.g., ketoconazole,
erythromycin).
  For Zyrtec-D 12 Hour, see *Pseudoephedrine* for additional remarks.
  Dosage adjustment is recommended in renal or hepatic impairment (see p. 948).

CHARCOAL, ACTIVATED

See Chapter 2

CHLORAL HYDRATE

Noctec, Aquachloral Supprettes
Sedative, hypnotic

Yes   1   C

Caps: 500 mg
Syrup: 250, 500 mg/5 mL
Suppository: 324, 500, 648 mg

Children:
  Sedative: 25–50 mg/kg/24 hr PO/PR ÷ Q6–8 hr; **max. dose:** 500 mg/dose
    Sedation for procedures: 25–100 mg/kg/dose PO/PR; **max. dose:** 1 g/dose
(infants); 2 g/dose (children)

Continued

CHLORAL HYDRATE *continued*

Adult:
  Sedative: 250 mg/dose TID PO/PR
  Hypnotic: 500–1000 mg/dose PO/PR; **max. dose:** 2 g/24 hr

> **Contraindicated** in patients with hepatic or renal disease. May cause GI irritation, paradoxical excitement, hypotension, and myocardial/respiratory depression. Chronic administration in neonates can lead to accumulation of active metabolites. Requires same monitoring as other sedatives.
> Not analgesic. Peak effects occur within 30-60 min. Do not exceed 2 weeks of chronic use. Sudden withdrawal may cause delirium tremens.
> **For additional information see Chapter 27.**

CHLORAMPHENICOL
Chloromycetin and others
Antibiotic   Yes   3   C

Caps: 250 mg
Inj: 1 g (2.25 mEq Na/1 g)
Otic solution: 0.5% (15 mL)
Ophthalmic solution: 0.5% (2.5, 7.5, 15 mL)
Ophthalmic ointment: 1% (3.5 g)
Powder for ophthalmic solution: 25 mg with 15 mL diluent (preservative-free)
Topical cream: 1% (30 g)

> *Neonates IV:*
>   *Loading dose:* 20 mg/kg
>   *Maintenance dose:*
>   ≤7 *days:* 25 mg/kg/24 hr QD
>   >7 *days:*
>   ≤2 *kg:* 25 mg/kg/24 hr QD
>   >2 *kg:* 50 mg/kg/24 hr ÷ Q12 hr
> The first maintenance dose should be given 12 hr after the loading dose
> *Infants/children/adults:* 50–75 mg/kg/24 hr IV/PO ÷ Q6 hr
>   *Meningitis:* 75–100 mg/kg/24 hr IV ÷ Q6 hr
>   **Max. dose:** 4 g/24 hr
> *Ophthalmic:* 1–2 drops or ribbon of ointment in each eye Q3–6 hr
> *Otic:* 2–3 drops in affected ear TID
> *Topical:* Apply to affected area TID-QID

> Dose recommendations are just guidelines for therapy; monitoring of blood levels is essential in neonates and infants. Follow hematologic status for dose-related or idiosyncratic marrow suppression. "Gray baby" syndrome may be seen with

Continued

CHLORAMPHENICOL *continued*

levels >50 mg/L. Use with **caution** in G6PD deficiency, renal or hepatic dysfunction, and neonates.

Concomitant use of phenobarbital and rifampin may lower chloramphenicol serum levels. Phenytoin may increase chloramphenicol serum levels. Chloramphenicol may increase phenytoin levels, reduce metabolism of oral anticoagulants, and decrease absorption of vitamin B_{12}. Chloramphenicol is an inhibitor of CYP 450 2C9.

Therapeutic levels: 15–25 mg/L for meningitis; 10–20 mg/L for other infections. *Trough:* 5–15 mg/L for meningitis; 5–10 mg/L for other infections. *Recommended serum sampling time:* Trough (IV/PO) within 30 min prior to next dose; peak (IV) 30 min after the end of infusion; peak (PO) 2 hr after oral administration. *Time to achieve steady-state:* 2-3 days for newborns; 12-24 hrs for children and adults. NOTE: Higher serum levels may be achieved using the oral, rather than the IV route.

CHLOROQUINE HCl/PHOSPHATE

Aralen
Amebicide, antimalarial   Yes   1   C

Tabs: 250, 500 mg as phosphate (150, 300 mg base, respectively)
Suspension: 16.67 mg/mL as phosphate (10 mg/mL base)
Inj: 50 mg/mL as HCl (40 mg/mL base) (5 mL)

Doses expressed in mg of chloroquine base:
Malaria prophylaxis (start 1 week prior to exposure and continue for 4 weeks after leaving edemic area):
Children: 5 mg/kg/dose PO Q week; **max. dose:** 300 mg/dose
Adult: 300 mg/dose PO Q week
Malaria treatment (chloroquine-sensitive strains):
Children: 10 mg/kg/dose (**max. dose:** 600 mg/dose) PO × 1; followed by 5 mg/kg/dose (**max. dose:** 300 mg/dose) 6 hours later and then once daily for 2 days
Adult: 600 mg/dose PO × 1; followed by 300 mg/dose 6 hours later and then once daily for 2 days

---

For treatment of malaria, consult with ID specialist or see the latest edition of the AAP *Red Book.* For IV use, consider safer alternatives such as quinidine or quinine.

Use with **caution** in liver disease, G6PD deficiency, or concomitant hepatotoxic drugs. May cause nausea, vomiting, blurred vision, retinal and corneal changes, headaches, confusion, and hair depigmentation.
Adjust dose in renal failure (see p. 948).

CHLOROTHIAZIDE

Diuril, Diurigen
Thiazide diuretic

Yes   1   D

Tabs: 250, 500 mg
Suspension: 250 mg/5 mL (237 mL)
Inj: 500 mg (5 mEq Na/1 g)

<6 mo: 20–40 mg/kg/24 hr ÷ Q12 hr PO/IV
≥6 mo: 20 mg/kg/24 hr ÷ Q12 hr PO/IV
Adults: 250–1000 mg/dose QD-QID PO/IV
Max. dose: 2 g/24 hr

Use with **caution** in liver and severe renal disease. May increase serum calcium, bilirubin, glucose, and uric acid. May cause alkalosis, pancreatitis, dizziness, hypokalemia, and hypomagnesemia.
Avoid IM or SC administration.

CHLORPHENIRAMINE MALEATE

Chlor-Trimeton and others
Antihistamine

No   ?   B

Tabs: 4 mg
Sustained-release caps and tabs: 8, 12 mg
Chewable tabs: 2 mg
Syrup: 2 mg/5 mL (120, 473 mL) (contains 5% alcohol)
Inj: 10 mg/mL

Children: 0.35 mg/kg/24 hr PO ÷ Q4–6 hr or dose based on age below
  2–6 yr: 1 mg/dose PO Q4–6 hr; **max. dose:** 6 mg/24 hr
  6–12 yr: 2 mg/dose PO Q4–6 hr; **max. dose** 12 mg/24 hr
  Sustained release (6–12 yr): 8 mg/dose PO Q12 hr
≥12 yrs/adults: 4 mg/dose Q4–6 hr PO; **max. dose:** 24 mg/24 hr
  Sustained release: 8–12 mg PO Q 12 hr
  IV/SC/IM: 5–20 mg × 1; **max. dose:** 40 mg/24 hr

Use with **caution** in asthma. May cause sedation, dry mouth, blurred vision, urinary retention, polyuria, and disturbed coordination. Young children may be paradoxically excited.
Doses may be administered PRN. Administer oral doses with food. Sustained-release forms are not recommended in children <6 yr.

CHLORPROMAZINE

Thorazine
Antiemetic, antipsychotic, phenothiazine derivative

No   3   C

Tabs: 10, 25, 50, 100, 200 mg
Extended-release caps: 30, 75, 150, 200, 300 mg
Syrup: 10 mg/5 mL (120 mL)
Suppository: 25, 100 mg
Oral concentrate: 30 mg/mL (120 mL), 100 mg/mL (60, 240 mL)
Inj: 25 mg/mL

Children >6 mo:
  IM or IV: 2.5–4 mg/kg/24 hr ÷ Q6–8 hr
  PO: 2.5–6 mg/kg/24 hr ÷ Q4–6 hr
PR: 1 mg/kg/dose Q6–8 hr
Max. IM/IV dose:
  <5 yr: 40 mg/24 hr
  5–12 yr: 75 mg/24 hr
Adult:
  IM/IV: Initial: 25 mg; repeat with 25–50 mg/dose, if needed, Q1–4 hr up to
  maximum of 400 mg/dose Q4–6 hr
  PO: 10–25 mg/dose Q4–6 hr; **max. dose:** 2 g/24 hr
  PR: 50–100 mg/dose Q6–8 hr

Adverse effects include drowsiness, jaundice, lowered seizure threshold,
extrapyramidal/anticholinergic symptoms, hypotension (more with IV), arrhythmias, agranulocytosis, and neuroleptic malignant syndrome. May potentiate
effect of narcotics, sedatives, and other drugs. Monitor BP closely. ECG changes include prolonged PR interval, flattened T waves, and ST depression. **Do not simultaneously administer** oral liquid dosage form with carbamazepine oral suspension since
an orange rubbery precipitate may form.

CHOLESTYRAMINE

Questran, Questran Light, LoCHOLEST, LoCHOLEST Light,
Prevalite
Antilipemic, binding resin

No   ?   B

Powder: 4 g anhydrous resin per 9-g packet (9, 378 g)
  Questran Light: 4 g anhydrous resin per 5-g packet with aspartame (5, 5.7, 210,
  231, 239 g)
  LoCHOLEST Light: 4 g anhydrous resin per 5.7-g packet with aspartame
  (5.7, 240 g)
  Prevalite: 4 g anhydrous resin per 5.5-g packet with aspartame (5.5, 231 g)

Continued

CHOLESTYRAMINE *continued*

All doses based in terms of anhydrous resin.
Children: 240 mg/kg/24 hr ÷ TID. Give PO as slurry in water, juice, or milk before meals.
Adult: 3–4 g of cholestyramine BID-QID
Max. dose: 32 g/24 hr

In addition to the use for managing hypercholesterolemia, drug may be used for itching associated with elevated bile acids, and diarrheal disorders associated with excess fecal bile acids or *Clostridium difficile* (pseudomembraneous colitis). May cause constipation, abdominal distention, vomiting, vitamin deficiencies (A, D, E, K), and rash. Hyperchloremic acidosis may occur with prolonged use.

Give other oral medications 4–6 hr after cholestyramine or 1 hr before dose to avoid decreased absorption.

CHOLINE MAGNESIUM TRISALICYLATE

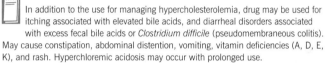

Trilisate and others
Nonsteroidal antiinflammatory agent

Yes   ?   C/D

Combination of choline salicylate and magnesium salicylate (1 : 1.24 ratio, respectively); strengths expressed in terms of mg salicylate:
Tabs: 500, 750, 1000 mg
Liquid: 500 mg/5 mL (237 mL)

Dose based on total salicylate content.
Children: 30–60 mg/kg/24 hr PO ÷ TID-QID
Adults: 500 mg–1.5 g/dose PO QD-TID

Avoid use in patients with suspected varicella or influenza because of concerns of Reye's syndrome. Use with **caution** in severe renal failure because of risk for hypermagnesemia, or in peptic ulcer disease. Less GI irritation than aspirin and other NSAIDs. No antiplatelet effects.

Pregnancy category changes to "D" if used during the third trimester.

Therapeutic salicylate levels, see *Aspirin.* 500 mg choline magnesium trisalicylate is equivalent to 650 mg aspirin.

CIMETIDINE

Tagamet, Tagamet HB [OTC]
Histamine-2-antagonist   Yes   1   B

Tabs: 100 (OTC), 200, 300, 400, 800 mg
Inj: 150 mg/mL
Syrup: 300 mg/5 mL (240, 470 mL) (contains 2.8% alcohol)

Neonates: 5–20 mg/kg/24 hr IM/PO/IV ÷ Q6–12 hr
Infants: 10–20 mg/kg/24 hr IM/PO/IV ÷ Q6–12 hr
Children: 20–40 mg/kg/24 hr IM/PO/IV ÷ Q6 hr
Adults (IM/PO/IV): 300 mg/dose QID or 400 mg/dose BID or 800 mg/dose QHS
Ulcer prophylaxis: 400–800 mg PO QHS
Max. dose: 2400 mg/24 hr

Diarrhea, rash, myalgia, confusion, neutropenia, gynecomastia, elevated LFTs, or dizziness may occur.

Inhibits cytochrome P-450 oxidase system; therefore, increases levels and effects of hepatically metabolized drugs (e.g., theophylline, phenytoin, lidocaine, diazepam, warfarin). Cimetidine may decrease the absorption of iron, ketoconazole, and tetracyclines. **Adjust dose in renal failure (see p. 948).**

CIPROFLOXACIN

Cipro, Ciloxan ophthalmic, Cipro HC Otic
Antibiotic, quinolone   Yes   1   C

Tabs: 100, 250, 500, 750 mg
Oral suspension: 250, 500 mg/5 mL (100 mL)
Inj: 10 mg/mL
Ophthalmic solution: 3.5 mg/mL (2.5, 5 mL)
Ophthalmic ointment: 3.3 mg/g (3.5 g)
Otitic suspension (Cipro HC Otic): 2 mg/mL
ciprofloxacin + 10 mg/mL hydrocortisone (10 mL)

Children:
   PO: 20–30 mg/kg/24 hr ÷ Q12 hr; **max. dose:** 1.5 g/24 hr
   IV: 10–20 mg/kg/24 hr ÷ Q12 hr; **max. dose:** 800 mg/24 hr
Cystic fibrosis:
   PO: 40 mg/kg/24 hr ÷ Q12 hr; **max. dose:** 2 g/24 hr
   IV: 30 mg/kg/24 hr ÷ Q8 hr; **max. dose:** 1.2 g/24 hr
Adults:
   PO: 250–750 mg/dose Q12 hr
   IV: 200–400 mg/dose Q12 hr
Ophthalmic solution: 1–2 drops Q2 hr while awake × 2 days, then 1–2 gtts Q4 hr while awake × 5 days

Continued

For explanation of icons, see p. 572.

CIPROFLOXACIN *continued*

Ophthalmic ointment: Apply 0.5-inch ribbon TID × 2, then BID × 5 days
Otitic:
> *>1 yr and adults:* 3 drops to affected ear(s) BID × 7 days

Can cause GI upset, renal failure, seizures. GI symptoms, headache, restlessness, and rash are common side effects. Like other quinolones, ciprofloxacin has caused arthropathy in immature animals; use with **caution** in children <18 yr. Do not use otic suspension with perforated tympanic membranes.

Inhibits CYP 450 1A2. Ciprofloxacin can increase effects and/or toxicity of theophylline, warfarin, and cyclosporine.

Do not administer antacids or other divalent salts with or within 2–4 hr of oral ciprofloxacin dose. **Adjust dose in renal failure (see p. 941).**

CISAPRIDE-LIMITED ACCESS PROTOCOL IN U.S.

Propulsid
GI stimulant, prokinetic agent

No   1   C

Suspension: 1 mg/mL (450 mL)
Tabs: 10, 20 mg
Medication available in the United States via a limited-access protocol only (1-877-795-4247)

Neonates: 0.1–0.2 mg/kg/dose Q6–12 hr PO
Infants and children: 0.2–0.3 mg/kg/dose TID-QID PO; **max. dose:** 10 mg/dose
Adults: 10 mg QID, administer 15 min AC and QHS PO; **max. dose:** 20 mg/dose

---

Contraindicated in patients taking medications that inhibit cytochrome P-450 3A4 to increase serum cisapride levels (potentially resulting in fatal cardiac arrhythmias); and in patients with electrolyte disorders (hypokalemia, hypocalcemia, and hypomagnesmia). These medications include ketoconazole, itraconazole, miconazole, fluconazole, erythromycin, clarithromycin, troleandomycin, nefazodone, indinavir, and ritonavir. **Do not use** in patients with cardiac disease (especially torsades de pointes, long QT syndrome [QTc >450 msec], sinus node dysfunction, and second- or third-degree AV block). **Avoid** concomitant use of drugs known to prolong the QT interval (e.g., quinidine, procainamide, sotalol, tricyclic antidepressants, maprotiline, phenothiazines, astemizole, and sparfloxacin).

A 12-lead ECG should be obtained before starting therapy. Serum electrolytes should be assessed in diuretic-treated patients before starting therapy and periodically thereafter.

Use in premature infants is controversial because of concerns of immature drug metabolism, leading to increased risk for toxicity.

Frequent adverse reactions are headaches and GI disturbance. Cisapride can decrease the absorption of digoxin.

CITRATE MIXTURES
Alkalinizing agent, electrolyte supplement

No   ?   C

Each mL contains (mEq):

	Na⁺	K⁺	Citrate or HCO₃
Polycitra or Cytra-3 (120, 480 mL)	1	1	2
*Polycitra-LC or Cytra-LC (120, 480 mL)	1	1	2
Polycitra-K or Cytra-K (120, 480 mL)	0	2	2
Bicitra or Cytra-2 (120, 480 mL)	1	0	1
Oracit (500 mL)	1	0	1

* LC = Low calorie (contains no sucrose, sorbitol, glycerin).

Dilute in water or juice and administer doses after meals and at bedtime.
All mEq doses based on citrate
Children: 5–15 mL/dose Q6–8 hr PO or 2–3 mEq/kg/24 hr PO ÷ Q6–8 hr
Adult: 15–30 mL/dose Q6–8 hr PO or 100–200 mEq/24 hr ÷ Q6–8 hr

Contraindicated in severe renal impairment and acute dehydration. Use with caution in patients already receiving potassium supplements or who are sodium restricted. May have laxative effect and cause hypocalemia and metabolic alkalosis.

Adjust dose to maintain desired pH. 1 mEq of citrate is equivalent to 1 mEq HCO₃ in patients with normal hepatic function.

CLARITHROMYCIN
Biaxin, Biaxin XL
Antibiotic, macrolide

Yes   2   C

Film tabs: 250, 500 mg
Extended-release tabs: 500 mg
Granules for suspension: 125, 250 mg/5 mL (50, 100 mL)

Children:
Acute otitis media, pharyngitis/tonsillitis, pneumonia, acute maxillary sinusitis, or uncomplicated skin infections: 15 mg/kg/24 hr PO ÷ Q12 hr
M. avium complex prophylaxis: 15 mg/kg/24 hr PO ÷ Q12 hr
Max. dose: 1 g/24 hr
Adult:
Pharyngitis/tonsillitis, acute maxillary sinusitis, bronchitis, pneumonia, or uncomplicated skin infections: 250–500 mg/dose Q12 hr PO (Biaxin XL, 1 g/24 hr PO ÷ Q12–24 hr, may be used to treat mild to moderate community-acquired pneumonia)
M. avium complex prophylaxis: 500 mg/dose Q12 hr PO

Continued

CLARITHROMYCIN *continued*

 Contraindicated in patients allergic to erythromycin. As with other macrolides, clarithromycin has been associated with QT prolongation and ventricular arrhythmias, including ventricular tachycardia and torsades de pointes. May cause cardiac arrhythmias in patients also receiving terfenadine, astemizole, and cisapride. Side effects include diarrhea, nausea, abnormal taste, dyspepsia, abdominal discomfort (less than erythromycin but greater than azithromycin), and headache. May increase carbamazepine, theophylline, cyclosporin, and tacrolimus levels. Inhibits CYP 450 3A4.

Adjust dose in renal failure (see p. 941). Doses, regardless of dosage form, may be administered with food.

CLEMASTINE

Tavist
Antihistamine

No   2   B

Available as clemastine fumarate salt:
Tabs: 1.34 mg (1 mg base) (OTC), 2.68 mg (2 mg base)
Syrup: 0.67 mg/5 mL (0.5 mg/5 mL base) (120, 480 mL) (contains 5.5% alcohol)

Doses expressed as clemastine base
Infants and children <6 yr: 0.05 mg/kg/24 hr ÷ BID–TID PO; **max. dose:** 1 mg/24 hr
6–12 yr: 0.5 mg BID PO; **max. dose:** 3 mg/24 hr
>12 yr: 1 mg BID PO dose, if needed, may increase dose up to a **maximum** of 6 mg/24 hr

Contraindicated in narow-angle glaucoma, bladder neck obstruction, stenosing peptic ulcer. May cause dizziness, drowsiness, dry mouth, and constipation. Doses may be taken with food.

CLINDAMYCIN

Cleocin-T, Cleocin, and others
Antibiotic

No   1   B

Caps: 75, 150, 300 mg
Oral solution: 75 mg/5 mL (100 mL)
Inj: 150 mg/mL (contains 9.45 mg/mL benzyl alcohol)
Solution, topical: 1% (30, 60, 480 mL)
Gel: 1% (7.5, 30 g)
Lotion: 1% (60 mL)
Vaginal cream: 2% (40 g)

Continued

CLINDAMYCIN *continued*

 Neonates: IV/IM: 5 mg/kg/dose
  ≤7 days:
    ≤2 kg: Q12 hr
   >2 kg: Q8 hr
  >7 days:
    <1.2 kg: Q12 hr
    1.2–2 kg: Q8 hr
    >2 kg: Q6 hr
Children:
  PO: 10–30 mg/kg/24 hr ÷ Q6–8 hr
  IM/IV: 25–40 mg/kg/24 hr ÷ Q6–8 hr
Adults:
  PO: 150–450 mg/dose Q6–8 hr; max dose: 1.8 g/24 hr
  IM/IV: 1200–1800 mg/24 hr IM/IV ÷ Q6–12 hr; **max. dose:** 4.8 g/24 hr
Topical: Apply to affected area BID

Not indicated in meningitis; CSF penetration is poor.
Pseudomembranous colitis may occur up to several weeks after cessation of
therapy. May cause diarrhea, rash, Stevens-Johnson syndrome, granulocytopenia, thrombocytopenia, or sterile abscess at injection site.
Clindamycin may increase the neuromuscular blocking effects of tubocurarine,
and pancuronium. **Do not exceed** IV infusion rate of 30 mg/min because hypotension,
and cardiac arrest have been reported with rapid infusions.

CLONAZEPAM

Klonopin
Benzodiazepine

No   3   D

Tabs: 0.5, 1, 2 mg
Suspension: 100 mcg/mL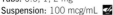

 Children: <10 yr or <30 kg:
  Initial: 0.01–0.03 mg/kg/24 hr ÷ Q8 hr PO
  Increment: 0.25–0.5 mg/24 hr Q3 days, up to **maximum** maintenance dose of
    0.1–0.2 mg/kg/24 hr ÷ Q8 hr
Children ≥10 yr or ≥30 kg and adults:
  Initial: 1.5 mg/24 hr PO ÷ TID
  Increment: 0.5–1 mg/24 hr Q3 days; **max. dose:** 20 mg/24 hr

 Contraindicated in severe liver disease and acute narrow-angle glaucoma.
Drowsiness, behavior changes, increased bronchial secretions, GI, CV, GU,
and hematopoietic toxicity (thrombocytopenia, leukopenia) may occur. Use

Continued

CLONAZEPAM *continued*

with **caution** in patients with renal impairment. Do not discontinue abruptly.
$T_{1/2}$ = 24–36 hr.

Therapeutic levels: 20–80 ng/mL. *Recommended serum sampling time:* Obtain trough level within 30 min prior to an oral dose. Steady-state is typically achieved after 5–8 days continuous therapy using the same dose.

Carbamazepine, phenytoin, and phenobarbital may decrease clonazepam levels and effect. Drugs that inhibit cytochrome P-450 3A4 isoenzymes (e.g., erythromycin) may increase clonazepam levels and effects/toxicity.

CLONIDINE
Catapres, Catapres TTS
Central alpha-adrenergic agonist, antihypertensive

No   ?   C

Tabs: 0.1, 0.2, 0.3 mg
Transdermal patch: 0.1, 0.2, 0.3 mg/24 hr (7 day)
Inj, epidural: 100, 500 mcg/mL (preservative free, 10 mL)

Children (PO): 5–7 mcg/kg/24 hr PO ÷ Q6–12 hr; if needed, increase at 5–7 day intervals to 5–25 mcg/kg/24 hr PO ÷ Q6 hr; **max. dose:** 0.9 mg/24 hr
Adult (PO): 0.1 mg BID initially; increase in 0.1 mg/24 hr increments at weekly intervals until desired response is achieved, **max. dose:** 2.4 mg/24 hr
Transdermal patch, adults: Initial 0.1 mg/24 hr patch for first week. May increase dose of patch to 0.3 mg/24 hr PRN. Patches last for 7 days.

Side effects: Dry mouth, dizziness, drowsiness, fatigue, constipation, anorexia, arrhythmias, and local skin reactions with patch. **Do not abruptly discontinue;** signs of sympathetic overactivity may occur; taper gradually over >1 wk.

Beta-blockers may exacerbate rebound hypertension during and following the withdrawal of clonidine. If patient is receiving both clonidine and a beta-blocker and clonidine is to be discontinued, the beta-blocker should be withdrawn several days prior to tapering the clonidine. If converting from clonidine to a beta-blocker, introduce the beta-blocker several days after discontinuing clonidine (following taper).

$T_{1/2}$: 44–72 hr (neonates), 6–20 hr (adults). Onset of action: 0.5–1 hr for oral route, 2–3 days for transdermal route. Applying >2 of the 0.3 mg/24 hr patches does not provide additional benefit.

CLOTRIMAZOLE
Lotrimin, Gyne-Lotrimin 3, Gyne-Lotrimin 7, Mycelex, Mycelex-7
Antifungal

No   ?   B

Cream: 1% (12, 15, 24, 30, 45 g)
Solution: 1% (10, 30 mL)

Continued

CLOTRIMAZOLE *continued*

Vaginal suppository: 200 mg
Vaginal cream: 1% (15, 30, 45 g), 2% (21 g)
Oral troche: 10 mg
Lotion: 1% (20, 30 mL)
Combination packs:
  Mycelex-8 combination Pack: Vaginal suppository 100 mg (7) and vaginal cream 1% (7 g)
  Gyne-Lotrimin 3 Combination Pack: Vaginal suppository 200 mg (3) and vaginal cream 1% (7 g)

Topical: Apply to skin BID × 4–8 wks
Vaginal candidiasis: (vaginal suppositories)
  100 mg/dose QHS × 7 days, or
200 mg/dose QHS × 3 days, or
1 applicator dose (5 g) of 1% vaginal cream QHS × 7–14 days, or
1 applicator dose of 2% vaginal cream QHS × 3 days
>3 yr-adult:
Thrush: Dissolve slowly (15–30 minutes) one troche in the mouth 5 times/24 hr × 14 days

May cause erythema, blistering, or urticaria with topical use. Liver enzyme elevation, nausea, and vomiting may occur with troches.

CLOXACILLIN

Tegopen, Cloxapen
Antibiotic, penicillin (penicillinase resistant)

No   ?   B

Caps: 250, 500 mg
Oral solution: 125 mg/5 mL (100, 200 mL)
Sodium content:
  250 mg tab = 0.6 mEq
  125 mg suspension = 0.48 mEq

Infant/child: 50–100 mg/kg/24 hr PO ÷ Q6 hr
Adults: 250–500 mg/dose PO Q6 hr
Max. dose: 4 g/24 hr

Contraindicated in patients with a history of penicillin allergy. Use with **caution** in cephalosporin hypersensitivity. May cause nausea, vomiting, and diarrhea. Administer doses on an empty stomach.

CODEINE

Various brands
Narcotic, analgesic, antitussive

Yes   1   C/D

Tabs: 15, 30, 60 mg
Inj: 30, 60 mg/mL
Oral solution: 15 mg/5 mL (500 mL)

Analgesic:
    Children: 0.5–1 mg/kg/dose Q4–6 hr IM, SC, or PO; **max. dose:** 60 mg/dose
    Adults: 15–60 mg/dose Q4–6 hr IM, SC, or PO
Antitussive (all doses PRN): 1–1.5 mg/kg/24 hr ÷ Q4–6 hr; alternatively dose by age
Children (2–6 yr): 2.5–5 mg/dose Q4–6 hr; **maximum** 30 mg/24 hr
Children (6–12 yr): 5–10 mg/dose Q4–6 hr; **maximum** 60 mg/24 hr
Adults: 10–20 mg/dose Q4–6 hr; **maximum** 120 mg/24 hr

Do not use in children <2 yr as antitussive. Not intended for IV use because of large histamine release and cardiovascular effects. *Side effects:* CNS and respiratory depression, constipation, cramping, hypotension, pruritis. May be habit forming.

For analgesia, use with acetaminophen orally. **See p. 894 for equianalgesic dosing. Adjust dose in renal failure (see p. 948).**

Pregnancy risk factor changes to a "D" if used for prolonged periods or in high doses at term.

CODEINE AND ACETAMINOPHEN

Tylenol #1, #2, #3, #4, and others
Narcotic analgesic combination product

Yes   1   C/D

Elixir (7% alcohol and saccharin), suspension, solution:
Acetaminophen 120 mg and codeine 12 mg/5 mL (120, 473 mL)
Caps: Acetaminophen 325 + 15 mg codeine
    Acetaminophen 325 + 30 mg codeine
    Acetaminophen 325 + 60 mg codeine
Tabs: (all contain 300 mg acetaminophen per tab)
    Tylenol #1: 7.5 mg codeine
    Tylenol #2: 15 mg codeine
    Tylenol #3: 30 mg codeine
    Tylenol #4: 60 mg codeine
Tabs:
    Acetaminophen 650 mg + codeine 30 mg
    Acetaminophen 500 mg + codeine 30 mg

Continued

CODEINE AND ACETAMINOPHEN *continued*

See Acetaminophen and Codeine for additional dosing information:
Children: 0.5–1 mg codeine/kg/dose PO Q4–6 hrs PRN
Using elixir:
3–6 yrs: 5 mL PO Q6–8 hr PRN
7–12 yrs: 10 mL PO Q6–8 hr PRN
≥12 yrs: 15 mL PO Q4 hr PRN
Adult: 1–2 tablets PO Q4 hr PRN; **max. codeine dose:** 120 mg /24 hr,
max. acetaminophen dose: 4 g/24 hr

See *Acetaminophen and Codeine.* Pregnancy category is "C" (changing to "D" if used for prolonged periods or in high doses at term) for codeine. **Do not use** combination product in renal impairment because codeine requires dosage adjustment; consider using each drug separately with proper dose adjustments.

COLFOSCERIL PALMITATE
See Surfactant, pulmonary

CORTICOTROPIN
ACTH, Corticotropin, Acthar, H.P.
Gel: Acthar, ACTH-80
Adrenocorticotropic hormone

No ? C

Aqueous (inj): 25, 40 U/vial
Gel: 40, 80 U/mL (1, 5 mL)
1 unit = 1 mg

Antiinflammatory:
Aqueous: 1.6 U/kg/24 hr IV, IM, or SC ÷ Q6–8 hr
Gel: 0.8 U/kg/24 hr ÷ Q12–24 hr IM
Infantile spasms: Many regimens exist
Gel: 20–40 U/24 hr IM QD × 6 weeks or 150 U/m^2/24hr ÷ BID for 2 weeks;
followed by a gradual taper.

Contraindicated in acute psychoses, CHF, Cushing's disease, TB, peptic ulcer, ocular herpes, fungal infections, recent surgery, sensitivity to porcine products.
IV administration for diagnostic purposes only. Gel dosage form is only for the IM route.
Can have hypersensitivity reaction. Similar adverse effects as corticosteroids.

CORTISONE ACETATE

Cortone acetate
Corticosteroid

No   ?   D

Tabs: 5, 10, 25 mg
Inj: 25, 50 mg/mL (IM only)

Antiinflammatory/immunosuppressive:
PO: 2.5–10 mg/kg/24 hr ÷ Q6–8 hr
IM: 1–5 mg/kg/24 hr ÷ Q12–24 hr
Physiologic replacement: see p. 907 for dosing

May produce glucose intolerance, Cushing's syndrome, edema, hypertension, adrenal suppression, cataracts, hypokalemia, skin atrophy, peptic ulcer, osteoporosis, and growth suppression.
See p. 907 for doses based on body surface area and other uses. IM form slowly absorbed over several days.

CO-TRIMOXAZOLE

Trimethoprim-sulfamethoxazole, TMP-SMX; Bactrim, Septra,
Sulfatrim, others
Antibiotic, sulfonamide derivative

Yes   1   C

Tabs (regular strength): 80 mg TMP/400 mg SMX
Tabs (double strength): 160 mg TMP/800 mg SMX
Suspension: 40 mg TMP/200 mg SMX per 5 mL (20, 100, 150, 200, 480 mL)
Inj: 16 mg TMP/mL and 80 mg SMX/mL; some preparations may contain propylene glycol and benzyl alcohol (5, 10, 20, 30 mL)

Doses based on TMP component.
Minor infections (PO or IV):
Child: 8–10 mg/kg/24 hr ÷ BID
Adult (>40 kg): 160 mg/dose BID
UTI prophylaxis: 2–4 mg/kg/24 hr PO QD
Severe infections and Pneumocystis carinii pneumonitis (PO or IV): 20 mg/kg/24 hr ÷ Q6–8 hr
Pneumocystis prophylaxis (PO or IV): 5–10 mg/kg/24 hr ÷ BID or 150 mg/m²/24 hr ÷ BID for 3 consecutive days/wk; **max. dose:** 320 mg/24 hr

Not recommended for use with infants <2 mo. **Contraindicated** in patients with sulfonamide or trimethoprim hypersensitivity, or megaloblastic anemia caused by folate deficiency. May cause kernicterus in newborns; may cause blood dyscrasias, crystalluria, glossitis, renal or hepatic injury, GI irritation, rash,

Continued

CO-TRIMOXAZOLE *continued*

Stevens-Johnson syndrome, hemolysis in patients with G6PD deficiency. Hyperkalemia may appear in HIV/AIDS patients. **Do not use drug at term during pregnancy.** Use with caution in renal and hepatic impairment.

Reduce dose in renal impairment (see p. 942). See p. 368 for PCP prophylaxis guidelines.

CROMOLYN

Intal, Nasalcrom, Gastrocrom, Crolom, Opticrom
Antiallergic agent

No   ?   B

Nebulized solution: 10 mg/mL (2 mL)
Aerosol inhaler: 800 mcg/spray (112 inhalations, 8.1g; 200 inhalations, 14.2 g)
Oral concentrate: 100 mg/5 mL
Ophthalmic solution: 4% (2.5, 10, 15 mL)
Nasal spray (OTC): 4% (5.2 mg/spray) (100 sprays, 13 mL; 200 sprays, 26 mL)

Nebulization: 20 mg Q6–8 hr
Nasal: 1 spray each nostril TID-QID
Aerosol inhaler:
  Children: 1–2 puffs TID-QID
  Adult: 2–4 puffs TID-QID
Ophthalmic: 1–2 gtts 4–6 times/24 hr
Food allergy/inflammatory bowel disease:
  Children >2 yr: 100 mg PO QID; give 15–20 min AC and QHS; **max. dose:** 40 mg/kg/24 hr
  Adults: 200–400 mg PO QID; give 15–20 min AC and QHS
Systemic mastocytosis:
  <2 yr: 20 mg/kg/24 hr ÷ QID PO;
    max. dose: 30 mg/kg/24 hr
  2–12 yr: 100 mg PO QID; **max. dose:** 40 mg/kg/24 hr
  Adults: 200 mg PO QID

May cause rash, cough, bronchospasm, nasal congestion. May cause headache, diarrhea with oral use. Use with **caution** in patients with renal or hepatic dysfunction. Bronchospasm and pharyngeal irritation may occur when using spinhaler product.

Therapeutic response often occurs within 2 weeks; however, a 4- to 6-week trial may be needed to determine maximum benefit. For exercise induced asthma, give no longer than 1 hr before activity. Oral concentrate can only be diluted in water. Nebulized solution can be mixed with albuterol nebs.

For explanation of icons, see p. 572.

CYANOCOBALAMIN/VITAMIN B$_{12}$

Cyanoject, Cyomin, VITAMIN B$_{12}$, and others
Vitamin (synthetic), water soluble   No   1   A/C

Tabs (OTC): 25, 50, 100, 250, 500, 1000, 5000 mcg
Lozenges (OTC): 100, 250, 500 mcg
Inj: 30, 100, 1000 mcg/mL; some preparations may contain benzyl alcohol

US RDA: See pp. 460–461.
Vitamin B$_{12}$ deficiency, treatment (administered IM or deep SC):
   Children: 100 mcg/24 hr × 10–15 days
   Maintenance: At least 60 mcg/mo
   Adults: 30–100 mcg/24 hr × 5–10 days
   Maintenance: 100–200 mcg/mo
Pernicious anemia (administered IM or deep SC):
   Children: 30–50 mcg/24 hr for at least 14 days to total dose of 1000–5000 mcg
   Maintenance: 100 mcg/month
   Adults: 100 mcg/24 hr × 7 days, followed by 100 mcg/dose QOD × 14 days, then
   100 mcg/dose Q 3–4 days until remission is complete.
   Maintenance: 100 mcg/mo

Contraindicated in optic nerve atrophy. May cause hypokalemia, hypersensitivity, pruritus, and vascular thrombosis. Pregnancy category changes to "C" if used in doses above the RDA.

Protect product from light. Oral route of administration is generally not recommended for pernicious anemia and B$_{12}$ deficiency because of poor absorption. IV route of administration is not recommended because of a more rapid elimination.
See pp. 463–465 for multivitamin preparations.

CYCLOPENTOLATE

Cyclogyl and others
Anticholinergic, mydriatic agent   No   ?   C

Ophthalmic solution: 0.5%, 1%, 2% (2, 5, 15 mL)

Infant: 1 drop of 0.5% OU 5–10 min before examination
Children: 1 drop of 0.5–1% OU, followed by repeat drop, if necessary, in 5 min
   Adult: 1 drop of 1% OU followed by another drop OU in 5 min; use 2% solution
for heavily pigmented iris

Do not use in narrow-angle glaucoma. May cause a burning sensation, behavioral disturbance, tachycardia, loss of visual accommodation. To minimize absorption, apply pressure over nasolacrimal sac for at least 2 min. CNS and cardiovascular side effects are common with the 2% solution in children.

Onset of action: 15–60 min. Observe patient closely for at least 30 min after dose.

CYCLOPENTOLATE/PHENYLEPHRINE

Cyclomydril
Anticholinergic/sympathomimetic, mydriatic agent

No   ?   C

Ophthalmic solution: 0.2% cyclopentolate/1% phenylephrine (2, 5 mL)

1 drop OU Q5–10 min; **max. dose:** 3 drops per eye

Used to induce mydriasis. See *Cyclopentolate* for comments.

CYCLOSPORINE, CYCLOSPORINE MICROEMULSION

Sandimmune, Gengraf, Neoral
Immunosuppressant

No   X   C

Inj: 50 mg/mL; contains 32.9% alcohol and 650 mg/mL polyoxyethylated castor oil
Oral solution: 100 mg/mL (50 mL); contains 12.5% alcohol
Caps: 25, 50, 100 mg; contains 12.7% alcohol
Neoral caps: 25, 100 mg
Neoral solution: 100 mg/mL (50 mL)
Neoral products contain 11.9% alcohol

Neoral manufacturer recommends a 1:1 conversion ratio with Sandimmune. Due to its better absorption, however, lower doses of Neoral may be required.
Oral: 15 mg/kg as a single dose given 4–12 hr pretransplant; give same daily dose for 1–2 wk posttransplant, then reduce by 5% per wk to 5–10 mg/kg/24 hr ÷ Q12–24 hr
IV: 5–6 mg/kg as a single dose given 4–12 hr pretransplant; administer over 2–6 hr; give same daily dose posttransplant until patient able to tolerate oral form

May cause nephrotoxicity, hepatotoxicity, hypomagnesemia, hyperkalemia, hyperuricemia, hypertension, hirsutism, acne, GI symptoms, tremor, leukopenia, sinusitis, gingival hyperplasia, and headache. Encephalopathy, convulsions, vision and movement disturbances, and impaired consciousness have been reported, especially in liver transplant patients. Use **caution** with concomitant use of other nephrotoxic drugs, such as amphotericin B and aminoglycosides.
Plasma concentrations increased with the use of fluconazole, ketoconazole, erythromycin, verapamil, carvedilol, and corticosteroids. Plasma concentrations decreased with the use of carbamazepine, rifampin, phenobarbital, and phenytoin. Cyclosporine is a substrate for CYP450 3A4.
Children may require dosages 2–3 times higher than adults. Plasma half-life 6–24 hrs.

Continued

CYCLOSPORINE, CYCLOSPORINE MICROEMULSION *continued*

Monitor trough levels (just prior to a dose at steady-state). Steady-state is generally achieved after 3–5 days of continuous dosing. Interpretation will vary based on treatment protocol and assay methodology (RIA monoclonal vs. RIA polyclonal vs. HPLC) as well as whole blood vs. serum sample.

CYPROHEPTADINE
Periactin
Antihistamine

No ? B

Tabs: 4 mg
Syrup: 2 mg/5 mL (473 mL); contains 5% alcohol

Antihistaminic uses:
Children: 0.25–0.5 mg/kg/24 hr ÷ Q8–12 hr PO
  Adult: Start with 12 mg/24 hr ÷ TID PO; dosage range: 12–32 mg/24 hr ÷ TID PO
Max. dose:
  2–6 yr: 12 mg/24 hr
  7–14 yr: 16 mg/24 hr
  Adults: 0.5 mg/kg/24 hr
Migraine prophylaxis:
0.25–0.4 mg/kg/24 hr ÷ BID–TID PO up to following **max. doses:**
  2–6 yr: 12 mg/24 hr
  7–14 yr: 16 mg/24 hr
  Adults: 0.5 mg/kg/24 hr

Contraindicated in neonates, patients currently on MAO inhibitors, and patients suffering from asthma, glaucoma, or GI/GU obstruction. May produce anticholinergic side effects including appetite stimulation.
Allow 4 to 8 weeks of continuous therapy for assessing efficacy in migraine prophylaxis.

DANTROLENE
Dantrium
Skeletal muscle relaxant

No ? C

Caps: 25, 50, 100 mg
Inj: 20 mg (3 g mannitol/20 mg drug)
Suspension: 5 mg/mL

Continued

DANTROLENE *continued*

Chronic spasticity:
Children: (<5 yr)
Initial: 0.5 mg/kg/dose PO BID
Increment: Increase frequency to TID-QID at 4- to 7-day intervals, then increase doses by 0.5 mg/kg/dose
Max. dose: 3 mg/kg/dose PO BID-QID, up to 400 mg/24 hr
Malignant hyperthermia:
Prevention:
PO: 4–8 mg/kg/24 hr ÷ Q6 hr × 1–3 days before surgery
IV: 2.5 mg/kg over 1 hr beginning 1.25 hr before anesthesia, additional doses PRN
Treatment: 1 mg/kg IV, repeat PRN to **maximum cumulative dose** of 10 mg/kg, then continue 4–8 mg/kg/24 hr PO ÷ Q6 hr for 1–3 days

Contraindicated in active hepatic disease. Monitor transaminases for hepatotoxicity. Use with **caution** in children with cardiac or pulmonary impairment. May cause change in sensorium, weakness, diarrhea, constipation, incontinence, and enuresis.

Avoid unnecessary exposure of medication to sunlight. Avoid extravasation into tissues. A decrease in spasticity sufficient to allow daily function should be therapeutic goal. Discontinue if benefits are not evident in 45 days.

DAPSONE

Avlosulfon
Antibiotic, sulfone derivative

Yes   1   C

Tabs: 25, 100 mg
Suspension: 2 mg/mL ; also see remarks

Pneumocystis carinii prophylaxis:
Children ≥1 mo: 2 mg/kg/24 hr PO QD; **max. dose:** 100 mg/24 hr
Adult: 100 mg/24 hr PO ÷ QD-BID; other combination regimens with pyrimethamine and leucovorin can be used (See www.hivatis.org/trtgdlns.html# Opportunistic)
Leprosy:
Children: 1–2 mg/kg/24 hr PO QD for a minimum of 3 yr; **max. dose:** 100 mg/24 hr
Adult: 50–100 mg PO QD for 3–10 years (in combination with Rifampin 600 mg PO QD × first 6 mo is recommended)

May cause hemolysis in G6PD deficiency, or methemoglobin reductase deficiency (primarily results in methemoglobinemia), or hemoglobin M. Side effects include hemolytic anemia (dose related), agranulocytosis, aplastic anemia,

Continued

For explanation of icons, see p. 572.

DAPSONE *continued*

nausea, vomiting, hyperbilirubinemia, headache, nephrotic syndrome, and hypersensitivity reaction (sulfone syndrome).

Didanosine and rifampin decrease dapsone levels. Trimethoprim increases dapsone levels. Pyrimethamine, nitrofurantoin, and primaquine increase risk for hematological side effects.

Suspension may not be absorbed as well as tablets. 2 mg/mL suspension product is also available via an IND for PCP prophylaxis from Jacobus Pharmaceutical Company (609) 921-7447.

DEFEROXAMINE MESYLATE

Desferal Mesylate
Chelating agent

No ? C

Injection: 500 mg

Acute iron poisoning:
Children:
  IV: 15 mg/kg/hr or
  IM: 50 mg/kg/dose Q6 hr
  Max. dose: 6 g/24 hr
Adult:
  IV: 15 mg/kg/hr
  IM: 1 g × 1, then 0.5 g Q4 hr × 2; may repeat 0.5 g Q4–12 hr
  Max. dose: 6 g/24 hr
Chronic iron overload:
  Children:
    IV: 15 mg/kg/hr
    SC: 20–40 mg/kg/dose QD as infusion over 8–12 hr
  Adult:
    IM: 0.5–1 g/dose QD
    SC: 1–2 g/dose QD as infusion over 8–24 hr

Contraindicated in anuria. Not approved for use in primary hemochromatosis. May cause flushing, erythema, urticaria, hypotension, tachycardia, diarrhea, leg cramps, fever, cataracts, hearing loss, nausea, and vomiting. Iron mobilization may be poor in children <3 yr.

High doses and concomitant low ferritin levels have also been associated with growth retardation. Growth velocity may resume to pretreatment levels by reducing the dosage. Acute respiratory distress syndrome has been reported following treatment with excessively high intravenous doses in patients with acute iron intoxication or thalassemia.

Maximum IV infusion rate: 15 mg/kg/hr. SC route is via a portable controlled-infusion device and is not recommended in acute iron poisoning.

DELAVIRDINE

Rescriptor, DLV
Antiviral, nonnucleoside reverse transcriptase inhibitor

No 3 C

Tabs: 100, 200 mg

>*12 yr and adults:* 400 mg PO TID; 600 mg PO BID is currently being studied

Use with **caution** in hepatic disease; drug is primarily metabolized by the liver. Incidence of rash has been reported as high as 50% and occurs within 1–3 weeks after initiation of therapy. Dose titration does not significantly reduce the incidence of rash. Other major side effects include headache, fatigue, and GI complaints.

Delavirdine inhibits the CYP450 3A4 and 2C9 drug metabolizing isoenzymes. Do not administer with astemizole, terfenadine, alprazolam, midazolam, triazolam, calcium channel blockers, ergot alkaloid dervatives, amphetamines, cisapride, and warfarin (increase risk of toxicity of these drugs). Antacids, H_2 antagonists, rifabutin, rifampin, carbamazepine, phenytoin, and phenobarbital may decrease delavirdine's efficacy. Ketoconazole, fluoxetine, and clarithromycin may increase delavirdine levels and effects. When administered with protease inhibitors, delavirdine can increase the effects of saquinavir and indinivir. **Carefully review the patient's drug profile for other drug interactions each time delavirdine is initiated or when a new drug is added to a regimen containing delavirdine.**

Adolescent dosing: Patients in early puberty (Tanner I-II) should be dosed with pediatric regimens and those in late puberty (Tanner V) should be dosed with adult regimens. Adolescents who are at the midst of their growth spurt (Tanner III females and Tanner IV males) can be dosed by either pediatric or adult regimen with close monitoring of efficacy and toxicity.

Doses may be administered with or without food. Doses of antacids and didanosine should be administered 1 hr before or 1 hr after taking delavirdine. Only the 100-mg tablets can be dissolved in water (four 100 mg tablets in ≥3 oz of water) to make a dispersion to be taken immediately. 200 mg tablets do not dissolve well in water.

Noncompliance can quickly promote resistant HIV Strains.

DESMOPRESSIN ACETATE

DDAVP, Stimate
Vasopressin analog, synthetic; hemostatic agent

No 2 B

Tabs: 0.1, 0.2 mg
Nasal solution: DDAVP, 100 mcg/mL (2.5 mL); Stimate, 1500 mcg/mL (2.5 mL); both preparations contain 9 mg NaCl/mL
Inj: 4 mcg/mL (1, 10 mL) (contains 9 mg NaCl/mL); 15 mcg/mL (1, 2 mL)

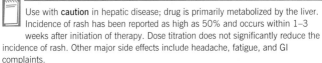

Continued

DESMOPRESSIN ACETATE *continued*

Nasal spray: 100 mcg/mL, 10 mcg/spray (50 sprays, 5 mL); contains 7.5 mg NaCl/mL
Conversion: 100 mcg = 400 IU arginine vasopressin

Diabetes insipidus:
  Oral:
    Children: Start with 0.05 mg/ dose QD–BID; titrate to effect
    Adult: Start with 0.05 mg/dose QD–BID; titrate dose to effect; usual dose range:
    0.1–0.2 mg/24 hr ÷ BID-TID
  Intranasal:
    3 mo–12 yr: 5–30 mcg/24 hr ÷ QD-BID
    Adults: 10–40 mcg/24 hr ÷ QD-TID; titrate dose to achieve control of excessive
    thirst and urination; **max. intranasal dose:** 40 mcg/24 hr
  IV/SC: 2–4 mcg/24 hr ÷ BID
Hemophilia A and von Willebrand's disease:
  Intranasal: 2–4 mcg/kg/dose
  IV: 0.2–0.4 mcg/kg/dose over 15–30 min
Nocturnal enuresis (>6 yr):
  Oral: 0.2 mg at bedtime, titrated to a **maximum** of 0.6 mg to achieve desired effect
  Intranasal: 20 mcg at bedtime, range 10–40 mcg; divide dose by 2 and administer
  each one-half dose in each nostril.

Use with **caution** in hypertension and coronary artery disease. May cause
headache, nausea, seizures, blood pressure changes, hyponatremia, nasal
congestion, abdominal cramps, and hypertension.
  Injection may be used SC or IV at approximately 10% of intranasal dose. Adjust fluid
intake to decrease risk of water intoxication.
  If switching stablized patient from intranasal route to IV/SC route, use 10% of
intranasal dose. *Peak effects:* 1–5 hr with intranasal route; 1.5–3 hr with IV route;
and 2–7 hr with PO route.
  For hemophilia A and von Willebrand's disease, administer dose intranasally, 2 hr
before procedure; IV, 30 min before procedure.

DEXAMETHASONE
Decadron and other brand names
Corticosteroid

No   ?   C

Tabs: 0.25, 0.5, 0.75, 1, 1.5, 2, 4, 6 mg
Inj: 4, 10, 20, 24 mg/mL (sodium phosphate; some preparations contain benzyl
alcohol)
IM inj: 8, 16 mg/mL (acetate)
Elixir: 0.5 mg/5 mL (some preparations contain 5% alcohol)
Oral solution: 0.1, 1 mg/mL (some preparations contain 30% alcohol)
Oral inhalation: 84 mcg/metered dose (170 sprays; 12.6 g)

Continued

DEXAMETHASONE *continued*

Nasal spray: 84 mcg/metered dose (170 sprays; 12.6 g)
Ophthalmic ointment: 0.05% (3.5 g)
Ophthalmic solution: 0.1% (5 mL)
Ophthalmic suspension: 0.1% (5, 15 mL)

Cerebral edema:
  Loading dose: 1–2 mg/kg/dose IV/IM × 1
  Maintenance: 1–1.5 mg/kg/24 hr ÷ Q4–6 hr; **max. dose:** 16 mg/24 hr
Airway edema: 0.5–2 mg/kg/24 hr IV/IM ÷ Q6 hr (begin 24 hr before extubation and continue for 4–6 doses after extubation)
Croup: 0.6 mg/kg/dose PO/IV/IM × 1 (use sodium phosphate injection)
Antiemetic:
  Initial: 10 mg/m^2/dose IV; **max. dose:** 20 mg
  Subsequent: 5 mg/m^2/dose Q6 hr IV
Antiinflammatory:
  Children: 0.08–0.3 mg/kg/24 hr PO, IV, IM ÷ Q6–12 hr
  Adults: 0.75–9 mg/24 hr PO, IV, IM ÷ Q6–12 hr
Spinal cord compression with neurological abnormalities:
  Children: 2 mg/kg/24 hr IV ÷ Q6 hr
Hib meningitis:
  >6 weeks: 0.6 mg/kg/24 hr IV ÷ Q6 hr × 2 days; initiate prior to or with the first dose of antibiotic
Ophthalmic use (children and adults):
  Ointment: Apply a thin coating of ointment to the conjunctival sac of the affected eye(s) TID–QID. When a favorable response is achieved reduce daily dosage to BID and later to QD as a maintenance dose sufficient to control symptoms.
  Solution: Instill 1 to 2 drops into the conjunctival sac of the affected eye(s) Q1 hr during the day and Q2 hr during the night as initial therapy. When a favorable response is achieved, reduce dosage to 1 drop Q4 hr. Further dose reduction to 1 drop TID–QID may be sufficient to control symptoms.
  Suspension: Shake well before using. Instill 1–2 drops in the conjunctival sacs of the affected eye(s). For severe disease, drops may be Q1 hr, being tapered to discontinuation as inflammation subsides. For mild disease, drops may be used ≤4 to 6 times/24 hr.

Toxicity: same as for prednisone without mineralocorticoid effects. **Contraindicated** in active untreated infections; and fungal, viral, and mycobacterial ocular infections. Use with **caution** in corneal/scleral thinning and glaucoma. Use ophthalmic preparation only in consultation with an ophthalmologist. Ophthalmic solution/suspension may be used in otitis externa.

Use in meningitis (other than Hib) is controversial. Consult ID specialist or latest edition of Red Book.

Oral peak serum levels occur 1–2 hr and within 8 hr following IM administration. **For other uses, doses based on body surface area, and dose equivalence to other steroids, see Chapter 28.**

For explanation of icons, see p. 572.

DEXTROAMPHETAMINE ± AMPHETAMINE

Dexedrine, Dexedrine Spansules, and many other brand names; in combination with amphetamine: Adderall

CNS stimulant

No   X   C

Tabs: 5, 10 mg
Sustained-release caps (Dexedrine Spansules): 5, 10, 15 mg
In combination with amphetamine (Adderall):
Tabs: 5, 7.5, 10, 12.5, 15, 20, 30 mg (available as 1 : 1 : 1 : 1 mixture of dextroamphetamine sulfate, dextroamphetamine saccharate, amphetamine aspartate, and amphetamine sulfate salts; for example, the 5-mg tablet contains 1.25 mg dextroamphetamine sulfate, 1.25 mg dextroamphetamine saccharate, 1.25 mg amphetamine aspartate, and 1.25 mg amphetamine sulfate)

> Dosages are in terms of mg of dextroamphetamine when using Dexedrine (dextroamphetamine alone) OR in terms of mg of the total dextroamphetamine and amphetamine salts when using Adderall.

Attention deficit hyperactivity disorder:
> *3–5 yr:* 2.5 mg/24 hr QAM; increase by 2.5 mg/24 hr at weekly intervals to a **max. dose** of 40 mg/24 hr ÷ QD-TID
> *≥6 yr:* 5 mg/24 hr QAM; increase by 5 mg/24 hr at weekly intervals to a **max. dose** of 40 mg/24 hr ÷ QD-TID

Narcolepsy:
> *6–12 yr:* 5 mg/24 hr ÷ QD-TID; increase by 5 mg/24 hr at weekly intervals to a **max. dose** of 60 mg/24 hr
> *>12 yr:* 10 mg/24 hr ÷ QD-TID; increase by 10 mg/24 hr at weekly intervals to a **max. dose** of 60 mg/24 hr

> Use with **caution** in presence of hypertension or cardiovascular disease. Not recommended for children <3 yr. Medication should generally not be used in children <5 yr because diagnosis of ADHD in this age group is extremely difficult (use in consultation with a specialist). Interrupt administration occasionally to determine need for continued therapy. Many side effects, including insomnia (avoid dose administration within 6 hr of bedtime), restlessness, anorexia, psychosis, headache, vomiting, abdominal cramps, dry mouth, and growth failure. Tolerance develops. (Same guidelines as for methylphenidate apply.) Do not give with MAO inhibitors, general anesthetics.

DIAZEPAM

Valium and others
Benzodiazepine; anxiolytic, anticonvulsant

No   3   D

Tabs: 2, 5, 10 mg
Oral solution: 1 mg/mL, 5 mg/mL (contains 19% alcohol)

Continued

DIAZEPAM *continued*

Inj: 5 mg/mL (contains 40% propylene glycol, 10% alcohol, and 1.5% benzyl alcohol)
Emulsified injection (Dizac, Diazemuls): 5 mg/mL
Sustained-release caps: 15 mg
Pediatric rectal gel (Diastat): 2.5, 5, 10 mg (5 mg/mL concentration with 4.4-cm rectal tip delivery system)
Adult rectal gel (Diastat): 10, 15, 20 mg (5 mg/mL concentration with 6-cm rectal tip delivery system)

Sedative/muscle relaxant:
  Children:
    IM or IV: 0.04–0.2 mg/kg/ dose Q2–4 hr
    Max. dose: 0.6 mg/kg within an 8-hr period
    PO: 0.12–0.8 mg/kg/24 hr ÷ Q6–8 hr
  Adults:
    IM or IV: 2–10 mg/dose Q3–4 hr PRN
    PO: 2–10 mg/dose Q6–12 hr PRN
Status epilepticus:
  Neonate: 0.3–0.75 mg/kg/dose IV Q15–30 min × 2–3 doses
  >1 mo: 0.2–0.5 mg/kg/dose IV Q15–30 min
    Max. total dose: <5 yr: 5 mg; ≥5 yr: 10 mg
  Adults: 5–10 mg/dose IV Q10–15 min
    Max. total dose: 30 mg
  Rectal dose (using IV dosage form): 0.5 mg/kg/dose followed by 0.25 mg/kg/dose in 10 min PRN
  Rectal gel: All doses rounded to the nearest available dosage strength; repeat dose in 4–12 hrs PRN
    2–5 yr: 0.5 mg/kg/dose
    6–11 yr: 0.3 mg/kg/dose
    ≥12 yr: 0.2 mg/kg/dose
Diazepam IV emulsion:
  Status epilepticus and severe recurrent seizures:
    >30 days old–5 yr: 0.2–0.5 mg slow IV Q2–5 min PRN up to a **total max. dose** of 5 mg
    Children ≥5 yr: 1 mg slow IV Q2–5 min PRN up to a **total max. dose** of 10 mg
    Adult: 5–10 mg slow IV × 1; if needed repeat in 10–15 min intervals up to a **total max. dose** of 30 mg (therapy may be repeated in 2–4 hrs with caution)
  Tetanus spasms (respiratory assistance should be available):
    Infants >30 days old: 1–2 mg slow IV Q3–4 hr PRN
    ≥5 yr: 5–10 mg slow IV Q3–4 hr PRN

Hypotension and respiratory depression may occur. Use with **caution** in glaucoma, shock, and depression. **Do not use** in combination with protease inhibitors. Concurrent use with CNS depressants, cimetidine, erythromycin, itraconazole, and valproic acid may enhance the effects of diazepam.

Administer the conventional IV product undiluted no faster than 2 mg/min. Do not mix with IV fluids.

Continued

DIAZEPAM *continued*

The injectable emulsion product must always be handled with strict aseptic technique because it is an excellent growth medium for microorganisms. Doses of this product must be injected slowly (no faster than 5 mg/min) and must not be administered through filters with pore sizes <5 microns or via polyvinyl chloride infusion sets.

In status epilepticus, diazepam must be followed by long-acting anticonvulsants. Onset of anticonvulsant effect: 1–3 min with IV route; 2–10 min with rectal route. **For management of status epilepticus, see pp. 16–17. For management of neonatal seizures, see pp. 427–429.**

DIAZOXIDE

Hyperstat IV, Proglycem
Antihypertensive agent, antihypoglycemic agent

No ? C

Inj: 15 mg/mL (20 mL)
Caps: 50 mg
Suspension: 50 mg/mL (30 mL); contains 7.25% alcohol

Hypertensive crisis: 1–3 mg/kg IV up to a **maximum** of 150 mg/dose; repeat Q5–15 min PRN, then Q4–24 hr
Hyperinsulinemic hypoglycemia (due to insulin-producing tumors):
Newborns and infants: 8–15 mg/kg/24 hr ÷ Q8–12 hr PO
Children and adults: 3–8 mg/kg/24 hr ÷ Q8–12 hr PO (start at lowest dose)

May cause hyponatremia, salt and water retention, GI disturbances, ketoacidosis, rash, hyperuricemia, weakness, hypertrichosis, and arrhythmias. Monitor BP closely for hypotension. Hyperglycemia occurs in majority of patients. Hypoglycemia should be treated initially with IV glucose; diazoxide should be introduced only if refractory to glucose infusion.

Peak antihypertensive effect with IV administration occurs within 5 min, with a duration of 3–12 hr. Hyperglycemic effect with PO administration occurs within 1 hr, with a duration of 8 hr.

DICLOXACILLIN SODIUM

Dycill, Dynapen, Pathocil, and others
Antibiotic, penicillin (penicillinase-resistant)

No ? B

Caps: 250, 500 mg; contains 0.6 mEq Na/250 mg
Oral suspension: 62.5 mg/5 mL (100, 200 mL; contains 2.9 mEq Na/62.5 mg)

Continued

DICLOXACILLIN SODIUM continued

Children (<40 kg):
  Mild/moderate infections: 12.5–25 mg/kg/24 hr PO ÷ Q6 hr
  Severe infections: 50–100 mg/kg/24 hr PO ÷ Q6 hr
Adults (≥40 kg): 125–500 mg/dose PO Q6 hr; **max. dose:** 4 g/24 hr

Toxicity and side effects similar to cloxacillin. Limited experience in neonates and very young infants. Higher doses (50–100 mg/kg/24 hr) are indicated following IV therapy for osteomyelitis.

Administer 1–2 hr before meals or 2 hr after meals. Use of the oral suspension dosage form may be limited by the resultant dose volume of the 62.5 mg/5 mL concentration.

DIDANOSINE

Videx, Videx EC, Dideoxyinosine, ddI
Antiviral agent, nucleoside analogue reverse transcriptase inhibitor

Yes   3   B

Tabs (buffered, chewable/dispersable): 25, 50, 100, 150, 200 mg; contains 11.5 mEq sodium, 15.7 mEq magnesium, and phenylalanine per tablet
Caps (delayed release, enteric coated): 125, 200, 250, 400 mg
Oral powder, buffered (single-dose packets for solution): 100, 167, 250, 375 mg; contains 60 mEq sodium per packet
Oral pediatric powder (for 10 mg/mL solution): 2, 4 g

Neonates and Infants <3 months: 100 mg/m^2/24 hr ÷ Q12 hr PO
Children <13 yr:
  Usual dose (in combination with other antiretrovirals): 180 mg/m^2/24 hr ÷ Q12 hr PO
  Dose range: 180–300 mg/m^2/24 hr ÷ Q12 hr; higher dose may be required for CNS disease
Alternative pediatric dosing based on 200 mg/m^2/24 hr, see table below.

ALTERNATIVE PEDIATRIC DOSING

BSA(m^2)	Chewable Tablets*	Pediatric Powder Dose
<0.4	25 mg Q12 hr	31 mg Q12 hr
0.5–0.7	50 mg Q12 hr	62 mg Q12 hr
0.8–1	75 mg Q12 hr	94 mg Q12 hr
1.1–1.4	100 mg Q12 hr	125 mg Q12 hr

*Use at least 2 tablets to assure adequate buffering capacity (e.g., give two 25-mg tablets for a 50-mg dose).

Continued

DIDANOSINE *continued*

Adolescent/adult (see remarks for additional adolescent dosing information):
  <60 kg:
    Tabs: 125 mg Q12 hr PO
    Buffered oral solution: 167 mg Q12 hr PO
    Caps (delayed release, enteric coated): 250 mg Q24 hr PO
  ≥60 kg:
    Tabs: 200 mg Q12 hr PO
    Buffered oral solution: 250 mg Q12 hr PO
    Caps (delayed release, enteric coated): 400 mg Q24 hr PO

Side effects include headaches, diarrhea, abdominal pain, nausea, vomiting, peripheral neuropathy (dose related), electrolyte abnormalities, hyperuricemia, increased liver enzymes, retinal depigmentation, CNS depression, rash/pruritus, myalgia, and pancreatitis (dose related, more in adults). Fatal lactic acidosis has been reported in pregnant women taking didanosine in combination with stavudine. Use with **caution** in patients on sodium restriction (11.5 mEq Na/buffered tablet, 60 mEq Na/single-dose packet) and with phenylketonuria (phenylalanine in tablets).

Adolescent dosing: Patients in early puberty (Tanner I-II) should be dosed with pediatric regimens and those in late puberty (Tanner V) should be dosed with adult regimens. Adolescents who are at the midst of their growth spurt (Tanner III females and Tanner IV males) can be dosed by either pediatric or adult regimen with close monitoring of efficacy and toxicity.

Reduce dose in renal impairment (see package insert). Delayed-release capsules should not be used for patients <60 kg with GFR <10 mL/min.

Administer all doses on empty stomach. Videx EC should be swallowed intact. Impairs absorption of drugs requiring an acidic environment and drugs that have impaired absorption impaired in the presence of divalent ions (e.g., ketoconazole and fluoroquinolones, respectively). Separate dosing when used in combination with the following drugs: 1 hr before or after ddI (indinavir); 2 hrs before or after ddI (delavirdine, ritonavir, fluoroquinolones, ketoconazole, itraconazole, tetracyclines, and dapsone).

Consult package insert for additional details.

DIGOXIN

Lanoxin, Lanoxicaps
Antiarrhythmic agent, inotrope

Yes   1   C

Caps: 50, 100, 200 mcg
Tabs: 125, 250, 500 mcg
Elixir: 50 mcg/mL (60 mL); may contain 10% alcohol
Inj: 100, 250 mcg/mL; may contain propylene glycol and alcohol

Continued

DIGOXIN continued

Digitalizing: Total digitalizing dose (TDD) and maintenance doses in mcg/kg/ 24 hr (see table below):

DIGOXIN DIGITALIZING AND MAINTENANCE DOSES

	TDD		Maintenance	
Age	PO	IV/IM	PO	IV/IM
Premature	20	15	5	3–4
Full term	30	20	8–10	6–8
<2 yr	40–50	30–40	10–12	7.5–9
2–10 yr	30–40	20–30	8–10	6–8
>10 yr and <100 kg	10–15	8–12	2.5–5	2–3

TDD, total digitalizing dose.

Initial: ½ TDD, then ¼ TDD Q8–18 hr × 2 doses; obtain ECG 6 hr after dose to assess for toxicity
Maintenance:
   <10 yr: Give maintenance dose ÷ BID
   ≥10 yr: Give maintenance dose QD

Contraindicated in patients with ventricular dysrhythmias. Use with **caution** in renal failure. May cause AV block or dysrhythmias. In the patient treated with digoxin, cardioversion or calcium infusion may lead to ventricular fibrillation (pretreatment with lidocaine may prevent this). Decreased serum potassium and magnesium, or increased magnesium and calcium may increase risk for digoxin toxicity. For signs and symptoms of toxicity, see p. 31.

Excreted via the kidney; **adjust dose in renal failure (see p. 948).** *Therapeutic concentration:* 0.8–2 ng/mL. Higher doses may be required for supraventricular tachycardia. Neonates, pregnant women, and patients with renal, hepatic, or heart failure may have falsely elevated digoxin levels because of the presence of digoxin-like substances.

$T_{1/2}$: Premature infants, 61–170 hr; full-term neonates, 35–45 hr; infants, 18–25 hr; and children, 35 hr.

Recommended serum sampling at steady-state: Obtain a single level from 6 hr post dose to just before the next scheduled dose following 5–8 days of continuous dosing. Levels obtained prior to steady-state may be useful in preventing toxicity.

DIGOXIN IMMUNE FAB (OVINE)

Digibind
Antidigoxin antibody

No   ?   C

Inj: 38 mg

Continued

DIGOXIN IMMUNE FAB (OVINE) *continued*

First, determine total body digoxin load (TBL):
TBL (mg) = serum digoxin level (ng/mL) × 5.6 × wt (kg) ÷ 1000, **OR** TBL (mg)
= mg digoxin ingested × 0.8
Then, calculate digoxin immune Fab dose:
Dose in number of digoxin immune Fab vials: # vials = TBL ÷ 0.5
Infuse IV over 15–30 min (through 0.22 micron filter).

Contraindicated if there is hypersensitivity to sheep products, or renal or cardiac
failure. May cause rapidly developing severe hypokalemia, decreased cardiac
output, rash, and edema. Digoxin therapy may be reinstituted in 3–7 days,
when toxicity has been corrected. See p. 31 for additional information.

DIHYDROTACHYSTEROL

DHT, Hytakerol, DHT Intensol
Fat-soluble vitamin D analog

No   ?   A/D

Solution: 0.2 mg/mL (20% alcohol) (30 mL)
Caps: 0.125 mg
Tabs: 0.125, 0.2, 0.4 mg
1 mg = 120,000 IU vitamin D_2

Hypoparathyroidism:
Neonates: 0.05–0.1 mg/24 hr PO
Infants/young children: Initial, 1–5 mg/24 hr PO × 4 days, then 0.5–1.5 mg/
24 hr PO
Older children/adults: Initial, 0.75–2.5 mg/24 hr PO × 4 days, then 0.2–1.5 mg/
24 hr PO
Nutritional rickets: 0.5 mg × 1 PO, or 13–50 mcg/24 hr PO QD until healing
Renal osteodystrophy:
Children/adolescents: 0.1–0.5 mg/24 hr PO
Adults: 0.1–0.6 mg/24 hr PO

Use with **caution** in patients with renal stones, renal failure, and heart disease.
Monitor serum Ca^{++} and PO_4. Toxicities include hypercalcemia or hypervita-
minosis D. May cause nausea, vomiting, anorexia, and renal damage.
Activated by 25-hydroxylation in liver; does not require 1-hydroxylation in kidney.
More potent than vitamin D_2 but more rapidly inactivated (half-life is hours vs. weeks).
Titrate dose with patient response. Oral Ca^{++} supplementation may be required.
Pregnancy category changes to "D" if used in doses above RDA.

DILTIAZEM

Cardizem, Cardizem SR, Cardizem CD, Dilacor XR, Tiazac, and others
Calcium channel blocker, antihypertensive

No   1   C

Tabs: 30, 60, 90, 120 mg
Extended-release tabs: 120, 180, 240 mg
Extended-release caps:
Cardizem SR: 60, 90, 120 mg
Cardizem CD: 120, 180, 240, 300, 360 mg
Dilacor XR: 120, 180, 240 mg
Tiazac: 120, 180, 240, 300, 360, 420 mg
Inj: 5 mg/mL (5, 10 mL)

Children: 1.5–2 mg/kg/24 hr PO ÷ TID-QID; **max. dose:** 3.5 mg/kg/24 hr
Adolescents:
Immediate release: 30–120 mg/dose PO TID-QID; usual range 180–360 mg/24 hr
Extended release: 120–300 mg/24 hr PO ÷ QD-BID (BID dosing with Cardizem SR; QD dosing with Cardizem CD, Dilacor XR, Tiazac)

Contraindicated in acute MI with pulmonary congestion, second- or third-degree heart block, and sick sinus syndrome. Dizziness, headache, edema, nausea, vomiting, heart block, and arrhythmias may occur.

Diltiazem is a substrate and inhibitor of the cytochrome P-450 3A4 enzyme system. May increase levels and/or effect of cyclosporin, carbamazepine, fentanyl, digoxin, quinidine, benzodiazepines, and beta-blockers. Cimetidine may increase diltiazem serum levels. Rifampin may decrease diltiazem serum levels.

Maximal antihypertensive effect seen within 2 weeks.

DIMENHYDRINATE

Dramamine, Children's Dramamine, and other brand names
Antiemetic, antihistamine

No   ?   B

Tabs: 50 mg
Chewable tabs: 50 mg (aspartame)
Inj: 50 mg/mL (benzyl alcohol and propylene glycol)
Solution: 12.5 mg/4 mL, 12.5 mg/5 mL, 15.62 mg/5 mL (some preparations may contain 5% alcohol)

Continued

DIMENHYDRINATE *continued*

Children (<12 yr): 5 mg/kg/24 hr ÷ Q6 hr PO/IM/IV
Adult: 50–100 mg/dose Q4–6 hr PRN PO/IM/IV
Max. PO doses:
2–6 yr: 75 mg/24 hr
6–12 yr: 150 mg/24 hr
Adults: 400 mg/24 hr
Max. IM dose: 300 mg/24 hr

Causes drowsiness and anticholinergic side effects. May mask vestibular symptoms and cause CNS excitation in young children. Use **caution** when taken with ototoxic agents or history of seizures. **Use should be limited to management of prolonged vomiting of known etiology.** Not recommended in children <2 yr. Toxicity resembles anticholinergic poisoning.

DIMERCAPROL

BAL, British anti-Lewisite
Heavy metal chelator (arsenic, gold, mercury, lead)

No   ?   D

Inj (in oil): 100 mg/mL; contains peanut oil (3 mL)

Give all injections deep IM.
Lead poisoning: Administer BAL with Ca-EDTA. See pp. 36–38 for details.
Arsenic or gold poisoning:
Days 1 and 2: 2.5–3 mg/kg/dose Q6 hr
Day 3: 2.5–3 mg/kg/dose Q12 hr
Days 4–14: 2.5–3 mg/kg/dose Q24 hr
Mercury poisoning: 5 mg/kg × 1, then 2.5 mg/kg/dose QD–BID × 10 days

Contraindicated in hepatic or renal insufficiency. May cause hypertension, tachycardia, GI disturbance, headache, fever (30% of children), nephrotoxicity, and transient neutropenia. Symptoms are usually relieved by antihistamines. Urine should be kept alkaline to protect the kidneys. Use cautiously in patients with G6PD deficiency. **Do not use** concomitantly with iron. See pp. 36–38 for additional information.

DIPHENHYDRAMINE

Benadryl and other brand names
Antihistamine

Yes   ?   B

Elixir (14% alcohol): 12.5 mg/5 mL
Syrup (some contain 5% alcohol): 12.5 mg/5 mL
Liquid: 12.5 mg/5 mL

Continued

DIPHENHYDRAMINE *continued*

Caps/tabs: 25, 50 mg
Chewable tabs: 12.5 mg (aspartame, phenylalanine)
Inj: 10, 50 mg/mL
Cream: 1, 2%
Lotion: 1% (75 mL)
Topical spray: 1%

Children: 5 mg/kg/24 hr ÷ Q6 hr PO/IM/IV
Max. dose: 300 mg/24 hr
Adult: 10–50 mg/dose Q4–8 hr PO/IM/IV
Max. dose: 400 mg/24 hr
For anaphylaxis or phenothiazine overdose: 1–2 mg/kg IV slowly

Contraindicated with concurrent MAO inhibitor use, acute attacks of asthma, and GI or urinary obstruction. Use with **caution** in infants and young children, and do not use in neonates due to potential CNS effects. Side effects include sedation, nausea, vomiting, xerostoma, blurred vision and other reactions common to antihistamines. CNS side effects more common than GI disturbances. May cause paradoxical excitement in children. **Adjust dose in renal failure (see p. 948).**

DISOPYRAMIDE PHOSPHATE

Norpace and others
Antiarrhythmic agent, class Ia   Yes   1   C

Caps: 100, 150 mg
Extended-release caps (CR): 100, 150 mg
Suspension: 1 mg/mL, 10 mg/mL 🖉

<1 yr: 10–30 mg/kg/24 hr ÷ Q6 hr PO
1–4 yr: 10–20 mg/kg/24 hr ÷ Q6 hr PO
4–12 yr: 10–15 mg/kg/24 hr ÷ Q6 hr PO
12–18 yr: 6–15 mg/kg/24 hr ÷ Q6 hr PO
Adult:
   <50 kg: 100 mg/dose Q6 hr PO or 200 mg (extended-release) Q12 hr PO
   ≥50 kg: 150 mg/dose Q6 hr PO or 300 mg (extended-release) Q12 hr PO
   Max. dose: 1.6 g/24 hr

Contraindicated in second- or third-degree heart block. May cause decreased cardiac output. Anticholinergic effects may occur. Causes dose-related AV block, wide QRS, increased QTc, ventricular dysrhythmias. **Adjust dose in renal (see p. 949) or hepatic failure.**
   Drug is metabolized by cytochrome P450 3A4 isoenzyme. Clarithromycin and erythromycin may increase serum levels. Phenytoin, phenobarbital, and rifampin may decrease serum levels. *Therapeutic levels:* 3–7 mg/L.
   Use limited in neurally mediated syncope.

DIVALPROEX SODIUM
Depakote, Depakote ER
Anticonvulsant

No   1   D

Extended/delayed-release tabs: 125, 250, 500 mg
Sprinkle caps: 125 mg

 Dose: See Valproic Acid

 See Valproic Acid. Preferred over valproic acid for patients on ketogenic diet.

DOBUTAMINE
Dobutrex
Sympathomimetic agent

No   ?   C

Inj: 12.5 mg/mL (contains sulfites) (20 mL)

 Continuous IV infusion: 2.5–15 mcg/kg/min;
Max. dose: 40 mcg/kg/min
To prepare infusion: See inside front cover

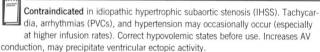 **Contraindicated** in idiopathic hypertrophic subaortic stenosis (IHSS). Tachycardia, arrhythmias (PVCs), and hypertension may occasionally occur (especially at higher infusion rates). Correct hypovolemic states before use. Increases AV conduction, may precipitate ventricular ectopic activity.

Dobutamine has been shown to increase cardiac output and systemic pressure in pediatric patients of every age group. However, in premature neonates, dobutamine is less effective than dopamine in raising systemic blood pressure without causing undue tachycardia, and dobutamine has not been shown to provide any added benefit when given to such infants already receiving optimal infusions of dopamine.

Monitor BP and vital signs. $T_{1/2}$: 2 min. Peak effects in 10–20 min.

DOCUSATE
Colace, Surfak, and others
Stool softener, laxative

No   ?   C

Caps: 50, 100, 240, 250 mg
Tabs: 100 mg

Continued

DOCUSATE *continued*

Syrup: 16.7 mg/5 mL, 20 mg/5 mL
Oral liquid: 10 mg/mL

PO: (take with liquids)
   <3 yr: 10–40 mg/24 hr ÷ QD-QID
   3–6 yr: 20–60 mg/24 hr ÷ QD-QID
  6–12 yr: 40–150 mg/24 hr ÷ QD-QID
   >12 yr: 50–400 mg/24 hr ÷ QD-QID
Rectal: Older children and adults: Add 50–100 mg of oral solution to enema fluid.

Oral dosage effective only after 1–3 days of therapy. Incidence of side effects is exceedingly low. Oral liquid is bitter; give with milk, fruit juice, or formula to mask taste.

A few drops of the 10 mg/mL oral liquid may be used in the ear as a cerumenolytic. Effect is usually seen within 15 min.

DOPAMINE

Intropin, and others
Sympathomimetic agent

No ? C

Inj: 40, 80, 160 mg/mL (5, 10, 20 mL)
Prediluted in D$_5$W: 0.8, 1.6, 3.2 mg/mL (250, 500 mL)

Low dose: 2–5 mcg/kg/min IV; increases renal blood flow; minimal effect on heart rate and cardiac output
  Intermediate dose: 5–15 mcg/kg/min IV; increases heart rate, cardiac contractility, cardiac output, and to a lesser extent, renal blood flow.
High dose: >20 mcg/kg/min IV; alpha-adrenergic effects are prominent; decreases renal perfusion
Max. dose recommended: 20–50 mcg/kg/min IV
To prepare infusion: See inside front cover

Do not use in pheochromocytoma, tachyarrhythmias, or hypovolemia. Monitor vital signs and blood pressure continuously. Correct hypovolemic states.

Tachyarrhythmias, ectopic beats, hypertension, vasoconstriction, and vomiting may occur. Use cautiously with phenytoin because hypotension and bradycardia may be exacerbated.

Newborn infants may be more sensitive to the vasoconstrictive effects of dopamine.

Should be administered through a central line or large vein. Extravasation may cause tissue necrosis; treat with phentolamine. **Do not** administer into an umbilical arterial catheter.

DORNASE ALFA/DNASE

Pulmozyme
Inhaled mucolytic

No ? B

Solution: 1 mg/mL (2.5 mL)

Children > 5 yr: 2.5 mg via nebulizer QD. Some may benefit from 2.5 mg BID

Contraindicated in patients with hypersensitivity to epoetin alfa. Voice alteration, pharyngitis, laryngitis may result. These are generally reversible without dose adjustment.

Should not mix with other nebulized drugs. A beta-agonist may be useful before administration to enhance drug distribution. Chest physiotherapy should be incorporated into treatment regimen. Use of the "Sidestream" nebulizer cup can significantly reduce the medication administration time.

DOXAPRAM HCl

Dopram
CNS stimulant

No ? B

Inj: 20 mg/mL (20 mL)
Contains 0.9% benzyl alcohol

Methylxanthine-refractory neonatal apnea: Load with 2.5–3 mg/kg over 15 min, followed by a continuous infusion of 1 mg/kg/hr titrated to the lowest effective dose; **max. dose:** 2.5 mg/kg/hr

Hypertension occurs with higher doses (>1.5 mg/kg/hr). May also cause tachycardia, arrhythmias, seizure, hyperreflexia, hyperpyrexia, and sweating. Avoid extravasation into tissues.

Do not use with general anesthetic agents that can sensitize the heart to catecholamines (e.g., halothane, cyclopropane, and enflurane) to reduce the risk of cardiac arrhythmias, including ventricular tachycardia and ventricular fibrillation. **Do not** initiate doxapram until the general anesthetic agent has been completely excreted.

DOXYCYCLINE
Vibramycin, Periostat, and others
Antibiotic, tetracycline derivative

No 2 D

Caps: 20 (Periostat), 50, 100 mg
Tabs: 20 (Periostat), 50, 100 mg
Syrup: 50 mg/5 mL (60 mL)
Suspension: 25 mg/5 mL (60 mL)
Inj: 100, 200 mg

Initial:
  ≤*45 kg:* 5 mg/kg/24 hr ÷ BID PO/IV × 1 day to **max. dose** of 200 mg/24 hr
    >*45 kg:* 100 mg BID PO/IV × 1 day
Maintenance:
  ≤*45 kg:* 2.5–5 mg/kg/24 hr ÷ QD-BID PO/IV
  >*45 kg:* 100–200 mg/24 hr ÷ QD-BID PO/IV
Max. adult dose: 300 mg/24 hr
PID: see p. 365.
Malaria prophylaxis (start 1–2 days prior to exposure and continue for 4 weeks after leaving edemic area):
  >*8 yr:* 2 mg/kg/24 hr PO QD; **max. dose:** 100 mg/24 hr
Adult: 100 mg PO QD
Periodontitis:
  Adults: 20 mg BID PO × ≤9 mo

Use with **caution** in hepatic and renal disease. May cause increased intracranial pressure. Generally not recommended for use in children <8 yr because of risk for tooth enamel hypoplasia and discoloration. However, the AAP *Red Book* recommends doxycycline as the drug of choice for rickettsial disease regardless of age. May cause GI symptoms, photosensitivity, hemolytic anemia, rash, and hypersensitivity reactions.

Doxycycline is approved for the treatment of anthrax *(Bacillus anthracis)* regardless of the route of exposure. See www.cdc.gov for additional information.

Rifampin, barbiturates, phenytoin, and carbamazepine may increase clearance of doxycycline. Doxycycline may enhance the hypoprothrombinemic effect of warfarin. See *Tetracycline* for additional drug/food interactions and comments.

Infuse IV over 1–4 hr. Avoid prolonged exposure to direct sunlight.

For periodontitis, take capsules ≥1 hr prior to meals; and take tablets ≥1 hr prior or 2 hours after meals.

DRONABINOL
Tetrahydrocannabinol, THC, Marinol
Antiemetic

No   ?   C

Caps: 2.5, 5, 10 mg (contains sesame oil)

Antiemetic:
  Children and adult (PO): 5 mg/m^2/dose 1–3 hr prior to chemotherapy, then
    Q2–4 hr up to a **maximum** of 6 doses/24 hr; doses may be gradually increased
by 2.5 mg/m^2/dose increments up to a **maximum** of 15 mg/m^2/dose if needed and
tolerated
Appetite stimulant:
  Adult (PO): 2.5 mg BID 1 hr before lunch and dinner; if not tolerated, reduce dose
  to 2.5 mg QHS.
  Max. dose: 20 mg/24 hr (Use **caution** when increasing doses because of increased
risk of dose-related adverse reactions at higher dosages)

Contraindicated in patients with history of substance abuse and mental illness,
allergy to sesame oil. Use with **caution** in heart disease, seizures, hepatic
disease (reduce dose if severe). Side effects include euphoria, dizziness, difficulty
concentrating, anxiety, mood change, sedation, hallucinations, ataxia, paresthesia,
hypotension, excessively increased appetite, and habit forming potential.
  Onset of action: 0.5–1 hr. Duration of psychoactive effects 4–6 hr, appetite
stimulation 24 hr.

DROPERIDOL
Inapsine
Sedative, antiemetic

No   ?   C

Inj: 2.5 mg/mL

Antiemetic/sedation:
  Children: 0.03–0.07 mg/kg/dose IM or IV over 2–5 min; if needed, may give
  0.1–0.15 mg/kg/dose; **max. dose:** 2.5 mg/dose
    Dosage interval:
      Antiemetic: PRN Q4–6 hr
      Sedation: Repeat dose in 15–30 min if necessary
  Adult: 2.5–5 mg IM or IV over 2–5 min
    Dosage interval:
      Antiemetic: PRN Q3–4 hr
      Sedation: Repeat dose in 15–30 min if necessary

Continued

DROPERIDOL *continued*

Side effects include hypotension, tachycardia, extrapyramidal side effects such as dystonia, feeling of motor restlessness, laryngospasm, and bronchospasm.
May lower seizure threshold. **Fatal arrhythmias and QT interval prolongation have been associated with use.**

Onset in 3–10 min. Peak effects within 10–30 min. Duration of 2–4 hr. Often given as adjunct to other agents.

EDROPHONIUM CHLORIDE

Tensilon, Enlon, Reversol
Anticholinesterase agent, antidote for neuromuscular blockade   Yes   ?   C

Inj: 10 mg/mL (1, 10, 15 mL) (contains phenol and sulfites)

Test for myasthenia gravis (IV):
Neonates: 0.1 mg single dose
Infants and children:
Initial: 0.04 mg/kg/dose × 1
Max. dose: 1 mg for <34 kg, 2 mg for ≥34 kg
If no response after 1 min, may give 0.16 mg/kg/dose for a total of 0.2 mg/kg
Total max. dose: 5 mg for <34 kg, 10 mg for ≥34 kg
Adult: 2-mg test dose IV; if no reaction, give 8 mg after 45 sec

May precipitate cholinergic crisis, arrhythmias, and bronchospasm. Keep atropine available in syringe and have resuscitation equipment ready. Hypersensitivity to test dose (fasciculations or intestinal cramping) is indication to stop giving drug. **Contraindicated** in GI or GU obstruction, or arrhythmias. Dose may need to be reduced in chronic renal failure.

Short duration of action with IV route (5–10 min). **Antidote:** Atropine 0.01–0.04 mg/kg/dose.

EDTA CALCIUM DISODIUM

Calcium disodium versenate
Chelating agent, antidote for lead toxicity   Yes   ?   C

Inj: 200 mg/mL (5 mL)

Lead poisoning: see pp. 35–38 for classification, treatment, and dosing.

Continued

EDTA CALCIUM DISODIUM *continued*

May cause renal tubular necrosis. **Do not use** if anuric. Follow urinalysis and
renal function. Monitor ECG continuously for arrhythmia when giving IV. Rapid
IV infusion may cause sudden increase in intracranial pressure in patients with
cerebral edema. May cause zinc and copper deficiency. Monitor Ca^{++} and PO_4.

IM route preferred. Give IM with 0.5% procaine.

EFAVIRENZ
Sustiva, DMP-266
Antiviral agent, nonnucleoside reverse transcriptase inhibitor   No   3   C

Caps: 50, 100, 200 mg

Children ≥3 yr and weighing ≥10 kg: daily PO dose administered QD (see table below)

Body Weight (kg)	Dose (mg)
10–<15	200
15–<20	250
20–<25	300
25–<32.5	350
32.5–<40	400
≥40	600

Adults: 600 mg/dose PO QD

Do not use as a single agent for HIV or added on as a sole agent to a failing
regimen. Therapy should always be initiated in combination with at least one
other antiretroviral agent to which the patient has not been previously exposed.

Dizziness, somnolence, insomnia, hallucinations, and euphoria are common side
effects. Skin rashes (usually mild to moderate maculopapular eruptions) may occur
within the first 2 weeks of initiating therapy and usually resolve (with continuing the
drug) within 1 mo. Rash is more common in children and more often of greater severity. Discontinue therapy in patients developing severe rash associated with blistering,
desquamation, mucosal involvement, or fever. Diarrhea, fever, cough, nausea,
vomiting, pancreatitis, and elevations in liver enzymes and serum lipids have
been reported. May cause false-positive urinary cannabinoid test (CEDIA DAU
multi-level THC assay).

Drug is a substrate and inducer of CYP 450 3A4; and may also inhibit other CYP
450 isoenzymes (2C9, 2C19, and 3A4). Monitor effect/serum levels of drugs
metabolized by the aforementioned CYP 450 isoenzymes (e.g., warfarin, rifampin).
Increases serum levels of nelfinavir and ritonavir; and decreases levels of indinavir
and saquinavir. Should **not** be administered with astemizole, cisapride, midazolam,
triazolam, or ergot derivatives because competition for CYP 450 3A4 may result in
inhibition of metabolism and toxicity of these drugs.

Continued

EFAVIRENZ *continued*

Adolescent dosing: Patients in early puberty (Tanner I-II) should be dosed with pediatric regimens and those in late puberty (Tanner V) should be dosed with adult regimens. Adolescents who are at the midst of their growth spurt (Tanner III females and Tanner IV males) can be dosed by either pediatric or adult regimen with close monitoring of efficacy and toxicity.

Pharmacokinetics in hepatic or renal impairment have not been adequately evaluated. Doses may be administered with or without food; however, avoid high-fat meals (increases absorption). Capsules may be opened and added to liquids or foods, but have a peppery taste; grape jelly may be used to disguise taste. Initiate dosing at bedtime for the first 2–4 weeks to reduce CNS side effects.

EMLA

Eutectic mixture of lidocaine and prilocaine
Topical analgesic

No   ?   B

Cream: Lidocaine 2.5% + prilocaine 2.5%; 5-g kit (with dressings); 30-g tube
Topical anesthetic disc: Lidocaine 2.5% + prilocaine 2.5%; 1 g (contact surface ~ 10 cm^2) (box of 2s or 10s)

See p. 893 for general use information.
Newborns ≥ 37 weeks gestation, children, and adults:
  Minor procedures: 2.5 g/site for at least 60 min
Painful procedures: 2 g/10 cm^2 of skin for at least 2 hr
See table below for maximum dose and application information.

Age and Weight	Maximum Total EMLA Dose (g)	Maximum Application Area (cm^2)	Maximum Application Time (hr)
Birth–3 mo or <5 kg	1	10	1
*3–12 mo and >5 kg	2	20	4
1–6 yr and >10 kg	10	100	4
7–12 yr and >20 kg	20	200	4

*If patient is >3 mo and is not >5 kg, use the maximum total dose that corresponds to the patient's weight.

Should not be used in neonates <37 weeks gestation nor in infants <12 mo receiving treatment with methemoglobin-inducing agents (e.g., sulfa drugs, acetaminophen, nitrofurantoin, nitroglycerin, nitroprusside, phenobarbital, phenytoin). Use with **caution** in patients with G6PD deficiency and in patients with renal and hepatic impairment. Prilocaine has been associated with methemoglobinemia. Long duration of application, large treatment area, small patients, or impaired elimination may result in high blood levels.

Apply topically to intact skin and cover with occlusive dressing; avoiding mucous membranes or the eyes. Wipe cream off before procedure.

ENALAPRIL MALEATE, ENALAPRILAT

Vasotec, Vasotec IV
Angiotensin converting enzyme inhibitor, antihypertensive   Yes   1   C/D

Tabs: 2.5, 5, 10, 20 mg (Enalapril)
Oral suspension: 1 mg/mL
Inj: 1.25 mg/mL (Enalaprilat); contains benzyl alcohol

Infants and children:
  PO: 0.1 mg/kg/24 hr ÷ QD–BID; increase PRN over 2 weeks
  Max. dose: 0.5 mg/kg/24 hr
  IV: 0.005–0.01 mg/kg/dose Q8–24 hr
Adult:
  PO: 2.5–5 mg/24 hr QD initially to **max. dose** of 40 mg/24 hr ÷ QD-BID
  IV: 0.625–1.25 mg/dose IV Q6 hr

Use with **caution** in bilateral renal artery stenosis. **Avoid use** with dialysis with high-flux membranes because anaphylactoid reactions have been reported.

Side effects include nausea, diarrhea, headache, dizziness, hyperkalemia, hypoglycemia, hypotension, and hypersensitivity. Cough is a reported side effect of ACE inhibitors.

Enalapril (PO) is converted to its active form (Enalaprilat) by the liver. Administer IV over 5 min. **Adjust dose in renal impairment (see p. 949).**

Pregnancy category is "C" during the first trimester but changes to "D" during the second and third trimester (fetal injury and death have been reported).

ENOXAPARIN

Lovenox
Anticoagulant, low-molecular-weight heparin   Yes   ?   B

Inj (ampules): 30 mg/0.3 mL
Inj (pre-filled syringes with 27-gauge × ½-inch needle): 30 mg/0.3 mL, 40 mg/0.4 mL, 60 mg/0.6 mL, 80 mg/0.8 mL, 100 mg/1 mL, 90 mg/0.6 mL, 120 mg/0.8 mL, 150 mg/1 mL
Approximate anti-factor Xa activity: 100 IU per 1 mg

DVT treatment:
  Infants <2 mo: 1.5 mg/kg/dose Q12 hr SC
  Infants ≥2 mo–adults: 1 mg/kg/dose Q12 hr SC

Continued

ENOXAPARIN continued

Dosage adjustment to achieve target anti-factor Xa levels of 0.5–1 units/mL (see table below):

Anti-Factor Xa Level (units/mL)	Hold Next Dose?	Dose Change	Repeat Anti-Factor Xa Level ?
<0.35	No	Increase by 25%	4 hrs post next new dose
0.35–0.49	No	Increase by 10%	4 hrs post next new dose
0.5–1	No	No	Next day, then 1 week later at 4 hrs post dose
1.1–1.5	No	Decrease by 20%	4 hrs post next new dose
1.6–2	3 hr	Decrease by 30%	4 hrs post next new dose
>2	Until anti-factor Xa reaches 0.5 U/mL (level can be measured Q12 hr until it reaches ≤0.5 U/mL)	When anti-factor Xa reaches 0.5 U/mL, dose may be restarted at a dose 40% less than originally prescribed	4 hrs post next new dose

DVT prophylaxis:
Infants <2 mo: 1 mg/kg/dose Q12 hr SC
Infants ≥2 mo up to children 18 yr: 0.5 mg/kg/dose Q12 hr SC
Adults: 30 mg BID SC × 7–10 days; initiate therapy 12–24 hr after hip or knee replacement surgery provided hemostasis is established. Doses of 40 mg QD SC × 7–12 days initiated 2 hr prior to abdominal surgery have also been used.

Inhibits thrombosis by inactivating factor Xa without significantly affecting bleeding time, platelet function, PT, or APTT at recommended doses. Dosages of enoxaparin, heparin, or other low-molecular-weight heparins **cannot** be used interchangeably on a unit-for-unit (or mg-for-mg) basis because of differences in pharmacokinetics and activity. Peak anti-factor Xa activity is achieved 4 hr after a dose.

Contraindicated in major bleeding and drug-induced thrombocytopenia. Use with **caution** in uncontrolled arterial hypertension, bleeding diathesis, history of recurrent GI ulcers, diabetic retinopathy, and severe renal dysfunction (consider dose reduction if GFR <30 mL/min). **Concurrent use with spinal or epidural anesthesia, or spinal puncture has resulted in long-term or permanent paralysis; potential benefits must be weighed against the risks.** May cause fever, confusion, edema, nausea, hemorrhage, thrombocytopenia, hypochromic anemia, and pain/erythema at injection site. **Protamine sulfate is the antidote;** 1 mg protamine sulfate neutralizes 1 mg enoxaparin.

Recommended anti-factor Xa levels obtained 4 hr after subcutaneous dose:
DVT treatment: 0.5–1 units/mL
DVT prophylaxis: 0.2–0.4 units/mL
Administer by deep SC injection by having the patient lie down. Alter administration between the left and right anterolateral and left and right posterolateral abdominal wall.
Continued

ENOXAPARIN *continued*

See package insert for detailed SC administration recommendations. To minimize bruising, do not rub the injection site. IV or IM route of administration is not recommended.

For additional information, see Chest 2001;119:344S-370S.

EPINEPHRINE HCl

Adrenalin and others
Sympathomimetic agent

No   ?   C

1:1000 (Aqueous):
  Inj: 1 mg/mL (1, 30 mL vials; 2 mL prefilled syringe)
1:200 (Sus-phrine suspension):
  Inj: 5 mg/mL (0.3, 5 mL)
1:10,000 (Aqueous):
  Inj: 0.1 mg/mL (3, 10 mL prefilled syringe)
1:100,000 (Epinephrine Pediatric, Aqueous):
  Inj: 0.01 mg/mL (5 mL)
Epi-pen: 0.3 mg autoinjection (2 mL of 1:1000 solution)
Epi-pen Jr: 0.15 mg autoinjection (2 mL of 1:2000 solution)
Aerosol: 0.16, 0.2 mg epinephrine base/spray (15, 22.5 mL)
Oral inhalation solution: 0.1% (1 mg/mL or 1:1000) (30 mL), 1% (10 mg/mL or 1:100) (7.5 mL)
Ophthalmic solution: 0.1% (1 mL); 0.5% (15 mL); 1% (10, 15 mL); 2% (10, 15 mL)
Nasal solution: 0.1% (1 mg/mL or 1:1000) (30 mL)
Some preparations may contain sulfites.

Cardiac uses:
  Neonate:
    Asystole and bradycardia: 0.1–0.3 mL/kg of 1:10,000 solution (0.01–0.03 mg/kg) IV/ET Q3–5 min
  Infants and children:
    Bradycardia/asystole and pulseless arrest: **see inside front cover and algorithms on inside back cover**
    Bradycardia, asystole, and pulseless arrest:
      First dose: 0.01 mg/kg of 1:10,000 solution (0.1 mL/kg) IO/IV; **max. dose:** 1 mg (10 mL). For ET route see below.
      Subsequent doses and all ET doses: 0.1 mg/kg of 1:1000 solution (0.1 mL/kg) IO/IV/ET Q3–5 min. If doses are not effective, increase dose to 0.2 mg/kg of 1:1000 solution (0.2 mL/kg).
  Adults:
    Asystole: 1 mg IV/ET Q3–5 min; if unresponsive, 1–5 mg IV/ET Q3–5 min
  IV drip (all ages): 0.1–1 mcg/kg/min; titrate to effect; to prepare infusion, see inside front cover

Continued

EPINEPHRINE HCl *continued*

Respiratory uses:
  Bronchodilator:
  1:1000 (Aqueous)
    Infants and children: 0.01 mL/kg/dose SC (**max. single dose** 0.5 mL); repeat
    Q15 min × 3–4 doses or Q4 hr PRN
    Adults: 0.3–0.5 mL/dose
  1:200 (Sus-phrine suspension)
    Infants and children: 0.005 mL/kg/dose SC (**max. single dose** 0.15 mL); repeat
    Q8–12 hr PRN
    Adults: 0.1–0.3 mL/dose
  Inhalation: 1–2 puffs Q4 hr PRN
  Nebulization: (alternative to racemic epinephrine): 0.5 mL/kg of 1:1000 solution
  diluted in 3 mL NS; **max. doses:** ≤4 yr: 2.5 mL/dose; >4 yr: 5 mL/dose
Hypersensitivity reactions (see remarks for IV dosing):
  Children: 0.01 mg/kg/dose IM/SC up to a **maximum** of 0.5 mg/dose Q20 min–4 hr
  PRN. If using EpiPen or EpiPen Jr, administer only via the IM route using the
  following dosage:
    <30 kg: 0.15 mg
    ≥30 kg: 0.3 mg
  Adults: Start with 0.1–0.5 mg IM/SC Q20 minutes–4 hr PRN; doses may be
  increased if necessary to a **single max. dose** of 1 mg

> *Hypersensitivity reactions:* For bronchial asthma and certain allergic manifesta-
> tions (e.g., angioedema, urticaria, serum sickness, anaphylactic shock) use
> epinephrine SC. The adult IV dose for hypersensitivity reactions or to relieve
> bronchospasm usually ranges from 0.1 to 0.25 mg injected slowly over 5–10 min
> Q5–15 min as needed. Neonates may be given a dose of 0.01 mg/kg body weight;
> for the infant, 0.05 mg is an adequate initial dose and this may be repeated at 20- to
> 30-min intervals in the management of asthma attacks.
>   May produce arrhythmias, tachycardia, hypertension, headaches, nervousness,
> nausea, and vomiting. Necrosis may occur at site of repeated local injection.
>   Concomitant use of noncardiac selective beta-blockers or tricyclic antidepressants
> may enhance epinephrine's pressor effect. Chlorpromazine may reverse the pressor
> effect.
>   ETT doses should be diluted with NS to a volume of 3–5 mL before administration.
> Follow with several positive pressure ventilations.
>   EpiPen and EpiPen Jr should be administered IM into the anterolateral aspect of the
> thigh.

EPINEPHRINE, RACEMIC

Asthmanefrin, MicroNefrin, Nephron, S-2
Sympathomimetic agent

No   ?   C

Solution: 2.25% (1.25% epinephrine base) (15, 30 mL)
Contains sulfites

For explanation of icons, see p. 572.

Continued

EPINEPHRINE, RACEMIC *continued*

<4 yr:
Croup (using 2.25% solution): 0.05 mL/kg/dose up to a **maximum** of 0.5 mL/dose diluted to 3 mL with NS. Given via nebulizer over 15 min PRN, but not more frequently than Q1–2 hr.
≥4 yrs: 0.5 mL/dose via nebulizer over 15 minutes Q3–4 hr PRN

Tachyarrhythmias, headache, nausea, and palpitations have been reported. Rebound airway edema may occur. Cardiorespiratory monitoring should be considered if administered more frequently than Q1–2 hr.

EPOETIN ALFA

Erythropoietin, Epogen, Procrit
Recombinant human erythropoietin

No ? C

Inj: 2000, 3000, 4000, 10,000, 20,000 U/mL
Contains 2.5 mg albumin per 1 mL; only multidose vials contain 1% benzyl alcohol.

Renal failure: SC/IV
Initial: 50–100 U/kg 3 times per week; may increase dose if hematocrit does not rise by 5–6 percent after 8 weeks; maintenance doses are individualized
AZT-treated HIV patients: SC/IV
100 U/kg/dose 3 times per week for 8 weeks; the dose may be increased by 50–100 U/kg/dose given 3 times per week; **max. dose** 300 U/kg/dose given 3 times per week
Anemia of prematurity:
25–100 U/kg/dose SC 3 times per week; alternatively, 200–300 U/kg/dose IV/SC 3–5 times per week for 2–6 weeks (**total dose per week** is 600–1400 U/kg)

Evaluate serum iron, ferritin, TIBC before therapy. Iron supplementation recommended during therapy unless iron stores are already in excess. Monitor Hct, BP, clotting times, platelets, BUN, and serum creatinine. Peak effect in 2–3 weeks. Reduce dose when target Hct is reached, or when Hct increases >4% in any 2-week period. May cause hypertension, seizure, hypersensitivity reactions, headache, edema, and dizziness. SC route provides sustained serum levels compared to IV route.

ERGOCALCIFEROL

Drisdol, Calciferol
Vitamin D$_2$

No ? A/D

Caps/tabs: 50,000 IU (1.25 mg)
Inj: 500,000 IU/mL

Continued

ERGOCALCIFEROL *continued*

Drops: 8000 IU/mL (200 mcg/mL) (60 mL)
1 mg = 40,000 IU vitamin D activity

Dietary supplementation:
  Preterm: 400–800 IU/24 hr PO
    Infants/children: 400 IU/24 hr PO; please refer to p. 460 for details.
Renal failure:
  Children: 4000–40,000 IU/24 hr PO
  Adult: 20,000 IU/24 hr PO
Vitamin D–dependent rickets:
  Children: 3000–5000 IU/24 hr PO; **max. dose:** 60,000 IU/24 hr
  Adults: 10,000–60,000 IU/24 hr PO; some may require 500,000 IU/24 hr
Nutritional rickets:
  Adults and children with normal GI absorption: 2000–5000 IU/24 hr PO ×
  6–12 weeks
  Malabsorption:
    Children: 10,000–25,000 IU/24 hr PO
    Adults: 10,000–300,000 IU/24 hr PO
Vitamin D–resistant rickets (with phosphate supplementation):
  Children: Initial dose 40,000–80,000 IU/24 hr PO; increase daily dose by
  10,000–20,000 IU PO Q3–4 mo if needed
  Adults: 10,000–60,000 IU/24 hr PO
Hypoparathyroidism (with calcium supplementation):
  Children: 50,000–200,000 IU/24 hr PO
  Adults: 25,000–200,000 IU/24 hr PO

Monitor serum Ca^{++}, PO_4, and alkaline phosphate. Serum Ca^{++}, PO_4 product
should be <70 mg/dL to avoid ectopic calcification. Titrate dosage to patient
response. Watch for symptoms of hypercalcemia: weakness, diarrhea, polyuria, metastatic calcification, and nephrocalcinosis. Vitamin D_2 is activated by
25-hydroxylation in liver and 1-hydroxylation in kidney.

Oral route is preferred. May use IM route in cases of fat malabsorption. **Injectable
for IM administration only.**

Pregnancy category changes to "D" if used in doses above the RDA.

ERGOTAMINE TARTRATE

Cafergot and others
Ergot alkaloid

No   X   X

Tabs: 1 mg and 100 mg caffeine
Sublingual tabs: 2 mg
Suppository: 2 mg and 100 mg caffeine
Drug also available in combinations with belladonna alkaloids and/or phenobarbital.

Continued

ERGOTAMINE TARTRATE *continued*

Older children and adolescents:
PO/SL: 1 mg at onset of migraine attack, then 1 mg Q30 min PRN up to **maximum** of 3 mg.

Adults:
PO/SL: 2 mg at onset of migraine attack, then 1–2 mg Q30 min up to 6 mg per attack.
Suppository: 2 mg at first sign of attack; follow with second dose (2 mg) after 1 hr, **max. dose** 4 mg per attack, not to exceed 10 mg/week.

Use with **caution** in renal or hepatic disease. May cause paresthesias, GI disturbance, angina-like pain, rebound headache with abrupt withdrawal, or muscle cramps. **Contraindicated** in pregnancy and breastfeeding. Concurrent administration with protease inhibitors, clarithromycin, or erythromycin is not recommended due to risk of ergotism (nausea, vomiting, vasospastic ischemia).

ERYTHROMYCIN ETHYLSUCCINATE AND ACETYLSULFISOXAZOLE

Yes   1   C

Pediazole, Eryzole, and others
Antibiotic, macrolide + sulfonamide derivative

Suspension: 200 mg erythromycin and 600 mg sulfa/5 mL (100, 150, 200, 250 mL)

Otitis media: 50 mg/kg/24 hr (as erythromycin) and 150 mg/kg/24 hr (as sulfa) ÷ Q6 hr PO, or give 1.25 mL/kg/24 hr ÷ Q6 hr PO
Max. dose: 2 g erythromycin, 6 g sulfisoxasole/24 hr

See adverse effects of erythromycin and sulfisoxazole. **Not** recommended in infants <2 mo. **Do not use** in renal impairment because dosage adjustments are inconsistent for sulfisoxazole and erythromycin.

ERYTHROMYCIN PREPARATIONS

Erythrocin, Pediamycin, E-Mycin, Ery-Ped, and others
Antibiotic, macrolide

Yes   1   B

Erythromycin base:
Tabs: 250, 333, 500 mg
Delayed-release tabs: 250, 333, 500 mg
Delayed-release caps: 250 mg
Topical ointment: 2% (25 g)

Continued

ERYTHROMYCIN PREPARATIONS *continued*

Topical gel: 2% (30, 60 g)
Topical solution: 1.5%, 2% (60 mL)
Topical swab: 2% (60s)
Ophthalmic ointment: 0.5% (3.5, 3.75 g)

Erythromycin Ethyl Succinate (EES):
Suspension: 200, 400 mg/5 mL (60, 100, 200, 480 mL)
Oral drops: 100 mg/2.5 mL (50 mL)
Chewable tabs: 200 mg
Tabs: 400 mg

Erythromycin Estolate:
Suspension: 125, 250 mg/5 mL
Oral drops: 100 mg/mL (10 mL)
Chewable tabs: 125, 250 mg
Tabs: 500 mg
Caps: 125, 250 mg

Erythromycin Stearate:
Tabs: 250, 500 mg

Erythromycin Gluceptate:
Inj: 1000 mg

Erythromycin Lactobionate:
Inj: 500, 1000 mg

Oral:
Neonates:
<1.2 kg: 20 mg/kg/24 hr ÷ Q12 hr PO
≥1.2 kg:
0–7 days: 20 mg/kg/24 hr ÷ Q12 hr PO
>7 days: 30 mg/kg/24 hr ÷ Q8 hr PO
Chlamydial conjunctivitis and pneumonia: 50 mg/kg/24 hr ÷ Q6 hr PO × 14 days
Children:
30–50 mg/kg/24 hr ÷ Q6–8 hr; **max. dose:** 2 g/24 hr
Adults: 1–4 g/24 hr ÷ Q6 hr; **max. dose:** 4 g/24 hr
Parenteral:
Children: 20–50 mg/kg/24 hr ÷ Q6 hr IV
Adults: 15–20 mg/kg/24 hr ÷ Q6 hr IV
Max. dose: 4 g/24 hr
Rheumatic fever prophylaxis: 500 mg/24 hr ÷ Q12 hr PO
Ophthalmic: Apply 0.5-inch ribbon to affected eye BID-QID
Pertussis: Estolate salt: 50 mg/kg/24 hr ÷ Q6 hr PO × 14 days
Preoperative bowel prep: 20 mg/kg/dose PO erythromycin base × 3 doses, with
neomycin, 1 day before surgery

Avoid IM route (pain, necrosis). GI side effects common (nausea, vomiting,
abdominal cramps). Use with **caution** in liver disease. Estolate may cause
cholestatic jaundice, although hepatotoxicity is uncommon (2% of reported
cases). Inhibits CYP 450 1A2, 3A3/4 isoenzymes. May produce elevated digoxin,
theophylline, carbamazapine, clozapine, cyclosporine, and methylprednisolone levels.

Continued

For explanation of icons, see p. 572.

ERYTHROMYCIN PREPARATIONS *continued*

Contraindicated in combination with astemizole, cisapride, or terfenadine. Hypertrophic pyloric stenosis in neonates receiving prophylactic therapy for pertussis has been reported.

Oral therapy should replace IV as soon as possible. Give oral doses after meals. Because of different absorption characteristics, higher oral doses of EES are needed to achieve therapeutic effects. May produce false positive urinary catecholamines. Formulations of IV lactobionate dosage form may contain benzyl alcohol.

Adjust dose in renal failure (see p. 942).

ERYTHROPOIETIN

See Epoietin Alfa

ESMOLOL HCl

Brevibloc
Beta-1-selective adrenergic blocking agent, antihypertensive No ? C
agent, class II antiarrhythmic

Inj: 10, 250 mg/mL (10 mL) 250 mg/mL concentration contains 25% alcohol and 25% propylene glycol

---

 Titrate to individual response.
Loading dose: 100–500 mcg/kg IV over 1 min
Maintenance dose: 25–100 mcg/kg/min as infusion
If inadequate response, may readminister loading dose above, and/or increase maintenance dose by 25–50 mcg/kg/min in increments of Q5–10 min
Usual maintenance dose range: 50–500 mcg/kg/min

 $T_{1/2}$ = 9 minutes. May cause bronchospasm, CHF, hypotension (at doses >200 mcg/kg/min), nausea, and vomiting. May increase digoxin level by 10%–20%. Morphine may increase esmolol level by 46%.
Do not administer the 250 mg/mL concentration undiluted; concentration for administration must be ≤10 mg/mL. Administer **only** in a monitored setting.

ETANERCEPT

Enbrel
Antirheumatic, immunomodulatory agent, tumor necrosis factor No 3 B
receptor p75 Fc fusion protein

Inj: 25 mg with diluent (1 mL bacteriostatic water containing 0.9% benzyl alcohol)
Contains mannitol, sucrose, tromethamine

Continued

ETANERCEPT *continued*

Children 4–17 yrs: 0.4 mg/kg/dose SC twice weekly administered 72–96 hours apart; **max. dose:** 25 mg
Adult: 25 mg SC twice weekly administered 72–96 hours apart

Contraindicated in serious infections, sepsis, or hypersensitivity to any of medication components. Use with **caution** in patients with history of recurrent infections or underlying conditions that may predispose them to infections, CNS demyelinating disorders, malignancies, immune-related diseases, and latex allergy. Common adverse effects in children include headache, abdominal pain, vomiting, and nausea. Injection-site reactions (e.g., discomfort, itching, swelling), rhinitis, dizziness, rash, depression, infections (varicella, systemic bacterial infections, and aseptic meningitis), bone marrow suppression, and vertigo have also been reported.

Do not administer live vaccines concurrently with this drug. In JRA, it is recommended that the patient be brought up to date with all immunizations in agreement with current immunization guidelines prior to initiating therapy.

Onset of action is 1–4 weeks, with peak effects usually within 3 mo.

Patients must be properly instructed on preparing and administering the medication. Drug requires reconstitution by gently swirling its contents with the supplied diluent (do not shake or vigorously agitate) because some foaming will occur. Reconstituted solutions should be clear and colorless and used within 6 hr.

Drug is administered SC by rotating injection sites (thigh, abdomen, or upper arm). Administer new injections ≥1 inch from an old site and never where the skin is tender, bruised, red, or hard.

ETHAMBUTOL HCl

Myambutol
Antituberculosis drug

Yes   1   B

Tabs: 100, 400 mg

Tuberculosis:
Infants, children, adolescents, and adults: 15–25 mg/kg/dose PO QD or 50 mg/kg/dose PO twice weekly
Max. dose: 2.5 g/24 hr
Nontuberculous mycobacterial infection:
Children, adolescents, and adults: 15–25 mg/kg/24 hr PO; **max. dose:** 1 g/24 hr
M. avium complex prophylaxis in AIDS (use in combination with other medications):
Infants, children, adolescents, and adults: 15 mg/kg/dose PO QD; **max. dose:** 900 mg/dose

May cause reversible optic neuritis, especially with larger doses. Obtain baseline ophthalmologic studies before beginning therapy and then monthly. Follow visual acuity, visual fields, and (red-green) color vision. Do not use in children

Continued

ETHAMBUTOL HCl *continued*

whose visual acuity cannot be assessed. **Discontinue** if any visual deterioration occurs. Monitor uric acid, liver function, heme status, and renal function. May cause GI disturbances. Give with food. **Adjust dose with renal failure (see p. 942).**

ETHOSUXIMIDE
Zarontin
Anticonvulsant

Yes   1   C

Caps: 250 mg
Syrup: 250 mg/5 mL

Children:
Oral:
  ≤6 yr: Initial: 15 mg/kg/24 hr ÷ BID; **max. dose:** 500 mg/24 hr; increase as needed Q4–7 days. Usual maintenance dose: 15–40 mg/kg/24 hr ÷ BID
  >6 yr and adults: 250 mg BID; increase by 250 mg/24 hr as needed Q4–7 days; usual maintenance dose: 20–40 mg/kg/24 hr ÷ BID
  Max. dose: 1500 mg/24 hr

Use with **caution** in hepatic and renal disease. Ataxia, anorexia, drowsiness, sleep disturbances, rashes, and blood dyscrasias are rare idiosyncratic reactions.
  May cause lupus-like syndrome; may increase frequency of grand mal seizures in patients with mixed type seizures. Drug of choice for absence seizures. Carbamazepine may decrease ethosuximide levels.
  Therapeutic levels: 40–100 mg/L. $T_{1/2}$ = 24–42 hr. *Recommended serum sampling time at steady-state:* Obtain trough level within 30 min prior to the next scheduled dose after 5-10 days of continuous dosing.
  To minimize GI distress, may administer with food or milk. Abrupt withdrawal of drug may precipitate absence status.

FAMCICLOVIR
Famvir
Antiviral

Yes   ?   B

Tabs: 125, 250, 500 mg

≥18 yrs:
Herpes zoster: 500 mg Q8hr PO × 7 days; initiate therapy promptly as soon as diagnosis is made.
Genital herpes simplex: 125 mg Q12hr PO × 5 days
Suppression of recurrent genital herpes: 250 mg Q12 hr PO up to 1 year
Recurrent mucocutaneous herpes in HIV: 500 mg Q12 hr PO × 7 days

Continued

FAMCICLOVIR *continued*

Drug is converted to its active form (penciclovir). Better absorption than PO acyclovir. May cause headache, diarrhea, nausea, and abdominal pain.

Concomitant use with probenecid and other drugs eliminated by active tubular secretion may result in decreased penciclovir clearance. **Adjust dose in renal impairment (see p. 942).**

Safety and efficacy in suppression of recurrent genital herpes have not been established beyond 1 yr. May be administered with or without food.

FAMOTIDINE

Pepcid, Pepcid AC (OTC), Pepcid Complete (OTC), Pepcid RPD
Histamine-2-receptor antagonist

Yes   1   B

Inj: 10 mg/mL (multidose vials contain 0.9% benzyl alcohol)
Premixed inj: 20 mg/50 mL in iso-osmotic sodium chloride
Liquid: 40 mg/5 mL (contains parabens)
Tabs: 10 (OTC), 20, 40 mg
Gel caps: 10 mg (OTC)
Disintegrating oral tabs: 20, 40 mg (contains aspartame)
Chewable tabs: 10 mg (OTC)

Neonate: 0.5 mg/kg/dose IV Q 24 hr
Children:
  IV: Initial: 0.6–0.8 mg/kg/24 hr ÷ Q8–12 hr up to a **max.** of 40 mg/24 hr
  PO: Initial: 1–1.2 mg/kg/24 hr ÷ Q8–12 hr up to a **max.** of 40 mg/24 hr
Adult:
  Duodenal ulcer:
    PO: 20 mg BID or 40 mg QHS × 4–8 weeks, then maintenance therapy at
    20 mg QHS
    IV: 20 mg BID
  Esophagitis and GERD: 20 mg BID PO

A Q12-hr dosage interval is generally recommended; however, infants and young children may require a Q8-hr interval because of enhanced elimination.

Headaches, dizziness, constipation, diarrhea, and drowsiness have occurred.
Dosage adjustment is required in severe renal failure (see p. 949).

Shake oral suspension well prior to each use. Disintegrating oral tablets should be placed on the tongue to be disintegrated and subsequently swallowed. Doses may be administered with or without food.

FELBAMATE
Felbatol
Anticonvulsant

No   ?   C

Tabs: 400, 600 mg
Suspension: 600 mg/5 mL

Lennox-Gastaut for children 2–14 yr (adjunctive therapy):
Start at 15 mg/kg/24 hr PO ÷ TID-QID; increase dosage by 15 mg/kg/24 hr-increments at weekly intervals up to a **maximum** of 45 mg/kg/24 hr or 3600 mg/24 hr. See remarks.

Children ≥14 yr–adults:
Adjunctive therapy: Start at 1200 mg/24 hr PO ÷ TID-QID; increase dosage by 1200 mg/24 hr at weekly intervals up to a **maximum** of 3600 mg/day. See remarks.
Monotherapy (as initial therapy): Start at 1200 mg/24 hr PO ÷ TID-QID. Increase dose under close clinical supervision at 600-mg increments Q2 weeks to 2400 mg/24 hr. **Max. dose:** 3600 mg/24 hr.
Conversion to monotherapy: Start at 1200 mg/24 hr ÷ PO TID-QID for 2 weeks; then increase to 2400 mg/24 hr for 1 week. At week 3 increase to 3600 mg/24 hr. See remarks for dose-reduction instructions of other antiepileptic drugs.

Drug should be prescribed under strict supervision by a specialist. **Contraindicated** in blood dyscrasias or hepatic dysfunction (prior or current); and hypersensitivity to meprobamate. Aplastic anemia and hepatic failure leading to death have been associated with drug. May cause headache, fatigue, anxiety, GI disturbances, gingival hyperplasia, increased liver enzymes, and bone marrow suppression. **Obtain serum levels of concurrent anticonvulsants.** Monitor liver enzymes, bilirubin, CBC with differential, platelets at baseline and every 1–2 weeks.

When initiating adjunctive therapy (all ages), doses of other antiepileptic drugs (AEDs) are reduced by 20% to control plasma levels of concurrent phenytoin, valproic acid, phenobarbital and carbamazepine. Further reductions of concomitant AED dosages may be necessary to minimize side effects caused by drug interactions.

When converting to monotherapy, reduce other AEDs by ⅓ at start of felbamate therapy. Then after 2 weeks and at the start of increasing the felbamate dosage, reduce other AEDs by an additional ⅓. At week 3, continue to reduce other AEDs as clinically indicated.

Carbamazepine levels may be decreased; whereas phenytoin and valproic acid levels may be increased. Phenytoin and carbamazepine may increase felbamate clearance; valproic acid may decrease its clearance.

Doses can be administered with or without food.

FENTANYL

Sublimaze, Duragesic, Fentanyl Oralet, Actiq
Narcotic; analgesic, sedative

Yes　1　B/D

Inj: 50 mcg/mL
SR patch (Duragesic): 25, 50, 75, 100 mcg/hr
Oralet lozenge:
　Fentanyl Oralet: 100, 200, 300, 400 mcg
　Actiq: 200, 400, 600, 800, 1200, 1600 mcg

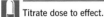 Titrate dose to effect.
　IV/IM: 1–2 mcg/kg/dose Q30–60 min PRN
　　Continuous IV infusion: 1 mcg/kg/hr; titrate to effect; usual infusion range
1–3 mcg/kg/hr
To prepare infusion, use the following formula:

$$50 \times \frac{\text{Desired dose (mcg/kg/hr)}}{\text{Desired infusion rate (mL/hr)}} \times \text{Wt (kg)} = \frac{\text{mcg Fentanyl}}{50 \text{ mL fluid}}$$

PO (Fentanyl Oralet): Sedation: 10–15 mcg/kg/dose up to **maximum** of 400 mcg/dose
Transdermal: Safety and efficacy have not been established in pediatrics.
See p. 894 for equianalgesic dosing and p. 897 for PCA dosing.

Use with **caution** in bradycardia, respiratory depression, and increased intracranial pressure. **Adjust dose in renal failure (see p. 949).** Highly lipophilic and may deposit into fat tissue. IV onset of action 1–2 min with peak effects in 10 min. IV duration of action 30–60 min. Give IV dose over 3–5 min. Rapid infusion may cause respiratory depression and chest-wall rigidity. Respiratory depression may persist beyond the period of analgesia. Transdermal onset of action 6–8 hr with a 72-hr duration of action. Fentanyl Oralet is **contraindicated** in children <10 kg. Actiq is indicated only for the management of breakthrough cancer pain. See p. 894 for pharmacodynamic information with transmucosal and transdermal routes.
　Fentanyl is a substrate for the cytochrome P-450 3A4 enzyme. Be aware of medications that inhibit or induce this enzyme because it may increase or decrease the effects of fentanyl, respectively.
　Pregancy category changes to "D" if drug is used for prolonged periods or in high doses at term.

FERROUS SULFATE

See Iron Preparations

FEXOFENADINE
Allegra
Antihistamine, less sedating

Yes   1   C

Tabs: 30, 60, 180 mg
Caps: 60 mg
Extended-release tab in combination with pseudoephedrine (PE):
  Allegra-D: 60 mg fexofenadine + 120 mg pseudoephedrine

Fexofenadine:
  6–11 yr: 30 mg PO BID
    ≥12 yr–adult: 60 mg PO BID; 180 mg PO QD may be used in seasonal rhinitis
Extended-release tabs of fexofenadine and pseudoephedrine:
  ≥12 yr–adult:
    Allegra-D: 1 tab PO BID

May cause drowsiness, fatigue, headache, dyspepsia, nausea, and dysmenorrhea. Has **not** been implicated in causing cardiac arrhythmias when used
with other drugs that are metabolized by hepatic microsomal enzymes (e.g.,
ketoconazole, erythromycin). **Reduce dose to 60 mg PO QD if CrCl <40 mL/min.**
  Medication as the single agent may be administered with or without food. Do not
administer antacids with or within 2 hr of fexofenadine dose. The extended-release
combination product should be swallowed whole without food.

FILGRASTIM
Neupogen, G-CSF
Colony stimulating factor

No   ?   C

Inj: 300 mcg/mL (1, 1.6 mL)

IV/SC: 5–10 mcg/kg/dose QD × 14 days or until ANC >10,000/mm^3. Dosage
may be increased by 5 mcg/kg/24 hr if desired effect is not achieved within
7 days.
Discontinue therapy when ANC >10,000/mm^3.

Individual protocols may direct dosing. May cause bone pain, fever, and rash.
Monitor CBC, uric acid, and LFTs. Use with **caution** in patients with malignancies with myeloid characteristics. **Contraindicated** for patients sensitive to
E. coli-derived proteins.
  SC routes of administration are preferred because of prolonged serum levels over IV
route. If used via IV route and G-CSF final concentration <15 mcg/mL, add 2 mg
albumin/1 mL of IV fluid to prevent drug adsorption to the IV administration set.

FLECAINIDE ACETATE

Tambocor
Antiarrhythmic, class Ic

Yes 1 C

Tabs: 50, 100, 150 mg
Suspension: 5, 20 mg/mL

Children: Initial: 1–3 mg/kg/24 hr ÷ Q8 hr PO; usual range: 3–6 mg/kg/24 hr ÷ Q8 hr PO, monitor serum levels to adjust dose if needed
Adults:
Sustained V tach: 100 mg PO Q12 hr; may increase by 50 mg Q12 hr every 4 days to **max. dose** of 600 mg/24 hr
Paroxysmal SVT/paroxysmal AF: 50 mg PO Q12 hr; may increase dose by 50 mg Q12 hr every 4 days to **max. dose** of 300 mg/24 hr

May aggravate LV failure, sinus bradycardia, and preexisting ventricular arrhythmias. May cause AV block, dizziness, blurred vision, dyspnea, nausea, headache, and increased PR or QRS intervals. **Reserve for life-threatening cases.** Reduce dosage in renal failure.

Flecainide is a substrate for the cytochrome P-450 2D6 enzyme. Be aware of medications that inhibit or induce this enzyme because it may increase or decrease the effects of flecainide, respectively.

Therapeutic trough level: 0.2–1 mg/L. *Recommended serum sampling time at steady-state:* Obtain trough level within 30 min prior to the next scheduled dose after 2–3 days of continuous dosing for children; after 3–5 days for adults.

Adjust dose in renal failure (see p. 949).

FLUCONAZOLE

Diflucan
Antifungal agent

Yes 1 C

Tabs: 50, 100, 150, 200 mg
Inj: 2 mg/mL (100, 200 mL); contains 9 mEq Na/2 mg drug
Oral suspension: 10 mg/mL, 40 mg/mL

Neonates:
Loading dose: 6-12 mg/kg IV/PO, then maintenance (see table on p. 708)

Continued

FLUCONAZOLE *continued*

NEONATAL MAINTENANCE DOSING

Postconceptional Age (weeks)	Postnatal Age (days)	Dose (mg/kg/dose)	Dosing Interval (hr) and Time (hr) to Start First Maintenance Dose After Load
≤29	0–14	5–6	72
	>14	5–6	48
30–36	0–14	3–6	48
	>14	3–6	24
37–44	0–7	3–6	48
	>7	3–6	24
≥45	>0	3–6	24

Children:
  Loading dose: 10 mg/kg IV/PO, then
  Maintenance: (begin 24 hr after loading dose) 3–6 mg/kg/24 hr IV/PO QD
  Max. dose: 12 mg/kg/24 hr
Adults:
  Oropharyngeal and esophageal candidiasis: Loading dose of 200 mg PO/IV followed by 100 mg QD beginning 24 hr after; doses up to **max. dose** of 400 mg/24 hr may be used for esophageal candidiasis
  Systemic candidiasis: Loading dose of 400 mg PO/IV, followed by 200 mg QD beginning 24 hr later
  Cryptococcal meningitis: Loading dose of 400 mg PO/IV, followed by 200–400 mg QD 24 hr later
  Bone marrow transplant prophylaxis: 400 mg PO/IV Q24hr
  Vaginal candidiasis: 150 mg PO × 1

Cardiac arrhythmias may occur when used with cisapride, terfenadine, astemizole. Concomitant administration of fluconazole with any of these drugs is **contraindicated**. May cause nausea, headache, rash, vomiting, abdominal pain, hepatitis, cholestasis, and diarrhea. Neutropenia, agranulocytosis, and thrombocytopenia have been reported.

PO and IV doses are equivalent. Loading doses (mg/kg or mg amounts) are twice the maintenance dose amount.

Inhibits CYP 450 2C9/10 and CYP 450 3A3/4 (weak inhibitor). May increase effects, toxicity, or levels of cyclosporin, midazolam, phenytoin, rifabutin, tacrolimus, theophylline, warfarin, oral hypoglycemics, and AZT. Rifampin increases fluconazole metabolism.

Adjust dose in renal failure (see p. 942).

FLUCYTOSINE

Ancobon, 5-FC, 5-Fluorocytosine
Antifungal agent

Yes 3 C

Caps: 250, 500 mg
Oral liquid: 10 mg/mL

> *Neonates:* 80–160 mg/kg/24 hr ÷ Q6 hr PO
> *Children and adults:* 50–150 mg/kg/24 hr ÷ Q6 hr PO

> Monitor CBC, BUN, serum creatinine, alkaline phos, AST, and ALT. Common side effects include nausea, vomiting, diarrhea, rash, CNS disturbance, anemia, leukopenia, and thrombocytopenia.
>
> *Therapeutic levels:* 25–100 mg/L. *Recommended serum sampling time at steady-state:* Obtain peak level 2-4 hr after oral dose following 4 days of continuous dosing. Peak levels of 40-60 mg/L have been recommended for systemic candidiasis. Prolonged levels above 100 mg/L can increase risk for bone marrow suppression.
>
> Flucytosine interferes with creatinine assay tests using the dry-slide enzymatic method (Kodak Ektachem analyzer). **Adjust dose in renal failure (see p. 942).**

FLUDROCORTISONE ACETATE

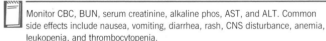

Florinef acetate, 9-Fluorohydrocortisone, Fluohydrisone
Corticosteroid

No 3 C

Tabs: 0.1 mg

> *Infants:* 0.05–0.1 mg/24 hr QD PO
> *Children and adults:* 0.05–0.2 mg/24 hr QD PO

> **Contraindicated** in CHF and systemic fungal infections. Has primarily mineralocorticoid activity. May cause hypertension, hypokalemia, acne, rash, bruising, headaches, GI ulcers, and growth suppression.
>
> Monitor BP and serum electrolytes. See p. 913 for steroid potency comparison.
>
> *Drug interactions:* Drug's hypokalemic effects may induce digoxin toxicity; phenytoin and rifampin may increase fludrocortisone metabolism.
>
> Doses 0.2–2 mg/24 hr has been used in the management of severe orthostatic hypotension in adults.

FLUMAZENIL

Romazicon
Benzodiazepine antidote

No ? C

Inj: 0.1 mg/mL (5, 10 mL)

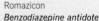 *Children, IV;* Reversal of benzodiazepine sedation:
Initial dose: 0.01 mg/kg (**max. dose:** 0.2 mg), then 0.005–0.01 mg/kg (**max. dose:** 0.2 mg) given Q 1 min to a **max. total cumulative dose** of 1 mg. Doses may be repeated in 20 min up to a **maximum** of 3 mg in 1 hr.

Does not reverse narcotics. Onset of benzodiazepine reversal occurs in 1–3 min. Reversal effects of flumazenil ($T_{1/2}$ approx 1 hr) may wear off sooner than benzodiazepine effects. If patient does not respond after cummulative 1–3 mg dose, suspect cause other than benzodiazepines.

May precipitate seizures, especially in patients taking benzodiazepines for seizure control or in patients with tricyclic antidepressant overdose.

See p. 27 for complete management of suspected ingestions.

FLUNISOLIDE

Nasalide, Nasarel, Aerobid, Aerobid-M
Corticosteroid

No ? C

Nasal solution: 25 mcg/spray (200 sprays/bottle) (25 mL)
Oral aerosol inhaler: 250 mcg/dose (100 doses/inhaler) (7 g); Aerobid-M contains menthol flavoring

 For all dosage forms, reduce to lowest effective maintenance dose to control symptoms
Nasal solution:
Children (6–14 yr):
Initial: 1 spray per nostril TID or 2 sprays per nostril BID; **max. dose:** 4 sprays per nostril/24 hr
Adults:
Initial: 2 sprays per nostril BID; **max. dose:** 8 sprays per nostril/24 hr
Inhaler:
Children (6-15 yr): 2 puffs BID
Adults: 2 puffs BID
Max. dose: 8 puffs/24 hr
NIH-National Heart Lung and Blood Institute recommendations: see pp. 911–912.

Continued

FLUNISOLIDE *continued*

Stop gradually after 3 weeks if no clinical improvement is seen. Shake inhaler well before use. Spacer devices may enhance drug delivery of inhaled form.
Rinse mouth after administering drug by inhaler to prevent thrush. Patients using nasal solution should clear nasal passages before use.

FLUORIDE

Luride, Fluoritab, Pediaflor, and others
Mineral

No   ?   C

Concentrations and strengths based on fluoride ion:
Drops: 0.125 mg/drop, 0.25 mg/drop, 0.5 mg/mL
Oral solution: 0.2 mg/mL
Chewable tabs: 0.25, 0.5, 1 mg
Tabs: 1 mg
Lozenges: 1 mg
See pp. 463–465 for fluoride-containing multivitamins.

All doses/24 hr (see table below): Recommendations from American Academy of Pediatrics and American Dental Association.

Age	Concentration of Fluoride in Drinking Water (ppm)		
	<0.3	0.3–0.6	>0.6
Birth–6 mo	0	0	0
6 mo–3 yr	0.25 mg	0	0
3–6 yr	0.5 mg	0.25 mg	0
6–16 yr	1 mg	0.5 mg	0

Contraindicated in areas where drinking water fluoridation is >0.7 ppm. **Acute overdose:** GI distress, salivation, CNS irritability, tetany, seizures, hypocalcemia, hypoglycemia, and cardiorespiratory failure. Chronic excess use may result in mottled teeth or bone changes.
Take with food, but **not** milk, to minimize GI upset. The doses have been decreased due to concerns over dental fluorosis.

FLUOXETINE HYDROCHLORIDE

Prozac, Prozac Weekly, Sarafem
Antidepressant, selective serotonin reuptake inhibitor (SSRI)

No   3   B

Liquid: 20 mg/5 mL; contains 0.23% alcohol
Caps: 10, 20, 40 mg

Continued

FLUOXETINE HYDROCHLORIDE *continued*

Delayed-released caps (Prozac Weekly): 90 mg
Tabs: 10 mg

Depression:
Children >5 yr:
　5–10 mg QD PO.
　Max. dose: 20 mg/24 hr
Adults: Start at 20 mg QD PO. May increase after several weeks by 20 mg/24 hr increments to **maximum** of 80 mg/24 hr. Doses >20 mg/24 hr should be divided BID.
Bulimia:
　Adults: 60 mg QAM PO; it is recommended to titrate up to this dose over several days.
Premenstrual dysphoric disorder:
　Adults: Start at 20 mg QD PO using the Sarafem product. **Max. dose:** 80 mg/24 hr. Systematic evaluation has shown that efficacy is maintained for periods of 6 mo at a dose of 20 mg/day. Reassess patients periodically to determine the need for continued treatment.

Contraindicated in patients taking MAO inhibitors because of possibility of seizures, hyperpyrexia, and coma. May increase the effects of tricyclic antidepressants. May cause headache, insomnia, nervousness, drowsiness, GI disturbance, and weight loss. Increased bleeding diathesis with unaltered prothrombin time may occur with warfarin. May displace other highly protein-bound drugs. Inhibits CYP 450 2C19, 2D6, and 3A3/4 drug metabolism isoenzymes, which may increase the effects or toxicity of drugs metabolized by these enzymes.

Delayed-release capsule is currently indicated for depression and is dosed at 90 mg Q7 days. It is unknown if weekly dosing provides the same protection from relapse as does daily dosing.

FLUTICASONE PROPIONATE

Flonase, Cutivate, Flovent, Flovent Rotadisk
Corticosteroid

No　？　C

Nasal spray: 50 mcg/actuation (9, 16 g)
Topical cream: 0.05% (15, 30, 60 g)
Topical ointment: 0.005% (15, 60 g)
Aerosol inhaler (MDI): 44 mcg/actuation, 110 mcg/actuation, 220 mcg/actuation (7.9 g = 60 doses/inhaler, 13 g = 120 doses/inhaler)
Dry powder inhalation (DPI) (all strengths come in a package of 15 rotadisks in which each rotadisk provides 4 doses for a total of 60 doses per package):
　50 mcg/dose, 100 mcg/dose, 250 mcg/dose

Continued

FLUTICASONE PROPIONATE *continued*

Intranasal (allergic rhinitis):
≥4 yr and adolescents: 1 spray (50 mcg) per nostril QD. Dose can be increased
to 2 sprays (100 mcg) per nostril QD if inadequate response or severe
symptoms. Reduce to 1 spray per nostril QD once symptoms are controlled.
   Max. dose: 2 sprays (100 mcg) per nostril/24 hr
Adults: Initial 200 mcg/24 hr (2 sprays [100 mcg] per nostril QD **OR** 1 spray
[50 mcg] per nostril BID). Reduce to 1 spray per nostril QD once symptoms are
controlled
   Max. dose: 2 sprays (100 mcg) per nostril/24 hr
Oral Inhalation: **Divide all 24-hr doses BID.** Reduce to the lowest effective dose when
asthma symptoms are controlled.
   Converting from other asthma regimens (see table below).

CONVERSION FROM OTHER ASTHMA REGIMENS TO FLUTICASONE

Age	Previous Use of Bronchodilators Only (max. dose)	Previous Use of Inhaled Corticosteroid (max. dose)	Previous Use of Oral Corticosteroid (max. dose)
Children (4–11 yr)	MDI: 88 mcg/24 hr (176 mcg/24 hr) DPI: 100 mcg/24 hr (200 mcg/24 hr)	MDI: 88 mcg/24 hr (176 mcg/ 24 hr) DPI: 100 mcg/24 hr (200 mcg/ 24 hr)	Dose not available
≥12 yr and adults	MDI: 176 mcg/24hr (880 mcg/24hr) DPI: 200 mcg/24 hr (1000 mcg/24 hr)	MDI: 176—440 mcg/ 24hr (880 mcg/ 24hr) DPI: 200—500 mcg/24 hr (1000 mcg/24 hr)	MDI: 1760 mcg/24hr (1760 mcg/24hr) DPI: 2000 mcg/24 hr (2000 mcg/24 hr)

MDI = Aerosol Inhaler; DPI = Dry Powder Inhalation

NIH-National Heart Lung and Blood Institute recommendations: see pp. 911–912.
Topical:
   ≥3 mo and adults: Apply to affected areas BID, then reduce to a less potent topical
   agent when symptoms are controlled. See pp. 908–909 for topical steroid
   comparisons.

Intranasal: Clear nasal passages prior to use. May cause epistaxis and nasal
irritation, which are usually transient. Taste and smell alterations, rare hypersensitivity reactions (angioedema, pruritis, urticaria, wheezing, dyspnea), and
nasal septal perforation have been reported in postmarketing studies.
   Oral inhalation: Rinse mouth after each use. May cause dysphonia, oral thrush, and
dermatitis. Compared to beclomethasone, has been shown to have less of an effect on
suppresing linear growth in asthmatic children. Eosinophilic conditions may occur with
the withdrawal or decrease of oral corticosteroids after the initiation of inhaled
fluticasone.
   Topical use: Avoid application/contact to face, eyes, and open skin. Occlusive
dressings are not recommended.

For explanation of icons, see p. 572.

FLUTICASONE PROPIONATE AND SALMETEROL

Advair Diskus

No   ?   C

Corticosteroid and long-acting beta-2 adrenergic agonist

Dry powder inhalation (DPI; Diskus):

    100 mcg fluticasone propionate + 50 mcg salmeterol per inhalation
    (28, 60 inhalations)
    250 mcg fluticasone propionate + 50 mcg salmeterol per inhalation
    (28, 60 inhalations)
    500 mcg fluticasone propionate + 50 mcg salmeterol per inhalation
    (28, 60 inhalations)

Conversion from other inhaled steroids (see table below):

Inhaled Corticosteroid	Current Daily Dose	Recommended Strength of Fluticasone Propionate + Salmeterol Diskus Administered at One Inhalation BID
Beclomethasone dipropionate	≤420 mcg	100 mcg + 50 mcg
	462–840 mcg	250 mcg + 50 mcg
Budesonide	≤400 mcg	100 mcg + 50 mcg
	800–1200 mcg	250 mcg + 50 mcg
	1600 mcg	500 mcg + 50 mcg
Flunisolide	≤1000 mcg	100 mcg + 50 mcg
	1250–2000 mcg	250 mcg + 50 mcg
Fluticasone propionate aerosol (MDI)	≤176 mcg	100 mcg + 50 mcg
	440 mcg	250 mcg + 50 mcg
	660–880 mcg	500 mcg + 50 mcg
Fluticasone propionate dry powder (DPI)	≤200 mcg	100 mcg + 50 mcg
	500 mcg	250 mcg + 50 mcg
	1000 mcg	500 mcg + 50 mcg
Triamcinolone	≤1000 mcg	100 mcg + 50 mcg
	1100–1600 mcg	250 mcg + 50 mcg

Max. dose: 500 mcg fluticasone propionate + 50 mcg salmeterol BID

See *Fluticasone propionate and salmeterol* for remarks. Titrate to the lowest effective strength after asthma is adequately controlled. Proper patient education, including dosage administration technique, is essential; see patient package insert for detailed instructions. Rinse mouth after each use.

FLUVOXAMINE

Luvox
Antidepressant, selective serotonin reuptake inhibitor (SSRI)

No   3   C

Tabs: 25, 50, 100 mg

Obsessive compulsive disorder:
>8 yr: Start at 25 mg PO QHS. Dose may be increased by 25 mg/24 hr Q 4–7 days up to a **maximum** of 200 mg/24 hr. Total daily doses >50 mg/24 hr should be divided BID.
Adults: Start at 50 mg PO QHS. Dose may be increased by 50 mg/24 hr Q4–7 days up to a **maximum** of 300 mg/24 hr. Total daily doses >100 mg/24 hr should be divided BID.

Contraindicated with coadministration of astemizole, cisapride, pimozide, terfenadine, or MAO inhibitors. Use with **caution** in hepatic disease; drug is extensively metabolized by the liver.

Inhibits CYP 450 1A2, 2C19, 2D6, and 3A3/4 which may increase the effects or toxicity of drugs metabolized by these enzymes. When used with warfarin, may increase warfarin plasma levels by 98% and prolong PT. May increase toxicity and/or levels of theophylline, caffeine, and tricyclic antidepressants. Side effects include headache, insomnia, somnolence, nausea, diarrhea, dyspepsia, and dry mouth.

Titrate to lowest effective dose.

FOLIC ACID

Folvite and others
Water-soluble vitamin

No   1   A

Tabs: 0.4, 0.8, 1 mg
Oral solution: 50 mcg/mL, 1 mg/mL
Inj: 5 mg/mL; contains 1.5% benzyl alcohol

For RDA, see pp. 460–461.
Folic acid deficiency PO, IM, IV, SC (see table below)

FOLIC ACID DEFICIENCY (PO, IM, IV, SC)		
Infants	Children (1–10 yr)	Adults (>11 yr)
INITIAL DOSE		
15 mcg/kg/ dose; **max. dose** 50 mcg/24 hr	1 mg/dose	1–3 mg/dose ÷ QD–TID
MAINTENANCE		
30–45 mcg/24 hr QD	0.1–0.4 mg/ 24 hr QD	0.5 mg/24 hr QD; pregnant/lactating women: 0.8 mg/24 hr QD

Continued

FOLIC ACID *continued*

Normal levels: see p. 552. May mask hematologic effects of vitamin B_{12} deficiency, but will not prevent progression of neurologic abnormalities. High-dose folic acid may decrease the absorption of phenytoin.

Women of child-bearing age considering pregnancy should take at least 0.4 mg QD before and during pregnancy to reduce risk of neural tube defects in the fetus.

FOMEPIZOLE

Antizol
Antidote for ethylene glycol or methanol toxicity   Yes   ?   C

Inj: 1 g/ mL (1.5 mL)

Adults not requiring hemodialysis (IV, all doses administered over 30 min):
Load: 15 mg/kg/dose × 1
   Maintenance: 10 mg/kg/dose Q12 hr × 4 doses, then 15 mg/kg/dose Q12 hr until ethylene glycol level decreases to <20 mg/dL and the patient is asymptomatic with normal pH

Adults requiring hemodialysis (IV following the above recommended doses at the intervals indicated below. All doses administered over 30 min):
   Dosing at the beginning of hemodialysis:
      If <6 hr since last fomepizole dose: Do not administer dose
      If ≥6 hr since last fomepizole dose: Administer next scheduled dose
   Dosing during hemodialysis: Administer Q4 hr
   Dosing at the time hemodialysis is completed (based on the time between last dose and end of hemodialysis):
      <1 hr: Do not administer dose at end of hemodialysis
      1–3 hr: Administer ½ of next scheduled dose
      >3 hr: Administer next scheduled dose
   Maintenance dose off hemodialysis: Give next scheduled dose 12 hr from last dose administered

Works by competitively inhibiting alcohol dehydrogenase. Safety and efficacy in pediatrics have not been established. **Contraindicated** in hypersensitivity to any components or other pyrazole compounds. Most frequent side effects include headache, nausea, and dizziness. Fomepizole is extensively eliminated by the kidneys (use with **caution** in renal failure) and removed by hemodialysis.

Drug product may solidify at temperatures <25° C (77° F); vial can be liquefied by running it under warm water (efficacy, safety, and stability are not affected). All doses must be diluted with at least 100 mL of D_5W or NS to prevent vein irritation. See pp. 25–26 for additional information.

FOSCARNET

Foscavir
Antiviral agent

Yes 3 C

Inj: 24 mg/mL (250, 500 mL)

Adolescents and adults, IV:
CMV retinitis:
Induction: 180 mg/kg/24 hr ÷ Q8 hr × 14–21 days
Maintenance: 90–120 mg/kg/24 hr QD
Acyclovir-resistant herpes simplex: 40 mg/kg/dose Q8 hr or 40–60 mg/kg/dose
Q12 hr for up to 3 weeks or until lesions heal

Use with **caution** in patients with renal insufficiency. **Discontinue** use if serum
Cr ≥2.9 mg/dL. **Adjust dose in renal failure (see p. 942).**
May cause peripheral neuropathy, seizures, hallucinations, GI disturbance,
increased LFTs, hypertension, chest pain, ECG abnormalities, coughing, dyspnea,
bronchospasm, and renal failure (adequate hydration may reduce risk). Hypocalcemia
(increased risk if given with pentamidine), hypokalemia, and hypomagnesemia may
also occur.

FOSPHENYTOIN

Cerebyx
Anticonvulsant

Yes 1 D

Inj: 50 mg phenytoin equivalent (75 mg fosphenytoin)/1 mL (2, 10 mL)
1 mg phenytoin equivalent provides 0.0037 mmol phosphate

All doses are expressed as phenytoin sodium equivalents (PE):
Children: See phenytoin and use the conversion of 1 mg phenytoin = 1 mg PE
Adults:
Loading dose:
  Status epilepticus: 15–20 mg PE/kg IV
  Nonemergent loading: 10–20 mg PE/kg IV/IM
Initial maintenance dose: 4–6 mg PE/kg/24 hr IV/IM

All doses should be prescribed and dispensed in terms of mg phenytoin
sodium equivalents (PE) to avoid medication errors. Safety in pediatrics has **not**
been fully established.
Use with **caution** in patients with porphyria, consider amount of phosphate delivered
by fosphenytoin in patients with phosphate restrictions. Drug is also metabolized to
liberate small amounts of formaldehyde, which is considered clinically insignificant
with short-term use (e.g., 1 week). Side effects include hypokalemia (with rapid IV

Continued

FOSPHENYTOIN *continued*

administration), slurred speech, dizziness, ataxia, rash, exfoliative dermatitis, nystagmus, diplopia, tinnitus. Increased unbound phenytoin concentrations may occur in patients with renal disease or hypoalbuminemia; measure "free" or "unbound" phenytoin levels in these patients.

Abrupt withdrawal may cause status epilepticus. BP and ECG monitoring should be present during IV loading dose administration. **Maximum IV infusion rate:** 3 mg PE/kg/min up to a maximum of 150 mg PE/min. Administer IM via 1 or 2 injection sites; IM route is **not recommended** in status epilepticus.

Therapeutic levels: 10–20 mg/L (free and bound phenytoin) OR 1–2 mg/L (free only). Recommended peak serum sampling times: 4 hours following an IM dose or 2 hours following an IV dose.

See phenytoin remarks for drug interactions.

FUROSEMIDE

Furomide, Lasix, and others
Loop diuretic

Yes ? C

Tabs: 20, 40, 80 mg
Inj: 10 mg/mL (2, 4, 10 mL)
Oral liquid: 10 mg/mL (contains 11.5% alcohol) (60, 120 mL), 40 mg/5 mL (contains 0.2% alcohol) (5, 10, 500 mL)

IM, IV, PO:
   Neonates: 0.5–1 mg/kg/dose Q8–24 hr; **max. PO dose:** 6 mg/kg/dose, **max. IV dose:** 2 mg/kg/dose
   Infants and children: 0.5–2 mg/kg/dose Q6–12 hr; **max. dose:** 6 mg/kg/dose
   Adults: 20–80 mg/24 hr ÷ Q6–12 hr; **max. dose:** 600 mg/24 hr
Continuous IV infusion:
   Children and adults: 0.05 mg/kg/hr, titrate to effect

Contraindicated in anuria and hepatic coma. Use with **caution** in hepatic disease. Ototoxicity may occur in presence of renal disease, especially when used with aminoglycosides. May cause hypokalemia, alkalosis, dehydration, hyperuricemia, and increased calcium excretion. Prolonged use in premature infants may result in nephrocalcinosis.

Furosemide-resistant edema in pediatric patients may benefit from the addition of metolazone. Some of these patients may have an exaggerated response leading to hypovolemia, tachycardia, and orthostatic hypotension requiring fluid replacement. Severe hypokalemia has been reported, with a tendency for diuresis persisting for up to 24 hr after discontinuing metolazone.

Max. rate of intermittent IV dose administration: 0.5 mg/kg/min.

GABAPENTIN

Neurontin
Anticonvulsant

Yes   ?   C

Caps: 100, 300, 400 mg
Tablets: 600, 800 mg
Oral solution: 250 mg/5 mL (480 mL)

3–12 yr (PO, see remarks):
 Day 1: 10-15 mg/kg/24 hr ÷ TID, then gradually titrate dose upward to the
  following dosages over a 3-day period:
  3–4 yr: 40 mg/kg/24 hr ÷ TID
  ≥5 yr: 25–35 mg/kg/24 hr ÷ TID
  Max. dose: 50 mg/kg/24 hr
>12 yr and adults (PO, see remarks):
 Day 1: 300 mg at bedtime
 Day 2: 300 mg BID
 Day 3: 300 mg TID
Usual effective doses: 900–1800 mg/24 hr ÷ TID
Doses as high as 3.6 g/24 hr have been tolerated

Generally used as adjunctive therapy for partial and secondary generalized
seizures, and neuropathic pain. Side effects include somnolence, dizziness,
ataxia, fatigue, and nystagmus. **Do not** withdraw medication abruptly. Drug is
not metabolized by the liver and is primarily excreted in the urine unchanged.
 May be taken with or without food. In TID dosing schedule, **interval between doses
should not exceed 12 hr. Adjust dose in renal impairment (see p. 949).**

GANCICLOVIR

Cytovene
Antiviral agent

Yes   ?   C

Inj: 500 mg; contains 4 mEq Na per 1 g drug
Caps: 250, 500 mg

Cytomegalovirus (CMV) infections:
 Children >3 mo and adults:
  Induction therapy (duration 14–21 days): 10 mg/kg/24 hr ÷ Q12 hr IV
  Maintenance therapy: 5 mg/kg/dose QD IV or 6 mg/kg/dose QD IV for
  5 days/week
  Oral maintenance therapy following induction (adults): 1000 mg PO TID
  with food

Continued

GANCICLOVIR *continued*

Prevention of CMV in transplant recipients:
  Children and adults:
    Induction therapy (duration 7–14 days): 10 mg/kg/24 hr ÷ Q12 hr IV
    Maintenance therapy: 5 mg/kg/dose QD IV or 6 mg/kg/dose QD IV for
    5 days/week
    Oral maintenance therapy (adults): 1000 mg PO TID with food
Prevention of CMV in HIV-Infected individuals:
  Infants and Children: 5 mg/kg/dose QD IV
  Adolescent and adults:
    IV: 5–6 mg/kg/dose QD for 5–7 days/week
    PO: 1000 mg PO TID with food

Limited experience with use in children <12. Use with extreme caution. **Adjust dose in renal failure (see p. 942).** Oral absorption is poor; consider the more bioavailable pro-drug, valganciclovir, in adult patients. Common side effects include neutropenia, thrombocytopenia, retinal detachment, and confusion. Drug reactions alleviated with dose reduction or temporary interruption. Ganciclovir may increase didanosine and zidovudine levels, whereas didanosine and zidovudine may decrease ganciclovir levels.

Minimum dilution is 10 mg/mL and should be infused IV over ≥1 hr. IM and SC administration are **contraindicated** because of high pH (pH = 11).

GCSF
See Filgrastim

GENTAMICIN
Garamycin and others
Antibiotic, aminoglycoside

Yes   1   C

Inj: 10 mg/mL (2 mL), 40 mg/mL (2, 20 mL)
Ophthalmic ointment: 0.3% (3.5 g)
Ophthalmic drops: 0.3% (1, 5, 15 mL)
Topical ointment: 0.1% (15 g)
Topical cream: 0.1% (15 g)
Intrathecal inj: 2 mg/mL

Continued

GENTAMICIN continued

Parenteral (IM or IV):
Neonate/infant (see table below):

NEONATAL/INFANT GENTAMICIN DOSING (IM, IV)

Postconceptional Age (weeks)	Postnatal Age (days)	Dose (mg/kg/ dose)	Interval (hr)
≤29*	0–28	2.5	24
	>28	3	24
30–36	0–14	3	24
	>14	2.5	12
≥37	0–7	2.5	12
	>7	2.5	8

*Or significant asphyxia.

Children: 6–7.5 mg/kg/24 hr ÷ Q8 hr
Adults: 3–6 mg/kg/24 hr ÷ Q8 hr
Cystic fibrosis: 7.5–10.5 mg/kg/24 hr ÷ Q8 hr
Intrathecal/intraventricular:
  >3 mo: 1–2 mg QD
  Adult: 4–8 mg QD
Ophthalmic ointment: Apply Q6–8 hr
Ophthalmic drops: 1–2 drops Q4 hr

Use with **caution** in patients receiving anesthetics or neuromuscular blocking agents, and in patients with neuromuscular disorders. May cause nephrotoxicity and ototoxicity. Ototoxicity may be potentiated with the use of loop diuretics. Eliminated more quickly in patients with cystic fibrosis, neutropenia, and burns. **Adjust dose in renal failure (see p. 943).** Monitor peak and trough levels.

Therapeutic peak levels:
  6–10 mg/L general
  8–10 mg/L in pulmonary infections, neutropenia, and severe sepsis
Therapeutic trough levels: <2 mg/L. *Recommended serum sampling time at steady-state:* Trough within 30 min prior to the third consecutive dose and peak 30–60 min after administration of the third consecutive dose.

GLUCAGON HCl
GlucaGen, Glucagon Emergency Kit
Antihypoglycemic agent

No   ?   B

Inj: 1 mg vial (requires reconstitution)
1 unit = 1 mg

Continued

GLUCAGON HCI *continued*

Hypoglycemia, IM, IV, SC:
Neonates, infants, and children <20 kg: 0.5 mg/dose (or 0.02–0.03 mg/kg/dose) Q20 min PRN
Children ≥20 kg and adults: 1 mg/dose Q20 min PRN
For beta-blocker and calcium channel blocker overdose, see pp. 27–28.

Drug product is genetically engineered and identical to human glucagon. High doses have cardiac stimulatory effect and have had some success in beta-blocker and calcium channel blocker overdose. May cause nausea, vomiting, urticaria, and respiratory distress. Do **not** delay glucose infusion; dose for hypoglycemia is 2–4 mL/kg of dextrose 25%.
Onset of action: IM: 8–10 min; IV: 1 min. Duration of action: IM: 12–27 min; IV: 9–17 min.

GLYCERIN

Fleet Babylax, Sani-Supp, and others
Osmotic laxative

No   ?   C

Rectal solution: 4 mL per application (6 doses)
Suppository:
   Infant/pediatric (10s, 12s, 25s)
   Adult (10s, 12s, 24s, 25s, 48s, 50s, 100s)

Constipation:
Neonate: 0.5 mL/kg/dose rectal solution PR as an enema QD–BID PRN
Children <6 yr: 2–5 mL rectal solution PR as an enema or 1 infant suppository PR QD–BID PRN
>6 yr–adult: 5–15 mL rectal solution PR as an enema or 1 adult suppository PR QD–BID PRN

Onset of action: 15-30 min. May cause rectal irritation, abdominal pain, bloating, and dizziness. Insert suppository high into rectum and retain for 15 min.

GLYCOPYRROLATE

Robinul
Anticholinergic agent

Yes   ?   B

Tabs: 1, 2 mg
Inj: 0.2 mg/mL (1, 2, 5, 20); some multidose vials contain 0.9% benzyl alcohol

Continued

GLYCOPYRROLATE *continued*

Respiratory antisecretory:
  IM/IV:
    Children: 0.004–0.01 mg/kg/dose Q4–8 hr
    Adults: 0.1–0.2 mg/dose Q4–8 hr
    Max. dose: 0.2 mg/dose or 0.8 mg/24 hr
  Oral:
    Children: 0.04–0.1 mg/kg/dose Q4–8 hr
    Adults: 1–2 mg/dose BID-TID
Reverse neuromuscular blockade:
  Children and adults: 0.2 mg IV for every 1 mg neostigmine or 5 mg pyridostigmine

Use with **caution** in hepatic and renal disease, ulcerative colitis, asthma, glaucoma, ileus, or urinary retention. Atropine-like side effects include tachycardia, nausea, constipation, confusion, blurred vision, and dry mouth. These may be potentiated if given with other drugs with anticholinergic properties. IV dosage form may be used orally.

Onset of action: PO: within 1 hr; IM/SC: 15–30 min; IV: 1 min. *Duration of antisialogogue effect:* PO: 8–12 hr; IM/SC/IV: 7 hr.

GRANISETRON

Kytril
Antiemetic agent, 5-HT$_3$ antagonist

No ? B

Inj: 1 mg/mL (1, 4 mL); 4-mL vials contain benzyl alcohol
Tabs: 1 mg
Oral liquid: 0.05, 0.2 mg/mL

Chemotherapy-induced nausea and vomiting:
  IV:
    Children ≥2 yr and adults: 10–20 mcg/kg/dose 15–60 min before chemotherapy; the same dose may be repeated 2–3 times at ≥10-min intervals following chemotherapy (within 24 hrs after chemotherapy) as a treatment regimen. Alternatively, a single 40 mcg/kg/dose 15–60 min before chemotherapy has been used.
  PO:
    Adults: 2 mg/24 hr ÷ QD-BID; initiate first dose 1 hr prior to chemotherapy
Postoperative nausea and vomiting prevention:
  Adults:
    IV: 20–40 mcg/kg/dose prior to anesthesia induction
    PO: 2–4 mg 1 hr prior to surgery
Radiation-induced nausea and vomiting prevention:
  Adults: 2 mg QD PO administered within 1 hr of radiation

Continued

For explanation of icons, see p. 572.

GRANISETRON *continued*

Use with **caution** in liver disease. May cause hypertension, hypotension, arrythmias, agitation, and insomnia. Inducers or inhibitors of the cytochrome P-450 3A3/4 drug metabolizing enzymes may increase or decrease, respectively, the drug's clearance.

Onset of action: IV: 4–10 min. *Duration of action:* IV: ≤24 hr

GRISEOFULVIN

Grifulvin V, Grisactin, Fulvicin
Antifungal agent

No   ?   C

Microsize:
    Tabs: 250, 500 mg
    Caps: 125, 250 mg
    Suspension: 125 mg/5 mL (120 mL); contains 0.2% alcohol
Ultramicrosize:
    Tabs: 125, 165, 250, 330 mg
    250 mg ultra is approximately 500 mg micro

Microsize:
    Children >2 yr: 20-25 mg/kg/24 hr PO ÷ QD-BID; give with milk, eggs, fatty foods
    Adult: 500–1000 mg/24 hr PO ÷ QD-BID
    Max. dose: 1 g/24 hr
Ultramicrosize:
    Children >2 yr: 15 mg/kg/24 hr PO ÷ QD-BID
    Adults: 330–750 mg/24 hr PO ÷ QD-BID
    Max. dose: 750 mg/24 hr

Contraindicated in porphyria or hepatic disease. Monitor hematologic, renal, and hepatic function. May cause leukopenia, rash, headache, paresthesias, and GI symptoms. Possible cross-reactivity in penicillin-allergic patients. Usual treatment period is 8 weeks for tinea capitis and 4–6 mo for tinea unguium. Photosensitivity reactions may occur. May reduce effectiveness or decrease level of oral contraceptives, warfarin, and cyclosporin. Phenobarbital may enhance clearance of griseofulvin. Coadministration with fatty meals will increase the drug's absorption.

HALOPERIDOL

Haldol and others
Antipsychotic agent

No   3   C

Inj (IM use only):
    Lactate: 5 mg/mL (1, 2, 2.5, 10 mL)

Continued

HALOPERIDOL *continued*

Decanoate (long acting): 50, 100 mg/mL (1, 5 mL); in seasame oil with
1.2% benzyl alcohol
Tabs: 0.5, 1, 2, 5, 10, 20 mg
Solution: 2 mg/mL

Children 3–12 yr:
(PO): Initial dose at 0.025–0.05 mg/kg/24 hr ÷ BID-TID. If necessary, increase
daily dosage by 0.25–0.5 mg/24 hr Q5–7 days PRN up to a **maximum** of
0.15 mg/kg/24 hr. Usual maintenance doses for specific indications include the
following:
Agitation: 0.01–0.03 mg/kg/24 hr QD PO
Psychosis: 0.05–0.15 mg/kg/24 hr ÷ BID-TID PO
Tourette's syndrome: 0.05–0.075 mg/kg/24 hr ÷ BID-TID PO; may increase daily
dose by 0.5 mg Q5–7 days.
IM, as lactate, for 6–12 yr: 1–3 mg/dose Q4–8 hr; **max. dose:** 0.15 mg/kg/24 hr
>12 yr:
Acute agitation: 2–5 mg/dose IM as lactate or 1–15 mg/dose PO; repeat in
1 hr PRN
Psychosis: 2–5 mg/dose Q4–8 hr IM PRN or 1–15 mg/24 hr ÷ BID-TID PO
Tourette's: 0.5–2 mg/dose BID-TID PO

Use with **caution** in patients with cardiac disease because of the risk of
hypotension and in patients with epilepsy because the drug lowers the seizure
threshold. Extrapyramidal symptoms, drowsiness, headache, tachycardia, ECG
changes, nausea, and vomiting can occur.
Drug is metabolized by cytochrome P-450 1A2, 2D6, and 3A3/4 isoenzymes. May
also inhibit cytochrome P-450 2D6 and 3A3/4 isoenzymes. Serotonin selective
reuptake inhibitors (e.g., fluoxetine) may increase levels and effects of haloperidol.
Carbamazepine and phenobarbital may decrease levels and effects of haloperidol.
Acutely aggravated patients may require doses as often as Q60 min. **Decanoate salt
is given every 3–4 weeks in doses that are 10 to 15 times the individual patient's
stablized oral dose.**

HEPARIN SODIUM

Various trade names
Anticoagulant

No 1 B

Inj:
Beef lung: 1000, 5000, 10,000, 20,000, 40,000 U/mL
Porcine intestinal mucosa: 1000, 2000, 2500, 5000, 7500, 10,000, 20,000,
40,000 U/mL (some products may be preservative-free)
Lock flush solution (porcine based): 10, 100 U/mL (some products may be
preservative-free)

Continued

HEPARIN SODIUM *continued*

Injection for IV infusion (porcine based):

D_5W: 40 U/mL (500 mL), 50 U/mL (200, 250, 500 mL), 100 U/mL (100, 200, 250 mL)

NS (0.9% NaCl): 2 U/mL (500, 1000 mL)

0.45% NaCl: 50 U/mL (250, 500 mL), 100 U/mL (250 mL)

120 U = approximately 1 mg

Anticoagulation **(see pp. 299–300 for dosage adjustments):**
Infants and children:
  Initial: 50 U/kg IV bolus
  Maintenance: 10–25 U/kg/hr as IV infusion or 50–100 U/kg/dose Q4 hr IV
Adults:
  Initial: 50–100 U/kg IV bolus
  Maintenance: 15–25 U/kg/hr as IV infusion or 75–125 U/kg/dose Q4 hr IV
See remarks
DVT prophylaxis:
  Adults: 5000 U/dose SC Q8–12 hr until ambulatory
Heparin flush (dose should be less than heparinizing dose):
  Younger children: Lower doses should be used to **avoid** systemic heparinization
  Older children and adults:
    Peripheral IV: 1–2 mL of 10 U/mL solution Q4 hr
    Central lines: 2–3 mL of 100 U/mL solution Q24 hr
    TPN (central line) and arterial line: Add heparin to make final concentration of 0.5–1 U/mL

Adjust dose to give PTT 1.5–2.5 times control value. PTT is best measured 6–8 hr after initiation or changes in infusion rate. For intermittent injection, PTT is measured 3.5–4 hrs after injection. Signs of toxicity include bleeding, allergy, alopecia, thrombocytopenia.

Use preservative-free heparin in neonates. **Note:** Heparin flush doses may alter PTT in small patients; consider using more dilute heparin in these cases.

Antidote: Protamine sulfate (1 mg per 100 U heparin in previous 4 hr). For low-molecular-weight heparin, see *Enoxaparin.*

HYALURONIDASE

Wydase
Antidote, extravasation

No   ?   C

Inj: 150 U/mL
Powder for injection: 150, 1500 U
📇: Pharmacy can make a 15 U/mL dilution.

Infants and children: Dilute to 15 U/mL; give 1 mL (15 U) by 5 separate injections of 0.2 mL (3 U) at borders of extravasation site SC or intradermal using a 25- or 26-gauge needle

Continued

HYALURONIDASE *continued*

Contraindicated in dopamine and alpha-agonist extravasation. May cause urticaria. Patients receiving large amounts of salicylates, cortisone, or antihistamines may decrease the effects of hyaluronidase (larger doses may be necessary). Administer as early as possible (minutes to 1 hr) after IV extravasation.

HYDRALAZINE HCl

Apresoline
Antihypertensive, vasodilator

Yes   1   C

Tabs: 10, 25, 50, 100 mg
Inj: 20 mg/mL
Oral liquid: 1.25, 2, 4 mg/mL
Some dosage forms may contain tartrazines or sulfites.

Hypertensive crisis (may result in severe and prolonged hypotension, see p. 14 for alternatives):
  Children: 0.1–0.2 mg/kg/dose IM or IV Q4–6 hr PRN; **max. dose:** 20 mg/dose
  Adults: 10–40 mg IM or IV Q4–6 hr PRN
Chronic hypertension:
  Infants and children: Start at 0.75–1 mg/kg/24 hr PO ÷ Q6–12 hr (**max. dose:** 25 mg/dose). If necessary, increase dose over 3–4 weeks up to a **max. dose** of 5 mg/kg/24 hr for infants and 7.5 mg/kg/24 hr for children; or 200 mg/24 hr
  Adults: 10–50 mg/dose PO QID; **max. dose:** 300 mg/24 hr

Use with **caution** in severe renal and cardiac disease. Slow acetylators, patients receiving high-dose chronic therapy and those with renal insufficiency are at highest risk of lupus-like syndrome (generally reversible). May cause reflex tachycardia, palpitations, dizziness, headaches, and GI discomfort. MAO inhibitors and beta-blockers may increase hypotensive effects. Indomethacin may decrease hypotensive effects.

Drug undergoes first-pass metabolism. *Onset of action:* PO: 20–30 min; IV: 5–20 min. *Duration of action:* PO: 2–4 hr; IV: 2–6 hr. **Adjust dose in renal failure (see p. 949).**

HYDROCHLOROTHIAZIDE

Esidrix, Hydro-Par, Hydrodiuril, Oretic, and others
Diuretic, thiazide

Yes   1   D/B

Tabs: 25, 50, 100 mg
Caps: 12.5 mg
Solution: 10 mg/mL

Continued

HYDROCHLOROTHIAZIDE *continued*

Neonates and infants <6 mo: 2–4 mg/kg/24 hr ÷ BID PO; **max. dose:** 37.5 mg/24 hr

≥*6 mo and children:* 2 mg/kg/24 hr ÷ BID PO; **max. dose:** 100 mg/24 hr
Adults: 25–100 mg/24 hr ÷ QD-BID PO; **max. dose:** 200 mg/24 hr

See *Chlorothiazide.* May cause fluid and electrolyte imbalances, and hyper-uricemia. Drug may not be effective when creatinine clearance is less than 25–50 mL/min.

Hydrochlorothiazide is also available in combination with potassium-sparing diuretics (e.g., spironolactone), ACE inhibitors, angiotensin II receptor antagonists, hydralazine ± reserpine, and beta-blockers.

Pregnancy category is a "D" during the first trimester (increased risk of congenital defects) and changes to a "B" in the later trimesters.

HYDROCORTISONE

Solu-cortef, Hydrocortone, Cortef, and others
Corticosteroid

No   ?   C

Hydrocortisone base:
  Tabs: 5, 10, 20 mg
  Rectal cream: 1%, 2.5%
  Topical ointment: 0.5%, 1%, 2.5%
  Topical cream: 0.5%, 1%, 2.5%
  Topical lotion: 0.25%, 0.5%, 1%, 2%, 2.5%
Cypionate (Cortef):
  Suspension: 10 mg/5 mL (120 mL)
Na Phosphate (Hydrocortone Phosphate):
  Inj: 50 mg/mL (2, 10 mL); contains sulfites
Na Succinate (Solu-Cortef):
  Inj: 100, 250, 500, 1000 mg/vial
Acetate (Hydrocortone):
  Inj: 25, 50 mg/mL; may contain 0.9% benzyl alcohol
  Topical ointment: 0.5%, 1%
  Topical cream: 0.5%, 1%, 2.5%
  Suppository: 25 mg
  Rectal foam aerosol: 10% (90 mg/dose) (20 g)

Status asthmaticus:
  Children:
    Load (optional): 4–8 mg/kg/dose IV; **max. dose:** 250 mg
    Maintenance: 8 mg/kg/24 hr ÷ Q6 hr IV
  Adults: 100–500 mg/dose Q6 hr IV
Physiologic replacement: see p. 907 for dosing

Continued

HYDROCORTISONE *continued*

Antiinflammatory/immunosuppressive:
   Children:
      PO: 2.5–10 mg/kg/24 hr ÷ Q6–8 hr
      IM/IV: 1–5 mg/kg/24 hr ÷ Q12–24 hr
   Adolescents and adults:
      PO/IM/IV: 15–240 mg/dose Q12 hr
Acute adrenal insufficiency: see p. 907 for dosing
Topical use:
   Children and adults: Apply to affected areas TID–QID

> For doses based on body surface area and topical preparations, see pp. 907–910. Na succinate used for IV, IM dosing. Na phosphate may be give IM, SC, or IV. **Acetate form recommended for intraarticular, intralesional, soft tissue use only, but not for IV use.**
> See pp. 908–909 for topical steroid comparisons.

HYDROMORPHONE HCl

Dilaudid, Dilaudid-HP, and others
Narcotic, analgesic

          Yes   ?   B/D

Tabs: 2, 4, 8 mg
Inj: 1, 2, 4, 10 mg/mL (may contain benzyl alcohol and/or parabens)
Suppository: 3 mg
Oral liquid: 1 mg/mL

> *Analgesia, titrate to effect:*
> *Children:*
>   *IV:* 0.015 mg/kg/dose Q4–6 hr PRN
>   *PO:* 0.03–0.08 mg/kg/dose Q4–6 hr PRN; **max. dose:** 5 mg/dose
> *Adolescents and adults:*
>   *IM, IV, SC:* 1–2 mg/dose Q4–6 hr PRN
>   *PO:* 1–4 mg/dose Q4–6 hr PRN

> Refer to p. 894 for equianalgesic doses and p. 897 for patient-controlled analgesia dosing. Less pruritus than morphine. Similar profile of side effects to other narcotics. Use with **caution** in infants and young children, and **do not use** in neonates because of potential CNS effects. Dose reduction recommended in renal insufficiency or severe hepatic impairment. Pregnancy category changes to "D" if used for prolonged peroids or in high doses at term.

HYDROXYZINE

Atarax, Vistaril
Antihistamine, anxiolytic

No ? C

Tabs (HCl): 10, 25, 50, 100 mg
Caps (pamoate): 25, 50, 100 mg
Syrup (HCl): 10 mg/5 mL
Suspension (pamoate): 25 mg/5 mL
Injection (HCl): 25, 50 mg/mL; may contain benzyl alcohol

Oral:
  Children: 2 mg/kg/24 hr ÷ Q6–8 hr
  Adult: 25–100 mg/dose Q4–6 hr PRN; **max. dose:** 600 mg/24 hr
IM:
  Children: 0.5–1 mg/kg/dose Q4–6 hr PRN
  Adult: 25–100 mg/dose Q4–6 hr PRN; **max. dose:** 600 mg/24 hr

May potentiate barbiturates, meperidine, and other CNS depressants. May cause dry mouth, drowsiness, tremor, convulsions, blurred vision, and hypotension. May cause pain at injection site.

Onset of action: Within 15–30 min. *Duration of action:* 4–6 hr. **IV administration is not recommended.**

IBUPROFEN

Motrin, Advil, Nuprin, Medipren, Children's Advil, Children's Motrin, and others
Nonsteroidal antiinflammatory agent

Yes 1 B/D

Oral suspension (OTC): 100 mg/5 mL (60, 120, 480 mL)
Oral drops (OTC): 40 mg/mL (7.5, 15 mL)
Chewable tabs (OTC): 50, 100 mg
Caplets: 100 mg
Tabs: 100 (OTC), 200 (OTC), 300, 400, 600, 800 mg
Caps (OTC): 200 mg

Children:
  Analgesic/antipyretic: 5–10 mg/kg/dose Q6–8 hr PO; **max. dose:** 40 mg/kg/24 hr PO
  JRA: 30–50 mg/kg/24 hr ÷ Q6 hr PO; **max. dose:** 2400 mg/24 hr
Adults:
  Inflammatory disease: 400–800 mg/dose Q6–8 hr PO
  Pain/fever/dysmenorrhea: 200–400 mg/dose Q4–6 hr PRN PO
  Max. dose: 800 mg/dose or 3.2 g/24 hr

Continued

IBUPROFEN *continued*

Contraindicated with active GI bleeding and ulcer disease. Use **caution** with aspirin hypersensitivity, or hepatic/renal insufficiency, dehydration, and in patients receiving anticoagulants. GI distress (lessened with milk), rashes, ocular problems, granulocytopenia, and anemia may occur. Inhibits platelet aggregation. Consumption of more than three alcoholic beverages per day may increase risk for GI bleeding.

May increase serum levels and effects of digoxin, methotrexate, and lithium. May decrease the effects of antihypertensives, furosemide, and thiazide diuretics. Pregnancy category changes to "D" if used in third trimester or near delivery.

IMIPENEM-CILASTATIN

Primaxin IV, Primaxin IM
Antibiotic, carbapenem

Yes ? C

Inj:
Primaxin IV: 250, 500 mg; contains 3.2 mEq Na/g drug
Primaxin IM: 500, 750 mg; contains 2.8 mEq Na/g drug

Neonates:
0–4 weeks and <1.2 kg: 50 mg/kg/24 hr ÷ Q12 hr IV
<1 week and ≥1.2 kg: 50 mg/kg/24 hr ÷ Q12 hr IV
≥1 week and ≥1.2 kg: 75 mg/kg/24 hr ÷ Q8 hr IV
Children (4 weeks–3 mo): 100 mg/kg/24hr ÷ Q6 hr IV
Children (>3 mo): 60–100 mg/kg/24 hr ÷ Q6 hr IV; **max. dose:** 4 g/24 hr
Adults: 250–1000 mg/dose Q6–8 hr IV; **max. dose:** 4 g/24 hr or 50 mg/kg/24 hr, whichever is less

For IV use, give slowly over 30–60 min. Adverse effects include pruritus, urticaria, GI symptoms, seizures, dizziness, hypotension, elevated LFTs, blood dyscrasias, and penicillin allergy. CSF penetration is variable but best with inflamed meninges.

Do not administer with probenecid (increases imipenem/cilastatin levels) and ganciclovir (increase risk for seizures).

Higher doses of 90 mg/kg/24 hr have been used in older children with cystic fibrosis. **Adjust dose in renal insufficiency (p. 943).**

IMIPRAMINE

Tofranil, Tofranil-PM, Janimine
Antidepressant, tricyclic

No 3 D

Tabs (HCl): 10, 25, 50 mg
Caps (Tofranil-PM, pamoate): 75, 100, 125, 150 mg
Inj (HCl): 12.5 mg/mL (2 mL)

Continued

IMIPRAMINE *continued*

Antidepressant:
Children:
  Initial: 1.5 mg/kg/24 hr ÷ TID PO; Increase 1–1.5 mg/kg/24 hr Q3–4 days to **maximum** of 5 mg/kg/24 hr
Adolescent:
  Initial: 25–50 mg/24 hr ÷ QD-TID PO; dosages exceeding 100 mg/24 hr are generally not necessary
Adult:
  Initial: 75–100 mg/24 hr ÷ TID PO/IM; **max. initial IM dose:** 100 mg/24 hr
  Maintenance: 50–300 mg/24 hr QHS PO; **max. PO dose:** 300 mg/24 hr
Enuresis (≥6 yr):
  Initial: 10–25 mg QHS PO
  Increment: 10–25 mg/dose at 1- to 2-week intervals until maximum dose for age or desired effect achieved. Continue × 2–3 mo, then taper slowly
  Max. dose:
    6–12 yr: 50 mg/24 hr
    12–14 yr: 75 mg/24 hr
Augment analgesia for chronic pain:
  Initial: 0.2–0.4 mg/kg/dose QHS PO; increase 50% every 2–3 days to **maximum** of 1–3 mg/kg/dose QHS PO

Contraindicated in narrow-angle glaucoma and patients who used MAO inhibitors within 14 days. See p. 44 for management of toxic ingestion. Side effects include sedation, urinary retention, constipation, dry mouth, dizziness, drowsiness, and arrhythmia. QHS dosing during first weeks of therapy will reduce sedation. Monitor ECG, BP, CBC at start of therapy and with dose changes. Tricyclics may cause mania.

Therapeutic reference range (sum of imipramine and desipramine) = 150–250 ng/mL. Levels >1000 ng/mL are toxic; however, toxicity may occur at >300 ng/mL. *Recommended serum sampling times at steady-state:* Obtain trough level within 30 min prior to the next scheduled dose after 5–7 days of continuous therapy. Carbamazepine may reduce imipramine levels; cimetidine, fluoxetine, fluvoxamine, labetolol, and quinidine may increase imipramine levels.

PO route preferred. May be given IM. **Do not** discontinue abruptly in patients receiving long-term high-dose therapy.

IMMUNE GLOBULIN

Yes   ?   C

IM preparations:
  BayGam: 150–180 mg/mL
  Gammar-P IM: 150–180 mg/mL
IV preparations:
  Gamimune-N: 5%, 10% solution
  Gammagard S/D: 2.5, 5, 10 g; dilute to 5% or 10%

Continued

IMMUNE GLOBULIN
continued

Gammar-P IV: 1, 2.5, 5, 10 g (contains 1 g sucrose per 1 g Ig); dilute to 5%
Iveegam: 5 g; dilute to 5%
Panglobulin: 6, 12 g (contains 1.67 g sucrose per 1 g Ig); dilute to 3%, 6%, or 12%
Polygam S/D: 2.5, 5, 10 g; dilute to 5% or 10%
Sandoglobulin: 1, 3, 6, 12 g (contains 1.67 g sucrose per 1 g Ig); dilute to 3%, 6% or 12%
Venoglobulin S: 5%, 10% solution

See indications and doses on pp. 307–310.
General guidelines for administration (see package insert of specific products):
Begin infusion at 0.01 mL/kg/min, double rate every 15–30 min, up to maximum of 0.08 mL/kg/min. If adverse reactions occur, stop infusion until side effects subside; may restart at rate that was previously tolerated.

May cause flushing, chills, fever, headache, hypotension. Hypersensitivity reaction may occur when IV form is administered rapidly. Gamimune-N contains maltose and may cause an osmotic diuresis. May cause **anaphylaxis** in IgA-deficient patients due to varied amounts of IgA. Some products are IgA depleted. Consult a pharmacist.

IV preparations containing sucrose have been associated with renal dysfunction, including acute renal failure. If used, it is recommended that the rate of infusion of these products **does not exceed** 3 mg sucrose/kg/min.

Delay MMR and varicella immunizations after IVIG (see *Red Book*).

INDINAVIR

Crixivan, IDV
Antiviral agent, protease inhibitor

No   3   C

Caps: 100, 200, 333, 400 mg

Children:
  Usual dose: 500 mg/m²/dose PO Q8 hr; **max. dose:** 800 mg/dose
  Patients with small body surface areas: 300–400 mg/m²/dose PO Q8 hr
Adolescents and adults:
  Usual dose: 800 mg PO Q8 hr
  In combination with rifabutin or efavirenz: 1000 mg PO Q8 hr
  In combination with delavirdine, itraconazole, or ketoconazole: 600 mg PO Q8 hr

Reduce dose in mild to moderate hepatic impairment. May cause GI discomfort, headache, metallic taste, hyperbilirubinemia, dizziness, nephrolithiasis, hyperglycemia, and body fat redistribution. Should not be used in neonates due to risk of hyperbilirubinemia.

Continued

INDINAVIR continued

Like other protease inhibitors, indinavir inhibits the cytochrome P450-3A4 isoenzyme to increase the effects or toxicities of many drugs. Concomitant use with astemizole, terfenadine, cisapride, ergot alkaloid derivatives, pimozide, triazolam, and/or midazolam is **contraindicated**. Rifampin, rifabutin, efavirenz, and nevirapine can decrease indinavir levels, whereas ketoconazole or itraconazole can increase levels. **Carefully review the patient's medication profile for potential interactions!**

Adolescent dosing: Patients in early puberty (Tanner I-II) should be dosed with pediatric regimens and those in late puberty (Tanner V) should be dosed with adult regimens. Adolescents who are at the midst of their growth spurt (Tanner III females and Tanner IV males) can be dosed by either pediatric or adult regimen with close monitoring of efficacy and toxicity.

Administer doses on an empty stomach (1 hr before or 2 hrs after a meal) with adequate hydration (48 oz/24 hr in adults). If didanosine is included in the regimen, space 1 hr apart on an empty stomach. Capsules are sensitive to moisture and should be stored with a desiccant. **Noncompliance can quickly promote resistant HIV strains.**

INDOMETHACIN
Indocin
Nonsteroidal antiinflammatory agent

Yes   1   B/D

Caps: 25, 50 mg
Sustained-release caps: 75 mg
Inj: 1 mg
Suppositories: 50 mg
Suspension: 25 mg/5 mL

Antiinflammatory:
>*14 yr:* 1–3 mg/kg/24 hr ÷ TID-QID PO; **max. dose:** 200 mg/24 hr
Adults: 50–150 mg/24 hr ÷ BID-QID PO; **max. dose:** 200 mg/24 hr
Closure of ductus arteriosus:
Infuse intravenously over 20–30 min:

Age	Dose (mg/kg/dose Q12–24 hr)		
	#1	#2	#3
<48 hr	0.2	0.1	0.1
2–7 days	0.2	0.2	0.2
>7 days	0.2	0.25	0.25

In infants <1500 g, 0.1–0.2 mg/kg/dose IV Q24 hr may be given for an additional 3–5 days
Intraventricular hemorrhage prophylaxis: 0.1 mg/kg/dose IV Q24 hr × three doses, initiated at 6–12 hr of age

Continued

INDOMETHACIN *continued*

Contraindicated in active bleeding, coagulation defects, necrotizing enterocolitis, and renal insufficiency. May cause (especially in neonates) decreased urine output, platelet dysfunction, decreased GI blood flow, and reduce the antihypertensive effects of beta-blockers, hydralazine, and ACE inhibitors. **Fatal hepatitis** reported in treatment of JRA. Monitor renal and hepatic function before and during use.

Reduction in cerebral blood flow associated with rapid IV infusion; infuse all IV doses over 20–30 min.

Pregnancy category changes to "D" if used for >48 hours or after 34 weeks gestation or close to delivery.

INSULIN PREPARATIONS
Pancreatic hormone

Yes ? B

Many preparations, at concentrations of 40, 100, 500 U/mL
: Diluted concentrations of 1 U/mL or 10 U/mL may be necessary for neonates and infants.

Insulin preparations: See p. 913.
Hyperkalemia: See pp. 242–243.
DKA: See pp. 213–215.

When using insulin drip with new IV tubing, fill the tubing with the insulin infusion solution and wait for 30 min (prior to connecting tubing to the patient). Then flush the line and connect the IV line to the patient to start the infusion. This will ensure proper drug delivery. **Adjust dose in renal failure (see p. 949).**

IODIDE
See Potassium Iodide

IPECAC
Emetic agent

No ? C

Syrup: 70 mg/mL (15, 30, 473, 4000 mL); contains 1.5%–2% alcohol

Continued

IPECAC *continued*

See p. 22 for indications.
All doses are administered × 1 and may be repeated once if vomiting does not occur within 20–30 min:
6–12 mo: 5–10 mL Ipecac followed by 10–20 mL/kg water
1–12 yr: 15 mL Ipecac followed by 10–20 mL/kg or 120–240 mL water
≥12 yr and adults: 15–30 mL followed by 200–300 mL of water

Do not administer if patient is unconscious or potential for decline in mental status, lacks a gag reflex, has seizures, or has ingested corrosives, strong acids or bases, volatile oils. May cause GI irritation, cardiotoxicity, myopathy. **Do not** use ipecac fluid extract because it is 14 times more potent. **Do not** adminster with milk or carbonated beverages.

IPRATROPIUM BROMIDE
Atrovent
Anticholinergic agent

No   1   B

Aerosol: 18 mcg/dose (200 actuations per canister, 14 g)
Nebulized solution: 0.02% (500 mcg/2.5 mL, 25s, 60s)
Nasal spray: 0.03% (21 mcg per actuation, 30 mL); 0.06% (42 mcg per actuation, 15 mL)

Inhaler:
  <12 yr: 1–2 puffs TID-QID
  ≥12 yr: 2–3 puffs QID up to 12 puffs/24 hr
Nebulized treatments:
  Infants and children: 250 mcg/dose TID-QID
  >12 yr and adults: 250–500 mcg/dose TID-QID
Nasal spray:
  Allergic and nonallergic rhinitis:
  >6 yr and adults: 2 sprays of 0.03% strength (42 mcg) per nostril BID-TID
  Rhinitis associated with common cold:
  >5 yr and adults: 2 sprays of 0.06% strength (84 mcg) per nostril TID-QID × 4 days

Contraindicated in soy or peanut allergy (for aerosol inhaler) and atropine hypersensitivity. Use with **caution** in narrow-angle glaucoma or bladder neck obstruction, though ipratropium has fewer anticholinergic systemic effects than atropine. May cause anxiety, dizziness, headache, GI discomfort, and cough with inhaler or nebulized use. Epistaxis, nasal congestion, and dry mouth/throat have been reported with the nasal spray. Proven efficacy of nebulized solution in pediatrics is currently limited to reactive airway disease management in the emergency room and intensive care unit areas.

Continued

IPRATROPIUM BROMIDE *continued*

Bronchodilation onset of action is 1-3 min, with peak effects within 1.5-2 hr and duration of action of 4-6 hr.

Shake inhaler well prior to use with spacer. Nebulized solution may be mixed with albuterol.

Breastfeeding safety **extrapolated** from safety of atropine.

IRON DEXTRAN

InfeD, DexFerrum
Parenteral iron

No ? C

Inj: 50 mg/mL (50 mg elemental Fe/mL) (2 mL)
Products containing phenol 0.5% are only for IM administration; products containing sodium chloride 0.9% can be administered via the IM or IV route.

Inject test dose (see remarks)
Iron deficiency anemia: Total replacement dose of iron dextran (mL) = 0.0476 × wt (kg) × (desired Hgb [g/dL] − measured Hgb [g/dL]) + (1 mL per 5 kg body weight, up to maximum of 14 mL).
Acute blood loss: Total replacement dose of iron dextran (mL) = 0.02 × blood loss (mL) × hematocrit expressed as fraction. Assumes 1 mL of RBC = 1 mg elemental iron. If no reaction to test dose, give remainder of replacement dose ÷ over 2–3 daily doses.
Max. daily (IM) dose:
  <5 kg: 0.5 mL (25 mg)
  5–10 kg: 1 mL (50 mg)
  >10 kg: 2 mL (100 mg)

Oral therapy with iron salts is preferred; injectable routes may be painful. Numerous adverse effects including anaphylaxis, fever, hypotension, rash, myalgias, and arthralgias. Use "Z-track" technique for IM administration. **Inject test dose:** 25 mg (12.5 mg for infants).

May begin treatment dose after 1 hr. **Max. rate of IV infusion:** 50 mg/min. For IV infusion, diluting in NS may lower the incidence of phlebitis. Direct IV push administration is **not** recommended. **Not** recommended in infants <4 mo. Compatible with parenteral nutrition solutions.

IRON PREPARATIONS

Fergon, Fer-In-Sol, Ferralet, Feosol, Niferex, and others
Oral iron supplements

No ? A

Ferrous sulfate (20% elemental Fe):
  Drops (Fer-In-Sol): 75 mg (15 mg Fe)/0.6 mL (50 mL); 125 mg (25 mg Fe)/1 mL (50 mL)

For explanation of icons, see p. 572.

Continued

IRON PREPARATIONS *continued*

Syrup (Fer-In-Sol): 90 mg (18 mg Fe)/5 mL (5% alcohol)
Elixir (Feosol): 220 mg (44 mg Fe)/5 mL (5% alcohol)
Caps: 250 mg (50 mg Fe)
Tabs: 195 mg (39 mg Fe), 300 mg (60 mg Fe), 324 mg (65 mg Fe)
Ferrous gluconate (12% elemental Fe):
Elixir: 300 mg (34 mg Fe)/5 mL (7% alcohol)
Tabs: 240 mg (27 mg Fe, as Fergon), 300 mg (34 mg Fe), 320 mg (37 mg Fe), 325 mg (38 mg Fe)
Sustained-release caps: 320 mg (37 mg Fe)
Caps: 86 mg (10 mg Fe)
Ferrous sulfate, exsiccated/dried (30% elemental Fe):
Tabs: 200 mg (65 mg Fe)
Extended-release tabs: 160 mg (50 mg Fe)
Caps: 190 mg (60 mg Fe)
Extended-release caps: 159 mg (50 mg Fe)
Polysaccharide-Iron Complex (Niferex) (expressed in mg elemental Fe):
Tabs: 50 mg
Caps: 150 mg
Elixir: 100 mg/5 mL (10% alcohol)

Iron deficiency anemia:
Premature Infants: 2–4 mg elemental Fe/kg/24 hr ÷ QD-BID PO; **max. dose:** 15 mg elemental Fe/24 hr
Children: 3–6 mg elemental Fe/kg/24 hr ÷ QD-TID PO
Adult: 60 mg elemental Fe BID-QID
Prophylaxis:
Children: Give dose below PO ÷ QD-TID
Premature: 2 mg elemental Fe/kg/24 hr
Full-term: 1–2 mg elemental Fe/kg/24 hr
Max. dose: 15 mg elemental Fe/24 hr
Adults: 60 mg elemental Fe/24 hr PO ÷ QD-BID

Iron preparations are variably absorbed. Less GI irritation when given with or after meals. Vitamin C, 200 mg per 30 mg iron, may enhance absorption.
Liquid iron preparations may stain teeth. Give with dropper or drink through straw. May produce constipation, dark stools (false-positive guaiac is controversial), nausea, and epigastric pain. Iron and tetracycline inhibit each other's absorption. Antacids may decrease iron absorption.

ISONIAZID

INH, Nydrazid, Laniazid
Antituberculous agent

Yes   1   C

Tabs: 50, 100, 300 mg
Syrup: 50 mg/5 mL (473 mL)
Inj: 100 mg/mL (10 mL)

Continued

ISONIAZID *continued*

See the most recent edition of the AAP *Red Book* for details and length of therapy.
Prophylaxis:
 Infants and children: 10 mg/kg (**max. dose:** 300 mg) PO QD. After 1 mo of
daily therapy and in cases where daily compliance cannot be assured, may change
to 20–40 mg/kg (**max. dose:** 900 mg) per dose PO, given twice weekly.
 Adults: 300 mg PO QD
Treatment:
 Infants and children:
 10–15 mg/kg (**max. dose:** 300 mg) PO QD or 20–30 mg/kg (**max. dose:** 900 mg)
per dose twice weekly with rifampin for uncomplicated pulmonary tuberculosis in
compliant patients. Additional drugs are necessary in complicated disease.
 Adults:
 5 mg/kg (**max. dose:** 300 mg) PO QD or 15 mg/kg (**max. dose:** 900 mg) per dose
twice weekly with rifampin. Additional drugs are necessary in complicated disease.
For INH-resistant TB: Discuss with Health Dept., and consult ID specialist.
See most recent edition of the *AAP Red Book*.

Should **not** be used alone for treatment. Peripheral neuropathy, optic neuritis,
seizures, encephalopathy, psychosis, and hepatic side effects may occur with
higher doses, especially in combination with rifampin. Follow LFTs monthly.
Supplemental pyridoxine (1–2 mg/kg/24 hr) is recommended. May cause false-positive
urine glucose test. Inhibits hepatic microsomal enzymes; decrease dose of carbamazepine, diazepam, phenytoin, and prednisone. May be given IM (same as oral doses)
when oral therapy is not possible. **Adjust dose in renal failure (see p. 943).**

ISOPROTERENOL
Isuprel and others
Adrenergic agonist

No   ?   C

Isoproterenol HCl:
 Tabs: 10, 15 mg (sublingual)
 Solutions for nebulization:
  0.25% (2.5 mg/mL) (0.5 mL, 15 mL)
  0.5% (5 mg/mL) (0.5, 10, 60 mL)
  1% (10 mg/mL) (10 mL)
 Aerosol: 131 mcg/dose (300 metered doses per 15 mL; 10, 15, 22.5 mL)
 Inj: 0.2 mg/mL (1, 5, 10 mL)
Isoproterenol Sulfate:
 Aerosol 80 mcg/dose (300 metered doses per 15 mL; 15 mL)
 Contains sulfites

Aerosol: 1–2 puffs up to 6 per 24 hr
Nebulized solution:
 Children: 0.05 mg/kg/dose = 0.01 mL/kg/dose of 0.5% solution (**min. dose:**
0.5 mg; **max. dose:** 1.25 mg) diluted with NS to 2 mL Q4 hr PRN

Continued

ISOPROTERENOL *continued*

Adults: 2.5–5 mg/dose = 0.25–0.5 mL of 1% solution diluted with NS to 2 mL Q4 hr PRN

IV infusion:

Children: 0.05–2 mcg/kg/min; start at minimum dose and increase every 5–10 min by 0.1 mcg/kg/min until desired effect or onset of toxicity; **max. dose:** 2 mcg/kg/min

Adults: 2–20 mcg/kg/min

See inside front cover for preparation of infusion

Sublingual:

Children: 5–10 mg/dose Q3-4 hr; **max. dose:** 30 mg/24 hr

Adults: 10–20 mg/dose Q3-4 hr; **max. dose:** 60 mg/24 hr

Use with **caution** in CHF, ischemia, or aortic stenosis. May cause flushing, ventricular arrhythmias, profound hypotension, anxiety, and myocardial ischemia. Patients with continuous IV infusion should have heart rate, respiratory rate, and blood pressure monitored. **Not** for treatment of asystole or for use in cardiac arrests.

Continuous infusion for bronchodilation must be gradually tapered over a 24–48 hr period to prevent rebound bronchospasm. Tolerance may occur with prolonged use. Clinical deterioration, myocardial necrosis, CHF, and **death** have been reported with continuous infusion use in refractory asthmatic children.

ISOTRETINOIN

Accutane
Retinoic acid, vitamin A derivative

No   3   X

Caps: 10, 20, 40 mg; contains soybean oil, EDTA, and parabens

Cystic acne: 0.5–2 mg/kg/24 hr ÷ BID PO × 15–20 weeks
Dosages as low as 0.05 mg/kg/24 hr have been reported to be beneficial.

Contraindicated during pregnancy; known teratogen. **Caution** in females during child-bearing years. May cause conjunctivitis, xerosis, pruritus, epistaxis, anemia, hyperlipidemia, pseudotumor cerebri (especially in combination with tetracyclines; avoid this combination), cheilitis, bone pain, muscle aches, skeletal changes, lethargy, nausea, vomiting, elevated ESR, mental depression, and psychosis. To avoid additive toxic effects, **do not** take vitamin A concomitantly. Monitor CBC, ESR, triglycerides, and LFTs.

ITRACONAZOLE

Sporanox
Antifungal agent

Yes   3   C

Caps: 100 mg
Oral solution: 10 mg/mL (150 mL)
Inj: 10 mg/mL (25 mL)

Children (limited data): 3–5 mg/kg/24 hr PO ÷ QD-BID; dosages as high as 5–10 mg/kg/24 hr have been used for aspergillus prophylaxis in chronic granulomatous disease

Adults:

Blastomycosis and nonmeningeal histoplasmosis:
   PO: 200 mg QD up to a **maximum** of 400 mg/24 hr ÷ BID (**max. dose:** 200 mg/dose)
   IV: 400 mg/24 hr ÷ BID × 2 days, followed by 200 mg QD; switch to oral therapy as soon as possible

Aspergillosis and severe infections:
   PO: 600 mg/24 hr ÷ TID × 3–4 days, followed by 200–400 mg/24 hr ÷ BID; **max. dose:** 600 mg/24 hr ÷ TID
   IV: 400 mg/24 hr ÷ BID × 2 days, followed by 200 mg QD; switch to oral therapy as soon as possible

Empiric therapy in febrile, neutropenic patients: 400 mg/24 hr IV ÷ BID × 2 days, followed by 200 mg QD for up to 14 days; continue with the oral solution at 200 mg PO BID until resolution

Oral solution and capsule dosage form should **NOT** be used interchangeably. Only the oral solution has been shown to be effective for oral and/or esophageal candidasis. Use with **caution** in hepatic impairment. May cause GI symptoms, headaches, rash, liver enzyme elevation, hepatitis, and hypokalemia.

Like ketoconazole, it inhibits the activity of the cytochrome P-450 3A4 drug metabolizing isoenzyme. Thus the coadministration of terfenadine, astemizole, cisapride, and midazolam is **contraindicated**. See remarks in Ketoconazole for additional drug interaction information.

IV dosage form should **not** be used in patients with GFR <30 mL/min because the hydoxypropyl-beta-cyclodextrin excipient has reduced clearance in patients with renal failure. IV form should be diluted with NS (not compatible with D_5W or LR) and infused over 1 hr.

Administer oral solution on an empty stomach, but administer capsules with food. Achlorhydria reduces absorption of the drug.

IVERMECTIN

Stromectol
Antihelmintic

No   1   C

Tabs: 3, 6 mg

Cutaneous larva migrans or strongyloidiasis: 0.2 mg/kg/dose PO QD × 1-2 days; dosing by body weight (see first table below):
Scabies: 0.2 mg/kg/dose PO × 1; dosing by body weight (see table below):

CUTANEOUS LAVA MIGRANS, SCABIES, STRONGYLOIDIASIS

Weight (kg)	Oral Dose
15–24	3 mg
25–35	6 mg
36–50	9 mg
51–65	12 mg
66–79	15 mg
≥80	0.2 mg/kg

Onchocerciasis: 0.15 mg/kg PO × 1; dosing by body weight (see table below):

ONCHOCERCIASIS

Weight (kg)	Single Oral Dose
15–25	3 mg
26–44	6 mg
45–64	9 mg
65–84	12 mg
≥85	0.15 mg/kg

Dose may be repeated every 6–12 mo until asymptomatic

Adverse reactions experienced in strongyloidiasis include diarrhea, nausea, vomiting, pruritus, rash, dizziness, and drowsiness.

Adverse reactions experienced in onchocerciasis include cutaneous or systemic allergic/inflammatory reactions of varying severity (Mazzotti reaction) and ophthalmological reactions. Specific reactions may include arthralgia/synovitis, lymph node enlargement and tenderness, pruritus, edema, fever, orthostatic hypotension, and tachycardia. Therapy for postural hypotension may include oral hydration, recumbency, IV normal saline, and/or IV steroids. Antihistamines and/or aspirin have been used for most mild to moderate cases.

KANAMYCIN

Kantrex and others
Antibiotic, aminoglycoside

Yes   1   D

Caps: 500 mg
Inj: 37.5, 250, 333, 500 mg/mL; may contain sulfites

Neonatal IV/IM administration (see table below):

NEONATAL DOSING

Birthweight	<7 days	≥7 days
<2 kg	15 mg/kg/24 hr ÷ Q12 hr	22.5 mg/kg/24 hr ÷ Q8 hr
≥2 kg	20 mg/kg/24 hr ÷ Q12 hr	30 mg/kg/24 hr ÷ Q8 hr

Infants and children: IM/IV: 15–30 mg/kg/24 hr ÷ Q8–12 hr
Adults: IV/IM: 15 mg/kg/24 hr ÷ Q8–12 hr
PO administration for GI bacterial overgrowth: 150–250 mg/kg/24 hr ÷ Q6 hr;
max. dose: 4 g/24 hr

Renal toxicity and ototoxicity may occur. Give over 30 min if IV route is used.
Reduce dosage frequency with renal impairment. Poorly absorbed orally, PO
route used to treat GI bacterial overgrowth.
Therapeutic levels: Peak: 15–30 mg/L; trough: <5–10 mg/L. *Recommended serum
sampling time at steady-state:* Trough within 30 min prior to the third consecutive
dose and peak 30–60 min after the administration of the third consecutive dose.
Adjust dose in renal failure (see p. 943).

KETAMINE

Ketalar and others
General anesthetic

No   3   B

Inj: 10 mg/mL (20 mL), 50 mg/mL (10 mL), 100 mg/mL (5 mL);
contains benzethonium chloride

Children:
  Sedation:
    PO: 3–4 mg/kg × 1
    IM: 2–3 mg/kg × 1
Adults:
  Analgesia with sedation:
    IV (see remarks): 0.2–1 mg/kg
    IM: 0.5–4 mg/kg

Continued

KETAMINE *continued*

Contraindicated in elevated ICP, increased intraocular pressure, hypertension, aneurysms, thyrotoxicosis, CHF, angina, and psychotic disorders. May cause hypertension, hypotension, emergence reactions, tachycardia, laryngospasm, respiratory depression, and stimulation of salivary secretions. Intravenous use may induce general anesthesia. Benzodiazepine may be added to prevent emergence phenomenon. Anticholinergic agent may be added to decrease hypersalivation. Rate of IV infusion should **not** exceed 0.5 mg/kg/min and should not be administered in less than 60 sec. For additional information, including onset and duration of action, see p. 904.

KETOCONAZOLE

Nizoral and others
Antifungal agent

No   1   C

Tabs: 200 mg
Suspension: 100 mg/5 mL
Cream: 2% (15, 30, 60 g)
Shampoo: 1% [OTC] (207 mL), 2% (120 mL)

Oral:
Children ≥2 yr: 3.3–6.6 mg/kg/24 hr QD
Adult: 200–400 mg/24 hr QD
Max. dose: 800 mg/24 hr ÷ BID
Topical: 1–2 applications/24 hr
Shampoo: Twice weekly for 4 weeks with at least 3 days between applications; intermittently as needed to maintain control
Suppressive therapy against mucocutaneous candidiasis in HIV:
Children: 5–10 mg/kg/24 hr ÷ QD-BID PO
Adolescents and adults: 200 mg/dose QD PO

Monitor LFTs in long-term use. Drugs that decrease gastric acidity will decrease absorption. May cause nausea, vomiting, rash, headache, pruritus, and fever. Inhibits CYP 450 3A4. Cardiac arrhythmias may occur when used with cisapride, terfenadine, and astemizole. Concomitant administration of ketoconazole with any of these drugs is **contraindicated**. May increase levels/effects of phenytoin, digoxin, cyclosporin, corticosteroids, nevirapine, protease inhibitors, and warfarin. Phenobarbital, rifampin, isoniazid, H_2 blockers, antacids, and omeprazole can decrease levels of ketoconazole.

To use shampoo, wet hair and scalp with water, apply sufficient amount to scalp and gently massage for about 1 min. Rinse hair thoroughly, reapply shampoo and leave on the scalp for an additional 3 min; then rinse.

KETOROLAC

Toradol, Accular (ophth)
Nonsteroidal antiinflammatory agent

Yes   1   C/D

Inj: 15 mg/mL (1 mL), 30 mg/mL (1, 2 mL); contains 10% alcohol
Tabs: 10 mg
Ophthalmic: 0.5% (3, 5, 10 mL)

IM/IV:
 Children: 0.5 mg/kg/dose IM/IV Q6 hr. **Max. dose:** 30 mg Q6 hr or 120 mg/24 hr
 Adults: 30 mg IM/IV Q6 hr. **Max. dose:** 120 mg/24 hr
PO:
 Children >50 kg and adults: 10 mg PRN Q6 hr; **max. dose:** 40 mg/24 hr
Ophthalmic:
 Adults: Instill 1 drop in each affected eye QID for up to 7 days

Ketorolac therapy is **not** to exceed 5 days (IM, IV, PO). May cause GI bleeding, nausea, dyspepsia, drowsiness, decreased platelet function, and interstitial nephritis. **Not** recommended in patients at increased risk of bleeding. **Do not** use in hepatic or renal failure. The **IV** route of administration in children is **not** yet recommended by the manufacturer, although it is well supported in the literature and in practice.

Pregnancy category changes to "D" if used in the third trimester.

LABETALOL

Normodyne, Trandate, and others
Adrenergic antagonist (alpha and beta), antihypertensive

No   1   C/D

Tabs: 100, 200, 300 mg
Inj: 5 mg/mL; contains parabens
Suspension: 10, 40 mg/mL

Children:
 PO: Initial: 4 mg/kg/24 hr ÷ BID. May increase up to 40 mg/kg/24 hr
 IV: Hypertensive emergency (start at lowest dose and titrate to effect; see p. 14):
  Intermittent dose: 0.2–1 mg/kg/dose Q10 min PRN; **max. dose:** 20 mg/dose
  Infusion: 0.4–1 mg/kg/hr, to a **maximum** of 3 mg/kg/hr; may initiate with a 0.2–1 mg/kg bolus; **max. bolus:** 20 mg
Adults:
 PO: 100 mg BID, increase by 100 mg/dose Q2–3 days PRN to a **maximum** of 2.4 g/24 hr

Continued

LABETALOL *continued*

IV: Hypertensive emergency (start at lowest dose and titrate to effect):
Intermittent dose: 20–80 mg/dose (begin with 20 mg) Q10 min PRN;
max. dose: 300 mg
Infusion: 2 mg/min, increase to titrate to response

Contraindicated in asthma, pulmonary edema, cardiogenic shock, and heart block. May cause orthostatic hypotension, edema, CHF, bradycardia, AV conduction disturbances, bronchospasm, urinary retention, and skin tingling. Use with **caution** in hepatic disease and diabetes. LFT elevation, hepatic necrosis, hepatitis, and cholestatic jaundice have been reported. Patient should remain supine for up to 3 hr after IV administration. Pregnancy category changes to "D" if used in second or third trimesters.
Onset of action: PO: 1–4 hr; IV: 5–15 min.

LACTULOSE

Cephulac, Chronulac, and others
Ammonium detoxicant, hyperosmotic laxative

No ? B

Syrup: 10 g/15 mL; contains galactose, lactose, and other sugars

Chronic constipation:
Children: 7.5 mL/24 hr PO after breakfast
Adults: 15–30 mL/24 hr PO QD to **maximum** of 60 mL/24 hr
Portal systemic encephalopathy (adjust dose to produce 2–3 soft stools/day):
Infants: 2.5–10 mL/24 hr PO ÷ TID-QID
Children: 40–90 mL/24 hr PO ÷ TID-QID
Adults: 30–45 mL/dose PO TID-QID; acute episodes 30–45 mL Q1–2 hr until 2–3 soft stools/day
Rectal (adults): 300 mL diluted in 700 mL water or NS in 30–60 min retention enema; may give Q4–6 hr

Contraindicated in galactosemia. Use with **caution** in diabetes mellitus. GI discomfort and diarrhea may occur. For portal systemic encephalopathy, monitor serum ammonia, serum potassium, and fluid status.
Adjust dose to achieve 2–3 soft stools per day. **Do not use** with antacids.

LAMIVUDINE

Epivir, Epivir-HBV, 3TC
Antiviral agent, nucleoside analogue reverse transcriptase inhibitor

Yes   3   C

Tabs: 100 mg (Epivir-HBV), 150 mg
Oral solution: 5 mg/mL (Epivir-HBV), 10 mg/mL
In combination with zidovudine (AZT) as Combivir:
  Tabs: 150 mg lamivudine + 300 mg zidovudine
In combination with abacavir and zidovudine (AZT) as Trizivir:
  Tabs: 150 mg lamivudine + 300 mg abacavir + 300 mg zidovudine

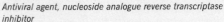

Neonate (<30 days): 2 mg/kg/dose PO BID
  Children (3 mo-12 yr): 4 mg/kg/dose PO BID; **max. dose:** 150 mg/dose
  Adolescents and adults:
 <50 kg: 2 mg/kg/dose PO BID
 ≥50 kg: 150 mg/dose PO BID
Needle stick prophylaxis: 150 mg/dose PO BID × 28 days. Use in combination with zidovudine (AZT) 200 mg/dose PO TID or 300 mg/dose PO BID, and indinavir 800 mg/dose PO TID × 28 days.
  Combivir: 1 tablet PO BID
  Trizivir (≥40 kg): 1 tablet PO BID
Chronic hepatitis B (see remarks):
  2–17 yrs: 3 mg/kg/dose PO QD up to a **maximum** of 100 mg/dose
  Adults: 100 mg/dose PO QD

May cause headache, fatigue, nausea, diarrhea, skin rash, pancreatitis, and abdominal pain. Peripheral neuropathy, decreased neutrophil count, and increased liver enzymes may occur in advanced disease with combination therapy. Lactic acidosis and severe hepatomegaly with steatosis, including fatal cases, have been reported. Concomitant use with cotrimoxazole (TMP/SMX) may result in increased lamivudine levels. Should **not** be used in combination with zalcitabine; may inhibit intracellular phosphorylation of one another.
  Adolescent dosing: Patients in early puberty (Tanner I-II) should be dosed with pediatric regimens and those in late puberty (Tanner V) should be dosed with adult regimens. Adolescents who are at the midst of their growth spurt (Tanner III females and Tanner IV males) can be dosed by either pediatric or adult regimen with close monitoring of efficacy and toxicity.
  CHRONIC HEPATITIS B: Use Epivir-HBV product for this indication. Safety and effectiveness beyond 1 yr have not been determined. Patients with both HIV and hepatitis B should use the higher HIV doses along with an appropriate combination regimen.
  May be administered with food. **Adjust dose in renal impairment, (p. 943).**

For explanation of icons, see p. 572.

LAMOTRIGINE

Lamictal
Anticonvulsant

Yes   3   C

Chewable tabs: 2, 5, 25 mg
Tabs: 25, 100, 150, 200 mg
Oral suspension: 1 mg/mL

Children 2–16 yr (see remarks):
WITH *enzyme-inducing antiepileptic drugs (AEDs)* **WITHOUT** *valproic acid:*
Weeks 1 and 2: 0.6 mg/kg/24 hr PO ÷ BID; rounded down to the nearest whole tablet
Weeks 3 and 4: 1.2 mg/kg/24 hr PO ÷ BID; rounded down to the nearest whole tablet
Usual maintenance dose: 5–15 mg/kg/24 hr PO ÷ BID titrated to effect; to achieve the usual maintenance dose, increase doses Q1–2 weeks by 1.2 mg/kg/24 hr (rounded down to the nearest whole tablet) as needed
Max. dose: 400 mg/24 hr ÷ BID
WITH *AEDs* **WITH** *valproic acid:*
Weeks 1 and 2: 0.15 mg/kg/24 hr PO ÷ QD-BID; rounded down to the nearest whole tablet (see table below)
Weeks 3 and 4: 0.3 mg/kg/24 hr PO ÷ QD-BID; rounded down to the nearest whole tablet (see table below)

Patient's Weight	Weeks 1 and 2	Weeks 3 and 4
6.7–14 kg	2 mg QOD	2 mg QD
14.1–27 kg	2 mg QD	4 mg/24 hr ÷ QD-BID
27.1–34 kg	4 mg/24 hr ÷ QD–BID	8 mg/24 hr ÷ QD-BID
34.1–40 kg	5 mg QD	10 mg/24 hr ÷ QD-BID

Usual maintenance dose: 1–5 mg/kg/24 hr PO ÷ QD-BID titrated to effect; to achieve the usual maintenance dose, increase doses Q1–2 weeks by 0.3 mg/kg/24 hr (rounded down to the nearest whole tablet) as needed
Max. dose: 200 mg/24 hr
≥12 yr and adults:
WITHOUT *valproic acid:*
Weeks 1 and 2: 50 mg QD PO
Weeks 3 and 4: 50 mg BID PO
Usual maintenance dose: 300–500 mg/24 hr ÷ BID PO titrated to effect; to achieve the usual maintenance dose, increase doses Q1–2 weeks by 100 mg/24 hr as needed. If adding lamotrigene to valproic acid alone, usual maintenance dose is 100–200 mg/kg/24 hr.
WITH *valproic acid:*
Weeks 1 and 2: 25 mg QOD PO
Weeks 3 and 4: 25 mg QD PO
Usual maintenance dose: 100–400 mg/24 hr ÷ QD-BID PO titrated to effect; to achieve the usual maintenance dose, increase doses Q1–2 weeks by 25–50 mg/24 hr as needed

Continued

LAMOTRIGINE *continued*

Converting from a single enzyme-inducing AED to lamotrigine monotherapy (titrate lamotrigine to maintenance dose, then gradually withdraw enzyme-inducing AED by 20% decrements over a 4-week period):

Weeks 1 and 2: 50 mg QD PO

Weeks 3 and 4: 50 mg BID PO

Usual maintenance dose: 500 mg/24 hr ÷ BID PO titrated to effect; to achieve the usual maintenance dose, increase doses Q1–2 weeks by 100 mg/24 hr as needed

Enzyme inducing antiepileptic drugs (AEDs) include carbamazepine, phenytoin, and phenobarbital. Stevens-Johnson syndrome, toxic epidermal necrolysis, and other potentially life-threatening rashes have been reported in children and adults (incidence higher in children). May cause fatigue, drowsiness, ataxia, rash (especially with valproic acid), headache, nausea, vomiting, and abdominal pain. Diplopia, nystagmus, and alopecia have also been reported.

Reduce maintenance dose in renal failure. Reduce all doses (initial, escalation, and maintenance) in liver dysfunction defined by the Child-Pugh grading system as follows:

Grade B: Moderate dysfunction, decrease dose by ~50%.

Grade C: Severe dysfunction, decrease dose by ~75%.

Withdrawal symptoms may occur if discontinued suddenly. A stepwise dose reduction over ≥2 weeks (~50% per week) is recommended unless safety concerns require a more rapid withdrawal.

Acetaminophen, carbamazepine, phenobarbital, and phenytoin may decrease levels of lamotrigine. Valproic acid may increase levels.

LEVALBUTEROL

Xopenex

Beta-2 adrenergic agonist

No 3 C

Prediluted nebulized solution: 0.31 mg in 3 mL, 0.63 mg in 3 mL, 1.25 mg in 3 mL (24s)

<6 yr: See remarks

6–11 yr: Start at 0.31 mg inhaled TID (Q6–8 hr) PRN; dose may be increased to 0.63 mg inhaled TID PRN

≥12 yr and adult: Start at 0.63 mg inhaled TID (Q6–8 hr) PRN; dose may be increased to 1.25 mg inhaled TID PRN

R-isomer of racemic albuterol. Side effects include tachycardia, palpitations, tremor, insomnia, nervousness, nausea, and headache.

Current clinical data in children indicate levalbuterol is as effective as albuterol with less cardiac side effects at equipotent doses (0.31–0.63 mg levalbuterol ~ 2.5 mg albuterol). Limited data from a single dose, randomized, double blind crossover study in children 2–11 yr indicate that 0.16–1.25-mg inhalations were used safely with clinical improvement.

More frequent dosing may be necessary in asthma exacerbation, but additional studies are required.

For explanation of icons, see p. 572.

LEVOTHYROXINE (T₄)

Synthroid, Levothroid
Thyroid product

No   1   A

Tabs: 25, 50, 75, 88, 100, 112, 125, 137, 150, 175, 200, 300 mcg
Inj: 200, 500 mcg
Suspension: 25 mcg/mL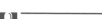

Children PO dosing:
  0–6 mo: 8–10 mcg/kg/dose QD
    6–12 mo: 6–8 mcg/kg/dose QD
  1–5 yr: 5–6 mcg/kg/dose QD
  6–12 yr: 4–5 mcg/kg/dose QD
  >12 yr: 2–3 mcg/kg/dose QD
IM/IV dose: 50%–75% of oral dose QD
Adults:
  PO:
  Initial: 12.5–50 mcg/dose QD
  Increment: Increase by 25–50 mcg/24 hr at intervals of Q2–4 wk until euthyroid
  Usual adult dose: 100–200 mcg/24 hr
IM/IV dose: 50% of oral dose QD
Myxedema coma or stupor: 200–500 mcg IV × 1, then 75–100 mcg IV QD; convert to oral therapy once patient is stabilized

Contraindications include acute MI, thyrotoxicosis, and uncorrected adrenal insufficiency. May cause hyperthyroidism, rash, growth disturbances, hypertension, arrythmias, diarrhea, and weight loss.
  Total replacement dose may be used in children unless there is evidence of cardiac disease; in that case, begin with ¼ of maintenance and increase weekly. Titrate dosage with clinical status and serum T₄ and TSH. Increases the effects of warfarin. Phenytoin and carbamazepine may decrease levothyroxine levels.
  100 mcg levothyroxine = 65 mg thyroid USP. Administer oral doses on an empty stomach. Excreted in low levels in breast milk; preponderance of evidence suggests no clinically significant effect in infants.

LIDOCAINE

Xylocaine and others
Antiarrhythmic class Ib, local anesthetic

No   1   C

Inj: 0.5%, 1%, 1.5%, 2%, 4%, 10%, 20% (1% sol = 10 mg/mL)
IV infusion (in D₅W): 0.2% (2 mg/mL) (500, 1000 mL); 0.4% (4 mg/mL) (250, 500 mL); 0.8% (8 mg/mL) (250, 500 mL)
Inj with 1:50,000 epinephrine: 2%
Inj with 1:100,000 epinephrine: 1%, 2%

Continued

LIDOCAINE *continued*

Inj with 1:200,000 epinephrine: 0.5%, 1%, 1.5%, 2%
Ointment: 2.5% (37.5 g), 5% (50 g)
Cream: 0.5% (120 g), 4% (5, 30 g)
Jelly: 2% (30 mL)
Liquid (topical): 2.5% (10 mL)
Liquid (viscous): 2% (20, 100 mL)
Solution (topical): 2% (15, 240 mL), 4% (50 mL)
Oral spray: 10% (26.8 mL aerosol)
Topical 2.5% (with 2.5% prilocaine): See *EMLA*, p. 675.

Anesthetic:
  Inj:
    Without epinephrine: **max. dose** of 4.5 mg/kg/dose (up to 300 mg)
    With epinephrine: **max. dose** of 7 mg/kg/dose (up to 500 mg); do not repeat within 2 hr
  Topical: 3 mg/kg/dose no more frequently than Q2 hr
Antiarrhythmic: Bolus with 1 mg/kg/dose slowly IV; may repeat in 10–15 min × 2;
max. total dose 3–5 mg/kg within the first hr
ETT dose = 2–2.5 × IV dose
Continuous infusion: 20–50 mcg/kg/min IV (do not exceed 20 mcg/kg/min for patients with shock or CHF); see inside cover for infusion preparation
Oral use:
  Adult: 15 mL swish and spit Q3 hr PRN up to a **maximum** of 8 doses/24 hr

Contraindicated in Stokes-Adams attacks, SA, AV, or intraventricular heart block without a pacemaker. Side effects include hypotension, asystole, seizures, and respiratory arrest.
  Decrease dose in hepatic failure or decreased cardiac output. **Do not** use topically for teething. Prolonged infusion may result in toxic accumulation of lidocaine, especially in infants. **Do not** use epinephrine-containing solutions for treatment of arrhythmias.
  Therapeutic levels: 1.5–5 mg/L. Toxicity occurs at >7 mg/L. Toxicity in neonates may occur at >5 mg/L.
  Elimination $T_{1/2}$: Premature infant: 3.2 hr; adult: 1.5–2 hr.
  For topical use, pregnancy category is a "B".

LINDANE

Kwell, Scabene, G-well, Gamma benzene hexachloride
Scabicidal agent, pediculocide

No   ?   B

Shampoo: 1% (30, 60, 473, 3800 mL)
Lotion: 1% (30, 60, 473, 3800 mL)

Continued

LINDANE *continued*

Scabies: Apply thin layer of lotion to skin. Bathe and rinse off medication in adults after 8–12 hr; children 6–8 hr. May repeat × 1 in 7 days PRN.
Pediculosis capitis: Apply 15–30 mL of shampoo, lather for 4–5 min, rinse hair and comb with fine comb to remove nits. May repeat × 1 in 7 days PRN.
Pediculosis pubis: May use lotion or shampoo (applied locally) as above.

Contraindicated in seizure disorders. **Avoid** contact with face, urethral meatus, damaged skin, or mucous membranes. Systemically absorbed. Risk of toxic effects is greater in young children; use other agents (permethrin) in infants, young children, and during pregnancy. May cause a rash; rarely may cause seizures or aplastic anemia. For scabies, change clothing and bedsheets after starting treatment and treat family members. For pediculosis pubis, treat sexual contacts.

LINEZOLID
Zyvox
Antibiotic, oxazolidinone

No ? C

Tabs: 400, 600 mg
Oral suspenion: 100 mg/5 mL (150 mL); contains phenylalanine
Inj: 2 mg/mL (100, 200, 300 mL)

Children (limited clinical data in children 1-17 yr with pneumonia; see remarks): 10 mg/kg/dose IV/PO Q8–12 hr
Adults:
MRSA Infections: 600 mg Q12 hr IV/PO
Vancomycin-resistant E. faecium: 600 mg Q12 hr IV/PO × 14–28 days
Community-acquired and nosocomial pneumonia, and bacteremia: 600 mg Q12 hr IV/PO × 10–14 days
Uncomplicated skin infections: 400 mg Q12 hr PO × 10–14 days

Pharmacokinetic studies in children indicate faster clearance in children <40 mo and suggest Q8 hr dosing interval for these patients.

Most common side effects include diarrhea, headache, and nausea. Anemia, leukopenia, pancytopenia, thrombocytopenia may occur in patients who are at risk for myelosuppression and who receive regimens >2 weeks. Complete blood count monitoring is recommended in these individuals. Pseudomembranous colitis has also been reported.

Use **caution** when using adrenergic (epinephrine, pseudoephedrine) agents or consuming large amounts of foods and beverages containing tyramine; may increase blood pressure. Dosing information in severe hepatic failure and renal impairment with multi-doses have not been completed.

Protect all dosage forms from light and moisture. Oral suspension product must be gently mixed by inverting the bottle 3-5 times prior to each use **(Do not shake).** All oral doses may be administered with or without food.

LITHIUM

Eskalith, Lithane, Lithonate, Lithotabs, Eskalith CR, Lithobid
Antimanic agent

Yes   X   D

Carbonate:
300 mg carbonate = 8.12 mEq lithium
Caps: 150, 300, 600 mg
Tabs: 300 mg
Controlled-release tabs: 450 mg
Slow-release tabs: 300 mg
Citrate:
Syrup: 8 mEq/5 mL (10, 480 mL); 5 mL is equivalent to 300 mg Li carbonate

Children:
Initial: 15–60 mg/kg/24 hr ÷ TID-QID PO. Adjust as needed (weekly) to achieve
therapeutic levels
Adolescents: 600–1800 mg/24 hr ÷ TID-QID PO (divided BID using controlled/slow-
release tablets)
Adults:
Initial: 300 mg TID PO. Adjust as needed to achieve therapeutic levels. Usual dose
is about 300 mg TID-QID. **Max. dose:** 2.4 g/24 hr or 900–1800 mg/24 hr with
controlled/slow-release tablets

Contraindicated in severe cardiovascular or renal disease. Increased sodium
intake will depress lithium levels. Decreased sodium intake or increased sodium
wasting will increase lithium levels. May cause goiter, nephrogenic diabetes
insipidus, hypothyroidism, arrhythmias, or sedation at therapeutic doses. Coadministration with thiazide diuretics or nonsteroidal antiinflammatory drugs may
increase risk for lithium toxicity. Iodine may increase risk for hypothyroidism.
Therapeutic levels: 0.6–1.5 mEq/L. In either acute or chronic toxicity, confusion, and
somnolence may be seen at levels of 2–2.5 mEq/L. Seizures or **death** may occur at levels
>2.5 mEq/L. *Recommended serum sampling:* Trough level within 30 min prior to the
next scheduled dose. Steady-state is achieved within 4–6 days of continuous dosing.
Adjust dose in renal failure (see p. 949).

LOPERAMIDE

Imodium, Imodium AD, and others
Antidiarrheal

No   1   B

Caps: 2 mg
Tabs: 2 mg
Caplets: 2 mg
Liquid: 1 mg/5 mL; may contain 0.5% alcohol (60, 90, 120 mL)
In combination with simethicone:
Chewable tabs: 2 mg loperamide and 125 mg simethicone

Continued

LOPERAMIDE *continued*

Active diarrhea:
Children (initial doses within the first 24 hrs):
   2–6 yr (13–20 kg): 1 mg PO TID
   6–8 yr (20–30 kg): 2 mg PO BID
   8–12 yr (>30 kg): 2 mg PO TID
   Max. single dose 2 mg
   Follow initial day's dose with 0.1 mg/kg/dose after each loose stool (not to exceed the above initial doses).
Adults: 4 mg/dose × 1, followed by 2 mg/dose after each stool up to **max. dose** of 16 mg/24 hr
Chronic diarrhea:
   Children: 0.08–0.24 mg/kg/24 hr ÷ BID-TID **max. dose:** 2 mg/dose

Contraindicated in acute dysentery. Rare hypersensitivity reactions, including anaphylactic shock, have been reported. May cause nausea, rash, vomiting, constipation, cramps, dry mouth, CNS depression, and rash. **Avoid** use in children <2 yr due to reports of necrotizing enterocolitis. **Discontinue** use if no clinical improvement is observed within 48 hr. Naloxone may be administered for CNS depression.

LOPINAVIR AND RITONAVIR

Kaletra, LPV/RTV
Antiviral, protease inhibitor combination

No   3   C

Caps: 133.3 mg lopinavir and 33.3 mg ritonavir
Oral solution: 80 mg lopinavir and 20 mg ritonavir/1 mL; contains 42.4% alcohol (160 mL)

6 mo–12 yr (administer all doses with food):
   NOT in combination with nevirapine or efavirenz: 230 mg/m^2/dose lopinavir and 57.5 mg/m^2/dose ritonavir BID PO up to a **maximum** of 400 mg lopinavir and 100 mg ritonavir/dose; **OR** use the following doses by weight (see table below):

Weight (kg)	Dose (Lopinavir and Ritonavir) BID PO
7–14	12 mg/kg/dose and 3 mg/kg/dose
15–40	10 mg/kg/dose and 2.75 mg/kg/dose
15–20	
21–25	
26–30	
31–35	
36–40	
>40	400 mg/dose and 100 mg/dose

Continued

LOPINAVIR AND RITONAVIR *continued*

In combination with nevirapine or efavirenz: 300 mg/m^2/dose lopinavir and 75 mg/m^2/dose ritonavir BID PO up to a **maximum** of 533 mg lopinavir and 133 mg ritonavir/dose; **OR** use the following doses by weight (see table below):

Weight (kg)	Dose (Lopinavir and Ritonavir) BID PO
7–14	13 mg/kg/dose and 3.25 mg/kg/dose
15–45	11 mg/kg/dose and 2.75 mg/kg/dose
>45	533 mg/dose and 133 mg/dose

Adolescent and adult (administer all doses with food):
   NOT in combination with nevirapine or efavirenz: 400 mg lopinavir and 100 mg ritonavir BID PO
   In combination with nevirapine or efavirenz: 533 mg lopinavir and 133 mg ritonavir BID PO

Do not administer with astemizole, cisapride, flecainide, propafenone, ergot alkaloids, pimozide, midazolam, terfenadine, and triazolam; may result in serious/life-threatening events. Use with **caution** in hepatic impairment, history of pancreatitis, diabetes, and hemophilia. May cause diarrhea, headache, asthenia, nausea, vomiting, increase in serum lipids, and rash (in combination with other antiretroviral agents).

Ritonavir is combined with lopinavir as an adjuvant for boosting lopinavir levels and not for its antiretroviral properties. Lopinavir/ritonavir is metabolized by CYP P450 3A drug metabolizing enzyme and inhibits CYP P450 2D6 and 3A. Efavirenz and nevirapine induces metabolism of lopinavir; higher doses of lopinavir/ritonavir are necessary. Carbamazepine, dexamethasone, phenobarbital, phenytoin, and rifampin may decrease lopinavir levels. Lopinavir/ritonavir may increase effects or toxicity of atorvastatin, cerivastatin, clarithromycin, rifabutin, lidocaine, quinidine, amiodarone, cyclosporin, tacrolimus, rapamycin, calcium channel blockers, ketoconazole, itraconazole, and metronidazole. Lopinavir can decrease the effectiveness of methadone, atovaquone, and birth control pills containing ethinyl estradiol (use alternative methods). **Always check the potential for other drug interactions when either initiating therapy or adding new drugs onto an existing regimen.**

Adolescent dosing: Patients in early puberty (Tanner I-II) should be dosed with pediatric regimens and those in late puberty (Tanner V) should be dosed with adult regimens. Adolescents who are at the midst of their growth spurt (Tanner III females and Tanner IV males) can be dosed by either pediatric or adult regimen with close monitoring of efficacy and toxicity.

Administer all doses with food. If didanosine is included in the regimen, administer didanosine 1 hr prior to or 2 hr after lopinavir/ritonavir. High-fat meal increases absorption (especially with liquid dosage form).

For explanation of icons, see p. 572.

LORACARBEF

Lorabid
Antibiotic, carbacephem

Yes   1   B

Susp: 100 mg/5 mL, 200 mg/5 mL (50, 75, 100 mL)
Caps: 200, 400 mg

Infants and children: (6 mo–12 yr):
Acute otitis media: 30 mg/kg/24 hr ÷ Q12 hr PO
Pharyngitis, impetigo, skin/soft tissue infection: 15 mg/kg/24 hr ÷ Q12 hr PO
≥*13 yr and adults:*
Uncomplicated cystitis: 200 mg PO Q24 hr
Sinusitis, uncomplicated pyelonephritis: 400 mg PO Q12 hr
Pharyngitis, skin/soft tissue infection: 200 mg PO Q12 hr
Lower respiratory infections: 200–400 mg PO Q12 hr

Use with **caution** in penicillin-allergic patients. **Adjust dose in renal impairment (see p. 943).** Use suspension for acute otitis media because of higher peak plasma levels. Adverse effects similar to other orally administered beta-lactam antibiotics. Administer on an empty stomach 1 hr before or 2 hr after meals.

LORATADINE

Claritin, Claritin RediTabs, Claritin-D 12 Hour, Claritin-D 24 Hour
Antihistamine, less sedating

Yes   1   B

Tabs: 10 mg
Disintegrating tabs (RediTabs): 10 mg
Syrup: 1 mg/mL (480 mL)
Time-release tabs in combination with pseudoephedrine (PE):
Claritin-D 12 Hour: 5 mg loritadine + 120 mg PE
Claritin-D 24 Hour: 10 mg loritadine + 240 mg PE

Loratadine:
2–5 yr: 5 mg PO QD
≥*6 yr and adults:* 10 mg PO QD

Continued

LORATADINE *continued*

Time-release tabs of loratidine and pseudoephedrine:
  ≥12 yr and adults:
    Claritin-D 12 Hour: 1 tablet PO BID
    Claritin-D 24 Hour: 1 tablet PO QD

May cause drowsiness, fatigue, dry mouth, headache, bronchospasm, palpitations, dermatitis, and dizziness. Has **not** been implicated in causing cardiac arrhythmias when used with other drugs that are metabolized by hepatic microsomal enzymes (e.g., ketoconazole, erythromycin). May be administered safely in patients who have allergic rhinitis and asthma.

In hepatic and renal function impairment (GFR <30 mL/min), prolong loratidine (single agent) dosage interval to QOD. For time-release tablets of the combination product (loratidine and pseudoephedrine), prolong dosage interval in renal impairment (GFR <30 mL/min) as follows: Claritin-D 12 Hour: 1 tablet PO QD; Claritin-D 24 Hour: 1 tablet PO QOD. **Do not** use the combination product in hepatic impairment because drugs cannot be individually titrated. **Adjust dose in renal failure (see p. 949).**

Administer doses on an empty stomach. For use of RediTabs, place tablet on tongue and allow it to disintegrate in the mouth with or without water. For Claritin-D, also see remarks under *Pseudoephedrine.*

LORAZEPAM

Ativan and others
Benzodiazepine anticonvulsant

No   3   D

Tabs: 0.5, 1, 2, mg
Inj: 2, 4 mg/mL (each contains 2% benzyl alcohol and propylene glycol)
Oral solution: 2 mg/mL

Status epilepticus:
  Neonates, infants, children, and adolescents:
    0.05–0.1 mg/kg/dose IV over 2–5 min. May repeat 0.05 mg/kg × 1 in 10–15 min.
      Max. dose: 4 mg/dose.
  Adult:
    4 mg/dose given slowly over 2–5 min. May repeat in 10–15 min. Usual **total max. dose** in 12-hr period is 8 mg.
Antiemetic adjunct therapy:
  Children:
    0.04–0.08 mg/kg/dose IV Q6 hr PRN
      Max. single dose: 4 mg

Continued

LORAZEPAM *continued*

Anxiolytic/sedation:
  Children:
    0.05 mg/kg/dose Q4–8 hr PO/IV; **max. dose:** 2 mg/dose
    May also give IM for preprocedure sedation
  Adults:
    1–10 mg/24 hr PO ÷ BID-TID

Contraindicated in narrow-angle glaucoma and severe hypotension. May cause respiratory depression, especially in combination with other sedatives. May also cause sedation, dizziness, mild ataxia, mood changes, rash, and GI symptoms. Significant respiratory depression and/or hypotension has been reported when used in combination with loxapine.

Injectable product may be given rectally. Benzyl alcohol and propylene glycol may be toxic to newborns at high doses.

Onset of action for sedation: PO, 20–30 min; IM, 30–60 min; IV, 1–5 min.
Duration of action: 6–8 hr. **Flumazenil is the antidote.**

LOW-MOLECULAR-WEIGHT HEPARIN
See *Enoxaparin*

MAGNESIUM CITRATE
Evac-Q-Mag, 16.17% Elemental Mg
Laxative/cathartic   Yes   1   B

Sol: (300 mL): 5 mL = 3.9–4.7 mEq Mg

Children:
  <6 yr: 2–4 mL/kg/24 hr PO ÷ QD-BID
  6–12 yr: 100–150 mL/24 hr PO ÷ QD-BID
  >12 yr: 150–300 mL/24 hr PO ÷ QD-BID

Use with **caution** in renal insufficiency and patients receiving digoxin. May cause hypermagnesemia, diarrhea, muscle weakness, hypotension, and respiratory depression. Up to about 30% of dose is absorbed. May decrease absorption of H_2 antagonists, phenytoin, iron salts, tetracycline, steroids, benzodiazepines, and ciprofloxacin.

FORMULARY

MAGNESIUM HYDROXIDE

Milk of Magnesia, 41.69% Elemental Mg
Antacid, laxative

Yes   1   B

Liquid: 390 mg/5 mL, 400 mg/5 mL (Milk of Magnesia)
Concentrated liquid: 800 mg/5 mL (Milk of Magnesia concentrate)
Susp: 2.5 g/30 mL
Chewable tabs: 311 mg
400 mg magnesium hydroxide is equivalent to 166.76 mg elemental magnesium
Combination product with aluminum hydroxide: See Aluminum hydroxide

All doses based on 400 mg/5 mL magnesium hydroxide
Laxative:
  Children:
  Dose/24 hr ÷ QD-QID PO
  <2 yr: 0.5 mL/kg
  2–5 yr: 5–15 mL
  6–12 yr: 15–30 mL
  ≥12 yr: 30–60 mL
Antacid:
  Children: 2.5–5 mL/dose QD-QID PO
  Adults:
    Liquid: 5–15 mL/dose QD-QID PO
    Concentrated liquid: 2.5–7.5 mL/dose QD-QID PO
    Tabs: 622–1244 mg/dose QD-QID PO

See *Magnesium citrate.*

MAGNESIUM OXIDE

Mag-Ox, Maox, Uro-Mag, and others, 60.32% Elemental Mg
Oral magnesium salt

Yes   1   B

Tabs: 400, 420, 500 mg
Caps: 140 mg
400 mg magnesium oxide is equivalent to 241.3 mg elemental Mg or 20 mEq Mg

Doses expressed in magnesium oxide salt
Magnesium suplementation:
  Children: 5–10 mg/kg/24 hr ÷ TID-QID PO
  Adults: 400–800 mg/24 hr ÷ BID-QID PO
Hypomagnesemia:
  Children: 65–130 mg/kg/24 hr ÷ QID PO
  Adults: 2000 mg/24 hr ÷ QID PO

Continued

For explanation of icons, see p. 572.

MAGNESIUM OXIDE *continued*

 See *Magnesium citrate.* For dietary recommended intake RDA for magnesium, see p. 462.

MAGNESIUM SULFATE

Epsom salts, and others, 9.9% Elemental Mg
Magnesium salt

Yes   1   B

Inj: 100 mg/mL (0.8 mEq/mL), 125 mg/mL (1 mEq/mL), 250 mg/mL (2 mEq/mL), 500 mg/mL (4 mEq/mL)
Oral solution: 50% (500 mg/mL)
Granules: Approximate 40 mEq Mg per 5 g (240 g)
500 mg magnesium sulfate is equivalent to 49.3 mg Elemental Mg or 4.1 mEq Mg

 All doses expressed in MgSO$_4$ salt
Cathartic:
   Child: 0.25 g/kg/dose PO Q4–6 hr
   Adult: 10–30 g/dose PO Q4–6 hr
Hypomagnesemia or hypocalcemia:
   IV/IM: 25–50 mg/kg/dose Q4–6 hr × 3–4 doses; repeat PRN. **Max. single dose:** 2 g
   PO: 100–200 mg/kg/dose QID PO
Daily maintenance:
   30–60 mg/kg/24 hr or 0.25–0.5 mEq/kg/24 hr IV
   Max. dose: 1 g/24 hr
Adjunctive therapy for moderate to severe reactive airway disease exacerbation (bronchodilation):
   Children: 25–75 mg/kg/dose (**max. dose:** 2 g) × 1 IV over 20 minutes
   Adult: 2 g/dose × 1 IV over 20 min

 When given IV, **beware of** hypotension, respiratory depression, complete heart block, and/or hypermagnesemia. Calcium gluconate (IV) should be available as **antidote.** Use with **caution** in patients with renal insufficiency and with patients on digoxin. **Serum level dependent toxicity** include the following: >3 mg/dL: CNS depression; >5 mg/dL: decreased deep tendon reflexes, flushing, somnolence; and >12 mg/dL: respiratory paralysis, heart block.
   Max. IV intermittent infusion rate: 1 mEq/kg/hr or 125 mg MgSO$_4$ salt/kg/hr.

MALATHION

Ovide
Pediculicide

No   ?   B

Lotion: 0.5% (59 mL); contains 79% isopropyl alcohol, terpineol, dipentene, and pine needle oil

Continued

MALATHION *continued*

Pediculosis capitis:
≥2 yr and adults: Sprinkle sufficient amounts of lotion onto dry hair and rub gently until the scalp is fully wet (pay special attention to the back of head and neck). Allow the hair to dry naturally; do not use hair dryer. After 8–12 hr, wash the hair with a nonmedicated shampoo, rinse, and use a fine-toothed comb to remove dead lice and eggs. If lice are still present, a second dose may be administered in 7–9 days.

DO NOT expose lotion and wet hair to open flame or electric heat, including hair dryers, because it contains flammable ingredients. For external use only.
Launder bedding and clothing. **Avoid** contact with eyes; flush eyes immediately with water if accidental exposure. May cause scalp irritation.

MANNITOL
Osmitrol, Resectisol, and others
Osmotic diuretic

Yes ? C

Inj: 50, 100, 150, 200, 250 mg/mL (5%, 10%, 15%, 20%, 25%)

Anuria/oliguria:
Test dose to assess renal function: 0.2 g/kg/dose IV; **max. dose:** 12.5 g over 3–5 min. If there is no diuresis within 2 hr, discontinue mannitol.
Initial: 0.5–1 g/kg/dose
Maintenance: 0.25–0.5 g/kg/dose Q4–6 hr IV
Cerebral edema:
0.25 g/kg/dose IV over 20–30 min. May increase gradually to 1 g/kg/dose if needed. (May give furosemide 1 mg/kg concurrently or 5 min before mannitol.)

Contraindicated in severe renal disease, active intracranial bleed, dehydration, and pulmonary edema. May cause circulatory overload and electrolyte disturbances. For hyperosmolar therapy, keep serum osmolality at 310–320 mOsm/kg.
Caution: May crystallize with concentration ≥20%; use in-line filter. May cause hypovolemia, headache, and polydipsia. Reduction in ICP occurs in 15 min and lasts 3–6 hr.

MEBENDAZOLE
Vermox
Anthelmintic

No 1 C

Chewable tabs: 100 mg (may be swallowed whole or chewed)

Continued

MEBENDAZOLE *continued*

Children and adults:
Pinworms (Entererobius):
   100 mg PO × 1, repeat in 2 weeks if not cured
Hookworms, roundworms (Ascaris), and whipworm (Trichuris):
   100 mg PO BID × 3 days. Repeat in 3–4 weeks if not cured. Alternatively, may administer 500 mg PO × 1.
Capillariasis:
   200 mg PO BID × 20 days
See latest edition of the AAP *Red Book* for additional information

Experience in children <2 yr is limited. May cause diarrhea and abdominal cramping in cases of massive infection. LFT elevations and hepatitis have been reported with prolonged courses; monitor hepatic function with prolonged therapy. Family may need to be treated as a group. Therapeutic effect may be decreased if administered to patients receiving carbamazepine or phenytoin. Administer with food.

MEDROXYPROGESTERONE ± ESTRADIOL

Amen, Curretab, Cycrin, Depo-Provera, Provera; in combination with estradiol: Lunelle

No   1   X

Contraceptive, progestin

Tabs: 2.5, 5, 10 mg
Inj, suspension as acetate (for IM use only): 100 mg/mL (5 mL), 150 mg/mL (1 mL), 400 mg/mL (1, 2.5, 10 mL)
In combination with estradiol:
Inj, suspension: 25 mg medroxyprogesterone acetate and 5 mg estradiol cypionate per 0.5 mL (0.5 mL); contains 4.28 mg Na/0.5 mL drug

Adolescents and adults:
   Contraception: 150 mg IM Q3 mo; initiate therapy during the first 5 days after onset of a normal menstrual period, within 5 days postpartum if not breast-feeding, or if breastfeeding, at 6 weeks postpartum.
   Amenorrhea: 5–10 mg PO QD × 5–10 days
   Abnormal uterine bleeding: 5–10 mg PO QD × 5–10 days initiated on the 16th or 21st day of the menstrual cycle
In combination with estradiol (Lunelle):
   Contraception: 0.5 mL IM Q month; initiate therapy during the first 5 days after onset of a normal menstrual period, no earlier than 4 weeks postpartum if not breastfeeding, or if breastfeeding, at 6 weeks postpartum.

Continued

MEDROXYPROGESTERONE ± ESTRADIOL *continued*

Contraindicated in pregnancy, breast or genital cancer, liver disease, missed abortion, thrombophlebitis, thromboembolic disorders, cerebral vascular disease, and undiagnosed vaginal bleeding. Use with **caution** in patients with family history of breast cancer, depression, diabetes, and fluid retention. May cause dizziness, headache, insomnia, fatigue, nausea, weight increase, appetite changes, amenorrhea, and breakthrough bleeding. Cholestatic jaundice and increased intracranial pressure have been reported.

Aminoglutethimide may decrease medroxyprogesterone levels. May alter thyroid and liver function, prothrombin time, factors VII, VIII, IX and X, and metyrapone test.

Injection is for IM use only. Shake IM injection vial well before use. Administer oral doses with food.

Estradiol concerns: Use with caution in smoking, hypertriglyceridemia, hypertension, and thrombosis.

MEFLOQUINE HCl

Lariam
Antimalarial

No   ?   C

Tabs: 250 mg (228 mg base)

Doses expressed in mg mefloquine HCl salt
Malaria prophylaxis (start 1 week prior to exposure and continue for 4 weeks after leaving edemic area):
Children (PO, administered Q weekly):
  <15 kg: 5 mg/kg
  15–19 kg: 62.5 mg (¼ tablet)
  20–30 kg: 125 mg (½ tablet)
  31–45 kg: 187.5 mg (¾ tablet)
  >45 kg: 250 mg (1 tablet)
Adult: 250 mg PO Q weekly
Malaria treatment:
  <45 kg: 15 mg/kg ×1 PO followed by 10 mg/kg × 1 PO 8–12 hrs later
  Adult: 750 mg × 1 PO followed by 500 mg × 1 PO 12 hrs later
See latest edition of the AAP *Red Book* for additional information

Use with **caution** in cardiac dysrhythmias and neurologic disease. May cause dizziness, headache, syncope, seizures, ocular abnormalities, GI symptoms, leukopenia, and thrombocytopenia. Monitor liver enzymes and ocular examinations for therapies greater than 1 yr. Mefloquine may reduce valproic acid levels. ECG abnormalities may occur when used in combination with quinine, quinidine, chloroquine, halofantrine, and beta blockers. If any of the aforementioned antimalarial drugs is used in the initial treatment of severe malaria, initiate mefloquine at least 12 hr after the last dose of any of these drugs.

Continued

MEFLOQUINE HCl *continued*

Do not take on an empty stomach. Administer with at least 240 mL (8 oz) water. Treatment failures in children may be related to vomiting of administered dose. If vomiting occurs less than 30 min after the dose, administer a second full dose. If vomiting occurs 30–60 min after the dose, administer an additional half-dose. If vomiting continues, monitor patient closely and consider alternative therapy.

MEPERIDINE HCl

Demerol and others
Narcotic, analgesic

Yes 1 B/D

Tabs: 50, 100 mg
Syrup, elixir: 50 mg/5 mL
Inj: 10, 25, 50, 75, and 100 mg/mL

PO, IM, IV, and SC:
Children:
    1–1.5 mg/kg/dose Q3–4 hr PRN
Max. dose: 100 mg
Adults:
    50–150 mg/dose Q3–4 hr PRN

See p. 894 for details of use and equianalgesic dosing. **Contraindicated** in cardiac arrhythmias, asthma, increased ICP. Potentiated by MAO inhibitors, tricyclic antidepressants, phenothiazines, other CNS-acting agents. Meperidine may increase the adverse effects of isoniazid. May cause nausea, vomiting, respiratory depression, smooth muscle spasm, pruritus, palpatations, hypotension, constipation, and lethargy.

Drug is metabolized by the liver and its metabolite (normeperidine) is renally eliminated. **Caution:** In renal failure, sickle cell disease, and seizure disorders, accumulation of normeperidine metabolite may precipitate seizures. **Adjust dose in renal failure (see p. 950).** Pregnancy category changes to "D" if used for prolonged periods or in high doses at term.

Onset of action: PO/IM/SC, 10–15 min; IV, 5 min.

MEROPENEM

Merrem
Carbapenem antibiotic

Yes ? B

Inj: 0.5, 1 g
Contains 3.92 mEq Na/g drug

Continued

MEROPENEM continued

Infants >3 mo and children:
Mild to moderate infections: 60 mg/kg/24 hr IV ÷ Q8 hr; **max. dose:** 3 g/24 hr
Meningitis and severe infections: 120 mg/kg/24 hr IV ÷ Q8 hr; **max. dose:**
6 g/24 hr

Adults:
Mild to moderate infections: 1.5–3 g/24 hr IV ÷ Q8 hr
Meningitis and severe infections: 6 g/24 hr IV ÷ Q8 hr

Contraindicated in patients sensitive to carbapenems, or with a history of anaphylaxis to beta-lactam antibiotics. Drug penetrates well into the CSF. May cause diarrhea, rash, vomiting, oral moniliasis, glossitis, pain and irritation at the IV injection site, and headache. Hepatic enzyme and bilirubin elevation, leukopenia, and neutropenia have been reported. **Adjust dose in renal impairment (see p. 943).**

MESALAMINE

Asacol, Pentasa, Rowasa, FIV-ASA, 5-aminosalicylic acid, 5-ASA
Salicylate, GI antiinflammatory agent

Yes   2   B

Caps, controlled release (Pentasa): 250 mg
Tabs, delayed release (Asacol): 400 mg
Suppository (Rowasa, FIV-ASA): 500 mg (12s)
Rectal suspension (Rowasa): 4 g/60 mL (7s); contains sulfites

Children:
Caps, controlled release: 50 mg/kg/24 hr ÷ Q6–12 hr PO
Tabs, delayed release: 50 mg/kg/24 hr ÷ Q8–12 hr PO

Adult:
Caps, controlled release: 1 g QID PO up to 8 weeks
Tabs, delayed release: 800 mg TID PO for 6 weeks; for ulcerative colitis remission, use 1.6 g/24 hr ÷ BID-QID PO up to 6 mo
Suppository: 500 mg BID PR × 3–6 weeks, retaining each dose in rectum for 1–3 hr
Rectal suspension: 60 mL (4 g) QHS × 3–6 weeks, retaining each dose for about 8 hr; lie on left side during administration to improve delivery to the sigmoid colon

Generally not recommended in children <16 yr with chickenpox or flu-like symptoms (risk of Reye's syndrome). **Contraindicated** in active peptic ulcer disease, severe renal failure, and salicylate hypersensitivity. Rectal suspension should not be used in patients with history of sulfite allergy. Use with **caution** in sulfasalazine hypersensitivity, renal insufficiency, pyloric stenosis, and concurrent thrombolytics. May cause headache, GI discomfort, pancreatitis, pericarditis, and Stevens-Johnson syndrome.

Do not administer with lactulose or other medications that can lower intestinal pH. Oral capsules are designed to release medication throughout the GI tract, and oral tablets release medication at the terminal ileum and beyond. 400 mg PO mesalamine is equivalent to 1 g sulfasalazine PO. Tablets should be swallowed whole.

For explanation of icons, see p. 572.

METAPROTERENOL

Metaprel, Alupent, and others
Beta-2-adrenergic agonist

No   ?   C

Syrup: 10 mg/5 mL
Tabs: 10, 20 mg
Inhaler: 650 mcg/actuation (5, 10 mL), approximately 100 actuations/5 mL
Inhalant solution: 5% (50 mg/mL) (10, 30 mL)
Single-dose inhalant solution: 0.4% (4 mg/mL), 0.6% (6 mg/mL) (2.5 mL)

Inhalation:
Aerosol:
    2–3 puffs Q3–4 hr to **max. dose** of 12 puffs/24 hr
Nebulized solution:
    Dilute 0.1–0.3 mL of 5% solution in 2.5 mL NS; administer Q4–6 hr PRN
Single-dose solutions:
    Infants: 2.5 mL of 0.4%
    Children: 2.5 mL of 0.6%
    Usual dose: Q4–6 hr. May give more frequently for acute bronchospasm.
Oral:
Children:
    <2 yr: 0.4 mg/kg/dose Q6–8 hr (Q8–12 hr for infants)
    2–6 yr: 0.33–0.85 mg/kg/dose Q6–8 hr
    6–9 yr: 10 mg/dose Q6–8 hr
    >9 yr and adults: 20 mg/dose Q6–8 hr

Contraindicated in cardiac arrhythmias or narrow-angle glaucoma. Adverse reactions as with other beta-adrenergic agents. Excessive use may result in cardiac arrhythmias and death. Also causes tachycardia, increased myocardial O_2 consumption, hypertension, nervousness, headaches, nausea, palpitations, and tremor. The use of tube spacers may enhance efficacy of administering doses via metered dose inhaler. Nebulizers may be given more frequently in the acute setting.

METFORMIN

Glucophage
Antidiabetic, biguanide

Yes   ?   B

Tabs: 500, 850, 1000 mg
Tabs, extended release: 500 mg

Children (see remarks)
Adults (see remarks):
    500 mg tabs: Start with 500 mg PO BID with morning and evening meals; may increase by 500 mg every week administered in divided doses up to a **maximum** of

Continued

METFORMIN *continued*

2500 mg/24 hr. Administer 2500 mg/24 hr doses by dividing daily dose TID with meals.

850 mg tabs: Start with 850 mg PO QD with morning meal; may increase by 850 mg every other week up to a **maximum** of 2550 mg/24 hr (first dosage increment: 850 mg PO BID with morning and evening meals; second dosage increment: 850 mg PO TID with meals).

Extended-release tabs: Start with 500 mg PO QD with evening meal; may increase by 500 mg every week up to a **maximum** of 2000 mg/24 hr (2000 mg PO QD or 1000 mg PO BID). If a dose >2000 mg is needed, switch to nonextended-release tablets in divided doses and increase dose to a **maximum** of 2550 mg/24 hr.

Contraindicated in renal impairment, CHF, metabolic acidosis, and during radiology studies using iodinated contrast media. Use with **caution** when transferring patients from chlorpropamide therapy (potential hypoglycemia risk), excessive alcohol intake, hypoxemia, dehydration, surgical procedures, hepatic disease, anemia, and thyroid disease.

Fatal lactic acidosis (diarrhea; severe muscle pain, cramping; shallow and fast breathing; unusual weakness and sleepiness) and decrease in vitamin B_{12} levels have been reported. May cause GI discomfort, anorexia and vomiting. Cimetidine, furosemide, and nifedipine may increase the effects/toxicity of metformin. In addition to monitoring serum glucose and glycosylated hemoglobin, monitor renal function and hematologic parameters (baseline and annual).

PEDIATRIC USE INFORMATION: A double-blind, placebo controlled trial with 77 children (39-drug/38-placebo) 10–16 years old (mean age: 13.6 yr) with type-2 diabetes used doses up to 2000 mg/24 hr for a duration up to 18 weeks, which resulted in significant reduction in fasting plasma glucose (adverse reactions were not reported). In a smaller double-blind, placebo controlled trial, 29 children (14-drug/15-placebo) 12–19 years old (mean age: 14.4 ± 0.6 yr) with type-2 diabetes used 500 mg PO BID for 6 mo. Results of this trial produced declines in fasting glucose and insulin levels. Transient abdominal discomfort or diarrhea occurred in 40% of patients receiving metformin. Pediatric pharmacokinetic data have not been completed.

Adult patients initiated on 500 mg PO BID may also have their dose increased to 850 mg PO BID after 2 weeks.

COMBINATION THERAPY WITH SULFONYLUREAS: If patient has not responded to 4 weeks of maximum doses of metformin monotherapy, consider gradual addition of an oral sulfonylurea with continued maximum metformin dosing (even if failure with sulfonylurea has occurred). Attempt to identify the minimum effective dosage for each drug (metformin and sulfonylurea) because the combination can increase risk for sulfonylurea-induced hypoglycemia. If patient does not respond to 1–3 mo of combination therapy with maximum metformin doses, consider discontinuing combination therapy and initiating insulin therapy.

Administer all doses with food.

For explanation of icons, see p. 572.

METHADONE HCl

Dolophine, Methadose, and others
Narcotic, analgesic

Yes   1   B/D

Tabs: 5, 10 mg
Tabs (dispersible): 40 mg
Solution: 5 mg/5 mL, 10 mg/5 mL
Concentrated solution: 10 mg/mL
Inj: 10 mg/mL

Children: 0.7 mg/kg/24 hr ÷ Q4–6 hr PO, SC, IM, or IV PRN pain. **Max. dose:** 10 mg/dose
Adults: 2.5–10 mg/dose Q3–4 hr PO, SC, IM, or IV PRN pain.
Detoxification or maintenance: See package insert

May cause respiratory depression, sedation, increased intracranial pressure, hypotension, and bradycardia. *Average $T_{1/2}$:* Children 19 hr, adults 35 hr. Oral duration of action is 6–8 hr initially and 22–48 hr after repeated doses. Respiratory effects last longer than analgesia. Accumulation may occur with continuous use, making it necessary to adjust dose. Nevirapine may decrease serum levels of methadone.

See p. 894 for equianalgesic dosing and onset of action. **Adjust dose in renal insufficiency (see p. 950).** Pregnancy category changes to "D" if used for prolonged period or in high doses at term.

METHICILLIN

Staphcillin
Antibiotic, penicillin (penicillinase-resistant)

Yes   ?   B

Inj: 1, 4, 6, 10 g
Contains 2.6–3.1 mEq Na/g drug

Neonates: IM/IV
≤7 days:
    <2 kg: 50–100 mg/kg/24 hr ÷ Q12 hr
    ≥2 kg: 75–150 mg/kg/24 hr ÷ Q8 hr
>7 days:
    <1.2 kg: 50–100 mg/kg/24 hr ÷ Q12 hr
    1.2–2 kg: 75–150 mg/kg/24 hr ÷ Q8 hr
    ≥2 kg: 100–200 mg/kg/24 hr ÷ Q6 hr
Infants >1 mo and children: 150–400 mg/kg/24 hr ÷ Q4–6 hr IV/IM
Adults: 4–12 g/24 hr ÷ Q4–6 hr IV/IM
Max. dose: 12 g/24 hr

Continued

METHICILLIN *continued*

 Allergic cross-reactivity with and same toxicity as penicillin. May cause bone marrow suppression, positive Coombs' test, hairy tongue, and phlebitis at infusion site. Methicillin has been associated with interstitial nephritis and hemorrhagic cystitis.

Use higher end of dosage range for serious infections and meningitis. **Adjust dose in patients with renal failure (see p. 943).** Alternative agents are oxacillin and nafcillin.

METHIMAZOLE

Tapazole
Anithyroid agent

No   1   D

Tabs: 5, 10 mg

Hyperthyroidism:
Children:
   Initial: 0.4–0.7 mg/kg/24 hr or 15–20 mg/m^2/24 hr PO ÷ Q8 hr
   Maintenance: ⅓–⅔ of initial dose PO ÷ Q8 hr
   Max. dose: 30 mg/24 hr
Adults:
   Initial: 15–60 mg/24 hr PO ÷ TID
   Maintenance: 5–15 mg/24 hr PO ÷ TID

Readily crosses placental membranes and distributes into breast milk (AAP considers it to be compatible with breastfeeding). Blood dyscrasias, dermatitis, hepatitis, arthralgias, CNS reactions, pruritus, nephritis, hypoprothrombinemia, agranulocytosis, headache, fever and hypothyroidism may occur.

May increase the effects of oral anticoagulants. When correcting hyperthyroidism, existing beta-blocker, digoxin, and theophylline doses may need to be reduced to avoid potential toxicities.

Switch to maintenance dose when patient is euthyroid. Administer doses with food.

METHSUXIMIDE

Celontin Kapseals
Anticonvulsant

Yes   ?   C

Caps: 150, 300 mg

Children PO:
10–15 mg/kg/24 hr ÷ Q6–8 hr. Increase weekly up to **maximum** 30 mg/kg/24 hr.

Continued

METHSUXIMIDE *continued*

Adults PO:
  Initial: 300 mg/24 hr ÷ BID-QID for 1 week. May increase by 300 mg/24 hr each week to **max. dose** of 1.2 g/24 hr ÷ BID-QID

GI symptoms, blood dyscrasias, mental status changes, periorbital edema, drowsiness, and Stevens-Johnson syndrome may occur. Use with **caution** in the presence of renal or liver disease (monitor levels). Follow CBC, LFTs, and urinalysis. Carbamazepine may decrease methsuximide levels. **Avoid** abrupt withdrawal.

Measure therapeutic range for metabolite, N-desmethylmethsuximide. *Therapeutic reference range:* 10–40 mg/L. *Recommended serum sampling time at steady-state:* Obtain trough level within 30 min of the next scheduled dose after 5–7 days of continuous dosing.

METHYLDOPA
Aldomet
Central alpha-adrenergic blocker, antihypertensive   Yes   1   C

Tabs: 125, 250, 500 mg
Inj: 50 mg/mL
Susp: 250 mg/5 mL

Hypertension:
  Children: 10 mg/kg/24 hr ÷ Q6–12 hr PO; increase PRN Q2 days.
    Max. dose: 65 mg/kg/24 hr or 3 g/24 hr, whichever is less.
  Adults: 250 mg/dose BID-TID PO. Increase PRN Q2 days to **maximum** of 3 g/24 hr
Hypertensive crisis:
  Children: 2–4 mg/kg/dose IV to **maximum** of 5–10 mg/kg/dose IV Q6–8 hr. **Max. dose** (whichever is less): 65 mg/kg/24 hr or 3 g/24 hr.
  Adults: 250–1000 mg IV Q6–8 hr. **Max. dose:** 4 g/24 hr

Contraindicated in pheochromocytoma and active liver disease. Use with **caution** if patient is receiving haloperidol, propranolol, lithium, or sympathomimetics. Positive Coombs' test rarely associated with hemolytic anemia. Fever, leukopenia, sedation, memory impairment, hepatitis, GI disturbances, orthostatic hypotension, black tongue, and gynecomastia may occur. May interfere with laboratory tests for creatinine, urinary catecholamines, uric acid, and AST.

Do not co-administer oral doses with iron; decreases methyldopa bioavailability.
Adjust dose in renal failure (see p. 950).

METHYLENE BLUE

Urolene Blue and others
Antidote, drug-induced methemoglobinemia, and cyanide toxicity

Yes ? C/D

Tabs: 65 mg
Inj: 10 mg/mL (1%) (1, 10 mL)

Methemoglobinemia:
Adults and children:
   1–2 mg/kg/dose or 25–50 mg/m²/dose IV over 5 min. May repeat in 1 hr if
needed.

At high doses, may cause methemoglobinemia. **Avoid** subcutaneous or
intrathecal routes of administration. Use with **caution** in G6PD deficiency
or renal insufficiency. May cause nausea, vomiting, dizziness, headache,
diaphoresis, stained skin, and abdominal pain. Causes blue-green discoloration of
urine and feces. Pregnancy category changes to "D" if injected intraamniotically.

METHYLPHENIDATE HCI

Ritalin, Ritalin SR, Methylin, Metadate CD, Metadate ER,
Methylin ER, Concerta, and others
CNS stimulant

No ? C

Tabs: 5, 10, 20 mg
Extended-release tabs:
   8-hr duration (Metadate ER, Methylin ER): 10, 20 mg
   24-hr duration (Concerta): 18, 36, 54 mg
Extended-release caps (Metadate CD): 20 mg
Sustained-release tabs:
   8-hr duration (Ritalin SR): 20 mg

Attention deficit hyperactivity disorder:
≥6 yr:
   Initial: 0.3 mg/kg/dose (or 2.5–5 mg/dose) given before breakfast and lunch.
   May increase by 0.1 mg/kg/dose PO (or 5–10 mg/24 hr) weekly until
   maintenance dose achieved. May give extra afternoon dose if needed.
   Maintenance dose range: 0.3–1 mg/kg/24 hr
   Max. dose: 2 mg/kg/24 hr or 60 mg/24 hr
Once daily dosing (Concerta), ≥6 yr:
   Patients new to methylphenidate: Start with 18 mg PO QAM; dosage may be
   increased at weekly intervals at 18-mg increments up to a **maximum** of 54 mg/
   24 hr

Continued

METHYLPHENIDATE HCl *continued*

Patients currently receiving methylphenidate: See table below

CONVERSION FROM METHYLPHENIDATE REGIMENS TO CONCERTA

Previous Methylphenidate Daily Dose	Recommended Concerta Dose
5 mg PO BID–TID or 20 mg SR PO QD	18 mg PO QAM
10 mg PO BID–TID or 40 mg SR PO QD	36 mg PO QAM
15 mg PO BID–TID or 60 mg SR PO QD	54 mg PO QAM

After a week of receiving the above-recommended Concerta dose, dose may be increased in 18-mg increments at weekly intervals up to a maximum of 54 mg/24 hr.

Contraindicated in glaucoma, anxiety disorders, motor tics, and Tourette's syndrome. Medication should generally not be used in children <5 yr because diagnosis of ADHD in this age group is extremely difficult and should be done only in consultation with a specialist. Use with **caution** in patients with hypertension and epilepsy. Insomnia, weight loss, anorexia, rash, nausea, emesis, abdominal pain, hypertension or hypotension, tachycardia, arrhythmias, palpitations, restlessness, headaches, fever, tremor, and thrombocytopenia may occur. Abnormal liver function, cerebral arteritis and/or occlusion, leukopenia and/or anemia, transient depressed mood, and scalp hair loss have been reported. High doses may slow growth and may cause appetite suppression.

May increase serum concentrations of tricyclic antidepressants, phenytoin, phenobarbital, and warfarin. Effect of methylphenidate may be potentiated by MAO inhibitors.

Extended/sustained-release dosage forms have either an 8- or 24-hour dosage interval (see above). Concerta dosage form delivers 22.2% of its dose as an immediate-release product with the remaining amounts as an extended-release product (e.g., 18 mg strength: 4 mg as immediate release and 14 mg as extended release).

METHYLPREDNISOLONE

Medrol, Solu-Medrol, Depo-Medrol, and others
Corticosteroid

No   ?   C

Tabs: 2, 4, 8, 16, 24, 32 mg
Tabs, dose pack: 4 mg (21s)
Inj., Na succinate (Solu-Medrol): 40, 125, 500, 1000, 2000 mg (IV/IM use)
Inj., Acetate (Depo-Medrol): 20, 40, 80 mg/mL (IM repository)

Antiinflammatory/immunosuppressive:
  PO/IM/IV: 0.5–1.7 mg/kg/24 hr ÷ Q6–12 hr
    Status asthmaticus:
Children: IM/IV:
  Loading dose: 2 mg/kg/dose × 1
  Maintenance: 2 mg/kg/24 hr ÷ Q6 hr
Adults: 10–250 mg/dose Q4–6 hr IM/IV

Continued

METHYLPREDNISOLONE *continued*

Acute spinal cord injury:
   30 mg/kg IV over 15 min followed in 45 min by a continuous infusion of 5.4 mg/
   kg/hr × 23 hr

See pp. 907–911 for relative steroid potencies and doses based on body surface area. Not all practitioners use loading dose for status asthmaticus. Acetate form may be used for intraarticular and intralesional injection; it should **not** be given IV. Like all steroids, may cause hypertension, pseudotumor cerebri, acne, Cushing's syndrome, adrenal axis suppression, GI bleeding, hyperglycemia, and osteoporosis.

Barbiturates, phenytoin, and rifampin may enhance methylprednisolone's clearance. Itraconazole may increase methylprednisone levels. Methylprednisolone may increase cyclosporine and tacrolimus levels.

METOCLOPRAMIDE
Clopra, Maxolon, Reglan, and others
Antiemetic, prokinetic agent

Yes   3   B

Tabs: 5, 10 mg
Inj: 5 mg/mL
Syrup (sugar-free): 5 mg/5 mL
Concentrated solution: 10 mg/mL

Gastroesophageal reflux (GER) or GI dysmotility:
   Infants and children: 0.1–0.2 mg/kg/dose up to QID IV/IM/PO; **max. dose:**
      0.8 mg/kg/24 hr
   Adult: 10–15 mg/dose QAC and QHS IV/IM/PO
Antiemetic:
   1–2 mg/kg/dose Q2–6 hr IV/IM/PO. Premedicate with diphenhydramine to
   reduce EPS.

Contraindicated in GI obstruction, seizure disorder, pheochromocytoma, or in patients receiving drugs likely to cause extrapyramidal symptoms (EPS). May cause EPS, especially at higher doses. Sedation, headache, anxiety, leukopenia, and diarrhea may occur.

For GER, give 30 min before meals and at bedtime. **Reduce dose in renal impairment (see p. 950).**

METOLAZONE

Zaroxolyn, Diulo, Mykrox
Diuretic, thiazide-like

No   1   D

Tabs: 0.5 (Mykrox), 2.5, 5, 10 mg
Susp: 1 mg/mL

Dosage based on Zaroxolyn (for Mykrox or oral suspension, see remarks):
Children: 0.2–0.4 mg/kg/24 hr ÷ QD-BID PO
Adults:
Hypertension: 2.5–5 mg QD PO
Edema: 5–20 mg QD PO

Contraindicated in patients with anuria or hepatic coma. Electrolyte imbalance, GI disturbance, hyperglycemia, marrow suppression, chills, hyperuricemia, chest pain, hepatitis and rash may occur. Mykrox and oral suspension have increased bioavailability; therefore lower doses may be necessary when using these dosage forms.

More effective than thiazide diuretics in impaired renal function; may be effective in GFRs as low as 20 mL/min. Furosemide-resistant edema in pediatric patients may benefit from the addition of metolazone.

METRONIDAZOLE

Flagyl, Protostat, Metro, and others
Antibiotic, antiprotozoal

Yes   3   B

Tabs: 250, 500 mg
Tabs, extended release: 750 mg
Caps: 375 mg
Susp: 20 mg/mL or 50 mg/mL
Inj: 500 mg; contains 830 mg mannitol/g drug
Ready to use inj: 5 mg/mL (100 mL); contains 28 mEq Na/g drug
Gel, topical: 0.75% (28, 45 g)
Cream, topical: 0.75% (45 g)
Gel, vaginal: 0.75% (70 g)

Amebiasis:
Children: 35–50 mg/kg/24 hr PO ÷ TID × 10 days
Adults: 750 mg/dose PO TID × 10 days
Anaerobic infection:
Neonates: PO/IV:
<7 days:
<1.2 kg: 7.5 mg/kg Q48 hr
1.2–2 kg: 7.5 mg/kg Q24 hr
≥2 kg: 15 mg/kg/24 hr ÷ Q12 hr

Continued

METRONIDAZOLE *continued*

≥7 days:
  <1.2 kg: 7.5 mg/kg Q48 hr
  1.2–2 kg: 15 mg/kg/24 hr ÷ Q12 hr
  ≥2 kg: 30 mg/kg/24 hr ÷ Q12 hr
Infants/children/adults:
  IV/PO: 30 mg/kg/24 hr ÷ Q6 hr
  Max. dose: 4 g/24 hr
Bacterial vaginosis:
  Adolescents and adults:
    PO: 500 mg BID × 7 days or 2 g × 1 dose
    Vaginal: 5 g (1 applicatorful) QD-BID × 5 days
Giardiasis:
  Children: 15 mg/kg/24 hr PO ÷ TID × 5 days
  Adults: 250 mg PO TID × 5 days
Trichomoniasis: Treat sexual contacts
  Children: 15 mg/kg/24 hr PO ÷ TID × 7 days
  Adolescents/adults: 2 g PO × 1 or 250 mg PO TID or 375 mg PO BID × 7 days
C. difficile infection:
  Children: 30 mg/kg/24 hr ÷ Q6 hr PO/IV (IV may be less efficacious) × 10 days
  Adults: 250–500 mg TID-QID × 10–14 days
Helicobacter pylori infection:
  Use in combination with amoxicillin and bismuth subsalicylate
  Children: 15–20 mg/kg/24 hr ÷ BID PO × 4 weeks
  Adults: 250–500 mg TID PO × 14 days
Inflammatory bowel disease (as alternative to sulfasalazine):
  Adults: 400 mg BID PO
Perianal disease: 20 mg/kg/24 hr PO in 3–5 divided doses
Topical use: Apply to affected areas BID

Avoid use in first-trimester pregnancy. Use with **caution** in patients with CNS disease, blood dyscrasias, severe liver or **renal disease (GFR <10 mL/min), see p. 943.** Nausea, diarrhea, urticaria, dry mouth, leukopenia, vertigo, metallic taste, and peripheral neuropathy may occur. Candidiasis may worsen. May discolor urine. Patients should **not** ingest alcohol for 24–48 hr after dose (disulfiram-type reaction).

May increase levels or toxicity of phenytoin, lithium, and warfarin. Phenobarbital and rifampin may increase metronidazole metabolism.

IV infusion must be given slowly over 1 hr. For intravenous use in all ages, some references recommend a 15 mg/kg loading dose.

MEZLOCILLIN

Mezlin
Antibiotic, penicillin (extended spectrum)

Yes 2 B

Inj: 1, 2, 3, 4, 20 g
Contains 1.85 mEq Na/g drug

Continued

MEZLOCILLIN *continued*

Neonates, IM/IV:
<1.2 kg: 150 mg/kg/24 hr ÷ Q12 hr
≥1.2 kg:
≤7 days: 150 mg/kg/24 hr ÷ Q12 hr
>7 days: 225 mg/kg/24 hr ÷ Q8 hr
Infants and children, IM/IV: 200–300 mg/kg/24 hr ÷ Q4–6 hr
Cystic fibrosis, IM/IV: 300–450 mg/kg/24 hr ÷ Q4–6 hr; **max. dose:** 24 g/24 hr
Adults, IM/IV: 1.5–4 g/dose Q4–6 hr; **max. dose:** 24 g/24 hr

Use with **caution** in biliary obstruction, penicillin allergy (10% cross-sensitivity) and **renal impairment (see p. 943).** May cause seizures, nausea, diarrhea, vomiting, bone marrow suppression, blood dyscrasias, elevated BUN/Cr, and elevated LFTs. Causes false-positive direct Coombs' test, urinary protein, prolonged bleeding time, and electrolyte abnormalities.

MICONAZOLE

Monistat
Antifungal agent

No ? C

Cream: 2% (15, 30, 90 g)
Lotion: 2% (30, 60 mL)
Ointment: 2% (28.4 g)
Topical solution: 2% with alcohol (7.4, 29.6 mL)
Vaginal cream: 2% (45 g)
Vaginal suppository: 100 mg (7s), 200 mg (3s)
Powder: 2% (45, 90 g)
Spray: 2% (105 mL)
Inj: 1% (10 mg/mL)

Topical: Apply BID × 2–4 weeks
Vaginal: 1 applicator full of cream or 100-mg suppository QHS × 7 days or 200 mg suppository QHS × 3 days
IV:
Neonates: 5–15 mg/kg/24 hr ÷ Q8–24 hr
Infants and children: 20–40 mg/kg/24 hr ÷ Q8 hr
Adult: 1.2–3.6 g/24 hr ÷ Q8 hr

Use with **caution** in liver disease. Side effects include phlebitis (IV route), pruritus, rash, nausea, vomiting, fever, drowsiness, diarrhea, anemia, lipemia, thrombocytopenia, anorexia, tremors, and flushing. CN XII palsy and arachnoiditis have been reported.
Systemic use may increase the effects of cyclosporine, phenytoin, and warfarin. Vaginal use with concomitant warfarin use has also been reported to increase warfarin's effect.

MIDAZOLAM

Versed
Benzodiazepine

Yes   3   D

Inj: 1, 5 mg/mL; may contain 1% benzyl alcohol
Oral syrup: 2 mg/mL

 Titrate to effect under controlled conditions.
See p. 902, for additional routes of administration.

Sedation for procedures:
Children:
   IV:
      6 mo–5 yr: 0.05–0.1 mg/kg/dose over 2–3 min. May repeat dose PRN in
      2–3 min intervals up to a **max. total dose** of 6 mg. A total dose up to
      0.6 mg/kg may be necessary for desired effect.
      6–12 yr: 0.025–0.05 mg/kg/dose over 2–3 min. May repeat dose PRN in
      2–3 min intervals up to a **max. total dose** of 10 mg. A total dose up to
      0.4 mg/kg may be necessary for desired effect.
      >12–16 yr: Use adult dose; up to a **max. total dose** of 10 mg
Adults:
   IV: 0.5–2 mg/dose over 2 min. May repeat PRN in 2–3 min intervals until desired
   effect. *Usual total dose:* 2.5–5 mg. **Max. total dose:** 10 mg.
Sedation with mechanical ventilation:
   Intermittent:
      Infants and children: 0.05–0.15 mg/kg/dose Q1–2 hr PRN
   Continuous IV infusion (initial doses, titrate to effect):
      Neonates:
         <32 weeks gestation: 0.5 mcg/kg/min
         ≥32 weeks gestation: 1 mcg/kg/min
      Infants and children: 1–2 mcg/kg/min
   See inside front cover for infusion preparation.
Refractory status epilepticus:
   >2 mo and children: Load with 0.15 mg/kg IV × 1 followed by a continuous
   infusion of 1 mcg/kg/min and titrate dose upward Q5 min to effect (mean dose of
   2.3 mcg/kg/min with a range of 1–18 mcg/kg/min has been reported).
   See inside front cover for infusion preparation.

 Contraindicated in patients with narrow-angle glaucoma and shock. Causes
respiratory depression, hypotension, and bradycardia. Cardiovascular monitoring
is recommended. Use lower doses when given in combination with narcotics or
in patients with respiratory compromise.
Drug is a substrate for CYP 450 3A4. Serum concentrations may be increased by
cimetidine, diltiazem, erythromycin, itraconazole, ketoconazole, and protease inhibitors. Sedative effects may be antagonized by theophylline. **Effects can be reversed by
flumazenil.** For pharmacodynamic information, see p. 902.
   Adjust dose in renal failure (see p. 950).

MILRINONE
Primacor
Inotrope

Yes ? C

Inj: 1 mg/mL (5, 10, 20 mL)
Premixed inj in D₅W: 200 mcg/mL (100, 200 mL)

Children (limited data): 50 mcg/kg IV bolus over 15 min, followed by a continuous infusion of 0.5–1 mcg/kg/min and titrated to effect.
Adults: 50 mcg/kg IV bolus over 10 min, followed by a continuous infusion of 0.375–0.75 mcg/kg/min and titrated to effect.

Contraindicated in severe aortic stenosis, severe pulmonic stenosis, acute MI. May cause headache, dysrhythmias, hypotension, hypokalemia, nausea, vomiting, anorexia, abdominal pain, hepatotoxicity, and thrombocytopenia. Pediatric patients may require higher mcg/kg/min doses because of a faster elimination $T_{1/2}$ and larger volume of distribution, when compared to adults. Hemodynamic effects can last up to 3–5 hr after discontinuation of infusion in children. Reduce dose in renal impairment.

MINERAL OIL
Kondremul and others
Laxative, lubricant

No ? C

Liquid: Various sizes
Rectal liquid: 133 mL
Emulsion, oral: 2.5 mL/5 mL, 2.75 mL/5 mL, 4.75 mL/5 mL
Jelly, oral: 2.75 mL/5 ML

Children 5–11 yr:
    PO: 5–15 mL/24 hr ÷ QD-TID
    Rectal: 30–60 mL as single dose
Children ≥12 yr and adults:
    PO: 15–45 mL/24 hr ÷ QD-TID
    Rectal: 60–150 mL as single dose

May cause lipid pneumonitis via aspiration, diarrhea, and cramps. Use as a laxative should **not** exceed >1 week. Onset of action is approximately 6–8 hr. Higher doses may be necessary to achieve desired effect. Do **not** give QHS dose, and use with **caution** in children <5 yr to minimize risk of aspiration. May impair the absorption of fat-soluble vitamins, calcium, phosphorus, oral contraceptives, and warfarin. Emulsified preparations are more palatable.
For disimpaction, doses up to 1 oz (30 mL) per year of age (**maximum** of 240 mL) BID can be given.

MINOCYCLINE

Minocin and others
Antibiotic, tetracycline derivative

Yes   2   D

Tabs: 50, 100 mg
Caps: 50, 75, 100 mg
Caps (pellet filled): 50, 100 mg
Oral susp: 50 mg/5 mL (60 mL); contains 5% alcohol
Inj: 100 mg

Children (8–12 yr): 4 mg/kg/dose × 1 PO/IV, then 2 mg/kg/dose Q12 hr PO/IV;
max. dose: 200 mg/24 hr
   Adolescents and adults: 200 mg/dose × 1 PO/IV, then 100 mg Q12 hr PO/IV
Acne: 50 mg PO QD-TID

Use with **caution** in renal failure; lower dosage may be necessary. Nausea, vomiting, allergy, increased intracranial pressure, photophobia and injury to developing teeth may occur. High incidence of vestibular dysfunction (30%–90%).
May be administered with food but **not** with milk or dairy products. See *Tetracycline*
for additional drug/food interactions and comments.

MINOXIDIL

Loniten, Rogaine, Rogaine Extra Strength for Men, Minoxidil
for Men
Antihypertensive agent, hair growth stimulant

No   1   C

Tabs: 2.5, 10 mg
Topical solution (Rogaine, Rogaine Extra Strength for Men, Minoxidil for Men): 2%,
5% (60 mL)

Children:
Start with 0.2 mg/kg/24 hr PO QD; **max. dose:** 5 mg/24 hr. Dose may be
increased in increments of 0.1–0.2 mg/kg/24 hr at 3-day intervals. *Usual*
effective range: 0.25–1 mg/kg/24 hr PO ÷ QD-BID; **max. dose:** 5 mg/kg/24 hr up to
50 mg/24 hr.
>12 yr and adults:
   Oral: Start with 5 mg QD. Dose may be gradually increased at 3-day intervals. *Usual*
   effective range: 10–40 mg/24 hr ÷ QD-BID; **max. dose:** 100 mg/24 hr.
   Topical (alopecia): Apply 1 mL to the total affected areas of the scalp BID (QAM and
   QHS). **Max. dose:** 2 mL/24 hr.

Contraindicated in acute MI, dissecting aortic aneurysm, pheochromocytoma.
Concurrent use with a beta-blocker and diuretic is recommended to prevent
reflex tachycardia and reduce water retention, respectively. May cause

Continued

MINOXIDIL *continued*

drowsiness, dizziness, CHF, pulmonary edema, pericardial effusion, pericarditis, thrombocytopenia, leukopenia, Stevens-Johnson syndrome, and hypertrichosis (reversible) with systemic use. Concurrent use of guanethidine may cause profound orthostatic hypotension; use with other antihypertensive agents may cause additive hypotension. Antihypertensive onset of action within 30 min and peak effects within 2–8 hr.

   TOPICAL USE: Local irritation, contact dermatitis may occur. Do **not** use in conjunction with other topical agents, including topical corticosteroids, retinoids, or petrolatum, or agents that are known to enhance cutaneous drug absorption. Onset of hair growth (topical use) is 4 mo.

MONTELUKAST
Singulair
Antiasthmatic, leukotriene receptor antagonist

No ? B

Chewable tabs: 4, 5 mg; contains phenylalanine
Tabs: 10 mg

   Children (2–5 yr): Chew 4 mg (chewable tablet) QHS
   Children (6–14 yr): Chew 5 mg (chewable tablet) QHS
   >15 yr and adults: 10 mg PO QHS

   Chewable tablet dosage form is **contraindicated** in phenylketonuric patients. Side effects include headache, abdominal pain, dyspepsia, fatigue, dizziness, cough, and elevated liver enzymes. Diarrhea, eosinophilia, hypersensitivity reactions, pharyngitis, nausea, otitis, sinusitis, and viral infections have been reported in children. Drug is a substrate for CYP 450 2A6, 2C9, and 3A3/4. Phenobarbital and rifampin may induce hepatic metabolism to increase the clearance of montelukast.
   Doses may be administered with or without food.

MORPHINE SULFATE
Roxanol, MS Contin, Oramorph SR, and many others
Narcotic, analgesic

Yes 1 B/D

Oral solution: 10, 20 mg/5 mL
Concentrated oral solution: 100 mg/5 mL
Caps/Tabs: 15, 30 mg
Controlled-release tabs (MS Contin, Oramorph SR): 15, 30, 60, 100, 200 mg
Controlled-release caps: 20, 30, 50, 60, 100 mg
Sustained-release tabs: 30, 60, 100 mg
Soluble tabs: 10, 15, 30 mg
Rectal suppository: 5, 10, 20, 30 mg
Inj: 0.5, 1, 2, 4, 5, 8, 10, 15, 25, 50 mg/mL

Continued

MORPHINE SULFATE *continued*

Titrate to effect
Analgesia/tetralogy (cyanotic) spells:
  Neonates: 0.05–0.2 mg/kg/dose IM, slow IV, SC Q4 hr
Neonatal opiate withdrawal: 0.08–0.2 mg/dose Q3–4 hr PRN
Infants and children:
  PO: 0.2–0.5 mg/kg/dose Q4–6 hr PRN (immediate release) or 0.3–0.6 mg/kg/dose
  Q12 hr PRN (controlled release)
  IM/IV/SC: 0.1–0.2 mg/kg/dose Q2–4 hr PRN; **max. dose:** 15 mg/dose
Adults:
  PO: 10–30 mg Q4 hr PRN (immediate release) or 15–30 mg Q8–12 hr PRN
  (controlled release)
  IM/IV/SC: 2–15 mg/dose Q2–6 hr PRN
Continuous IV infusion: (Dosing ranges, titrate to effect)
  Neonates: 0.01–0.02 mg/kg/hr
  Infants and children:
    Postoperative pain: 0.01–0.04 mg/kg/hr
    Sickle cell and cancer: 0.04–0.07 mg/kg/hr
  Adults: 0.8–10 mg/hr
To prepare infusion for neonates, infants, and children, use the following formula:

$$50 \times \frac{\text{Desired dose (mg/kg/hr)}}{\text{Desired infusion rate (mL/hr)}} \times \text{Wt (kg)} = \frac{\text{mg Morphine}}{\text{50 mL fluid}}$$

Dependence, CNS and respiratory depression, nausea, vomiting, urinary
retention, constipation, hypotension, bradycardia, increased ICP, miosis, biliary
spasm, and allergy may occur. **Naloxone may be used to reverse effects,**
especially respiratory depression. Causes histamine release resulting in itching and
possible bronchospasm. Neonates may require higher doses due to decreased amounts
of active metabolites. See p. 910, for equianalgesic dosing. Pregnancy category
changes to "D" if used for prolonged periods or in higher doses at term. Rectal dosing
is same as oral dosing but is not recommended due to poor absorption.

Controlled/sustained-released oral tablets must be administered whole. Controlled-
release oral capsules may be opened and the entire contents sprinkled on applesauce
immediately prior to ingestion. **Adjust dose in renal failure (see p. 950).**

MUPIROCIN

Bactroban
Topical antibiotic

No   ?   B

Ointment: 2% (15, 30 g); contains polyethylene glycol
Cream: 2% (15, 30 g)
Nasal ointment: 2% (1 g), as calcium salt

Continued

MUPIROCIN *continued*

 Topical: Apply small amount TID to affected area × 5–14 days
Intranasal: Apply small amount intranasally 2–4 times/24 hr for 5–14 days

 Avoid contact with the eyes. Do **not** use topical ointment preparation on open wounds due to concerns about systemic absorption of polyethylene glycol. May cause minor local irritation.

If clinical response is not apparent in 3–5 days with topical use, reevaluate infection. Intranasal administration may be used to eliminate carriage of *S. aureus,* including MRSA.

MYCOPHENOLATE MOFETIL
CellCept
Immunosuppressant agent

Yes ? C

Tabs: 500 mg
Caps: 250 mg
Oral suspension: 200 mg/mL (225 mL); contains phenylalanine (0.56 mg/mL) and methylparabens
Inj: 500 mg

 Children: 600 mg/m^2/dose PO BID up to a **max. dose** of 2000 mg/24 hr; alternatively, patients with body surface areas ≥1.25 m^2 may be dosed as follows:
1.25–1.5 m^2: 750 mg PO BID
>1.5 m^2: 1000 mg PO BID
Adults (in combination with corticosteroids and cyclosporine):
PO/IV: 2000–3000 mg/24 hr ÷ BID

Check specific transplantation protocol for specific dosage. Mycophenolate mofetil is a pro-drug for mycophenolic acid. Common side effects may include headache, hypertension, diarrhea, vomiting, bone marrow suppression, anemia, fever, opportunistic infections, and sepsis. May also increase the risk for lymphomas or other malignancies.

Use with **caution** in patients with active GI disease or renal impairment (GFR <25 mL/min/1.73 m^2) outside of the immediate post-transplant period. In adults with renal impairment, **avoid** doses >2 g/24 hr and observe carefully. No dose adjustment is needed for patients experiencing delayed graft function postoperatively.

Drug interactions: (1) Displacement of phenytoin or theophylline from protein binding sites will decrease total serum levels and increase free serum levels of these drugs. Salicylates displace mycophenolate to increase free levels of mycophenolate. (2) Competition for renal tubular secretion results in increased serum levels of acyclovir, ganciclovir, probenecid, and mycophenolate (when any of these are used together).

Continued

MYCOPHENOLATE MOFETIL *continued*

Administer oral doses on an empty stomach. Cholestyramine and antacid use may decrease mycophenolic acid levels. Infuse intravenous doses over 2 hr. Oral suspension may be administered via NG tube with a minimum size of 8 French.

NAFCILLIN

Unipen, Nafcil, Nallpen, and others
Antibiotic, penicillin (penicillinase resistant)

Yes   2   B

Tabs: 500 mg
Caps: 250 mg
Oral solution: 250 mg/5 mL (100 mL)
Inj: 0.5, 1, 2, 4, 10 g; contains 2.9 mEq Na/g

Neonates: IM/IV
  ≤7 days:
    <2 kg: 50 mg/kg/24 hr ÷ Q12 hr
    ≥2 kg: 75 mg/kg/24 hr ÷ Q8 hr
  >7 days:
    <1.2 kg: 50 mg/kg/24 hr ÷ Q12 hr
    1.2–2 kg: 75 mg/kg/24 hr ÷ Q8 hr
    ≥2 kg: 100 mg/kg/24 hr ÷ Q6 hr
Infants and children:
  PO: 50–100 mg/kg/24 hr ÷ Q6 hr
  IM/IV: (mild to moderate infections): 50–100 mg/kg/24 hr ÷ Q6 hr
    (Severe infections): 100–200 mg/kg/24 hr ÷ Q4–6 hr
    Max. dose: 12 g/24 hr
Adults:
  PO: 250–1000 mg Q4–6 hr
  IV: 500–2000 mg Q4–6 hr
  IM: 500 mg Q4–6 hr
  Max. dose: 12 g/24 hr

Allergic cross-sensitivity with penicillin. **Oral route not recommended** due to unpredictable absorption. High incidence of phlebitis with IV dosing. CSF penetration is poor unless meninges are inflamed. Use with **caution** in patients with combined renal and hepatic impairment (reduce dose by 33%-50%). Nafcillin may increase elimination of warfarin. Acute interstitial nephritis is rare. May cause rash and bone marrow suppression.

NALOXONE

Narcan
Narcotic antagonist

No   ?   B

Inj: 0.4, 1 mg/mL; some preparations may contain parabens
Neonatal inj: 0.02 mg/mL (2 mL)

Opiate intoxication (see remarks):
Neonates, infants, children <20 kg: IM/IV/SC/ETT: 0.1 mg/kg/dose. May repeat PRN Q2–3 min.
Children ≥20 kg or >5 yr: 2 mg/dose. May repeat PRN Q2–3 min.
Continuous infusion (children and adults): 0.005 mg/kg loading dose followed by infusion of 0.0025 mg/kg/hr has been recommended. A range of 0.0025–0.16 mg/kg/hr has been reported. Taper gradually to avoid relapse.
Adults: 0.4–2 mg/dose. May repeat PRN Q2–3 min. Use 0.1- to 0.2-mg increments in opiate dependent patients.

Short duration of action may necessitate multiple doses. For severe intoxication, doses of 0.2 mg/kg may be required. If no response is achieved after a cumulative dose of 10 mg, reevaluate diagnosis. **In the non-arrest situation, use the lowest dose effective (may start at 0.001 mg/kg/dose).** See p. 899 for additional information.

Will produce narcotic withdrawal syndrome in patients with chronic dependence. Use with **caution** in patients with chronic cardiac disease. Abrupt reversal of narcotic depression may result in nausea, vomiting, diaphoresis, tachycardia, hypertension, and tremulousness.

May be used simultaneously with opiates at lower dosages to abate opiate-related side effects. The neonatal concentration (0.02 mg/mL) is no longer recommended in most instances due to large volumes of administration (2 mg/100 mL).

NAPROXEN/NAPROXEN SODIUM

Naprosyn, Anaprox, EC-Naprosyn, Naprelan, Aleve (OTC), and others
Nonsteroidal antiinflammatory agent

Yes   1   B/D

Tabs (Naproxen): 250, 375, 500 mg
Delayed-release tabs (Naproxen; EC-Naprosyn): 375, 500 mg
Tabs (Naproxen sodium):
   Anaprox: 275 mg (250 mg base), 550 mg (500 mg base); contains 1 mEq, 2 mEq Na, respectively
   Aleve: 220 mg (200 mg base); contains 0.87 mEq Na
Controlled-release tabs (Naproxen sodium):
   Naprelan: 412.5 mg (375 mg base), 550 mg (500 mg base)
Susp: Naproxen 125 mg/5 mL; contains 0.34 mEq Na/1 mL and parabens

Continued

NAPROXEN/NAPROXEN SODIUM *continued*

All doses based on Naproxen base
Children >2 yr:
Analgesia: 5–7 mg/kg/dose Q8–12 hr PO
JRA: 10–20 mg/kg/24 hr ÷ Q12 hr PO
Usual max. dose: 1250 mg/24 hr
Rheumatoid arthritis, ankylosing spondylitis:
Adults:
Immediate-release forms: 250–500 mg BID PO
Delayed-release tabs (EC-Naprosyn): 375–500 mg BID PO
Controlled-release tabs (Naprelan): 750–1000 mg QD PO; **max. dose:**
1500 mg/24 hr
Dysmenorrhea:
500 mg × 1, then 250 mg Q6–8 hr PO; **max. dose:** 1250 mg/24 hr.

May cause GI bleeding, thrombocytopenia, heartburn, headache, drowsiness,
vertigo, and tinnitus. Use with **caution** in patients with GI disease, cardiac
disease, renal or hepatic impairment, and those receiving anticoagulants. See
Ibuprofen for other side effects.
Pregnancy category changes to "D" if used in third trimester or near delivery.
Administer doses with food or milk to reduce GI discomfort.

NEDOCROMIL SODIUM
Tilade, Alocril
Antiallergic agent

No   ?   B

Aerosol inhaler: 1.75 mg/actuation (112 actuations/inhaler, 16.2 g)
Ophthalmic solution (Alocril): 2% (5 mL)

Children ≥6 yr and adults:
2 puffs QID. May reduce dosage to BID-TID once clinical response is obtained.
Ophthalmic use:
≥3 yr–adults: 1-2 drops to affected eye(s) BID

May cause dry mouth/pharyngitis, unpleasant taste, cough, nausea, headache,
and rhinitis. Therapeutic response often occurs within 2 weeks, however, a
4–6 week trial may be needed to determine maximum benefit.
Use spacer device with MDI to improve drug delivery. Shake MDI well before each
use. When using a new canister of drug or if canister has not been used for >7 days,
prime the MDI with three actuations prior to use.
For ophthalmic use, remove contact lens.

NELFINAVIR

Viracept, NFV
Antiviral, protease inhibitor

No   3   B

Powder, oral: 200 mg/level teaspoonful or 50 mg/level scoop (50 mg/g powder); contains 11.2 mg phenylalanine/g powder)
Tabs: 250 mg

Neonates (investigational dose from ACTG 353): 40 mg/kg/dose PO BID
Children and adolescents (early puberty, Tanner I-II): 20–30 mg/kg/dose PO TID; **max. dose:** 750 mg/dose TID
Adolescents and adults: 750 mg PO TID or 1250 mg PO BID

Avoid use of oral powder dosage form in patients with phenylketonuria because it contains phenylalanine. Diarrhea is the most common side effect. Asthenia, abdominal pain, rash, hyperglycemia, and exacerbation of chronic liver disease may occur. Spontaneous bleeding episodes in hemophiliacs have been reported.

Nelfinavir is a substrate and inhibitor of CYP 450 3A4. The following drugs should **NOT** be coadministered with nelfinavir: terfenadine, astemizole, cisapride, midazolam, triazolam, ergot derviatives, amiodarone, or quinidine. Rifampin, phenobarbital, phenytoin, and carbamazepine can decrease nelfinavir levels. Nelfinavir can increase rifabutin levels; decrease delavirdine levels; and decrease oral contraceptive effectiveness (use alternative methods). When used in combination with other protease inhibitors (PI), nelfinavir and other PI levels may increase. **Always check the potential for other drug interactions when either initiating therapy or adding new drugs onto an existing regimen.**

Adolescent dosing: Patients in early puberty (Tanner I-II) should be dosed with pediatric regimens and those in late puberty (Tanner V) should be dosed with adult regimens. Adolescents who are at the midst of their growth spurt (Tanner III females and Tanner IV males) can be dosed by either pediatric or adult regimen with close monitoring of efficacy and toxicity.

Administer all doses with food; avoid mixing with acidic foods or juice. If didanosine is part of the antiviral regimen, nelfinavir should be administered at least 2 hr prior or 1 hr after didanosine. Oral powder dosage form may be mixed with water, milk, pudding, or formula (up to 6 hr). **Noncompliance can quickly promote resistant HIV strains.**

NEOMYCIN SULFATE

Mycifradin and others
Antibiotic, aminoglycoside; ammonium detoxicant

Yes   ?   C

Tabs: 500 mg
Solution: 125 mg/5 mL; contains parabens
Cream: 0.5% (15 g)
Ointment: 0.5% (15, 30 g)

Continued

NEOMYCIN SULFATE *continued*

Diarrhea:
Preterm and newborns: 50 mg/kg/24 hr ÷ Q6 hr PO
  Hepatic encephalopathy:
Infants and children: 50–100 mg/kg/24 hr ÷ Q6–8 hr PO × 5–6 days. **Max. dose:** 12 g/24 hr
Adults: 4–12 g/24 hr ÷ Q4–6 hr PO × 5–6 days
Bowel preparation:
  Children: 90 mg/kg/24 hr PO ÷ Q4 hr × 2–3 days
  Adults: 1 g Q1 hr PO × 4 doses, then 1 g Q4 hr PO × 5 doses (many other regimens exist)
Topical: Apply QD–TID to infected area

Contraindicated in ulcerative bowel disease or intestinal obstruction. Monitor for nephrotoxicity and ototoxicity. Oral absorption is limited, but levels may accumulate. Consider dosage reduction in the presence of renal failure. May cause itching, redness, edema, colitis, candidiasis, or poor wound healing if applied topically.

NEOMYCIN/POLYMYXIN B/± BACITRACIN

No   ?   C

Neosporin, Neosporin GU Irrigant, and others
Topical antibiotic

Cream: 3.5 mg neomycin sulfate, 10,000 U polymyxin B/g (0.94, 15 g)
Solution, genitourinary irrigant: 40 mg neomycin sulfate, 200,000 U polymyxin B/mL (1, 20 mL); contains methylparabens
In combination with bacitracin:
  Ointment (topical): 3.5 mg neomycin sulfate, 400 U bacitracin, 5000 U polymyxin B/g
  Ointment (ophthalmic): 3.5 mg neomycin sulfate, 400 U bacitracin, 10,000 U polymyxin B/g

Topical: Apply to minor wounds and burns QD-TID
Ophthalmic: Apply small amount to conjunctiva QD-QID
  Bladder irrigation:
Adults: Mix 1 mL in 1000 mL NS and administer via a three-way catheter at a rate adjusted to the patient's urine output. Do not exceed 10 days of continuous use.

Do **not** use for extended periods. May cause superinfection, delayed healing. See *Neomycin.* Ophthalmic preparation may cause stinging and sensitivity to bright light. **Avoid** use of bladder irrigant in patients with defects in the bladder mucosa or wall.

For explanation of icons, see p. 572.

NEOSTIGMINE

Prostigmin and others
Anticholinesterase (cholinergic) agent

Yes   ?   C

Tabs: 15 mg (bromide)
Inj: 0.25, 0.5, 1 mg/mL (methylsulfate); may contain parabens

Myasthenia gravis-diagnosis: Use with atropine (see comments).
  Children: 0.025–0.04 mg/kg IM × 1
  Adults: 0.022 mg/kg IM × 1
Treatment:
  Children:
    IM/IV/SC: 0.01–0.04 mg/kg/dose Q2–3 hr PRN
    PO: 2 mg/kg/24 hr ÷ Q3–4 hr
  Adults: IM/IV/SC: 0.5–2.5 mg/dose Q1–3 hr PRN
    PO: 15 mg/dose TID. May increase every 1–2 days. Dosage requirements may
    vary from 15–375 mg/24 hr
Reversal of nondepolarizing neuromuscular blocking agents: Administer with atropine
or glycopyrrolate
  Infants: 0.025–0.1 mg/kg/dose IV
  Children: 0.025–0.08 mg/kg/dose IV
  Adults: 0.5–2.5 mg/dose IV
  Max. dose: 5 mg/dose

Contraindicated in GI and urinary obstruction. **Caution** in asthmatics. May cause
cholinergic crisis, bronchospasm, salivation, nausea, vomiting, diarrhea, miosis,
diaphoresis, lacrimation, bradycardia, hypotension, fatigue, confusion,
respiratory depression, and seizures. Titrate for each patient, but **avoid** excessive
cholinergic effects.

For diagnosis of myasthenia gravis (MG), administer atropine 0.011 mg/kg/dose
IV immediately before or IM (0.011 mg/kg/dose) 30 min before neostigmine. For
treatment of MG, patients may need higher doses of neostigmine at times of greatest
fatigue.

Antidote: Atropine 0.01–0.04 mg/kg/dose. Atropine and epinephrine should be
available in the event of a hypersensitivity reaction.

Adjust dose in renal failure (see p. 950).

NEVIRAPINE

Viramune, NVP
Antiviral, nonnucleoside reverse transcriptase inhibitor

Yes   3   C

Tabs: 200 mg
Susp: 10 mg/mL (240 mL); contains parabens

Continued

NEVIRAPINE continued

Neonate-3 mo (investigational dose from ACTG 356): Start with 5 mg/kg/dose or 120 mg/m^2/dose QD PO × 14 days, followed by 120 mg/m^2/dose Q12 hr PO × 14 days, then 200 mg/m^2/dose Q12 hr PO

Children: Start with 120 mg/m^2/dose QD PO × 14 days, then increase dose to 120 mg/m^2/dose Q12 hr PO if no rash or other side effects. *Usual maintenance dose:* 120–200 mg/m^2/dose Q12 hr PO; **max. dose:** 200 mg/dose Q12 hr. Alternatively:

2 mo-8 yr: Start with 4 mg/kg/dose QD PO × 14 days, then increase dose to 4 mg/kg/dose Q12 hr PO if no rash or other side effects. *Usual maintenance dose:* 7 mg/kg/dose Q12 hr PO; **max. dose:** 200 mg/dose Q12 hr.

>8 yr: Start with 4 mg/kg/dose QD PO × 14 days, then increase dose to 4 mg/kg/dose Q12 hr PO if no rash or other side effects; **max. dose:** 200 mg/dose Q12 hr.

Adults: Start with 200 mg/dose QD PO × 14 days, then increase to 200 mg/dose Q12 hr if no rash or other side effects.

Use with **caution** in patients with hepatic or renal dysfunction. Most frequent side effects include skin rash (may be life-threatening, including Stevens-Johnson syndrome), fever, abnormal LFTs, headache, and nausea. **Discontinue** therapy if a severe rash or a rash with fever, blistering, oral lesions, conjunctivitis, or muscle aches occur. **Life-threatening** hepatotoxicity has been reported primarily during the first 12 weeks of therapy. Patients with increased serum transaminase or a history of hepatitis B or C infection prior to nevirapine are at greater risk for hepatotoxiciy. Monitor LFTs and CBCs.

Nevirapine induces the CYP450 3A4 drug metabolizing isoenzyme to cause an autoinduction of its own metabolism within the first 2-4 weeks of therapy and has the potential to interact with many drugs. The drug can decrease levels of itraconazole, ketoconazole, methadone, indinavir, ritonavir, saquinavir, and oral/other hormonal contraceptives. Rifampin and rifabutin can lower serum levels of nevirapine. Cimetidine, clarithromycin, erythromycin, ketoconazole can increase serum levels of nevirapine. **Carefully review the patients' drug profile for other drug interactions each time nevirapine is initiated or when a new drug is added to a regimen containing nevirapine.**

Adolescent dosing: Patients in early puberty (Tanner I-II) should be dosed with pediatric regimens and those in late puberty (Tanner V) should be dosed with adult regimens. Adolescents who are at the midst of their growth spurt (Tanner III females and Tanner IV males) can be dosed by either pediatric or adult regimen with close monitoring of efficacy and toxicity.

Doses can be administered with food and concurrently with didanosine. **Noncompliance can quickly promote resistant HIV strains.**

NIACIN/VITAMIN B$_3$

Niacor, Niaspan, Nicolor, Nicotinic acid, Vitamin B$_3$, and others
Vitamin, water soluble

No   ?   A/C

Tabs: 25, 50, 100, 250, 500 mg
Timed or extended-release tabs: 150, 250, 375, 500, 750, 1000 mg

Continued

NIACIN/VITAMIN B₃ *continued*

Timed-release caps: 125, 250, 300, 400, 500 mg
Elixir: 50 mg/5 mL (14% alcohol)
Inj: 100 mg/mL

US RDA: See pp. 460–461.
Pellagra PO/IM/IV/SC:
    Children: 50–100 mg/dose TID
    Adults: 50–100 mg/dose TID-QID
    Max. dose: 500 mg/24 hr

Contraindicated in hepatic dysfunction, active peptic ulcer, and severe hypotension. Adverse reactions of flushing, pruritus, or GI distress may occur with PO
administration. May cause hyperglycemia, hyperuricemia, blurred vision, abnormal LFTs, dizziness, and headaches. May cause false-positive urine catecholamines
(fluorometric methods) and urine glucose (Benedict's reagent).
   Pregnancy category changes to "C" if used in doses above the RDA.
See pp. 463–465 for multivitamin preparations.

NICARDIPINE
Cardene, Cardene SR
Calcium channel blocker, antihypertensive

Yes   3   C

Caps (immediate release): 20, 30 mg
Sustained-release caps: 30, 45, 60 mg
Inj: 2.5 mg/mL (10 mL)

Children (see remarks):
Hypertension: 0.5–5 mcg/kg/min via continuous IV infusion
Adult:
Hypertension:
   Oral:
      Immediate release: 20 mg PO TID, dose may be increased after 3 days to
      40 mg PO TID if needed.
      Sustained release: 30 mg PO BID, dose may be increased after 3 days to
      60 mg PO BID if needed.
   Continuous IV infusion: Start at 5 mg/hr, increase dose as needed by 2.5 mg/hr
   Q5–15 min up to a **maximum** of 15 mg/hr. Following attainment of desired BP,
   decrease infusion to 3 mg/hr and adjust rate as needed to maintain desired
   response.

Continued

NICARDIPINE *continued*

Reported use in children has been limited to a small number of preterm infants, infants, and children. **Contraindicated** in advanced aortic stenosis. Use with **caution** in hepatic or renal dysfunction by carefully titrating dose. The drug undergoes significant first-pass metabolism through the liver and is excreted in the urine (60%). May cause headache, dizziness, asthenia, peripheral edema, and GI symptoms. **See nifedipine for drug and food interactions.** Onset of action for PO administration is 20 min with peak effects in 0.5–2 hr. IV onset of action is 1 min. Duration of action following a single IV or PO dose is 3 hr. For additional information, see p. 14.

NIFEDIPINE

Adalat, Adalat CC, Procardia, Procardia XL, and others
Calcium channel blocker, antihypertensive

No   1   C

Caps: (Adalat, Procardia): 10 mg (0.34 mL), 20 mg (0.45 mL)
Sustained-release tabs: (Adalat CC, Procardia XL): 30, 60, 90 mg

Children (see remarks for precautions):
  Hypertension/hypertensive urgency: 0.25–0.5 mg/kg/dose Q4–6 hr PRN PO/SL.
    Max. dose: 10 mg/dose or 3 mg/kg/24 hr
  Hypertrophic cardiomyopathy: 0.5–0.9 mg/kg/24 hr ÷ Q6–8 hr PO/SL
Adults:
  Hypertension:
    Caps: Start with 10 mg/dose PO TID. May increase to 30 mg/dose PO TID-QID.
      Max. dose: 180 mg/24 hr
    Sustained release: Start with 30–60 mg PO QD. May increase to **max. dose:** 120 mg/24 hr

Use of immediate-release dosage form in children is controversial and has been abandoned by some. Use with **caution** in children with acute CNS injury due to increased risk for stroke, seizure, and altered level of consciousness. To prevent rapid decrease in blood pressure in children, an initial dose of ≤0.25 mg/kg is recommended.

Use with **caution** in patients with CHF and aortic stenosis. May cause severe hypotension, peripheral edema, flushing, tachycardia, headaches, dizziness, nausea, palpitations, and syncope. Although overall use in adults has been abandoned, the immediate-release dosage form is **contraindicated** in adults with severe obstructive coronary artery disease or recent MI, and hypertensive emergencies.

Nifedipine is a substrate for CYP 450 3A3/4, and 3A5–7. **Do not** administer with grapefruit juice; may increase bioavailability and effects. Itraconazole may increase nifedipine levels/effects. Nifedipine may increase phenytoin, cyclosporine, and digoxin levels. For hypertensive emergencies, see p. 14.

For sublingual administration, capsule must be punctured and liquid expressed into mouth. A small amount is absorbed via the SL route. The majority of effects are due to swallowing and oral absorption. **Do not** crush or chew sustained-release tablet dosage form.

NITROFURANTOIN

Furadantin, Macrodantin, Macrobid, and others
Antibiotic

Yes   1   B

Caps (Macrocrystals): 25, 50, 100 mg
Caps (dual release, Macrobid): 100 mg (25 mg macrocrystal/75 mg monohydrate)
Caps, extended release: 100 mg
Susp: 25 mg/5 mL (470 mL); contains saccharin

Children (>1 mo):
  Treatment: 5–7 mg/kg/24 hr ÷ Q6 hr PO; **max. dose:** 400 mg/24 hr
  UTI prophylaxis: 1–2 mg/kg/dose QHS PO; **max. dose:** 100 mg/24 hr
Adults:
  (Macrocrystals): 50–100 mg/dose Q6 hr PO
  (Dual-release): 100 mg/dose Q12 hr PO
  UTI prophylaxis (macrocrystals): 50–100 mg/dose PO QHS

Contraindicated in severe renal disease, G6PD deficiency, infants <1 mo, and pregnant women at term. May cause nausea, hypersensitivity reactions, vomiting, cholestatic jaundice, headache, hepatotoxicity, polyneuropathy, and hemolytic anemia. Causes false-positive urine glucose with Clinitest. Administer doses with food or milk.

NITROGLYCERIN

Tridil, Nitro-bid, Nitrostat, and others
Vasodilator, antihypertensive

No   ?   B

Inj: 0.5, 5, 10 mg/mL; may contain alcohol or propylene glycol
Prediluted injection in D_5W: 100 mcg/mL (250, 500 mL), 200 mcg/mL (250 mL), 400 mcg/mL (250, 500 mL)
Sublingual tabs: 0.3, 0.4, 0.6 mg
Buccal tabs (controlled release): 2, 3 mg
Sustained-release tabs: 9 mg
Sustained-release caps: 2.5, 6.5, 9 mg
Ointment, topical: 2% (30, 60 g)
Patch: 2.5 mg/24 hr (0.1 mg/hr), 5 mg/24 hr (0.2 mg/hr), 7.5 mg/24 hr (0.3 mg/hr), 10 mg/24 hr (0.4 mg/hr), 15 mg/24 hr (0.6 mg/hr), 20 mg/24 hr (0.8 mg/hr)
Spray, translingual: 0.4 mg per metered spray (14.48 g, delivers 200 doses per canister)

Children:
  Continuous IV infusion: Begin with 0.25–0.5 mcg/kg/min; may increase by 0.5–1 mcg/kg/min Q3–5 min PRN. Usual dose: 1–5 mcg/kg/min. **Max. dose:** 20 mcg/kg/min

Continued

NITROGLYCERIN *continued*

Adults:

Continuous IV infusion: 5 mcg/min IV, then increase Q3–5 min PRN by 5 mcg/min up to 20 mcg/min. If no response, increase by 10 mcg/min Q3–5 min PRN up to a **maximum** of 200 mcg/min.

To prepare infusion: See inside front cover

NOTE: The dosage units for adults are in mcg/min; compared to mcg/kg/min for children.

Sublingual: 0.2–0.6 mg Q5 min. **Maximum** of three doses in 15 min

Oral: 2.5–9 mg BID-TID; up to 26 mg QID

Ointment: Apply 1–2 inches Q8 hr, up to 4–5 inches Q4 hr

Patch: 0.2–0.4 mg/hr initially, then titrate to 0.4–0.8 mg/hr; apply new patch daily (tolerance is minimized by removing patch for 10–12 hr/24 hr)

Contraindicated in glaucoma and severe anemia. In small doses (1–2 mcg/kg/min) acts mainly on systemic veins and decreases preload. At 3–5 mcg/kg/min acts on systemic arterioles to decrease resistance. May cause headache, flushing, GI upset, blurred vision, and methemoglobinemia. Use with **caution** in severe renal impairment, increased ICP, and hepatic failure. IV nitroglycerin may antagonize anticoagulant effect of heparin.

Decrease dose gradually in patients receiving drug for prolonged periods to **avoid** withdrawal reaction. Must use polypropylene infusion sets to avoid adsorption of drug to plastic tubing.

Onset (duration) of action: IV: 1-2 min (3-5 min); sublingual: 1-3 min (30-60 min); PO sustained release: 40 min (4-8 hr); topical ointment: 20-60 min (2-12 hr); and transdermal patch: 40-60 min (18-24 hr).

NITROPRUSSIDE

Nipride and others
Vasodilator, antihypertensive

Yes   ?   C

Inj: 50 mg

Children and adults: IV, continuous infusion

Dose: Start at 0.3–0.5 mcg/kg/min, titrate to effect. Usual dose is 3–4 mcg/kg/min. **Max. dose:** 10 mcg/kg/min.

To prepare infusion: See inside front cover

Contraindicated in patients with decreased cerebral perfusion and in situations of compensatory hypertension (increased ICP). Monitor for hypotension and acidosis. Dilute with D_5W and protect from light.

Nitroprusside is nonenzymatically converted to cyanide, which is converted to thiocyanate. Cyanide may produce metabolic acidosis and methemoglobinemia; thiocyanate may produce psychosis and seizures. Monitor thiocyanate levels if used for >48 hrs or if dose ≥4 mcg/kg/min. **Thiocyanate levels should be <50 mg/L.**

Continued

NITROPRUSSIDE *continued*

Monitor **cyanide levels (toxic levels >2 mcg/mL)** in patients with hepatic dysfunction and thiocyanate levels in patients with renal dysfunction.

Onset of action is 2 min with a 1- to 10-min duration of effect.

NOREPINEPHRINE BITARTRATE
Levophed and others
Adrenergic agonist

No   ?   C

Inj: 1 mg/mL as norepinephrine base (4 mL); contains sulfites

Children: **Continuous IV infusion doses as norepinephrine base.** Start at 0.05–0.1 mcg/kg/min. Titrate to effect. **Max. dose:** 2 mcg/kg/min
To prepare infusion: See inside front cover

Adults: **Continuous IV infusion doses as norepinephrine base.** Start at 4 mcg/min and titrate to effect. Usual dosage range: 8–12 mcg/min.

NOTE: **The dosage units for adults are in mcg/min; compared to mcg/kg/min for children.**

May cause cardiac arrhythmias, hypertension, hypersensitivity, headaches, vomiting, uterine contractions, and organ ischemia. May cause decreased renal blood flow and urine output. Avoid extravasation into tissues; may cause severe tissue necrosis. If this occurs, treat locally with phentolamine.

NORFLOXACIN
Noroxin, Chibroxin
Antibiotic, quinolone

Yes   3   C

Tabs: 400 mg
Ophthalmic drops (Chibroxin): 3 mg/mL (5 mL)

Adults:

UTI: 400 mg PO Q12 hr (× 7–10 days for uncomplicated cases and × 10–21 days for complicated cases)

Prostatitis: 400 mg PO Q12 hr × 28 days

N. gonorrheae (uncomplicated): 800 mg PO × 1

Ophthalmic:

≥1 yr–adults: 1–2 drops QID × ≤7 days. May give up to Q2 hr for severe infections during the first day of therapy.

Like other quinolones, there is concern regarding development of arthropathy, which has been shown in immature animals. Norfloxacin does **not** adequately treat chlamydia co-infections. Use with **caution** in children <18 yr. Inhibits CYP

Continued

NORFLOXACIN *continued*

450 1A2. May increase serum theophylline levels. May prolong PT in patients on warfarin. See *Ciprofoxacin* for common side effects and drug interactions. Ophthalmic dosage form may cause local burning or discomfort, photophobia, and bitter taste. Administer oral doses on an empty stomach.

Adjust dose in renal failure with systemic use (see p. 943).

NORTRIPTYLINE HYDROCHLORIDE

Pamelor, Aventyl, and others
Antidepressant, tricyclic

No   3   D

Caps: 10, 25, 50, 75 mg
Solution: 10 mg/5 mL; contains up to 4% alcohol

Depression:
Children 6–12 yr: 1–3 mg/kg/24 hr ÷ TID-QID PO or 10–20 mg/24 hr ÷ TID-QID PO
Adolescents: 1–3 mg/kg/24 hr ÷ TID-QID PO or 30–50 mg/24 hr ÷ TID-QID PO
Adults: 75–100 mg/24 hr ÷ TID-QID PO
Max. dose: 150 mg/24 hr
Nocturnal enuresis:
6–7 yr (20–25 kg): 10 mg PO QHS
8–11 yr (25–35 kg): 10–20 mg PO QHS
>11 yr (35–54 kg): 25–35 mg PO QHS

See *Imipramine* for contraindications and common side effects. Less CNS and anticholinergic side effects than amitriptyline. Lower doses and slower dose titration is recommended in hepatic impairment. Therapeutic antidepressant effects occur in 7–21 days. **Do not** discontinue abruptly. Nortriptyline is a substrate for the cytochrome P450 1A2 and 2D6 drug metabolizing enzymes.

Therapeutic nortriptyline levels for depression: 50–150 ng/mL. *Recommended serum sampling time:* Obtain a single level 8 or more hr after an oral dose (following 4 days of continuous dosing for children and after 9–10 days for adults).

Administer with food to decrease GI upset.

NYSTATIN

Mycostatin, Nilstat, and others
Antifungal agent

No   1   B

Tabs: 500,000 U
Troches/pastilles: 200,000 U
Susp: 100,000 U/mL (60, 473 mL)

Continued

NYSTATIN *continued*

Cream/ointment: 100,000 U/g (15, 30 g)
Topical powder: 100,000 U/g (15 g)
Vaginal tabs: 100,000 U (15s, 30s)

Oral:
  Preterm infants: 0.5 mL (50,000 U) to each side of mouth QID
  Term infants: 1 mL (100,000 U) to each side of mouth QID
Children/adults:
  Susp: 4–6 mL (400,000–600,000 U) swish and swallow QID
  Troche: 200,000–400,000 U 4–5 ×/24 hr
Vaginal: 1 tab QHS × 14 days
Topical: Apply BID-QID

May produce diarrhea and GI side effects. Treat until 48–72 hr after resolution of symptoms. Drug is poorly absorbed through the GI tract. Do **not** swallow troches whole (allow to dissolve slowly). Oral suspension should be swished about the mouth and retained in the mouth as long as possible before swallowing.

OCTREOTIDE ACETATE

Sandostatin, Sandostatin LAR Depot
Somatostatin analog, antisecretory agent

Yes   ?   B

Inj (amps): 0.05, 0.1, 0.5 mg/mL (1 mL)
Inj (multi-dose vials): 0.2, 1 mg/mL (5 mL)
Inj, microspheres for suspension (Sandostatin LAR Depot): 10 mg/5 mL,
20 mg/5 mL, 30 mg/5 mL

Infants and children:
  Intractable diarrhea (IV/SC): 1–10 mcg/kg/24 hr ÷ Q12–24 hr. Dose may be increased within the recommended range by 0.3 mcg/kg/dose every 3 days as needed.
  Max. dose: 1500 mcg/24 hr

Cholelithiasis, hyperglycemia, hypoglycemia, nausea, diarrhea, abdominal discomfort, headache, and pain at injection site may occur. Growth hormone suppression may occur with long-term use. Cyclosporine levels may be reduced in patients receiving this drug.

Patients with severe renal failure requiring dialysis may require dosage adjustments due to an increase in half-life. The effects of hepatic dysfunction on octreotide have not been evaluated.

Sandostatin LAR Depot is administered once every 4 weeks **only** by the IM route and is currently indicated for use in adults who have been stabilized on IV/SC therapy. See package insert for details.

OFLOXACIN

Floxin, Floxin Otic, Ocuflox
Antibiotic, quinolone

Yes   1   C

Tabs: 200, 300, 400 mg
Inj: 4 mg/mL (10 mL)
Prediluted inj in D₅W: 200 mg/ 50 mL, 400 mg/100 mL
Otic solution (Floxin Otic): 0.3% (5 mL)
Ophthalmic solution (Ocuflox): 0.3% (1, 5 mL)

Adults:
   Lower respiratory tract, and skin infections: 400 mg PO/IV Q12 hr × 10 days
      Uncomplicated gonorrhea: 400 mg PO × 1, plus treatment for chlamydia.
   Nongonococcal (Chlamydia) urethritis, cervicitis: 300 mg PO/IV Q12 hr × 7 days
   PID: 400 mg PO BID × 10–14 days in combination with metronidazole
   UTI: 200 mg PO/IV Q12 hr × 3–10 days
   Prostatitis: 300 mg PO/IV Q12 hr × 6 weeks; **maximum** IV use at 10 days, convert
   to PO
Otitic use:
   Otitis externa:
      1–12 yr: 5 drops to affected ear(s) BID × 10 days
      >12 yr: 10 drops to affected ear(s) BID × 10 days
   Chronic suppurative otitis media:
      ≥12 yr: 10 drops to affected ear(s) BID × 14 days
   Acute otitis media with tympanostomy tubes:
      1–12 yr: 5 drops to affected ear(s) BID × 10 days
Ophthalmic use:
   >1 yr: 1 drop to affected eye(s) Q2–4 hr × 2 days, then QID for an additional 5 days

Like other quinolones, ofloxacin has caused arthropathy in immature animals;
use with **caution** in children <18 yr and in those with seizures. Common side
effects with systemic use include nausea, diarrhea, headache, insomnia and
dizziness. Rash, photosensitivity, pain, liver enzyme elevation, and neutropenia have
also been reported. Like most fluoroquinolones, drug may inhibit CYP 450 1A2 to
increase theophylline serum levels. Antacids, didanosine, sucralfate, and food may
impair oral absorption of ofloxacin. **Adjust dose in renal impairment (see p. 943).**
   Pruritus, local irritation, taste perversion, dizziness, and earache have been reported
with otic use. Ocular burning/discomfort is frequent with ophthalmic use.
   When using otic solution, warm solution by holding the bottle in the hand for
1-2 min. Cold solutions may result in dizziness. For otitis externa, patient should lie
with affected ear upward before instillation and remain in the same position after
dose administration for 5 min to enhance drug delivery. For acute otitis media with
tympanostomy tubes, patient should lie in the same position prior to instillation and
the tragus should be pumped four times after the dose to assist in drug delivery to the
middle ear.
   Administer oral doses on an empty stomach, 1 hr before or 2 hr after meals, and
avoid antacids containing magnesium or aluminum or products containing iron or zinc
within 4 hr before or 2 hr after dosing.
   Consult with ophthalmology in corneal ulcers.

For explanation of icons, see p. 572.

OLOPATADINE

Patanol
Antihistamine

No ? C

Ophthalmic solution: 0.1% (5 mL)

Allergic conjunctivitis:
≥3 yr and adults: 1–2 drops in affected eye(s) BID (spaced 6–8 hr apart)

DO NOT use while wearing contact lenses. Ocular side effects include burning or stinging, dry eye, foreign body sensation, hyperemia, keratitis, lid edema, and pruritis. May also cause headaches, asthenia, pharyngitis, rhinitis, and taste perversion.

OLSALAZINE

Dipentum, Di-mesalazine, Di-5-ASA
Salicylate, GI antiinflammatory agent

Yes 2 C

Caps: 250 mg

Ulcerative colitis:
Adult: 500 mg PO BID

Drug is converted to 5-aminosalicylic acid (mesalamine) by colonic bacteria. 1 g olsalazine generally delivers 0.9 g of mesalamine to the colon. Only 1% to 3% of olsalazine is systemically absorbed.

Contraindicated in salicylate hypersensitivity. Use with **caution** in severe liver disease, renal dysfunction, sulfasalazine hypersensitivity, and bronchial asthma. Diarrhea is the most common side effect. May also cause GI discomfort, headaches, rash, dizziness, and increased PT with warfarin use. Pancreatitis and hepatotoxicity in children have been reported. Monitor urinalysis and renal function.

Administer all doses with food to enhance efficacy.

Use in children (2-18 yr) has been limited to a trial in which olsalazine 30 mg/kg/ 24 hr (max. 2 g/24 hr) was found to be less efficacious than sulfasalazine 60 mg/kg/ 24 hr (max. 4 g/24 hr) in treating mild/moderate ulcerative colitis.

FORMULARY

OMEPRAZOLE

Prilosec
Gastric acid pump inhibitor

No   3   C

Caps, sustained release: 10, 20, 40 mg
Oral suspension: 2 mg/mL

Children:
Start at 0.6–0.7 mg/kg/dose PO QD. Dose may be increased to 0.6–0.7 mg/kg/dose PO BID if needed. Effective dosage range of 0.3–3.3 mg/kg/24 hr has been reported.

Adults:
Duodenal ulcer or GERD: 20 mg/dose PO QD × 4–8 weeks; may give up to 12 weeks for erosive esophagitis
Gastric ulcer: 40 mg/24 hr PO ÷ QD-BID × 4–8 weeks
Pathological hypersecretory conditions: Start with 60 mg/24 hr PO QD. If needed, dose may be increased up to 120 mg/24 hr PO ÷ TID. Daily doses >80 mg should be administered in divided doses.

Common side effects include headache, diarrhea, nausea, and vomiting. Allergic reactions, including anaphylaxis, have been reported. Drug induces CYP 450 1A2 (decreases theophylline levels) and is also a substrate and inhibitor of CYP 2C19. Increases $T_{1/2}$ of citalopram, diazepam, phenytoin, and warfarin. May decrease absorption of itraconazole, ketoconazole, iron salts, and ampicillin esters. May be used in combination with clarithromycin and amoxicillin for *H. pylori* infections.

Administer all doses before meals. Administer 30 min prior to sulcralfate. Capsules contain enteric-coated granules to ensure bioavailability. Do **not** chew or crush capsule. For doses unable to be divided by 10 mg, capsule may be opened and intact pellets may be administered in an acidic beverage (e.g., apple juice, cranberry juice) or apple sauce. The extemporaneously compounded oral suspension product may be less bioavailable due to the loss of the enteric coating.

ONDANSETRON

Zofran
Antiemetic agent, 5-HT₃ antagonist

No   ?   B

Inj: 2 mg/mL (2, 20 mL); contains parabens
Premix inj: 32 mg/50 mL
Tabs: 4, 8, 24 mg
Tabs, orally disintegrating: 4, 8 mg; contains aspartame
Oral solution: 4 mg/5 mL (50 mL)

Continued

ONDANSETRON *continued*

Preventing nausea and vomiting associated with chemotherapy:
Oral (give initial dose 30 min before chemotherapy):
  Children, dose based on body surface area:
    <0.3 m^2: 1 mg TID PRN nausea
    0.3–0.6 m^2: 2 mg TID PRN nausea
    0.6–1 m^2: 3 mg TID PRN nausea
    >1 m^2: 4–8 mg TID PRN nausea
  Dose based on age:
    <4 yr: Use dose based on body surface area from above.
    4–11 yr: 4 mg TID PRN nausea
    ≥12 yr and adults: 8 mg TID PRN nausea
  IV: Children and adults:
    Moderately emetogenic drugs: 0.15 mg/kg/dose at 30 min before, 4 and 8 hr after emetogenic drugs. Then same dose Q4 hr PRN nausea.
    Highly emetogenic drugs: 0.45 mg/kg/dose (max. 32 mg/dose) 30 min before emetogenic drugs. Then 0.15 mg/kg/dose Q4 hr PRN.
Preventing nausea and vomiting associated with surgery (see remarks):
  IV/IM (administered prior to anesthesia over 2-5 min.):
  Children (2-12 yr):
    ≤40 kg: 0.1 mg/kg/dose × 1
    >40 kg: 4 mg × 1
    Adults: 4 mg × 1
  PO:
    Adults: 16 mg × 1, 1 hr prior to induction of anesthesia
Preventing nausea and vomiting associated with radiation therapy (adults):
  Total body irradiation: 8 mg PO 1-2 hr prior to radiation QD
  Single high-dose fraction radiation to abdomen: 8 mg PO 1-2 hr prior to radiation with subsequent doses Q8 hr after first dose × 1-2 days after completion of radiation
  Daily fractionated radiation to abdomen: 8 mg PO 1-2 hr prior to radiation with subsequent doses Q8 hr after first dose for each day radiation is given

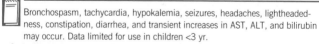

Bronchospasm, tachycardia, hypokalemia, seizures, headaches, lightheadedness, constipation, diarrhea, and transient increases in AST, ALT, and bilirubin may occur. Data limited for use in children <3 yr.

Ondansetron is a substrate for cytochrome P 450 1A2, 2D6, 2E1, and 3A3/4 drug metabolizing enzymes. It is likely that the inhibition/loss of one of the above enzymes will be compensated by others and may result in insignificant changes to ondansetron's elimination. Ondansetron's elimination may be affected by cytochrome P 450 enzyme inducers. Follow theophylline, phenytoin, or warfarin levels closely, if used in combination.

Additional postoperative doses for controlling nausea and vomiting may not provide any benefits.

In severe hepatic impairment, extend dosage interval up to QD and limit **max. dose** to 8 mg/dose.

Administer orally disintegrating tablet by placing it on the tongue and swallowing it with or without taking liquids.

OPIUM TINCTURE

Deodorized tincture of opium
Narcotic, analgesic

No　2　B/D

Liquid: 10% opium. Contains 17%–21% alcohol (1 mL equivalent to 10 mg morphine)

Dilute 25-fold with water to make a final concentration of 0.4 mg/mL morphine equivalent.
Neonatal opiate withdrawal:
Start with 0.2–0.3 mL/dose Q3–4 hr, increase dose by 0.05 mL/dose Q3–4 hr until symptoms abate; **max. dose:** 0.7 mL/dose

Use 25-fold dilution to treat neonatal abstinence syndrome (NAS). Follow neonatal abstinence scores. **Doses for the dilution are equivalent to paregoric doses.** Morphine may also be used to treat NAS. May cause respiratory depression, hypotension, bradycardia, and CNS depression. Pregnancy category changes to "D" if used for prolonged periods or in high doses at term.

OSELTAMIVIR PHOSPHATE

Tamiflu
Antiviral

Yes　?　C

Caps: 75 mg
Oral suspension: 12 mg/mL (100 mL); contains saccharin

Treatment of influenza (initiate therapy within 2 days of onset of symptoms):
Children 1–12 yr: See table below

Weight (kg)	Dosage for 5 Days	Volume of Oral Suspension (mL)
≤15	30 mg PO BID	2.5
15–23	45 mg PO BID	3.75
23–40	60 mg PO BID	5
>40	75 mg PO BID	6.25

>12 yr and adults: 75 mg PO BID × 5 days
Prophylaxis of influenza (see remarks):
≥13 yr and adults: 75 mg PO QD × 7 days; initiate therapy within 2 days of exposure

Continued

OSELTAMIVIR PHOSPHATE *continued*

Nausea and vomiting generally occuring within the first 2 days and are the most common adverse effects. Insomnia, vertigo, seizures, arrhythmias, rash, and toxic epidermal necrolysis have also been reported. Adjust treatment interval if GFR is 10–30 mL/min to 75 mg PO QD × 5 days (for >12 yr and adults).

PROPHYLAXIS USE: Oseltamivir is not a substitute for annual flu vaccination. Safety and efficacy have been demonstrated for ≤6 weeks; duration of protection lasts for as long as dosing is continued. Adjust prophylaxis interval if GFR is 10–30 mL/min to 75 mg PO QOD (for >12 yr and adults).

Dosage adjustments in hepatic impairment, severe renal disease, and dialysis have not been established for either treatment or prophylaxis use. The safety and efficacy of repeated treatment or prophylaxis courses have not been evaluated. Doses may be administered with or without food.

OXACILLIN

Bactocil, Prostaphlin
Antibiotic, penicillin (penicillinase resistant)

Yes   ?   B

Caps: 250, 500 mg
Oral solution: 250 mg/5 mL (100 mL); contains 0.8 mEq Na per 250 mg drug and may contain saccharin
Inj: 0.25, 0.5, 1, 2, 4, 10 g; contains 2.8-3.1 mEq Na per 1 g drug

Neonates, IM/IV: Doses are the same as for nafcillin.
Infants and children:
  Oral: 50–100 mg/kg/24 hr ÷ Q6 hr
  IM/IV: 100–200 mg/kg/24 hr ÷ Q4–6 hr
  Max. dose: 12 g/24 hr
Adults:
  Oral: 500–1000 mg/dose Q4–6 hr
  IM/IV: 250–2000 mg/dose Q4–6 hr

Side effects include allergy, diarrhea, nausea, vomiting, leukopenia, and hepatotoxicity. CSF penetration is poor unless meninges are inflamed. Acute interstitial nephritis has been reported. Hematuria and azotemia have occurred in neonates and infants with high doses. Use the lower end of the usual dosage range for patients with creatinine clearances <10 mL/min. Oral form should be administered on an empty stomach. **Adjust dose in renal failure (see p. 945).**

OXCARBAZEPINE

Trileptal
Anticonvulsant

Yes   ?   C

Tabs: 150, 300, 600 mg
Oral suspension: 300 mg/5 mL (250 mL); contains saccharin and ethanol

---

Children (4–16 yr, see remarks):
   Adjunctive therapy: Start with 8–10 mg/kg/24 hr PO ÷ BID up to a **maximum** of 600 mg/24 hr. Then gradually increase the dose over a 2-week period to the following maintenance doses:
     20–29 kg: 900 mg/24 hr PO ÷ BID
     29.1–39 kg: 1200 mg/24 hr PO ÷ BID
     >39 kg: 1800 mg/24 hr PO ÷ BID
Adults:
   Adjunctive therapy: Start with 600 mg/24 hr PO ÷ BID. Dose may be increased at weekly intervals, as clinically indicated, by a **maximum** of 600 mg/24 hr. Usual maintenance dose is 1200 mg/24 hr PO ÷ BID. Doses ≥2400 mg/24 hr are generally not well tolerated due to CNS side effects.
   Conversion to monotherapy: Start with 600 mg/24 hr PO ÷ BID and simultaneously initiate dosage reduction of concomitant AEDs. Dose may be increased at weekly intervals, as clinically indicated, by a **maximum** of 600 mg/24 hr to achieve a dose of 2400 mg/24 hr PO ÷ BID. Concomitant AEDs should be terminated gradually over approximately 3–6 weeks.
   Initiation of monotherapy: Start with 600 mg/24 hr PO ÷ BID. Then increase by 300 mg/24 hr every 3 days up to 1200 mg/24 hr PO ÷ BID.

Clinically significant hyponatremia may occur; generally seen within the first 3 mo of therapy. May also cause headache, dizziness, drowsiness, ataxia, fatigue, nystagmus, diplopia, abnormal gait, and GI discomfort. Approximately 25%-30% of patients with carbamazepine hypersensitivity will experience a cross reaction with oxcarbazepine.
   Inhibits CYP 450 2C19 and induces CYP 450 3A4/5 drug metabolizing enzymes. Carbamazepine, phenobarbital, phenytoin, valproic acid, and verapamil may decrease oxcarbazepine levels. Oxcarbazepine may increase phenobarbital and phenytoin levels. Oxcarbazepine can decrease the effects of oral contraceptives, felodipine, and lamotrigine.
   A median pediatric maintenance dose of 31 mg/kg/24 hr (range: 6–51 mg/kg/24 hr) was achieved in a clinical trial. Adjust dosage if GFR <30 mL/min by administering 50% of the normal starting dose (**max. dose:** 300 mg/24 hr) followed by a slower than normal increase in dose if necessary. No dosage adjustment is required in mild/moderate hepatic impairment.
   Doses may be administered with or without food.

OXYBUTYNIN CHLORIDE

Ditropan, Ditropan XL, and others
Anticholinergic agent, antispasmodic

Yes   ?   B

Tabs: 5 mg
Tabs, extended release (Ditropan XL): 5, 10, 15 mg
Syrup: 1 mg/mL (473 mL); contains parabens

Child ≤5 yr: 0.2 mg/kg/dose BID-QID PO; **max. dose:** 15 mg/24 hr
Child >5 yr: 5 mg/dose BID-TID PO; **max. dose:** 15 mg/24 hr
Adult:
Immediate release: 5 mg/dose BID-QID PO
Extended release (Ditropan XL): 5–10 mg/dose QD PO up to a **maximum** of 30 mg/
dose QD PO

Use with **caution** in hepatic or renal disease, hyperthyroidism, IBD, or
cardiovascular disease. Anticholinergic side effects may occur, including
drowsiness and hallucinations. **Contraindicated** in glaucoma, GI obstruction,
megacolon, myasthenia gravis, severe colitis, hypovolemia, and GU obstruction. May
increase atenolol and digoxin levels. May decrease haloperidol levels.
   Dosage adjustments for the extended-release dosage form should be made at weekly
intervals. Do not crush, chew, or divide the extended-release tablets.

OXYCODONE

Roxicodone, Oxycontin, and others
Narcotic, analgesic

Yes   2   B/D

Solution: 1 mg/mL (8% alcohol and saccharin), 20 mg/mL (saccharin)
Tabs: 5 mg
Controlled-release tabs (Oxycontin): 10, 20, 40, 80, 160 mg **(80 and 160 mg
strengths for opioid-tolerant patients only)**
Caps: 5 mg

Dose based on oxycodone salt:
Children: 0.05–0.15 mg/kg/dose Q4–6 hr PRN up to 5 mg/dose PO
Adults: 5–10 mg Q4–6 hr PRN PO; see remarks for use of controlled-release
tabs.

Abuse potential, CNS and respiratory depression, increased ICP, histamine
release, constipation, and GI distress may occur. Use with **caution** in severe
renal impairment. **Naloxone is the antidote.** See p. 894 for equianalgesic
dosing. Check dosages of acetaminophen or aspirin when using combination products

Continued

FORMULARY

OXYCODONE *continued*

(e.g., Tylox, Percodan). Aspirin is **not** recommended in children due to concerns of Reye's syndrome. Oxycodone is metabolized by the cytochrome P 450 2D6 isoenzyme.

When using controlled-release tablets (Oxycontin), determine patient's total 24-hr requirements and divide by two to administer on a Q12-hr dosing interval. Oxycontin 80 mg and 160 mg tablets are **USED ONLY** for opioid-tolerant patients; these strengths can cause fatal respiratory depression in opioid-naïve patients. Controlled-release dosage form **should not be used** as a PRN analgesic.

Pregnancy category changes to "D" if used for prolonged periods or in high doses at term.

OXYCODONE AND ACETAMINOPHEN

Tylox, Roxilox, Percocet, Endocet, Roxicet, and others
Combination analgesic with a narcotic   Yes   2   C

Capsule/Caplet: Acetaminophen 500 mg + oxycodone HCl 5 mg
Tabs:
   Most common strength: Acetaminophen 325 mg + oxycodone HCl 5 mg
   Other strengths: Acetaminophen 325 mg + oxycodone HCl 2.5 mg, acetaminophen 500 mg + oxycodone HCl 7.5 mg, acetaminophen 650 mg + oxycodone HCl 10 mg
Solution: Acetaminophen 325 mg + oxycodone HCl 5 mg/5 mL; contains 0.4% alcohol and saccharin

Dose based on amount of oxycodone and acetaminophen.

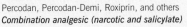

See *Oxycodone* and *Acetaminophen.*

OXYCODONE AND ASPIRIN

Percodan, Percodan-Demi, Roxiprin, and others
Combination analgesic (narcotic and salicylate)   Yes   2   D

Tabs:
   (Percodan or Roxiprin): Aspirin 325 mg, oxycodone HCl 4.5 mg, and oxycodone tereph 0.38 mg
   (Percodan-Demi): Aspirin 325 mg, oxycodone HCl 2.25 mg, and oxycodone tereph 0.19 mg

Dose based on amount of oxycodone (combined salts) and aspirin.

Continued

For explanation of icons, see p. 572.

OXYCODONE AND ASPIRIN *continued*

 See *Oxycodone* and *Aspirin.* Do **not** use in children <16 yr because of risk for Reye's syndrome.

OXYMETAZOLINE

Nasal: Afrin, Allerest 12 Hour Nasal, Nostrilla, and others
Ophthalmic: OcuClear, Visine LR
Nasal decongestant, vasoconstrictor

No ? C

Nasal drops (OTC): 0.025% (20 mL), 0.05% (15, 20 mL)
Nasal spray (OTC): 0.05% (15, 30 mL)
Ophthalmic drops (OTC): 0.025% (15, 30 mL)

Nasal decongestant (not to exceed 3 days in duration):
2–5 yr: 2–3 drops of 0.025% solution in each nostril BID
  ≥6 yr–adults: 2–3 sprays or 2–3 drops of 0.05% solution in each nostril BID
Ophthalmic:
  ≥6 yr–adults: Instill 1–2 drops in the affected eye(s) Q6 hr

Contraindicated in patients on MAO inhibitor therapy. Rebound nasal congestion may occur with excessive use (>3 days) via the nasal route. Systemic absorption may occur with either route of administration. Headache, dizziness, hypertension, transient burning, stinging, dryness, nasal mucosa ulceration, sneezing, blurred vision, and mydriasis have occurred. Do **not** use ophthalmic solution if it changes color or becomes cloudy.

PALIVIZUMAB

Synagis
Monoclonal antibody

No ? C

Inj: 50, 100 mg

RSV prophylaxis (see p. 339 and latest edition of the AAP Red Book for most recent indications):
  ≤2 yr with chronic lung disease, premature infants (≤28 weeks gestation) <12 mo, or premature infants (29–32 weeks gestation) <6 mo: 15 mg/kg/dose IM Q monthly just prior to and during the RSV season.

Continued

PALIVIZUMAB continued

RSV season is typically November through April in the northern hemisphere but may begin earlier or persist later in certain communities. Use with **caution** in patients with thrombocytopenia or any coagulation disorder because of IM route of administration. IM is currently the only route of administration. The following adverse effects have been reported at slightly higher incidences when compared to placebo: rhinitis, rash, pain, increased liver enzymes, pharyngitis, cough, wheeze, diarrhea, vomiting, conjunctivitis, and anemia.

Advantages over intravenous RSV Immune Globulin include smaller fluid volume of drug, ease of IM injection (compared to lengthy IV infusion), and does not interfere with the response to routine childhood vaccines.

Palivizumab is currently indicated for RSV prophylaxis only; currently being evaluated in congenital heart disease; and has not been evaluated in immunocompromised children.

Each dose should be administered IM in the anterolateral aspect of the thigh. It is recommended to divide doses with total injection volumes >1 mL. **Avoid** injection in the gluteal muscle because of risk for damage to the sciatic nerve. Reconstitute each vial with 1 mL sterile water for injection and gently swirl the contents. Dose should be administered within 6 hr of reconstitution.

PAMIDRONATE

Aredia
Bisphosphonate derivative, hypercalcemia antidote

Yes ? C

Inj: 30, 90 mg; contains mannitol

Hypercalcemia (dose may be repeated after 7 days, see remarks):
Children (limited data; see Journal Clin Oncology 17(6):1960; 1999):
  Mild hypercalcemia: 0.5–1 mg/kg/dose IV × 1
  Severe hypercalcemia: 1.5–2 mg/kg/dose IV × 1
Adults:
  Corrected serum Ca^{++} 12–13.5 mg/dL: 60 mg IV × 1 over 4 hr **OR** 90 mg IV × 1 over 24 hr
  Corrected serum Ca^{++} > 13.5 mg/dL: 90 mg IV × 1 over 24 hr
Osteogenesis imperfecta (limited data):
  Children: 0.5–1 mg/kg/dose IV QD × 3 days; may be repeated in 4–6 mo
Paget's disease:
  Adults: 30 mg IV over 4 hr QD × 3 days

May cause headache, hypertension, GI discomfort, uveitis, hyperpyrexia, and decrease in serum calcium, phosphorus, potassium, and magnesium. Use **caution** in renal impairment. Maintain adequate hydration and urinary output during treatment. Longer infusion times (2–24 hr) may decrease the risk of renal toxicity, especially in patients with renal insufficiency.

Continued

PAMIDRONATE *continued*

USE IN HYPERCALCEMIA: Correct serum Ca⁺⁺ for low serum albumin (a change in serum albumin of 1 g/dL changes serum Ca^{++} in the same direction by 0.8 mg/dL). Local redness, swelling, induration, or pain on palpation at the catheter site is common in patients receiving a 90-mg dose. Seizures have been reported.

PANCREATIC ENZYMES

No   ?   C

See p. 914, for description and contents of lipase, protease, and amylase.

Initial doses (actual requirements are patient specific):
Enteric-coated microspheres and microtabs:
  Infants: 2000–4000 U lipase per 120 mL formula or per breast feeding
  Children <4 yr: 1000 U lipase/kg/meal
  Children ≥4 yr: 500 U lipase/kg/meal
  Max. dose: 2500 U lipase/kg/meal
The total daily dose should include approximately three meals and two to three snacks per day. Snack doses are approximately half of meal doses.

May cause occult GI bleeding, allergic reactions to porcine proteins, hyperuricemia, and hyperuricosuria with high doses. Dose should be titrated to eliminate diarrhea and to minimize steatorrhea. Do **not** chew microspheres or microtabs. Concurrent administration with H_2 antagonists or gastric acid pump inhibitors may enhance enzyme efficacy. Doses higher than 6000 U lipase/kg/meal have been associated with colonic strictures in children <12 yr. Powder dosage form is not preferred due to potential GI mucosal ulceration. Avoid use of generic pancreatic enzyme products because they have been associated with treatment failures.

PANCURONIUM BROMIDE
Pavulon and others
Nondepolarizing neuromuscular blocking agent

Yes   ?   C

Inj: 1, 2 mg/mL (contains 1% benzyl alcohol)

Neonate:
Initial: 0.02 mg/kg/dose IV
  Maintenance: 0.05–0.1 mg/kg/dose Q 0.5–4 hr PRN
1 mo–adult:
  Initial: 0.04–0.1 mg/kg/dose IV
  Maintenance: 0.015–0.1 mg/kg/dose IV Q30–60 min
  Continuous IV infusion: 0.1 mg/kg/hr

Continued

PANCURONIUM BROMIDE *continued*

Onset of action is 1–2 min. May cause tachycardia, salivation, and wheezing. Drug effects may be accentuated by hypothermia, acidosis, neonatal age, decreased renal function, halothane, succinylcholine, hypokalemia, hyponatremia, hypocalcemia, clindamycin, tetracycline, and aminoglycoside antibiotics. Drug effects may be antagonized by alkalosis, hypercalcemia, peripheral neuropathies, diabetes mellitus, demyelinating lesions, carbamazepine, phenytoin, theophylline, anticholinesterases (e.g., neostigmine, pyridostigmine) and azathioprine.

Antidote is neostigmine (with atropine or glycopyrrolate). **Avoid** use in severe renal impairment (<10 mL/min).

PAREGORIC

Camphorated opium tincture
Narcotic, analgesic

No   2   B

Camphorated tincture: 2 mg (morphine equivalent)/5 mL (some preparations contain up to 45% alcohol)

Analgesia:
  Children: 0.25–0.5 mL/kg/dose PO QD-QID
  Adults: 5–10 mL/dose PO QD-QID
Neonatal opiate withdrawal:
  Start with 0.2–0.3 mL/dose Q3–4 hr, increase dose by 0.05 mL/dose Q3–4 hr until symptoms abate; **max. dose:** 0.7 mL/dose

Morphine or DTO is preferred over paregoric because of excipients found in paregoric. Each 5 mL of paregoric contains 2 mg morphine equivalent, 0.02 mL anise oil, 20 mg benzoic acid, 20 mg camphor, 0.2 mL glycerin and alcohol. The final concentration of morphine equivalent is 0.4 mg/mL. This is 25-fold less potent than undiluted deodorized tincture of opium (DTO: 10 mg morphine equivalent/mL). **If using DTO to treat neonatal abstinence, must dilute 25-fold prior to use.** Similar side effects to morphine. After symptoms are controlled for several days, dose for opiate withdrawal should be decreased gradually over a 2- to 4-week period (e.g., by 10% Q2–3 days). Monitor neonatal abstinence scores for NAS.

PAROMOMYCIN SULFATE

Humatin
Amebicide, antibiotic (aminoglycoside)

No   ?   C

Caps: 250 mg

Continued

see p. 572.

PAROMOMYCIN SULFATE *continued*

Intestinal amebiasis (Entamoeba histolytica), Dientamoeba fragilis, and Giardia lamblia infection:
  Children and adults: 25–35 mg/kg/24 hr PO ÷ Q8 hr × 7 days
Tapeworm (see remarks):
  Children: 11 mg/kg/dose PO Q15 min × 4 doses
  Adults: 1 g PO Q15 min × 4 doses
Tapeworm (Hymenolepis nana):
  Children and adults: 45 mg/kg/dose PO QD × 5–7 days
Cryptosporidial diarrhea:
  Children: 25–35 mg/kg/24 hr PO ÷ BID-QID; see latest edition of the AAP *Red Book*
  Adult: 1.5–3 g/24 hr PO ÷ 3–6 × daily. Duration varies from 10-14 days to 4–8 weeks. Maintenance therapy has also been used. Alternatively, 1 g PO BID × 12 weeks in conjunction with azithromycin 600 mg PO QD × 4 weeks has been used in patients with AIDS.

Tapeworms affected by short-duration therapy include *T. saginata, T. solium, D. latum,* and *D. caninum.* Drug is poorly absorbed and therefore not indicated for sole treatment of extraintestinal amebiasis. Side effects include GI disturbance, hematuria, rash, ototoxicity, and hypocholesterolemia. May decrease the effects of digoxin.

PAROXETINE

Paxil
Antidepressant, selective serotonin reuptake inhibitor (SSRI)   Yes   3   C

Tabs: 10, 20, 30, 40 mg
Oral suspension: 10 mg/5 mL (250 mL); contains saccharin and parabens

Children:
  Depression (limited data, in an open labeled trial of 45 children <14 yr—mean age 10.7 ± 2 yr): Start with 10 mg PO QD. If needed, adjust upwards. A mean dose of 16.2 mg/24 hr was used for an average of 8.4 mo in the open label trial. Additional studies are needed.
  Obesessive-compulsive disorder (limited data, based on a 12-week open labeled trial of 20 children 8–17 yr—mean age 11.1 ± 2.5 yr): Start with 10 mg PO QD. If needed, adjust upwards by increasing dose no more than 10 mg Q2 weeks up to a **maximum** of 60 mg/24 hr. A mean dose of 41.1 mg/24 hr was used resulting with a ≥30% reduction in OCD symptom severity (CY-BOCS score).
Adult:
  Depression: Start with 20 mg PO QAM × 4 weeks. If no clinical improvement, increase dose by 10 mg/24 hr Q7 days PRN up to a **maximum** of 50 mg/24 hr.
  Obsessive-compulsive disorder: Start with 20 mg PO QD; increase dose by 10 mg/24 hr Q 7 days PRN up to a **maximum** of 60 mg/24 hr. Usual dose is 40 mg PO QD.

Continued

FORMULARY

PAROXETINE *continued*

> *Panic disorder:* Start with 10 mg PO QD; increase dose by 10 mg/24 hr Q 7 days PRN up to a **maximum** of 60 mg/24 hr.
> *Social/generalized anxiety disorder:* 20 mg PO QAM

> **Contraindicated** in patients taking MAO inhibitors, within 14 days of discontinuing MAO inhibitors, or thioridazine. Common side effects include anxiety, nausea, anorexia, and decreased appetite. Paroxetine is an inhibitor and substrate for CYP 450 2D6. May increase the effects/toxicity of tricyclic antidepressants, theophylline, and warfarin. Cimetidine, ritonavir, MAO inhibitors (fatal serotonin syndrome), dextromethorphan, phenothiazines, and type 1C antiarrhythmics may increase the effect/toxicity of paroxetine. Weakness, hyperreflexia, and poor coordination have been reported when taken with sumatriptan.
>
> Patients with severe renal or hepatic impairment should initiate therapy at 10 mg/24 hr and increase dose as needed up to a **maximum** of 40 mg/24 hr. Do **not** discontinue therapy abruptly; may cause sweating, dizziness, confusion, and tremor. May be taken with or without food.

PEMOLINE
Cylert
CNS stimulant

Yes   ?   B

Tabs: 18.75, 37.5, 75 mg
Chewable tabs: 37.5 mg

> *Children ≥6 yr:*
> *Initial:* 37.5 mg QAM PO
> *Increment:* 18.75 mg/24 hr at weekly intervals
> *Maintenance:* 0.5–3 mg/kg/24 hr (*effective dose range:* 56.25–75 mg/24 hr)
> **Max. dose:** 112.5 mg/24 hr
> Effect may not be seen for 3–4 weeks. **Do not abruptly discontinue drug.**

> May cause insomnia, headache, seizures, anorexia, hypersensitivity, depression, abdominal pain, movement disorders, hepatotoxicity, and drug dependence.
> Use with **caution** in renal disease (~50% excreted in urine unchanged).
> **Contraindicated** in hepatic disease or abnormal LFTs and Tourette syndrome. Long-term use associated with growth inhibition. **Not recommended for children <6 yr.**
>
> Patients who fail to show substantial clinical benefit after completing the dose titration to the maximum daily dose should be withdrawn from therapy due to risk of hepatotoxicity. **Fatal hepatotoxicity** has been reported. Pemoline should be discontinued if serum ALT is increased more than two times the upper normal limit, or if clinical signs and symptoms suggest liver faliure. Baseline and periodic LFTs are recommended.

PENICILLAMINE

Cuprimine, Depen
Heavy metal chelator

Yes   ?   D

Tabs: 250 mg
Caps: 125, 250 mg
Suspension: 50 mg/mL

Lead chelation therapy (third-line therapy):
  Children: 30–40 mg/kg/24 hr or 600–750 mg/m^2/24 hr PO ÷ TID–QID.
    Max. dose: 1.5 g/24 hr
  Adults: 1–1.5 g/24 hr PO ÷ BID–TID
  Durations of treatment vary from 1–6 mo.
Wilson's disease (see remarks for titration information):
  Infants and children: 20 mg/kg/24 hr PO ÷ BID–QID. **Max. dose:** 1 g/24 hr
  Adults: 250 mg/dose PO QID. **Max. dose:** 2 g/24 hr
Arsenic poisoning:
  100 mg/kg/24 hr PO ÷ Q6 hr × 5 days. **Max. dose:** 1 g/24 hr
Cystinuria (see remarks for titration information):
  Infants and young children: 30 mg/kg/24 hr ÷ QID PO
  Older children and adults: 1–4 g/24 hr ÷ QID PO
Primary biliary cirrhosis (adults):
  Initial: 250 mg/24 hr PO; increase by 250 mg Q2 weeks to a total of 1 g/24 hr
  (given as 250 mg QID)
Juvenile rheumatoid arthritis:
  5 mg/kg/24 hr ÷ QD–BID PO × 2 mo, then 10 mg/kg/24 hr ÷ QD–BID PO × 4 mo

Dose should be given 1 hr before or 2 hr after meals. **AAP relegates this drug as a third-line agent for lead chelation indicated only after unacceptable reaction with oral succimer and calcium EDTA (see pp. 35–38).** If used, must be in lead-free environment because it can increase absorption of lead if present in GI tract. **Avoid** use if patient's creatinine clearance is <50 mL/min. Follow CBC, LFTs, and urinalysis. Can cause optic neuritis, fever, rash, nausea, altered taste, vomiting, lupus-like syndrome, nephrotic syndrome, peripheral neuropathy, leukopenia, eosinophilia, and thrombocytopenia. May reduce serum digoxin levels. **Avoid** concomitant administration with iron, antacids, and food.

Patients treated for Wilson's disease, rheumatoid arthritis, or cystinuria should be treated with pyridoxine 25–50 mg/24 hr. Titrate urinary copper excretion to >1 mg/24 hr for patients with Wilson's disease. Patients with cystinuria should have doses titrated to maintain urinary cystine excretion at <100–200 mg/24 hr.

PENICILLIN G PREPARATIONS—
AQUEOUS POTASSIUM AND SODIUM

Yes   ?   B

Various trade names
Antibiotic, aqueous penicillin

Inj (K⁺): 1, 5, 10, 20 million U (contains 1.7 mEq K and 0.3 mEq Na/1 million U Pen G)
Pre-mixed frozen inj (K⁺): 1 million U in 50 mL dextrose 4%; 2 million U in 50 mL dextrose 2.3%; 3 million U in 50 mL dextrose 0.7% (contains 1.7 mEq K and 0.3 mEq Na/1 million U Pen G)
Inj (Na⁺): 5 million U (contains 2 mEq Na/1 million U Pen G)
Conversion: 250 mg = 400,000 U

Neonates: IM/IV
  ≤7 days:
    ≤2 kg: 50,000–100,000 U/kg/24 hr ÷ Q12 hr
    >2 kg: 75,000–150,000 U/kg/24 hr ÷ Q8 hr
  >7 days:
    <1.2 kg: 50,000–100,000 U/kg/24 hr ÷ Q12 hr
    1.2–2 kg: 75,000–150,000 U/kg/24 hr ÷ Q8 hr
    ≥2 kg: 100,000–200,000 U/kg/24 hr ÷ Q6 hr
  Group B streptococcal meningitis:
    ≤7 days: 250,000–450,000 U/kg/24 hr ÷ Q8 hr
    >7 days: 450,000 U/kg/24 hr ÷ Q6 hr
Infants and children:
  IM/IV: 100,000–400,000 U/kg/24 hr ÷ Q4–6 hr; **max. dose:** 24 million U/24 hr
Adults:
  IM/IV: 4–24 million U/24 hr ÷ Q4–6 hr
Congenital syphilis, neurosyphilis: See pp. 358–359.

Use penicillin V potassium for oral use. Side effects include anaphylaxis, urticaria, hemolytic anemia, interstitial nephritis, Jarisch-Herxheimer reaction (syphilis). T₁/₂ = 30 min; may be prolonged by concurrent use of probenecid. For meningitis, use higher daily dose at shorter dosing intervals. For the treatment of anthrax *(Bacillus anthracis),* see www.cdc.gov for additional information. May cause false-positive or negative urinary glucose (Clinitest method), false-positive direct Coombs', and false-positive urinary and/or serum proteins.
Adjust dose in renal impairment (see p. 944).

PENICILLIN G PREPARATIONS— BENZATHINE

Permapen, Bicillin L-A   No   ?   B
Antibiotic, penicillin (very long-acting IM)

Inj: 300,000, 600,000 U/mL (contains parabens and povidone)
Injection should be IM only.

Group A streptococci:
Infants and children: 25,000–50,000 U/kg/dose IM × 1. **Max. dose:** 1.2 million U/dose
Or
>1 mo and <27 kg: 600,000 U/dose IM × 1
≥27 kg and adults: 1.2 million U/dose IM × 1
Rheumatic fever prophylaxis:
Infants and children: 25,000–50,000 U/kg/dose IM Q3–4 weeks. **Max. dose:** 1.2 million U/dose
Adults: 1.2 million U/dose IM Q3–4 weeks or 600,000 U/dose IM Q2 weeks
Syphilis: Early acquired and >1 yr duration: See p. 362.

Provides sustained levels for 2–4 weeks. Side effects same as for Penicillin G.
Do not administer intravenously; cardiac arrest and death may occur.

PENICILLIN G PREPARATIONS— PENICILLIN G BENZATHINE AND PENICILLIN G PROCAINE

Bicillin C-R, Bicillin C-R 900/300   No   ?   B
Antibiotic, penicillin (very long acting)

Bicillin CR:
  150,000 U PenG procaine + 150,000 U PenG benzathine/mL to provide 300,000 U penicillin per 1 mL (10 mL vial)
  300,000 U PenG procaine + 300,000 U PenG benzathine/mL to provide 600,000 U penicillin per 1 mL (1, 2 mL tubex, 4 mL syringe)
Bicillin CR (900/300): 150,000 U PenG procaine + 450,000 U PenG benzathine/mL (2 mL tubex)
All preparations contain parabens and povidone.
Injection should be for IM use only.

Acute streptococcal infection: Dose such that PenG benzathine is given in recommended amount (2000 AAP *Red Book,* p. 531). See doses for PenG benzathine.

Continued

For explanation of icons, see p. 572.

PENICILLIN G PREPARATIONS—PENICILLIN G BENZATHINE AND PENICILLIN G PROCAINE *continued*

This preparation provides early peak levels in addition to prolonged levels of penicillin in the blood. **Do not administer IV.** The addition of procaine penicillin has not been shown to be more efficacious than benzathine alone. However, it may reduce injection discomfort.

PENICILLIN G PREPARATIONS— PROCAINE

No ? B

Wycillin, Crysticillin A.S., Pfizerpen-AS
Antibiotic, penicillin (long-acting IM)

Inj: 300,000 (10 mL), 500,000 (1.2 mL), 600,000 U/ml (1, 2, 4 mL); may contain parabens, phenol, povidone, and formaldehyde
Contains 120 mg procaine per 300,000 U penicillin

Newborns (see remarks): 50,000 U/kg/24 hr IM QD
Infants and children: 25,000–50,000 U/kg/24 hr ÷ Q12–24 hr IM. **Max. dose:** 4.8 million U/24 hr
Adults: 0.6–4.8 million U/24 hr ÷ Q12–24 hr IM
Congenital syphilis, syphilis, neurosyphilis: See pp. 358–359.

Provides sustained levels for 2–4 days. Use with **caution** in neonates because of higher incidence of sterile abscess at injection site and risk of procaine toxicity. Side effects similar to Penicillin G. In addition, may cause CNS stimulation and seizures. **Do not administer IV;** neurovascular damage may result. Large doses may be administered in two injection sites. No longer recommended for empiric treatment of gonorrhea because of resistant strains.

PENICILLIN V POTASSIUM

Yes ? B

Pen Vee K, V-Cillin K, and others
Antibiotic, penicillin

Tabs: 125, 250, 500 mg
Oral solution: 125 mg/5 mL, 250 mg/5 mL; may contain saccharin
Contains 0.7 mEq potassium/250 mg drug
250 mg = 400,000 U

Continued

PENICILLIN V POTASSIUM *continued*

Children: 25–50 mg/kg/24 hr ÷ Q6–8 hr PO. **Max. dose:** 3 g/24 hr
Adults: 250–500 mg/dose PO Q6–8 hr
  Acute group A streptococcal pharyngitis:
Children: 250 mg PO BID–TID × 10 days
Adolescents and adults: 500 mg PO BID–TID × 10 days
Rheumatic fever/pneumococcal prophylaxis:
  ≤5 yr: 125 mg PO BID
  >5 yr: 250 mg PO BID

See *Penicillin G Preparations—Aqueous Potassium and Sodium* for side effects
and drug-lab interactions. GI absorption is better than penicillin G. Note: Must
be taken 1 hr before or 2 hr after meals. Penicillin will prevent rheumatic fever
if started within 9 days of the acute illness. The BID regimen for streptococcal pharyngitis should be used only if good compliance is expected. **Adjust dose in renal failure
(see p. 944).**

PENTAMIDINE ISETHIONATE
Pentam 300, NebuPent
Antibiotic, antiprotozoal   Yes   ?   C

Inj: 300 mg (Pentam 300)
Inhalation: 300 mg (NebuPent)

Treatment:
Pneumocystis carinii: 4 mg/kg/24 hr IM/IV QD × 14–21 days
  Trypanosomiasis (T. gambiense, T. rhodesiense): 4 mg/kg/24 hr IM QD ×
10 days
  Leishmaniasis (L. donovani): 2–4 mg/kg/dose IM QD or QOD × 15 doses
Prophylaxis:
  Pneumocystis carinii:
  IM/IV: 4 mg/kg/dose Q2–4 weeks
  Inhalation (≥5 yr): 300 mg in 6 ml H_2O via inhalation Q month (Respigard II
  nebulizer). See also p. 368 for indications.
  Trypanosomiasis (T. gambiense, T. rhodesiense): 4 mg/kg/24 hr IM q3–6 mo.
Max. single dose: 300 mg

Use with **caution** in ventricular tachycardia, Stevens Johnson syndrome, and
daily doses >21 days. May cause hypoglycemia, hyperglycemia, hypotension
(both IV and IM administration), nausea, vomiting, fever, mild hepatotoxicity,
pancreatitis, megaloblastic anemia, nephrotoxicity, hypocalcemia, and granulocytopenia. Additive nephrotoxicity with aminoglycosides, amphotericin B, cisplatin, and
vancomycin may occur. Aerosol administration may also cause bronchospasm, oxygen
desaturation, dyspnea, and loss of appetite. Infuse IV over 1-2 hr to reduce the risk
of hypotension. Sterile abscess may occur at IM injection site.
Adjust dose in renal impairment (see p. 944).

PENTOBARBITAL

Nembutal and others
Barbiturate

No ? D

Caps: 50, 100 mg
Suppository: 30, 60, 120, 200 mg
Inj: 50 mg/mL; contains prophylene glycol and 10% alcohol
Elixir: 18.2 mg/5 mL

Hypnotic
Children:
  PO/PR:
    <4 yr: 3–6 mg/kg/dose QHS
    ≥4 yr: 1.5–3 mg/kg/dose QHS
  IM: 2–6 mg/kg/dose. **Max. dose:** 100 mg
Preprocedure sedation
  Children:
    PO/PR/IM: 2–6 mg/kg/dose. **Max. dose:** 150 mg
    IV: 1–3 mg/kg/dose. **Max. dose:** 150 mg
Barbiturate coma
  Children and adults
    IV: Load: 10–15 mg/kg given slowly over 1–2 hr
    Maintenance: Begin at 1 mg/kg/hr. Dose range: 1–3 mg/kg/hr as needed

Contraindicated in liver failure, CHF, and hypotension. No advantage over phenobarbital for control of seizures. Adjunct in treatment of ICP. May cause drug-related isoelectric EEG. Do **not** administer for >2 weeks in treatment of insomnia. May cause hypotension, arrhythmias, hypothermia, respiratory depression, and dependence.
Onset of action: PO/PR: 15–60 min; IM: 10–15 min; IV: 1 min. *Duration of action:* PO/PR: 1–4 hr; IV: 15 min.
Administer IV at a rate of <50 mg/min. Suppositories should **not** be divided.
Therapeutic serum levels: Sedation: 1–5 mg/L; Hypnosis: 5–15 mg/L; Coma: 20–40 mg/L (steady state is achieved after 4–5 days of continuous IV dosing).

PERMETHRIN

Elimite, Acticin, Nix
Scabicidal agent

No ? B

Cream (Elimite, Acticin): 5% (60 g); contains 0.1% formaldehyde
Liquid cream rinse (Nix-OTC): 1% (60 mL); contains 20% isopropyl alcohol

Continued

PERMETHRIN *continued*

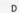
Pediculus capitis, Phthirus pubis:
Head lice: Saturate hair and scalp with 1% cream rinse after shampooing, rinsing, and towel drying hair. Leave on 10 min, then rinse. May repeat in 7–10 days. May be used for lice in other areas of the body (e.g., pubic lice) in same fashion.
Scabies (see remarks): Apply 5% cream from neck to toe (head to toe for infants and toddlers), wash off with water in 8–14 hr. May repeat in 7 days.

Ovicidal activity generally makes single-dose regimen adequate. **Avoid** contact with eyes during application. Shake well before using. May cause pruritus, hypersensitivity, burning, stinging, erythema, and rash. For either lice or scabies, instruct patient to launder bedding and clothing. For lice, treat symptomatic contacts only. For scabies, treat all contacts even if asymptomatic. The 5% cream has been used safely in children <1 mo with neonatal scabies (a 6-hour application time was utilized). Topical cream dosage form contains formaldehyde. Dispense 60 g per adult or two small children.

PHENAZOPYRIDINE HCl
Pyridium, Azo-Standard (OTC), and others
Urinary analgesic

Yes ? B

Tabs: 95 mg (OTC), 97.2 mg, 100 mg (OTC/Rx), 150 mg 200 mg
Oral suspension: 10 mg/mL

Children 6–12 yr: 12 mg/kg/24 hr ÷ TID PO until symptoms of lower urinary tract irritation are controlled or 2 days.
Adults: 100–200 mg TID PO until symptoms are controlled or 2 days.

May cause hepatitis, GI distress, vertigo, headache, renal insufficiency, methemoglobinemia, and hemolytic anemia. Colors urine orange; stains clothing. May also stain contact lenses and interfere with urinalysis tests based on spectrometry or color reactions. Give doses after meals.
Adjust dose in renal impairment (see p. 950).

PHENOBARBITAL
Luminal, Solfoton, and others
Barbiturate

Yes 2 D

Tabs: 8, 15, 16, 30, 32, 60, 65, 100 mg
Caps: 16 mg

Continued

PHENOBARBITAL *continued*

Elixir: 15, 20 mg/5 mL (contains alcohol)
Inj: 30, 60, 65, 130 mg/mL (some injectable products may contain 10% alcohol, benzyl alcohol, and propylene glycol)
Powder for inj: 120 mg

Status epilepticus:
Loading dose, IV:
   Neonates, infants, and children: 15–20 mg/kg/dose in a single or divided dose.
May give additional 5 mg/kg doses Q15–30 min to a **maximum** of 30 mg/kg.
Maintenance dose, PO/IV: Monitor levels.
   Neonates: 3–5 mg/kg/24 hr ÷ QD-BID
   Infants: 5–6 mg/kg/24 hr ÷ QD-BID
   Children 1–5 yr: 6–8 mg/kg/24 hr ÷ QD-BID
   Children 6–12 yr: 4–6 mg/kg/24 hr ÷ QD-BID
   >12 yr: 1–3 mg/kg/24 hr ÷ QD-BID
Hyperbilirubinemia: <12 yr: 3–8 mg/kg/24 hr PO ÷ BID-TID. Doses up to 12 mg/kg/24 hr have been used.
Preoperative sedation, children: 1–3 mg/kg/dose IM/IV/PO × 1. Give 60–90 min prior to procedure.

Contraindicated in porphyria, severe respiratory disease with dyspnea or obstruction. Use with **caution** in hepatic or renal disease (reduce dose). IV administration may cause respiratory arrest or hypotension. Side effects include drowsiness, cognitive impairment, ataxia, hypotension, hepatitis, skin rash, respiratory depression, apnea, megaloblastic anemia, and anticonvulsant hypersensitivity syndrome. Paradoxical reaction in children (not dose-related) may cause hyperactivity, irritability, insomnia. Induces several liver enzymes (CYP 450 1A2, 2B6, 2C8, 3A3/4, 3A5-7), thus decreases blood levels of many drugs (e.g., anticonvulsants). IV push **not to exceed** 1 mg/kg/min.

$T_{1/2}$ *is variable with age:* Neonates, 45–100 hr; infants, 20–133 hr; children, 37–73 hr. Due to long half-life, consider other agents for sedation for procedures.

Therapeutic levels: 15–40 mg/L. *Recommended serum sampling time at steady-state:* Trough level obtained within 30 min prior to the next scheduled dose after 10–14 days of continuous dosing.

Adjust dose in renal failure (see p. 951).

PHENTOLAMINE MESYLATE

Regitine
Adrenergic blocking agent (alpha); antidote, extravasation

No   ?   C

Inj: 5-mg vial; contains 25 mg mannitol

Continued

PHENTOLAMINE MESYLATE *continued*

 Treatment of alpha adrenergic drug extravasation (most effective within 12 hr of extravasation)

Neonates: Make a solution of 0.25–0.5 mg/mL with normal saline. Inject 1 mL (in 5 divided doses of 0.2 mL) SC around site of extravasation; **max. total dose:** 0.1 mg/kg or 2.5 mg total.

Infants, children, and adults: Make a solution of 0.5–1 mg/mL with normal saline. Inject 1–5 mL (in 5 divided doses) SC around site of extravasation; **max. total dose:** 0.1–0.2 mg/kg or 5 mg total.

Diagnosis of pheochromocytoma, IM/IV:
  Children: 0.05–0.1 mg/kg/dose up to a **maximum** of 5 mg
  Adults: 5 mg/dose

Hypertension, prior to surgery for pheochromocytoma, IM/IV:
  Children: 0.05–0.1 mg/kg/dose up to a **maximum** of 5 mg 1–2 hr prior to surgery, repeat Q2–4 hr PRN
  Adults: 5 mg/dose 1–2 hr prior to surgery, repeat Q2–4 hr PRN

 Contraindicated in MI, coronary insufficiency, and angina. Use with **caution** in hypotension, arrhythmias, and cerebrovascular spasm/occlusion.

For diagnosis of pheochromocytoma, patient should be resting in a supine position. A blood pressure reduction of more than 35 mm Hg systolic and 24 mm Hg diastolic is considered a positive test for pheochromocytoma. For treatment of extravasation, use 27- to 30-gauge needle with multiple small injections and monitor site closely because repeat doses may be necessary.

PHENYLEPHRINE HCl

Neo-Synephrine and others
Adrenergic agonist

No ? C

Nasal drops (OTC): 0.125, 0.16, 0.25, 0.5% (15, 30 mL)
Nasal spray (OTC): 0.25, 0.5, 1% (15, 30 mL)
NOTE: Neo-Synephrine 12 hours, see *Oxymetazoline*
Ophthalmic drops: 0.12% [OTC] (0.3, 15, 20 mL), 2.5% (2, 3, 5, 15 mL), 10% (2, 5 mL)
Inj: 10 mg/mL (1%) (1, 5 mL); may contain bisulfites

 Hypotension:
  Children:
    IM/SC: 0.1 mg/kg/dose Q1–2 hr PRN; **max. dose:** 5 mg
    IV bolus: 5–20 mcg/kg/dose Q10–15 min PRN
    IV drip: 0.1–0.5 mcg/kg/min; titrate to effect
  Adults:
    IM/SC: 2–5 mg/dose Q1–2 hr PRN; **max. dose:** 5 mg
    IV bolus: 0.1–0.5 mg/dose Q10–15 min PRN
    IV drip: Initial rate at 100–180 mcg/min; titrate to effect. Usual maintenance dose: 40–60 mcg/min.

Continued

PHENYLEPHRINE HCl *continued*

To prepare infusion: See inside front cover.
>   NOTE: The dosage units for adults are in mcg/min; compared to mcg/kg/min for children.

Nasal decongestant (in each nostril; give up to 3 days):
>   *Infants (>6 mo):* 1–2 drops of 0.16% solution Q3 hr PRN
>   *<6 yr:* 2–3 drops of 0.125% solution Q4 hr PRN
>   *6–12 yr:* 2–3 drops or 1–2 sprays of 0.25% solution Q4 hr PRN
>   *>12 yr–adult:* 2–3 drops or 1–2 sprays of 0.25% or 0.5% solution Q4 hr PRN

Pupillary dilation: 2.5% sol; 1 drop in each eye 15 min before examination

> Use **cautiously** in presence of arrhythmias, hyperthyroidism, or hyperglycemia. May cause tremor, insomnia, and palpitations. Metabolized by MAO. **Contraindicated** in pheochromocytoma and severe hypertension.

Nasal decongestants may cause rebound congestion with excessive use (>3 days). The 1% nasal spray can be used in adults with extreme congestion.

Injectable product may contain sulfites. NOTE: Phenylephrine is found in a variety of combination cough and cold products.

PHENYTOIN

Dilantin, Dilantin Infatab, and others
Anticonvulsant, class Ib antiarrhythmic

Yes   1   D

Chewable tabs: 50 mg (Infatab)
Prompt caps: 100 mg
Extended-release caps: 30, 100 mg
Oral suspension: 125 mg/5 mL (240 mL); contains ≤0.6% alcohol
Inj: 50 mg/mL; contains alcohol and propylene glycol

> *Status epilepticus:* See p. 17
> *Loading dose (all ages):* 15–20 mg/kg IV
>   **Max. dose:** 1500 mg/24 hr

Maintenance for seizure disorders:
>   *Neonates:* start with 5 mg/24 hr PO/IV ÷ Q12 hr; usual range 5–8 mg/kg/24 hr PO/IV ÷ Q8–12 hr
>   *Infants/children:* start with 5 mg/kg/24 hr ÷ BID-TID PO/IV; usual dose range (doses divided BID-TID):
>>   *6 mo–3 yr:* 8–10 mg/kg/24 hr
>>   *4–6 yr:* 7.5–9 mg/kg/24 hr
>>   *7–9 yr:* 7–8 mg/kg/24 hr
>>   *10–16 yr:* 6–7 mg/kg/24 hr
>>   NOTE: Use QD-BID dosing with extended-release caps.
>   *Adults:* Start with 100 mg/dose Q8 hr IV/PO and carefully titrate to 300–600 mg/24 hr (or 6–7 mg/kg/24 hr) ÷ Q8–24 hr IV/PO

Continued

PHENYTOIN *continued*

Antiarrhythmic (secondary to digitalis intoxication):
    Load (all ages): 1.25 mg/kg IV Q5 min up to a total of 15 mg/kg
    Maintenance:
        Children: IV/PO: 5–10 mg/kg/24 hr ÷ Q12 hr
        Adults: 250 mg PO QID × 1 day, then 250 mg PO Q12 hr × 2 days, then
        300–400 mg/24 hr ÷ Q6–24 hr

Contraindicated in patients with heart block or sinus bradycardia. IM administration is **not** recommended because of erratic absorption and pain at injection site. Side effects include gingival hyperplasia, hirsutism, dermatitis, blood dyscrasia, ataxia, lupus-like and Stevens-Johnson syndromes, lymphadenopathy, liver damage, and nystagmus. Many drug interactions; levels may be increased by cimetidine, chloramphenicol, INH, sulfonamides, trimethoprim, etc. Levels may be decreased by some antineoplastic agents. Phenytoin induces hepatic microsomal enzymes (CYP 450 3A4), leading to decreased effectiveness of oral contraceptives, quinidine, valproic acid, and theophylline.

Oral absorption reduced in neonates. $T_{1/2}$ is variable (7–42 hr) and dose-dependent. Drug is highly protein-bound; free fraction of drug will be increased in patients with hypoalbuminemia.

Therapeutic levels for seizure disorders: 10–20 mg/L (free and bound phenytoin) **OR** 1–2 mg/L (free only). Monitor free phenytoin levels in hypoalbuminemia or renal insufficiency. *Recommended serum sampling times:* Trough level (PO/IV) within 30 min prior to the next scheduled dose; peak or post load level (IV) 1 hr after the end of IV infusion. Steady state is usually achieved after 5–10 days of continuous dosing. For routine monitoring, measure trough.

IV push/infusion rate: **Not to exceed** 0.5 mg/kg/min in neonates, or 1 mg/kg/min infants, children, and adults with a **maximum** of: 50 mg/min; may cause cardiovascular collapse. Consider fosphenytoin in situations of tenuous IV access and risk for extravasation.

PHOSPHORUS SUPPLEMENTS

NeutraPhos, NeutraPhos-K, K-PHOS Neutral, K-PHOS M.F.,
K-PHOS No.2, Uro-KP-Neutral, Sodium Phosphate,
Potassium Phosphate

Yes   ?   C

Oral: (reconstitute in 75 mL H_2O per capsule or packet)
Na and K Phosphate:
    NeutraPhos; Caps, powder: 250 mg P, 7 mEq Na, 7 mEq K
    Uro-KP-Neutral; Tabs: 250 mg P, 10.9 mEq Na, 1.27 mEq K
    K-PHOS Neutral; Tabs: 250 mg P, 13 mEq Na, 1.1 mEq K
    K-PHOS M.F.; Tabs: 125.6 mg P, 2.9 mEq Na, 1.1 mEq K
    K-PHOS No.2; Tabs: 250 mg P, 5.8 mEq Na, 2.3 mEq K
K Phosphate:
    NeutraPhos-K; Caps, powder: 250 mg P, 14.25 mEq K

Continued

PHOSPHORUS SUPPLEMENTS *continued*

Inj:
Na Phosphate: 94 mg P, 4 mEq Na/mL
K Phosphate: 94 mg P, 4.4 mEq K/mL
Conversion: 31 mg P = 1 mM P

Acute hypophosphatemia: 5–10 mg/kg/dose IV over 6 hr
Maintenance/replacement:
   Children:
   IV: 15–45 mg/kg over 24 hr
   PO: 30–90 mg/kg/24 hr ÷ TID–QID
Adults:
   IV: 1.5–2 g over 24 hr
   PO: 3–4.5 g/24 hr ÷ TID–QID
Recommended infusion rate: ≤3.1 mg/kg/hr (0.1 mM/kg/hr) of phosphate. When potassium salt is used, the rate will be limited by the maximum potassium infusion rate. Do not co-infuse with calcium-containing products.

May cause tetany, hyperphosphatemia, hyperkalemia, and hypocalcemia. Use with **caution** in patients with renal impairment. Be aware of sodium and/or potassium load when supplementing phosphate. IV administration may cause hypotension and renal failure, or arrhythmias, heart block, cardiac arrest with potassium salt. PO dosing may cause nausea, vomiting, abdominal pain, or diarrhea. See p. 462 for daily requirements, and pp. 247–248 for additional information on hypophosphatemia and hyperphosphatemia.

PHYSOSTIGMINE SALICYLATE

Antilirium
Cholinergic agent

No   ?   C

Inj: 1 mg/mL (2 mL); contains 2% benzyl alcohol and 0.1% sodium bisulfite

For antihistamine overdose or anticholinergic poisoning, see p. 26.

Physostigmine antidote: Atropine always should be available. **Contraindicated** in asthma, gangrene, diabetes, cardiovascular disease, GI or GU tract obstruction, any vagotonic state, patients receiving choline esters or depolarizing neuromuscular blocking agents (e.g., decamethonium, succinylcholine).

PHYTONADIONE/VITAMIN K₁

Aqua-Mephyton, Mephyton

No 1 C

Tabs: 5 mg
Inj: 2, 10 mg/mL; may contain 0.9% benzyl alcohol

Neonatal hemorrhagic disease:
  Prophylaxis: 0.5–1 mg IM × 1
    Treatment: 1–2 mg/24 hr IM/SC/IV
Oral anticoagulant overdose:
  Infants: 1–2 mg/dose Q4–8 hr IM/SC/IV
  Children and adults: 2.5–10 mg/dose PO/IM/SC/IV
  Dose may be repeated 12–48 hr after PO dose or 6–8 hr after parenteral dose
Vitamin K deficiency:
  Infants and children:
    PO: 2.5–5 mg/24 hr
    IM/SC/IV: 1–2 mg/dose × 1
  Adults:
    PO: 5–25 mg/24 hr
    IM/SC/IV: 10 mg/dose × 1

Monitor PT/PTT. Large doses (10–20 mg) in newborns may cause hyperbilirubinemia and severe hemolytic anemia. Blood coagulation factors increase within
6–12 hr after oral doses and within 1–2 hr after parenteral administration.
  IV injection rate **not to exceed** 3 mg/m²/min or 1 mg/min. IV or IM doses may cause
flushing, dizziness, cardiac/respiratory arrest, hypotension, and anaphylaxis. IV or IM
administration is indicated only when other routes of administration are not feasible
(or in emergency situations).
  Mineral oil may decrease GI absorption of vitamin K with concurrent oral
administration. See pp. 464–465 for multivitamin preparations.

PILOCARPINE HCl

Akarpine, Isopto Carpine, Piligan, Ocusert Pilo, Salagen,
and others
Cholinergic agent

No ? C

Ophthalmic solution: 0.25%, 0.5%, 1%, 2%, 3%, 4%, 5%, 6%, 8%, 10%
Ophthalmic gel: 4% (3.5 g)
Ocular therapeutic system (Ocusert Pilo): 20, 40 mcg/hr for 1 week (8 units)
Tab (Salagen): 5 mg

Continued

PILOCARPINE HCl *continued*

For elevated intraocular pressure: 1–2 drops in each eye 4–6 per 24 hr; adjust concentration and frequency as needed.

Gel: 0.5-inch ribbon applied to lower conjunctival sac QHS. Adjust dose as needed.

Xerostomia:

Adults: 5 mg/dose PO TID, dose may be titrated to 10 mg/dose PO TID in patients who do not respond to lower dose and who are able to tolerate the drug.

Contraindicated in acute iritis or anterior chamber inflammation and uncontrolled asthma. May cause stinging, burning, lacrimation, headache, and retinal detachment with ophthalmic use. Use with **caution** in patients with corneal abrasion or significant cardiovascular disease. Use with topical NSAIDs (e.g., ketorolac) may decrease topical pilocarpine effects. Sweating, nausea, rhinitis, chills, flushing, urinary frequency, dizziness, asthenia, and headaches have also been reported with oral dosing.

PIPERACILLIN
Pipracil
Antibiotic, penicillin (extended spectrum)

Yes ? B

Inj: 2, 3, 4, 40 g
Contains 1.85 mEq Na/g drug

Neonates, IV:
≤7 *days:*
≤36 *weeks gestation:* 150 mg/kg/24 hr ÷ Q12 hr
>36 *weeks gestation:* 225 mg/kg/24 hr ÷ Q8 hr
>7 *days:*
≤36 *weeks gestation:* 225 mg/kg/24 hr ÷ Q8 hr
>36 *weeks gestation:* 300 mg/kg/24 hr ÷ Q6 hr
Infants and children:
200–300 mg/kg/24 hr IM/IV ÷ Q4–6 hr; **max. dose:** 24 g/24 hr
Cystic fibrosis:
350–600 mg/kg/24 hr IM/IV ÷ Q4–6 hr; **max. dose:** 24 g/24 hr
Adults: 2–4 g/dose IV Q4–6 hr or 1–2 g/dose IM Q6 hr; **max. dose:** 24 g/24 hr

Similar to penicillin. Like other penicillins, CSF penetration occurs only with inflamed meninges. May cause seizures, myoclonus, and fever. May falsely lower aminoglycoside serum levels if the drugs are infused close to one another; allow a minimum of 2 hr between infusions to prevent this interaction.

For IM use, drug may be diluted to 400 mg/mL with 0.5 or 1% lidocaine without epinephrine.

Adjust dose in renal impairment (see p. 944).

PIPERACILLIN/TAZOBACTAM

Zosyn

Antibiotic, penicillin (extended spectrum with beta-lactamase inhibitor)

Yes   ?   B

Inj: 2 g piperacillin, 0.25 g tazobactam; 3 g piperacillin, 0.375 g tazobactam; 4 g piperacillin, 0.5 g tazobactam (8:1 ratio of piperacillin to tazobactam)
Contains 2.35 mEq Na/g piperacillin

All doses based on piperacillin component
Infants <6 mo: 150–300 mg/kg/24 hr IV ÷ Q6–8 hr
Infants >6 mo and children: 300–400 mg/kg/24 hr IV ÷ Q6–8 hr
Adults: 3 g IV Q6 hr; doses as high as 18 g/24 hr IV ÷ Q4 hr have been used in nosocomial pneumonia.
Cystic fibrosis: See Piperacillin

Tazobactam is a beta-lactamase inhibitor, thus extending the spectrum of piperacillin. Like other penicillins, CSF penetration occurs only with inflammed meninges. See *Piperacillin* and *Penicillin* for additional comments.
Adjust dose in renal impairment, (see p. 944).

PIPERAZINE

Vermizine, Piperazine Citrate
Anthelmenthic

Yes   2   B

Tabs: 250 mg

Enterobius vermicularis (pinworm): Adults and children: 65 mg/kg/24 hr PO QD × 7 days. **Max. dose:** 2.5 g/24 hr. May repeat in 1 week if necessary.
Ascaris lumbricoides (roundworm):
Children: 75 mg/kg/24 hr PO QD × 2 days
Adults: 3.5 g PO QD × 2 days
Max. dose: 3.5 g/24 hr

Contraindicated in seizure disorders, and liver or renal impairment. Large doses may cause GI irritation, blurred vision, urticaria, and muscle weakness. Use with **caution** in anemia or when administering with chlorpromazine.
Mebendazole and pyrantel pamoate are considered first-line therapy for Ascaris and Enterobius infections. In cases of intestinal obstruction due to heavy worm load, piperazine may be given through NG tube at doses recommended (*Red Book,* 2000, pg. 177). **Pyrantel pamoate and piperazine should not be administered together because they are antagonistic.**
Breastfeeding mothers should take their doses immediately following feeding infant and then express and discard milk during the next 8 hr.

PIRBUTEROL ACETATE

Maxair
Beta-2-adrenergic agonist

No　?　C

Aerosol inhaler: 0.2 mg/actuation (25.6 g, 300 actuations)
AUTOHALER: 0.2 mg/actuation (13.7 g, 400 actuations; 2.8 g, 80 actuations)
2.8 g is sample pack

 Children ≥12 yr and adults: 1–2 inhalations Q4–6 hr PRN.
Max. dose: 12 inhalations/24 hr.

 See *Albuterol* for remarks. AUTOHALER is a breath-actuated inhaler. See package insert for directions. *Onset of action:* 5 min. *Duration:* 5 hr.

POLYCITRA

See Citrate Mixtures

POLYETHYLENE GLYCOL— ELECTROLYTE SOLUTION

GoLYTELY, Co-Lav, Colovage, CoLyte, GoEvac, NuLYTELY,
OCL, Miralax

No　?　C

Bowel evacuant, osmotic laxative

Powder for oral solution:
GoLYTELY: Polyethylene glycol 3350 236 g, Na sulfate 22.74 g, Na bicarbonate 6.74 g, NaCl 5.86 g, KCl 2.97 g. Contents vary somewhat. See package insert for contents of other products.
Miralax: Polyethylene glycol 3350 (255, 527 g)

 Bowel cleansing (patients should be NPO 3–4 hr prior to dosing):
Children:
　Oral/nasogastric: 25–40 mL/kg/hr until rectal effluent is clear
Adults:
　Oral: 240 mL PO Q10 min up to 4 L or until rectal effluent is clear
　Nasogastric: 20–30 mL/min (1.2–1.8 L/hr) up to 4 L until rectal effluent is clear
Constipation (Miralax):
　Children: (limited data in 20 children with chronic constipation, 18 mo–11 yr; see remarks): a mean effective dose of 0.84 mg/kg/24 hr PO ÷ BID for 8 weeks (range: 0.25–1.42 mg/kg/24 hr) was used to yield two soft stools per day.
　Adults: 17 g (1 heaping tablespoonful) mixed in 240 mL of water, juice, soda, coffee, or tea PO QD.

Continued

POLYETHYLENE GLYCOL—ELECTROLYTE SOLUTION *continued*

Contraindicated in polyethylene glycol hypersensitivity. Monitor electrolytes, BUN, serum glucose, and urine osmolality with prolonged administration.

BOWEL CLEANSING: **Contraindicated** in toxic megacolon, gastric retention, colitis, and bowel perforation. Use with **caution** in patients prone to aspiration or with impaired gag reflex. Effect should occur within 1–2 hr. Solution generally more palatable if chilled.

CONSTIPATION (Miralax): **Contraindicated** in bowel obstruction.

Children: Dilute powder using the ratio of 17 g powder to 240 mL of water, juice, or milk. An onset of action within 1 week in 12 of 20 patients, with the remaining 8 patients reporting improvement during the second week of therapy has been reported. Side effects reported in this trial included diarrhea, flatulence, and mild abdominal pain. See J Peds 139(3):428–432; 2001 for additional information.

Adults: 2 to 4 days may be required to produce a bowel movement. Most common side effects include nausea, abdominal bloating, cramping, and flatulence. Use beyond 2 weeks has not been studied.

POLYMYXIN B SULFATE AND BACITRACIN
See Bacitracin ± Polymyxin B

POLYMYXIN B SULFATE, NEOMYCIN SULFATE, HYDROCORTISONE
Cortisporin Otic and others
Topical antibiotic (otic preparations listed)

No   ?   C

Otic solution or suspension: Polymyxin B sulfate 10,000 U, Neomycin sulfate 5 mg, Hydrocortisone 10 mg/mL (10 mL)

Otitis externa:
≥2 yr–adults: 3–4 drops TID-QID × 7–10 days. If preferred, a cotton wick may be saturated and inserted into ear canal. Moisten wick with antibiotic every 4 hr. Change wick Q24 hr.

Shake suspension well before use. **Contraindicated** in patients with active varicella and herpes simplex. May cause cutaneous sensitization. **Do not use** in cases with perforated eardrum because of possible ototoxicity.

PORACTANT ALFA
See Surfactant, pulmonary

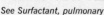

POTASSIUM IODIDE

Pima, Potassium Iodide Enseals, SSKI, Thyro Block, and others
Antithyroid agent

No   1   D

Tabs (Thyro Block): 130 mg
Syrup (Pima): 325 mg/5 mL (473 mL, 4000 mL)
Saturated solution (SSKI): 1000 mg/mL (30, 240 mL); 10 drops = 500 mg potassium iodide
Lugol's (Strong Iodine) solution: Iodine 50 mg and potassium iodide 100 mg per mL (120, 473 mL)

Neonatal Grave's disease: 1 drop strong iodine (Lugol's sol) PO Q8 hr
Thyrotoxicosis:
  Children: 50–250 mg PO TID (about 1–5 drops of SSKI TID)
  Adults: 50–500 mg PO TID (1–10 drops SSKI PO TID)
Sporotrichosis:
  Adults and children: 65–325 mg PO TID. Daily doses may be increased in increments of 150–250 mg/24 hr. **Max. dose:** increase to tolerance or 4.5–9 g/24 hr.

Contraindicated in pregnancy. GI disturbance, metallic taste, rash, salivary gland inflammation, headache, lacrimation, and rhinitis are symptoms of iodism. Give with milk or water after meals. Monitor thyroid function tests. *Onset of antithyroid effects:* 1–2 days.

Continue sporotrichosis treatment for 4–6 weeks after lesions have completely healed. Increase dose until either **maximum dose** is achieved or signs of intolerance appear.

POTASSIUM SUPPLEMENTS

Many brand names
Electrolyte

Yes   1   A

Potassium chloride:
  40 mEq K = 3 g KCl
  Sustained-release caps: 8, 10 mEq
  Sustained-release tabs: 6.7, 8, 10, 20 mEq
  Powder: 15, 20, 25 mEq/packet
  Solution: 10% (6.7 mEq/5 mL), 15% (10 mEq/5 mL), 20% (13.3 mEq/5 mL)
  Concentrated inj: 2 mEq/mL
Potassium gluconate:
  40 mEq K = 9.4 g K gluconate
  Tabs: 500 mg (2.15 mEq), 595 mg (2.56 mEq)
  Elixir: 20 mEq/15 mL

Continued

POTASSIUM SUPPLEMENTS *continued*

Potassium acetate:
   40 mEq K = 3.9 g K acetate
   Concentrated Inj: 2 mEq/mL
Potassium phosphate:
   See *Phosphorus supplements*

Normal daily requirements: See p. 233.
   Replacement: Determine based on maintenance requirements, deficit, and
   ongoing losses. See Chapter 10.
Hypokalemia:
   Oral:
      Children: 1–4 mEq/kg/24 hr ÷ BID-QID. Monitor serum potassium.
      Adults: 40–100 mEq/24 hr ÷ BID-QID
   IV: **MONITOR SERUM K CLOSELY**
      Children: 0.5–1 mEq/kg/dose given as an infusion of 0.5 mEq/kg/hr × 1–2 hr.
      Max. IV infusion rate: 1 mEq/kg/hr. This may be used in critical situations (e.g.,
      hypokalemia with arrhythmia).
      Adults:
         Serum K ≥2.5 mEq/L: Replete at rates up to 10 mEq/hr. Total dosage not to
         exceed 200 mEq/24 hr.
         Serum K <2 mEq/L: Replete at rates up to 40 mEq/hr. Total dosage not to
         exceed 400 mEq/24 hr.
   Maximum peripheral IV Sol conc: 40 mEq/L
   Maximum concentration for central line administration: 150–200 mEq/L

PO administration may cause GI disturbance and ulceration. Oral liquid
supplements should be diluted in water or fruit juice prior to administration.
   Sustained-release tablets must be swallowed whole, and **not** dissolved in the
mouth or chewed.
   Do **not** administer IV potassium undiluted. IV administration may cause irritation,
pain, phlebitis at the infusion site. **Rapid or central IV infusion may cause cardiac
arrhythmias.** Patients receiving infusion >0.5 mEq/kg/hr (>20 mEq/hr for adults)
should be placed on an ECG monitor.

PRALIDOXIME CHLORIDE
Protopam, 2-PAM
Antidote, organophosphate poisoning

Yes   ?   C

Autoinj: 300 mg/mL (2 mL)
Inj: 1000 mg

Use with atropine.
   Children: 20–50 mg/kg/dose × 1 IM/IV/SC. May repeat in 1–2 hr if muscle
   weakness is not relieved.

Continued

FORMULARY

PRALIDOXIME CHLORIDE *continued*

Adults: 1–2 g/dose × 1 IM/IV/SC. May repeat in 1–2 hr if muscle weakness is not relieved.
Continuous infusions have also been recommended; see package insert.

Do not use as an antidote for carbamate classes of pesticides. Removal of secretions and maintaining a patent airway is critical. May cause muscle rigidity, laryngospasm, and tachycardia after rapid IV infusion. Drug is generally ineffective if administered 36–48 hr after exposure. Additional doses may be necessary.

For IV administration, dilute to 50 mg/mL or less and infuse over 15–30 min (**not to exceed** 200 mg/min). Reduce dosage in renal impairment because 80% to 90% of the drug is excreted unchanged in the urine 12 hr after administration.

PRAZIQUANTEL
Biltricide
Anthelmintic

No ? B

Tabs: 600 mg (tri-scored)

Children and adults:
Schistosomiasis: 20 mg/kg/dose PO BID–TID × 1 day
Flukes: 25 mg/kg/dose PO Q8 hr × 1 day (× 2 days for *P. westermani*)
Cysticercosis: 50–100 mg/kg/24 hr PO ÷ Q8 hr × 15–30 days (dexamethasone may be added to regimen for 2–3 days to minimize inflammatory response)
Tapeworms: 5–10 mg/kg/dose PO × 1 dose (25 mg/kg/dose × 1 dose for *H. nana*)

Contraindicated in ocular cysticercosis and spinal cysticercosis. Use with **caution** in patients with severe hepatic disease or history of seizures. May cause dizziness, and drowsiness. Headache, seizures, intracranial hypertension, increased CSF protein, and hyperthermia have occurred in patients treated for neurocysticercosis. Carbamazepine, phenytoin, and chloroquine may decrease praziquantel's effects. Cimetidine may increase praziquantel's effects. Take with food. Do **not** chew tablets because of bitter taste.

PRAZOSIN HCl
Minipress
Adrenergic blocking agent (alpha-1), antihypertensive, vasodilator

No ? C

Caps: 1, 2, 5 mg

Continued

PRAZOSIN HCl *continued*

Children:
Initial: 5 mcg/kg PO test dose
Maintenance: 25–150 mcg/kg/24 hr PO ÷ Q6 hr
Max. dose: 15 mg/24 hr or 0.4 mg/kg/24 hr
Adults:
1 mg PO BID–TID initially. Increase PRN to **max. dose** of 20 mg/24 hr PO ÷ BID–TID

Contraindicated in hypersensitivty to quinazolines. May cause syncope, tachycardia, hypotension, dizziness, nausea, headache, drowsiness, fatigue, and anticholinergic effects. Marked orthostatic hypotension, syncope, and loss of consciousness may occur with first dose.

PREDNISOLONE
Delta-Cortef, Orapred, Prelone, Pediapred, and others
Corticosteroid

No   1   B

Tabs: 5 mg
Syrup (Orapred, Prelone): 15 mg/5 mL (240 mL); contains alcohol
Syrup (Pediapred, Prelone): 5 mg/5 mL (120 mL); Pediapred is alcohol and dye free
Inj (as acetate): 25, 50 mg/mL (not for IV use); may contain benzyl alcohol
Inj (as Na phosphate): 20 mg/mL
Inj (as tebutate): 20 mg/mL (not for IV use)
Ophthalmic suspension (as acetate): 0.12%, 0.125%, 1% (5, 10 mL)
Ophthalmic solution (as Na phosphate): 0.125%, 1% (5, 10, 15 mL)

See *Prednisone* (equivalent dosing)
Ophthalmic (consult ophthalmologist before use):
Children and adults: Start with 1–2 drops Q1 hr during the day and Q2 hr during the night until favorable response, then reduce dose to 1 drop Q4 hr. Dose may be further reduced to 1 drop TID-QID.

See *Prednisone* for remarks. See p. 913 for relative steroid potencies. Orapred product should be stored in the refrigerator.

PREDNISONE
Many brand names
Corticosteroid

No   1   B

Tabs: 1, 2.5, 5, 10, 20, 50 mg
Syrup/solution: 1 mg/mL (120, 240, 500 mL); contains 5% alcohol
Concentrated solution: 5 mg/mL (30 mL); contains 30% alcohol

Continued

PREDNISONE continued

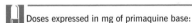

Children:

Antiinflammatory/immunosuppressive: 0.5–2 mg/kg/24 hr PO ÷ QD–BID

Acute asthma: 2 mg/kg/24 hr PO ÷ QD-BID × 5–7 days; **max. dose:** 80 mg/24 hr. Patients may benefit from tapering if therapy exceeds 5–7 days.

Nephrotic syndrome: Starting doses of 2 mg/kg/24 hr PO (**max. dose:** 80 mg/24 hr) are recommended. Further treatment plans are individualized. Consult a nephrologist.

See pp. 907–913, for physiologic replacement, relative steroid potencies, and doses based on body surface area. Methylprednisolone is preferable in hepatic disease because prednisone must be converted to methylprednisolone in the liver.

Side effects may include mood changes, seizures, hyperglycemia, diarrhea, nausea, abdominal distension, GI bleeding, HPA axis suppression, osteopenia, cushingoid effects, and cataracts with prolonged use. Prednisone is a cytochrome P 450 3A3/4 substrate and inducer. Barbiturates, carbamazepine, phenytoin, rifampin, and isoniazid, may reduce the effects of prednisone, whereas estrogens may enhance the effects.

PRIMAQUINE PHOSPHATE

Primaquine
Antimalarial

No   ?   C

Tabs: 26.3 mg (15 mg base)

Doses expressed in mg of primaquine base:

Malaria:

Prevention of relapses for P. vivax or P. ovale only (initiate therapy during the last 2 weeks of, or following a course of, suppression with chloroquine or comparible drug):

Children: 0.3 mg/kg/dose PO QD × 14 days

Adults: 15 mg PO QD × 14 days **OR** 45 mg PO Q7 days × 8 weeks.

Prevention of chloroquine-resistant strains (initiate 1 day prior to departure and continue until 2 days after leaving endemic area):

Children: 0.5 mg/kg/dose PO QD

Adults: 30 mg PO QD

Pneumocystis carinii pneumonia (in combination with clindamycin):

Adult: 30 mg PO QD × 21 days

Contraindicated in granulocytopenia (e.g., rheumatoid arthritis, lupus erythematosus) and bone marrow suppression. **Avoid** use with quinacrine and with other drugs that have a potential for causing hemolysis or bone marrow suppression. Use with **caution** in G6PD and NADH methemoglobin-reductase deficient patients due to increased risk for hemolytic anemia and leukopenia, respectively.

May cause headache, visual disturbances, nausea, vomiting, and abdominal cramps. Administer all doses with food to mask bitter taste.

For explanation of icons, see p. 572.

PRIMIDONE

Mysoline
Anticonvulsant, barbiturate

Yes 2 D

Tabs: 50, 250 mg
Susp: 250 mg/5 mL (240 mL); contains saccharin

Adjust dose in renal failure (see p. 951).

<8 yr	≥8 yr and Adults
DAY 1–3	
50 mg PO QHS	100–125 mg PO QHS
DAY 4–6	
50 mg PO BID	100–125 mg PO BID
DAY 7–9	
100 mg PO BID	100–125 mg PO TID
THEREAFTER	
125–250 mg PO TID or	250 mg PO TID-QID; **max. dose:** 2 g/24 hr
10–25 mg/kg/24 hr ÷ TID–QID	

Use with **caution** in renal or hepatic disease and pulmonary insufficiency. Primidone is metabolized to phenobarbital and has the same drug interactions and toxicities (see *Phenobarbital,* pp. 818–819). Additionally, primidone may cause vertigo, nausea, leukopenia, malignant lymphoma-like syndrome, diplopia, nystagmus, and systemic lupus-like syndrome. **Adjust dose in renal failure (see p. 951).**

Follow both primidone and phenobarbital levels. *Therapeutic levels:* 5–12 mg/L of primidone and 15–40 mg/L of phenobarbital. *Recommended serum sampling time at steady-state:* Trough level obtained within 30 min prior to the next scheduled dose after 1–4 days of continuous dosing.

PROBENECID

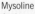

Benemid and others
Penicillin therapy adjuvant, uric acid–lowering agent

Yes ? B

Tabs: 500 mg

Use with penicillin
Children (2–14 yr): 25 mg/kg PO × 1, then 40 mg/kg/24 hr ÷ QID; **max. dose:** 500 mg/dose. Use adult dose if >50 kg.
Adults: 500 mg PO QID
Hyperuricemia:
Adults: 250 mg PO BID × 1 week, then 500 mg PO BID; may increase by 500 mg increments Q4 weeks PRN up to a **maximum** of 2–3 g/24 hr ÷ BID.

Continued

PROBENECID *continued*

Use with **caution** in patients with peptic ulcer disease. **Contraindicated** in children <2 yr and patients with renal insufficiency. **Do not use** if GFR <30 mL/min.

Increases uric acid excretion. Inhibits renal tubular secretion of acyclovir, ganciclovir, ciprofloxacin, organic acids, penicillins, cephalosporins, AZT, dapsone, methotrexate, nonsteroidal antiinflammatory agents, and benzodiazepines. Salicylates may decrease probenecid's activity. Alkalinize urine in patients with gout. May cause headache, GI symptoms, rash, anemia, and hypersensitivity. False-positive glucosuria with Clinitest may occur.

PROCAINAMIDE
Pronestyl, Procan SR, and others
Antiarrhythmic, class Ia

Yes   1   C

Tabs: 250, 375, 500 mg
Sustained-release tab: 250, 500, 750, 1000 mg
Caps: 250, 375, 500 mg
Inj: 100, 500 mg/mL; may contain benzyl alcohol and bisulfites
Suspension: 5, 50, 100 mg/mL

Children:
 Ventricular tachycardia with poor perfusion: Consider 15 mg/kg/dose IV × 1 over 30–60 min if cardioversion ineffective **(see inside back cover)**; follow with continuous infusion if effective (see below)
IM: 20–30 mg/kg/24 hr ÷ Q4–6 hr; **max. dose:** 4 g/24 hr (peak effect in 1 hr).
IV: Load: 2–6 mg/kg/dose over 5 min **(max. dose:** 100 mg/dose); repeat dose Q5–10 min PRN up to a total **maximum** of 15 mg/kg. **Do not exceed** 500 mg in 30 min.
 Maintenance: 20–80 mcg/kg/min by continuous infusion; **max. dose:** 2 g/24 hr
 To prepare infusion: See inside front cover
PO: 15–50 mg/kg/24 hr ÷ Q3–6 hr; **max. dose:** 4 g/24 hr
Adults:
IM: 50 mg/kg/24 hr ÷ Q3–6 hr
IV: Load: 50–100 mg/dose; repeat dose Q5 min PRN to **maximum** of 1000–1500 mg
 Maintenance: 1–6 mg/min by continuous infusion
PO: Usual dose: 50 mg/kg/24 hr
 Immediate release: 250–500 mg/dose Q3–6 hr
 Sustained release: 500–1000 mg/dose Q6 hr
Note: The IV infusion dosage units for adults are in mg/min; compared to mcg/kg/min for children.

Continued

PROCAINAMIDE *continued*

> Contraindicated in myasthenia gravis, complete heart block, SLE, torsade de pointes. Use with **caution** in asymtomatic premature ventricular contractions, digitalis intoxication, CHF, renal or hepatic dysfunction. **Adjust dose in renal failure (see p. 951).**

May cause lupus-like syndrome, positive Coombs' test, thrombocytopenia, arrhythmias, GI complaints, confusion. Increased LFTs and liver failure have been reported. Monitor BP, ECG when using IV. QRS widening by >0.02 sec suggests toxicity.

Cimetidine, ranitidine, amiodarone, beta-blockers, trimethoprim may increase procainamide levels. Procainamide may enhance the effects of skeletal muscle relaxants and anticholinergic agents. *Therapeutic levels:* 4–10 mg/L of procainamide or 10–30 mg/L of procainamide and NAPA levels combined.

Recommended serum sampling times:

IM/PO intermittent dosing: Trough level within 30 min prior to the next scheduled dose after 2 days of continuous dosing (steady-state).

IV continuous infusion: 2 and 12 hr after start of infusion and at 24-hour intervals thereafter.

PROCHLORPERAZINE

Compazine and others
Antiemetic, phenothiazine derivative

No   2   C

Tabs (as maleate): 5, 10, 25 mg
Slow-release caps (as maleate): 10, 15, 30 mg
Syrup (as edisylate): 5 mg/5 mL (120 mL)
Suppository: 2.5, 5, 25 mg (12s)
Inj (as edisylate): 5 mg/mL (2, 10 mL); may contain bisulfites and benzyl alcohol

> *Antiemetic doses:*
> *Children (>10 kg or >2 yr):*
>   *PO or PR:* 0.4 mg/kg/24 hr ÷ TID–QID
>   *IM:* 0.1–0.15 mg/kg/dose TID–QID
> *Adults:*
>   *PO:*
>   *Immediate release:* 5–10 mg/dose TID–QID
>   *Extended release:* 10 mg/dose BID or 15 mg/dose QD
>   *PR:* 25 mg/dose BID
>   *IM:* 5–10 mg/dose Q3–4 hr
>   *IV:* 2.5–10 mg/dose; may repeat Q3–4 hr
>   **Max. IM/IV dose:** 40 mg/24 hr

> Toxicity as for other phenothiazines (see *Chlorpromazine*). Extrapyramidal reactions (reversed by diphenhydramine) or orthostatic hypotension may occur. May cause false-positive test for phenylketonuria, urinary amylase,

Continued

PROCHLORPERAZINE *continued*

uroporphyrins, and urobilinogen. Do **not** use IV route in children. **Use only in management of prolonged vomiting of known etiology.**

PROMETHAZINE

Phenergan and others
Antihistamine, antiemetic, phenothiazine derivative

No   ?   C

Tabs: 12.5, 25, 50 mg
Syrup: 6.25 mg/5 mL, 25 mg/5 mL; contains alcohol
Suppository: 12.5, 25, 50 mg (12s)
Inj: 25, 50 mg/mL; may contain sulfites

Antihistaminic:
  Children >2 yr: 0.1 mg/kg/dose PO Q6 hr and 0.5 mg/kg/dose QHS PO PRN.
    Adults: 12.5 mg PO TID and 25 mg PO QHS
Nausea and vomiting PO/IM/IV/PR:
  Children >2 yr: 0.25–1 mg/kg/dose Q4–6 hr PRN
  Adults: 12.5–25 mg Q4–6 hr PRN
Motion sickness: (first dose 0.5–1 hr before travel):
  Children >2 yr: 0.5 mg/kg/dose Q12 hr PO PRN
  Adults: 25 mg PO BID PRN

Toxicity similar to other phenothiazines (see *Chlorpromazine*). Administer oral doses with meals to decrease GI irritation. May cause profound sedation, blurred vision, and dystonic reactions (reversed by diphenhydramine). May interfere with pregnancy tests (immunological reactions between hCG and anti-hCG). **For nausea and vomiting, use only in management of prolonged vomiting of known etiology.**

PROPRANOLOL

Inderal and others
Adrenergic blocking agent (beta), antiarrhythmic, class II

Yes   1   C/D

Tabs: 10, 20, 40, 60, 80, 90 mg
Extended-release caps: 60, 80, 120, 160 mg
Oral solution: 20, 40 mg/5 mL; contains parabens and saccharin
Concentrated solution: 80 mg/mL; alcohol and dye free
Inj: 1 mg/mL

Arrhythmias:
  Children:
    IV: 0.01–0.1 mg/kg/dose IV push over 10 min, repeat Q6–8 hr PRN.
    Max. dose: 1 mg/dose for infants; **Max. dose:** 3 mg/dose for children.

Continued

PROPRANOLOL *continued*

> *PO:* Start at 0.5–1 mg/kg/24 hr ÷ Q6–8 hr; increase dosage Q3–5 days PRN.
> *Usual dosage range:* 2–4 mg/kg/24 hr ÷ Q6–8 hr. **Max. dose:** 60 mg/24 hr or
> 16 mg/kg/24 hr.

Adults:

> *IV:* 1 mg/dose Q5 min up to total 5 mg
> *PO:* 10–20 mg/dose TID-QID. Increase PRN. Usual range 40–320 mg/24 hr ÷
> TID-QID.

Hypertension:

Children:

> *PO:* Initial: 0.5–1 mg/kg/24 hr ÷ Q6–12 hr. May increase dose Q3–5 days PRN;
> **max. dose:** 8 mg/kg/24 hr

Adults:

> *PO:* 40 mg/dose PO BID or 60–80 mg/dose (sustained-release capsule) PO QD.
> May increase 10–20 mg/dose Q3–5 days; **max. dose:** 640 mg/24 hr

Migraine prophylaxis:

Children:

> *<35 kg:* 10–20 mg PO TID
> *≥35 kg:* 20–40 mg PO TID

> *Adults:* 80 mg/24 hr ÷ Q6–8 hr PO; increase dose by 20–40 mg/dose Q3–4 weeks
> PRN. *Usual effective dose range:* 160–240 mg/24 hr.

Tetralogy spells:

> *IV:* 0.15–0.25 mg/kg/dose slow IV push. May repeat in 15 min × 1. See also
> p. 156.
> *PO:* Start at 2–4 mg/kg/24 hr ÷ Q6 hr PRN. *Usual dose range:* 4–8 mg/kg/24 hr ÷
> Q6 hr PRN. Doses as high as 15 mg/kg/24 hr have been used with careful
> monitoring.

Thyrotoxicosis:

Neonates: 2 mg/kg/24 hr PO ÷ Q6–12 hr

Adolescents and adults:

> *IV:* 1–3 mg/dose over 10 min. May repeat in 4–6 hr.
> *PO:* 10–40 mg/dose PO Q6 hr

Contraindicated in asthma, Raynaud's syndrome, heart failure, and heart block.
Use with **caution** in presence of obstructive lung disease, diabetes mellitus, renal
or hepatic disease. May cause hypoglycemia, hypotension, nausea, vomiting,
depression, weakness, impotence, bronchospasm, and heart block.

Therapeutic levels: 30–100 ng/mL. Drug is metabolized by CYP 450 1A2, 2C18,
2C19 and 2D6 isoenzymes. Concurrent administration with barbiturates,
indomethacin, or rifampin may cause decreased activity of propranolol. Concurrent
administration with cimetidine, hydralazine, flecainide, quinidine, chlorpromazine, or
verapamil may lead to increased activity of propranolol. **Avoid** IV use of propranolol
with calcium channel blockers; may increase effect of calcium channel blocker.

Pregnancy category changes to "D" if used in second or third trimesters.

PROPYLTHIOURACIL

PTU
Antithyroid agent

Yes   1   D

Tabs: 50 mg
Oral suspension: 5 mg/mL
100 mg PTU = 10 mg methimazole

Neonates: 5–10 mg/kg/24 hr ÷ Q8 hr PO
Children:

Initial: 5–7 mg/kg/24 hr ÷ Q8 hr PO, OR by age:

6–10 yr: 50–150 mg/24 hr ÷ Q8 hr PO

>10 yr: 150–300 mg/24 hr ÷ Q8 hr PO

Maintenance: Generally begins after 2 mo. Usually ⅓ to ⅔ the initial dose when the patient is euthyroid.

Adults:

Initial: 300–450 mg/24 hr ÷ Q8 hr PO; some may require larger doses of 600–1200 mg/24 hr

Maintenance: 100–150 mg/24 hr ÷ Q8–12 hr PO

May cause blood dyscrasias, fever, liver disease, dermatitis, urticaria, malaise, CNS stimulation or depression, arthralgias. Glomerulonephritis, interstitial pneumonitis, exfoliative dermatitis, and erythema nodosum have also been reported. May decrease the effectiveness of warfarin. Monitor thyroid function. Dosages should be adjusted as required to achieve and maintain T_4 and TSH levels in normal ranges.

For neonates, use suspension or crush tablets, weigh appropriate dose, and mix in formula/breast milk.

Adjust dose in renal impairment (see p. 951).

PROSTAGLANDIN E₁

See Alprostadil

PROTAMINE SULFATE

Antidote, heparin

No   ?   C

Inj: 10 mg/mL (5, 10, 25 mL)

Heparin antidote, IV:
1 mg protamine will neutralize 115 U porcine intestinal heparin or 90 U beef lung heparin.

Continued

PROTAMINE SULFATE *continued*

Consider time since last heparin dose:
  If <0.5 hr: Give 100% of above dose
  If within 0.5–1 hr: Give 50%–75% of above dose
  If within 1–2 hr: Give 37.5%–50% of above dose
  If ≥2 hr: Give 25%–37.5% of above dose
  Max. dose: 50 mg IV
  Max. infusion rate: 5 mg/min
  Max. IV concentration: 10 mg/mL
If heparin was administered by deep SC injection, give 1-1.5 mg protamine per
100 U heparin as follows:
  Load with 25–50 mg via slow IV infusion followed by the rest of the calculated dose
  via continuous infusion over 8–16 hr or the expected duration of heparin absorption.

> Risk factors for protamine hypersensitivity include known hypersensitivity to fish and exposure to protamine-containing insulin or prior protamine therapy. May cause hypotension, bradycardia, dyspnea, and anaphylaxis. Monitor aPTT or ACT. Heparin rebound with bleeding has been reported to occur 8–18 hr later.
> For neonates, reconstitute medication with preservative-free sterile water for injection.

PSEUDOEPHEDRINE
Sudafed, Efidac/24, and others
Sympathomimetic, nasal decongestant

Yes   1   C

Tabs: 30, 60 mg
Chewable tabs: 15 mg; contains phenylalanine
Extended-release tabs: 120 mg, 240 mg (Efidac/24)
Caps: 60 mg
Sustained-release caps: 120 mg
Liquid: 15, 30 mg/5 mL
Drops: 7.5 mg/0.8 mL

> *Children <12 yr:* 4 mg/kg/24 hr ÷ Q6 hr PO
> *Children ≥12 yr and adults:*
>   *Immediate release:* 30–60 mg/dose Q6–8 hr PO; **max. dose:** 240 mg/24 hr
>   *Sustained release:* 120 mg PO Q12 hr
>   *Efidac/24:* 240 mg PO Q24 hr

> **Contraindicated** with MAO inhibitor drugs and in severe hypertension and severe coronary artery disease. Use with **caution** in mild/moderate hypertension, hyperglycemia, hyperthyroidism, and cardiac disease. May cause dizziness, nervousness, restlessness, insomnia, and arrhythmias. Pseudoephedrine is a common component of OTC cough and cold preparations and is combined with several antihistamines. Because drug and active metabolite are primarily excreted renally, doses should be adjusted in renal impairment. May cause false-positive test for amphetamines (EMIT assay).

PSYLLIUM

Metamucil, Fiberall, Seruton, Konsyl, and many others
Bulk-forming laxative

No 1 B

Granules (OTC): 2.5 g/rounded teaspoonful (480 g), 4.03 g/rounded teaspoonful (100, 250 g)
Powder (OTC): 50% psyllium, 50% dextrose (sugar-free version available); 100% psyllium (6 g/rounded teaspoon; Konsyl)
Wafers (OTC): 3.4 g
Effervescent powder (OTC): 3.4 g/rounded teaspoonful (single-dose packet, 141 g, 261 g, 387 g, 621 g)
Chewable squares (OTC): 1.7 g, 3.4 g

Children (granules or powder must be mixed with a full glass of water or juice):
<6 yr: 1.25–2.5 g/dose PO QD-TID; **max. dose** 7.5 g/24 hr
6–11 yr: 2.5–3.75 g/dose PO QD-TID; **max. dose** 15 g/24 hr
≥12 yr: 2.5–7.5 g/dose PO QD-TID; **max. dose:** 30 g/24 hr

Contraindicated in cases of fecal impaction or GI obstruction. Use with **caution** in patients with esophageal strictures and rectal bleeding. Phenylketonurics should be aware that certain preparations may contain aspartame. Should be taken with a full glass of liquid. *Onset of action:* 12–72 hr.

PYRANTEL PAMOATE

Antiminth, Reese's Pinworm medicine, Pin-Rid, Pin-X
Anthelmintic

No ? C

Suspension: 50 mg/mL (60 mL)
Liquid: 50 mg/mL, 144 mg/mL (30 mL)
Caps: 180 mg

Adults and children:
Ascaris (roundworm) and Trichostrongylus: 11 mg/kg/dose PO × 1
Enterobius (pinworm): 11 mg/kg/dose PO × 1. Repeat same dose 2 weeks later.
Hookworm or eosinophilic enterocolitis: 11 mg/kg/dose PO QD × 3 days
Max. dose (all indications): 1 g/dose

May cause nausea, vomiting, anorexia, transient AST elevations, headaches, rash, and muscle weakness. Use with **caution** in liver dysfunction. **Do not use** in combination with piperazine because of antagonism. Drug may be mixed with milk or fruit juices and may be taken with food.

PYRAZINAMIDE

Pyrazinoic acid amide
Antituberculous agent

Yes ? C

Tabs: 500 mg
Suspension: 100 mg/mL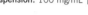

Use as part of a multi-drug regimen for tuberculosis.
Children:
  Daily dose: 20–40 mg/kg/24 hr PO ÷ QD-BID; **max. dose:** 2 g/24 hr
  Twice-weekly dose: 50 mg/kg/dose PO 2 × week; **max. dose:** 2 g/dose
Adults:
  Daily dose: 15–30 mg/kg/24 hr PO ÷ QD-QID; **max. dose:** 2 g/24 hr
  Twice-weekly dose: 50–70 mg/kg/dose PO 2 × week; **max. dose:** 4 g/dose

See the latest edition of the AAP's *Red Book* for recommended treatment for tuberculosis. **Contraindicated** in severe hepatic damage. Hepatoxicity is most common side effect. Hyperuricemia, maculopapular rash, arthralgia, fever, acne, porphyria, dysuria, and photosensitivity may occur. Use with **caution** in patients with renal failure (dosage reduction has been recommended), gout, or diabetes mellitus.

PYRETHRINS

A-200, Pyrinyl, Pronto, RID, and others
Pediculicide

No ? C

Available as gel, shampoo, and liquid, all in combination with piperonyl butoxide.
All products are available without a prescription.

Pediculosis: Apply to hair or affected body area for 10 min, then wash thoroughly; repeat in 7–10 days.

Contraindicated in ragweed hypersensitivity; drug is derived from the chrysanthemum flower. For topical use only. **Avoid** eye or facial contact and PO intake. **Avoid** repeat applications in <24 hr. Low ovicidal activity requires repeat treatment. Dead nits require mechanical removal. Wash bedding and clothing to eradicate infestation.

PYRIDOSTIGMINE BROMIDE

Mestinon, Regonol
Cholinergic agent

Yes   1   C

Syrup: 60 mg/5 mL (480 mL); contains 5% alcohol
Tabs: 60 mg
Sustained-release tabs: 180 mg
Inj: 5 mg/mL; may contain parabens and/or benzyl alcohol

Myasthenia gravis:
Neonates:
   PO: 5 mg/dose Q4–6 hr
   IM/IV: 0.05–0.15 mg/kg/dose Q4–6 hr; **max. single IM/IV dose:** 10 mg
Children:
   PO: 7 mg/kg/24 hr in 5–6 divided doses
   IM/IV: 0.05–0.15 mg/kg/dose Q4–6 hr; **max. single IM/IV dose:** 10 mg
Adults:
   PO (immediate release): 60 mg/dose TID. Increase Q48 hr PRN. *Usual effective dose:* 60–1500 mg/24 hr.
   PO (sustained release): 180–540 mg/dose QD-BID
   IM/IV: 2–5 mg/dose Q2–3 hr

Contraindicated in mechanical intestinal or urinary obstruction. Use with **caution** in patients with epilepsy, asthma, bradycardia, hyperthyroidism, arrhythmias, or peptic ulcer. May cause nausea, vomiting, diarrhea, rash, headache, and muscle cramps. Pyridostigmine is mainly excreted unchanged by the kidney. Therefore lower doses titrated to effect in renal disease may be necessary.
   Changes in oral dosages may take several days to show results. **Atropine is the antidote.**

PYRIDOXINE/VITAMIN B₆

Vitamin B₆
Vitamin, water soluble

No   1   A/C

Tabs (OTC): 25, 50, 100, 250, 500 mg
Tabs, extended release (OTC): 200, 500 mg
Inj: 100 mg/mL

Deficiency, IM/IV/PO (PO preferred):
   Children: 5–25 mg/24 hr × 3 weeks, followed by 1.5–2.5 mg/24 hr as maintenance therapy (via multivitamin preparation)
   Adult: 10–20 mg/24 hr × 3 weeks, followed by 2–5 mg/24 hr as maintenance therapy (via multivitamin preparation)

Continued

PYRIDOXINE/VITAMIN B₆ *continued*

Drug-induced neurititis, PO:
  Prophylaxis:
    Children: 1–2 mg/kg/24 hr
    Adults: 25–100 mg/24 hr
  Treatment:
    Children: 10–50 mg/24 hr
    Adults: 100–300 mg/24 hr
Sideroblastic anemia:
  Adult: 200–600 mg/24 hr PO × 1–2 mo. If adequate response, dose may be
  reduced to 30–50 mg/24 hr.
Pyridoxine-dependent seizures:
  Neonate/infant:
    Initial: 50–100 mg/dose IM or rapid IV × 1
    Maintenance: 50–100 mg/24 hr PO
Recommended daily allowance: See pp. 460–461.

Use **caution** with concurrent levodopa therapy. Chronic administration has been
associated with sensory neuropathy. Nausea, headache, increased AST,
decreased serum folic acid level, and allergic reaction may occur. May lower
phenytoin levels. See pp. 427–429 for management of neonatal seizures. Pregnancy
category changes to "C" if used in doses above the RDA.

PYRIMETHAMINE ± SULFADOXINE

Daraprim; in combination with sulfadoxine-Fansidar
Antiparasitic agent ± sulfonamide antibiotic

Yes   1   C

Tabs: 25 mg
Suspension: 2 mg/mL
In combination with sulfadoxine:
  Tabs: Pyrimethamine 25 mg and sulfadoxine 500 mg

PYRIMETHAMINE:
Congenital toxoplasmosis (administer with sulfadiazine):
  Load: 2 mg/kg/24 hr PO ÷ Q12 hr × 2 days
  Maintenance: 1 mg/kg/24 hr PO QD × 2–6 mo, then 1 mg/kg/24 hr 3 ×/week to
  complete total 12 mo of therapy.
Toxoplasmosis (administer with sulfadiazine or trisulfapyrimidines)
  Children:
    Load: 2 mg/kg/24 hr PO ÷ BID × 3 days; **max. dose:** 100 mg/24 hr
    Maintenance: 1 mg/kg/24 hr PO ÷ QD-BID × 4 weeks; **Max. dose:** 25 mg/
    24 hr
  Adults: 25–100 mg/24 hr × 3–4 weeks depending on response. After response,
  decrease dose by 50% and continue for an additional 4–5 weeks.

Continued

PYRIMETHAMINE ± SULFADOXINE *continued*

PYRIMETHAMINE AND SULFADOXINE:

Malaria treatment (single dose on the last day of quinine therapy):
2–11 mo: ¼ tab
1–3 yr: ½ tab
4–8 yr: 1 tab
9–14 yr: 2 tabs
>14 yr and adults: 3 tabs

Malaria prophylaxis (for areas of chloroquine-resistant P. falciparum used as a single dose for self-treatment of febrile illness when medical care is not immediately available):
2–11 mo: ¼ tab
1–3 yr: ½ tab
4–8 yr: 1 tab
9–14 yr: 2 tabs
>14 yr and adults: 3 tabs

Pyrimethamine is a folate antagonist. Supplementation with folinic acid leucovorin at 5–15 mg/24 hr is recommended. **Contraindicated** in megaloblastic anemia secondary to folate deficiency. Use with **caution** in G6PD deficiency, malabsorption syndromes, alcoholism, pregnancy, and renal or hepatic impairment. Pyrimethamine can cause glossitis, bone marrow suppression, seizures, rash, and photosensitivity. For congenital toxoplasmosis, see Clin Infect Dis 1994; 18:38–72. Administer doses with meals. Most cases of acquired toxoplasmosis **do not** require specific antimicrobial therapy.

PYRIMETHAMINE AND SULFADOXINE: Effective against certain strains of *P. falciparum* that are resistant to chloroquine. Resistance has been reported in Southeast Asia and the Amazon Basin. **Contraindicated** (in addition to above) in sulfa hypersensitivity, porphyria, severe renal impairment, and pregnancy at term. May cause (in addition to above) erythema multiforme, Stevens-Johnson syndrome, toxic epidermal necrolysis, elevated ALT and AST, and renal impairment. Administer doses with meals.

QUINIDINE

Many brand names
Antiarrhythmic, class Ia

Yes 1 C

As gluconate (62% quinidine):
Slow-release tabs: 324 mg
Inj: 80 mg/mL; contains phenol
As sulfate (83% quinidine):
Tabs: 200, 300 mg
Slow-release tabs: 300 mg
Susp: 10 mg/mL
As polygalacturonate (80% quinidine):
Tabs: 275 mg
Equivalents: 200 mg sulfate = 267 mg gluconate = 275 mg polygalacturonate

Continued

QUINIDINE *continued*

All doses expressed as salt forms.
Antiarrhythmic:
  Children (give PO as sulfate, give IM/IV as gluconate):
  Test dose: 2 mg/kg × 1 IM/PO; **max. dose:** 200 mg
  Therapeutic dose:
  IV (as gluconate): 2–10 mg/kg/dose Q3–6 hr PRN
  PO (as sulfate): 15–60 mg/kg/24 hr ÷ Q6 hr
  Adults (give PO as sulfate, give IM as gluconate):
  Test dose: 200 mg × 1 IM/PO.
  Therapeutic dose
  As sulfate:
    PO, immediate release: 100–600 mg/dose Q4–6 hr. Begin at 200 mg/dose
    and titrate to desired effect.
    PO, sustained release: 300–600 mg/dose Q 8–12 hr.
  As gluconate:
    IM: 400 mg/dose Q4–6 hr
    IV: 200–400 mg/dose, infused at a rate of ≤10 mg/min.
    PO: 324–972 mg Q8–12 hr
  As polygalacturonate:
    PO: 275 mg Q8–12 hr
Malaria:
  Children and adults (give IV as gluconate; see remarks):
  Loading dose: 10 mg/kg/dose (**max. dose:** 600 mg) IV over 1–2 hr followed by
  maintenance dose. Omit or decrease load if patient has received quinine or
  mefloquine.
  Maintenance dose: 0.02 mg/kg/min IV as continuous infusion until oral therapy
  can be initiated. If more than 48 hrs of IV therapy is required, reduce dose by
  ⅓ to ½.

Test dose is given to assess for idiosyncratic reaction to quinidine. Toxicity
indicated by increase of QRS interval by ≥0.02 sec (skip dose or stop drug). May
cause GI symptoms, hypotension, tinnitus, TTP, rash, heart block, and blood
dyscrasias. When used alone, may cause 1 : 1 conduction in atrial flutter leading to
ventricular fibrillation. May get idiosyncratic ventricular tachycardia with low levels,
especially when initiating therapy.

Quinidine is a substrate of cytochrome P 450 3A3/4 and 3A5-7 enzymes, and
inhibitor of cytochrome P 450 2D6 and 3A3/4 enzymes. Can cause increase in
digoxin levels. Quinidine potentiates the effect of neuromuscular blocking agents, beta-
blockers, anticholinergics, and warfarin. Amiodarone, antacids, delavirdine, diltiazem,
grapefruit juice, saquinavir, ritonavir, verapamil, or cimetidine may enhance the drug's
effect. Barbiturates, phenytoin, cholinergic drugs, nifedipine, sucralfate, or rifampin
may reduce quinidine's effect. Use with **caution** in renal insufficiency (15%-25% of
drug is eliminated unchanged in the urine).

Therapeutic levels: 3–7 mg/L. *Recommended serum sampling times at
steady-state:* Trough level obtained within 30 min prior to the next scheduled dose
after 1–2 days of continuous dosing (steady-state).

MALARIA USE: Continuous monitoring of ECG, blood pressure, and serum glucose
is recommended; especially in pregnant women and young children.

QUINUPRISTIN AND DALFOPRISTIN

Synercid
Antibiotic, streptogramin

No   ?   B

Inj: 500 mg (150 mg quinupristin and 350 mg dalfopristin)

Doses expressed in mg of combined quinupristin and dalfopristin.
Children <16 yr (limited data), ≥16 yr and adults:
Vancomycin-resistant Enterococcus faecium (VREF): 7.5 mg/kg/dose IV Q8 hr
Complicated skin infections: 7.5 mg/kg/dose IV Q12 hr for at least 7 days

Not active against *Enterococcus faecalis.* Use with **caution** in hepatic
impairment; dosage reduction may be necessary. Most common side effects
include pain, burning, inflammation, and edema at the IV infusion site;
thrombophlebitis, and thrombosis. Nausea, diarrhea, vomiting, rash, arthralgia,
myalgia, increased liver enzymes, hyperbilirubinemia, headache, pain, or pruritus
may also occur.

Drug is an inhibitor of the cytochrome P 450 3A4 isoenzyme. **Avoid** use with
cytochrome P 450 3A4 substrates that can prolong QTc interval (e.g., astemizole,
cisapride, and terfenadine). May increase the effects/toxicity of cyclosporine,
tacrolimus, sirolimus, delavirdine, nevirapine, indinavir, ritonavir, diazepam,
midazolam, carbamazepine, methylprednisolone, vinca alkaloids, docetaxel, paclitaxel,
quinidine, and some calcium channel blockers.
Pediatric pharmacokinetic studies have not been completed.

Drug is compatible with D_5W and incompatible with saline and heparin. Infuse
each dose over 1 hr using the following **maximum** IV concentrations: peripheral line:
2 mg/mL, central line: 5 mg/mL. If injection site reaction occurs, dilute infusion to
<1 mg/mL.

RANITIDINE HCl

Zantac, Zantac 75(OTC), and others
Histamine-2-antagonist

Yes   1   B

Tabs: 75 (OTC), 150, 300 mg
Effervescent tabs: 150 mg
Syrup: 15 mg/mL; contains 7.5% alcohol and parabens
Effervescent granules: 150 mg; contains phenylalanine and povidone
Carbohydrate-free oral solution: 5, 10 mg/mL (dissolve 150 mg effervescent granules
with 30 mL [5 mg/mL] or 15 mL [10 mg/mL] water; solution good for 24 hrs)
Caps, GELdose: 150, 300 mg
Inj: 25 mg/mL; contains 0.5% phenol
Inj (pre-mixed): 0.5 mg/mL (preservative-free in ½ normal saline, 100 mL)

Continued

RANITIDINE HCl *continued*

Neonates:
　PO: 2–4 mg/kg/24 hr ÷ Q8–12 hr
　IV: 2 mg/kg/24 hr ÷ Q6–8 hr
≥*1 mo-16 yr:*
　Duodenal/gastric ulcer (see remarks):
　　PO:
　　　Treatment: 2–4 mg/kg/24 hr ÷ Q12 hr; **max. dose:** 300 mg/24 hr
　　　Maintenance: 2–4 mg/kg/24 hr ÷ Q12 hr; **max. dose:** 150 mg/24 hr
　　IV/IM: 2–4 mg/kg/24 hr ÷ Q6–8 hr; **max. dose:** 150 mg/24 hr
　GERD/erosive esophagitis:
　　PO: 5–10 mg/kg/24 hr ÷ Q12 hr; GERD **max. dose:** 300 mg/24 hr; erosive
　　esophagitis **max. dose:** 600 mg/24 hr
　　IV/IM: 2–4 mg/kg/24 hr ÷ Q6–8 hr; **max. dose:** 150 mg/24 hr
Adults:
　PO: 150 mg/dose BID or 300 mg/dose QHS
　IM/IV: 50 mg/dose Q6–8 hr
　　Max. dose: 400 mg/24 hr
Continuous infusion, all ages: Administer daily IV dosage over 24 hr (may be added to
parenteral nutrition solutions)

May cause headache and GI disturbance, malaise, insomnia, sedation,
arthralgia, and hepatotoxicity. May increase levels of nifedipine. May decrease
levels of ketoconazole, itraconazole, and delavirdine. May cause false-positive
urine protein test (Multistix).

　Duodenal/gastric ulcer doses for ≥1 mo–16 yr are extrapolated from clinical
adult trials and pharmacokinetic data in children. Extemporaneously compounded
carbohydrate-free oral solution dosage form useful for patients receiving the
ketogenic diet.

　Adjust dose in renal failure (see p. 951).

RESPIRATORY SYNCYTIAL VIRUS IMMUNE GLOBULIN

Respigam　　　　　　　　　　　　　　　　　　　**No**　**?**　**C**
Immune globulin, RSV (high titer)

Inj: 50 mg/mL (1000 mg/20 mL, 2,500 mg/50 mL); contains 5% sucrose,
1% albumin (human) and 1–1.5 mEq Na/50 mL

*RSV prophylaxis (see pp. 338–339 and latest edition of Red Book for most
recent indications):*
　≤*2 yr with chronic lung disease, premature infants (≤28 weeks gestation)
　<12 mo, or premature infants (29–32 weeks gestation) <6 mo:* 750 mg/kg/dose
IV Q monthly just prior and during the RSV season. Gradually increase IV infusion

Continued

RESPIRATORY SYNCYTIAL VIRUS IMMUNE GLOBULIN *continued*

(if tolerated) by starting at 1.5 mL/kg/hr for 15 min, increase to 3 mL/kg/hr the next 15 min, then to 6 mL/kg/hr to the end of infusion.

RSV season is typically November through April in the northern hemisphere but may begin earlier or persist later in certain communities. **Contraindicated** in IgA deficiency. Should **not** be used in patients with cyanotic heart disease. Use with **caution** in patients with fluid restrictions. Frequent side effects include fever, respiratory distress, vomiting, and wheezing. Monitor heart rate, blood pressure, temperature, and respiratory rate. Live virus vaccines (e.g., MMR, varicella) should be deferred for 9–10 mo after the last dose of RSVIG. Some patients may benefit from premedications (e.g., diphenhydramine, acetaminophen).

RH$_O$ (D) IMMUNE GLOBULIN INTRAVENOUS (HUMAN)

WinRho-SDF

Immune globulin

No ? C

Inj: 600, 1500, 5000 IU
Conversion: 1 mcg = 5 IU

Immune thrombocytopenic purpura (nonsplenectomized Rho [D]-positive patients):

Initial dose (may given in two divided doses on separate days or as a single dose):

Hemoglobin ≥10 mg/dL: 250 IU/kg/dose IV × 1

Hemoglobin <10 mg/dL: 125–200 IU/kg/dose IV × 1

Additional doses: 125–300 IU/kg/dose IV; actual dose and frequency of adminstration is determined by the patient's response and subsequent hemoglobin level.

WinRho SDF is currently the only Rho (D) immune globulin product compatible with intravenous administration. **Contraindicated** in IgA deficiency. **Use with extreme caution in patients with a hemoglobin <8 mg/dL.** Adverse events associated with ITP include headache, chills, fever, and reduction in hemoglobin (due to the destruction of Rho [D] antigen-positive red cells). Intravascular hemolysis resulting in anemia and renal insufficiency has been reported. May interfere with immune response to live virus vaccines (e.g., MMR, varicella). Administer IV doses over 3–5 min.

RIBAVIRIN

Virazole, Rebetol
Antiviral agent

Yes   ?   X

Aerosol (Virazole): 6 g
Oral caps (Rebetol): 200 mg (only available in combination with Interferon Alfa-2b as a kit [Rebetron])

Inhalation:
Continuous: Administer 6 g by aerosol over 12–18 hr QD for 3–7 days. The 6-g ribavirin vial is diluted in 300 mL preservative-free sterile water to a final concentration of 20 mg/mL. Must be administered with Viratek Small Particle Aerosol Generator (SPAG-2).
Intermittent (for nonventilated patients): Administer 2 g by aerosol over 2 hr TID for 3–7 days. The 6-g ribavirin vial is diluted in 100 mL preservative-free sterile water to a final concentration of 60 mg/mL. Intermittent use is not recommended in patients with endotracheal tubes.
Hepatitis C:
Adults (in combination with interferon alfa-2b at 3 million units 3 ×/week SC):
≤75 kg (PO): 400 mg QAM and 600 mg QPM
>75 kg (PO): 600 mg BID

Use of ribavirin for RSV is controversial and not routinely indicated. Ribavirin aerosol therapy may be considered for selected infants and young children at high risk for serious RSV disease (see AAP recommendations in Pediatrics 1996; 97:137-40). Most effective if begun early in course of RSV infection, generally in the first 3 days. May cause worsening respiratory distress, rash, conjunctivitis, mild bronchospasm, hypotension, anemia, and cardiac arrest. **Avoid** unnecessary occupational exposure to ribavirin because of its teratogenic effects. Drug can precipitate in the respiratory equipment.

ORAL RIBAVIRIN: Contraindicated in pregnancy. With oral use, administer with **caution** in patients with creatinine clearance <50 mL/min; **not recommended in severe renal impairment.** Anemia (most common), insomnia, depression, irritability, and suicidal behavior have been reported with the oral route. Tinnitus, hearing loss, vertigo, and severe hypertriglyceridemia have been reported in combination with interferon. Reduce dose to 600 mg/24 hr if hemoglobin <10 g/dL but discontinue use of drug if hemoglobin drops below 8.5 g/dL.

RIBOFLAVIN/VITAMIN B$_2$

Vitamin B$_2$, Riobin, and others
Water-soluble vitamin

No   1   A/C

Tabs (OTC): 10, 25, 50, 100 mg

Continued

RIBOFLAVIN/VITAMIN B₂ *continued*

Riboflavin deficiency:
Children: 2.5–10 mg/24 hr ÷ QD-BID PO
Adults: 5–30 mg/24 hr ÷ QD-BID PO
RDA requirements: see pp. 460–461.

Hypersensitivity may occur. Administer with food. Causes yellow to orange discoloration of urine. For multi-vitamin information, see pp. 463–465. Pregnancy category changes to "C" if used in doses above the RDA.

RIFABUTIN
Mycobutin
Antituberculous agent

Yes   ?   B

Caps: 150 mg
Suspension: 10, 20 mg/mL

MAC prophylaxis for first episode of opportunistic disease in HIV:
Children:
 <6 yr: 5 mg/kg/24 hr PO QD; **max. dose:** 300 mg/24 hr
 ≥6 yr: 300 mg PO QD with food
Adolescents and adults: 300 mg PO QD or 150 mg PO BID with or without azithromycin.
MAC prophylaxis for recurrence of opportunistic disease in HIV (in combination with a multidrug regimen that includes a macrolide antibiotic):
 Infants and children: 5 mg/kg/24 hr PO QD; **max. dose:** 300 mg/24 hr
 Adolescents and adults: 300 mg PO QD or 150 mg PO BID with food
MAC treatment:
 Children: 5–10 mg/kg/24 hr PO QD; **max. dose:** 300 mg/24 hr as part of a multi-drug regimen.
 Adults: 300 mg PO QD; may be used in combination with azithromycin and ethambutol.
  In combination with nonnucleoside reverse transcriptase inhibitors:
   With efavirenz: 450 mg PO QD or 600 mg PO 2 × per week
   With nevirapine: 300 mg PO 2 × per week
  In combination with protease inhibitors:
   With amprenavir, indinavir, or nelfinavir: 150 mg PO QD or 300 mg PO 2 × per week.
   With ritonavir or lopinavir/ritonavir: 150 mg PO QOD
   With saquinavir/ritonavir: 150 mg PO 2–3 × per week or 300 mg PO Qweek

May cause GI distress, discoloration of skin and body fluids (brown-orange color), and marrow suppression. Use with **caution** in renal failure. **Adjust dose in renal impairment (see p. 944).** May permanently stain contact lenses. Uveitis

Continued

RIFABUTIN *continued*

can occur when using high doses (>300 mg/24 hr in adults) in combination with macrolide antibiotics.

Rifabutin is an inducer of cytochrome P 450 3A enzyme and is structurally similar to rifampin (similar drug interactions, see *Rifampin*). Clarithromycin, fluconazole, itraconazole, nevirapine, and protease inhibitors increase rifabutin levels. Efavirenz may decrease rifabutin levels. May decrease effectiveness of dapsone, delavirdine, nevirapine, amprenavir, indinavir, nelfinavir, saquinavir, itraconazole, warfarin, oral contraceptives, digoxin, cyclosporin, ketoconazole, and narcotics.

Doses may be administered with food if patient experiences GI intolerance.

RIFAMPIN

Rimactane, Rifadin, and others
Antibiotic, antituberculous agent

Yes   1   C

Caps: 150, 300 mg
Suspension: 10, 15 mg/mL
Inj: 600 mg

Tuberculosis: (see the latest edition of the AAP's *Red Book,* for duration of therapy and combination therapy). Twice weekly therapy may be used after 1–2 mo of daily therapy
Children:
    Daily therapy: 10–20 mg/kg/24 hr ÷ Q12–24 hr IV/PO
    Twice weekly therapy: 10–20 mg/kg/24 hr PO twice weekly
    Max. daily dose: 600 mg/24 hr
Adults:
    Daily therapy: 10 mg/kg/24 hr QD PO
    Twice weekly therapy: 10 mg/kg/24 hr QD twice weekly
    Max. daily dose: 600 mg/24 hr
Prophylaxis for N. meningitidis:
    0–1 mo: 10 mg/kg/24 hr ÷ Q12 hr PO × 2 days
    >1 mo: 20 mg/kg/24 hr ÷ Q12 hr PO × 2 days
    Adults: 600 mg PO Q12 hr × 2 days
    Max. dose (all ages): 1200 mg/24 hr

May cause GI irritation, allergy, headache, fatigue, ataxia, confusion, fever, hepatitis, blood dyscrasias, interstitial nephritis, and elevated BUN and uric acid.
Causes red discoloration of body secretions such as urine, saliva, and tears (which can permanently stain contact lenses). Induces hepatic enzymes (CYP 450 2C9, 2C19, and 3A4), which may decrease plasma concentration of digoxin, corticosteroids, buspirone, benzodiazepines, fentanyl, calcium channel blockers, beta-blockers, cyclosporine, tacrolimus, itraconazole, ketoconazole, oral anticoagulants, barbiturates, and theophylline. May reduce the effectiveness of oral contraceptives.
Adjust dose in renal failure (see p. 944). Reduce dose in hepatic impairment. Give 1 hr before or 2 hr after meals.

For *H. influenzae* prophylaxis, see latest edition of the AAP *Red Book.*

RIMANTADINE
Flumadine
Antiviral agent

Yes ? C

Syrup: 50 mg/ 5 mL (240 mL); contains saccharin and parabens
Tabs: 100 mg

Influenza A prophylaxis:
  Children <10 yr: 5 mg/kg/24 hr PO QD; **max. dose:** 150 mg/24 hr
  Children ≥10 yr and adults: 100 mg PO BID
Influenza A treatment (within 48 hr of illness onset):
  Children <10 yr: 5 mg/kg/24 hr PO ÷ QD-BID × 5–7 days; **max. dose:** 150 mg/ 24 hr
  Children ≥10 yr (<40 kg): 5 mg/kg/24 hr PO ÷ QD-BID × 5–7 days.
  Children ≥10 yr (≥40 kg) and adults: 100 mg PO BID × 5–7 days.

During influenza season, use prophylaxis for 2–3 weeks after influenza vaccination until patient develops protective antibody response. Alternatively, may be used for 10 days after patient has been exposed. May cause GI disturbance, dizziness, headache, and urinary retention. CNS disturbances are less than with amantadine. **Contraindicated** in amantadine hypersensitivity. Use with **caution** in renal or hepatic insufficiency; dosage reduction may be necessary. A dosage reduction of 50% has been recommended in severe hepatic or renal impairment.

RITONAVIR
Norvir
Antiviral, protease inhibitor

No 3 B

Caps, soft gel: 100 mg; contains alcohol
Oral solution: 80 mg/mL (240 mL); contains saccharin

Children ≤12 yr: Start at 250 mg/m^2/dose Q12 hr PO, then increase dose by 50 mg/m^2/dose Q12 hr increments over 5 days up to 400 mg/m^2/dose Q12 hr. *Dosage range:* 350–400 mg/m^2/dose Q12 hr.
  Max. dose: 600 mg/dose BID
Adolescents and adults: Start at 300 mg/dose Q12 hr PO. To minimize nausea and vomiting, increase by 100-mg increments up to 600 mg/dose Q12 hr over 5 days as tolerated. If used in combination with other protease inhibitors as a pharmacokinetic enhancer, 200–400 mg/dose Q12 hr PO.

Dose titration schedule is recommended to minimize risk for side effects. Use with **caution** in liver impairment.
  Most frequent side effects include nausea, vomiting, diarrhea, headache, abdominal pain, anorexia, and paresthesias. Increases in liver enzymes, triglycerides, cholesterol,

Continued

For explanation of icons, see p. 572.

RITONAVIR *continued*

and serum glucose may also occur. Spontaneous bleeding in hemophiliacs has been reported.

Inhibits and is metabolized by the CYP 3A4 microsomal enzyme to cause many drug interactions. **Do NOT use** concurrently with amiodarone, astemizole, bepridil, bupropion, cisapride, clozapine, dihydroergotamine, ergotamine, flecainide, encainide, meperidine, pimozide, piroxicam, propafenone, propoxyphene, quinidine, rifabutin, rifampin, terfenadine, and benzodiazepines (except for lorazepam). Drug may increase the levels of clarithromycin, calcium channel blockers, desipramine, warfarin, digoxin, and other protease inhibitors. Theopylline and digoxin levels may be reduced. **Always check the potential for other drug interactions when either initiating therapy or adding new drugs onto an existing regimen.**

Adolescent dosing: Patients in early puberty (Tanner I-II) should be dosed with pediatric regimens and those in late puberty (Tanner V) should be dosed with adult regimens. Adolescents who are in the midst of their growth spurt (Tanner III females and Tanner IV males) can be dosed by either pediatric or adult regimen with close monitoring of efficacy and toxicity.

Administer doses with food to assure absorption. If didanosine is included in the antiretroviral regimen, space the administration of two drugs by 2 hr. Store both capsules and oral solution in the refrigerator. Oral solution can be kept at room temperature if used within 30 days. Oral solution must be kept in original container. Administering doses with milk, chocolate milk, pudding, or ice cream can enhance compliance in children. **Noncompliance can quickly promote resistant HIV strains.**

When using in combination with saquinavir, doses >400 mg PO BID for either ritonavir or saquinavir may be associated with risk for increased adverse effects.

ROCURONIUM

Zemuron

Nondepolarizing neuromuscular blocking agent

No ? B

Inj: 10 mg/mL (5 mL)

Infants:
IV: 0.5 mg/kg/dose; may repeat Q 20–30 min PRN
Children and adults:
IV: Start with 0.6–1.2 mg/kg/dose × 1, if needed, maintenance doses at 0.1–0.2 mg/kg/dose Q 20–30 min.
Continuous IV infusion: Start at 10–12 mcg/kg/min and titrate to effect. Maintenance infusion rates have ranged from 4–16 mcg/kg/min in adults.
To prepare infusion: See inside front cover.

Use with **caution** in hepatic impairment. Hypertension, hypotension, arrhythmia, tachycardia, nausea, vomiting, bronchospasm, wheezing, hiccups, rash, and edema at the injection site may occur. Increased neuromuscular blockade may occur with concomitant use of aminoglycosides, clindamycin, tetracycline, magnesium sulfate, quinine, quinidine, succinylcholine, and inhalation anesthetics. Caffeine,

Continued

FORMULARY

ROCURONIUM *continued*

calcium, carbamazepine, phenytoin, phenylephrine, azathioprine, and theophylline may reduce neuromuscular blocking effects.

Peak effects occur in 0.5–1 min for children and in 1–3.7 min for adults. *Duration of action:* 30–40 min in children and 20–94 min in adults. Recovery time in children 3 mo to 1 yr is similar to adults. In obese patients, use actual body weight for dosage calculation.

SALMETEROL

Serevent, Serevent Diskus
Beta-2-adrenergic agonist (long acting)

No   ?   C

Aerosol metered-dose inhaler (MDI): 21 mcg/actuation (6.5 g, 13 g; 6.5 g = 60 actuations)
Dry powder inhalation (DPI; Diskus): 50 mcg/inhalation (28, 60 inhalations)
In combination with fluticasone: See *Fluticasone propionate and salmeterol*

Persistent asthma:
  MDI:
    Children: 1–2 puffs (21–42 mcg) Q12 hr
    >12 yr and adults: 2 puffs (42 mcg) Q12 hr
  DPI (>4 yr and adults): 1 inhalation (50 mcg) Q12 hr
Exercise-induced asthma (>12 yr):
  MDI: 2 puffs 30–60 min before exercise. Additional doses should not be used for another 12 hr.
  DPI: 1 inhalation 30–60 min before exercise. Additional doses should not be used for another 12 hr.

Should not be used to relieve symptoms of acute asthma. It is long acting and has its onset of action in 10–20 min with a peak effect at 3 hr. May be used QHS (1–2 MDI puffs or 1 DPI) for nocturnal symptoms. Salmeterol is a chronic medication and is **not** used in similar fashion to short-acting beta-agonists (e.g., albuterol). Patients already receiving salmeterol Q12 hr (MDI or DPI) should not use additional doses for prevention of exercise-induced bronchospasm; consider alternative therapy. Use of spacers or chambers may enhance the efficacy of MDIs. Proper patient education is essential. Side effects are similar to albuterol. Hypertension and arrhythmias have been reported. See pp. 513–515 for recommendations for asthma controller therapy.

SAQUINAVIR

Invirase (mesylate salt), Fortovase
Antiviral agent, protease inhibitor

No   3   B

Caps, hard gel: (Invirase): 200 mg
Caps, soft gel: (Fortovase): 200 mg

Continued

SAQUINAVIR *continued*

Children (investigational dose from ACTG 397):
Fortovase: 50 mg/kg/dose PO Q8 hr; if in combination with nelfinavir, use
33 mg/kg/dose PO Q8 hr
Adolescents and adults:
Single protease inhibitor regimen:
Fortovase: 1200 mg/dose PO TID OR 1600 mg/dose PO BID
In combination with ritonavir dosed at 400 mg PO BID:
Invirase or Fortovase: 400 mg/dose PO BID

Invirase and Fortovase are **not** bioequivalent and cannot be used interchangeably. Use Invirase only in combination with ritonavir. Most frequent adverse effects include diarrhea, GI discomfort, nausea, and headache. Spontaneous bleeding in hemophiliacs, hyperglycemia, and body fat redistribution without serum lipid abnormalities have been reported.

Drug inhibits and is metabolized by the CYP450 3A4 drug metabolizing enzyme. **Do not use** in combination with astemizole, terfenadine, cisapride, lovastatin, simvastatin, ergot alkaloids, and benzodiazepines (except lorazepam). Increased levels and/or toxicity may occur with the following concurrent medications: calcium channel blockers, clindamycin, dapsone, and quinidine. Rifampin, rifabutin, niverapine, carbamazepine, dexamethasone, phenobarbital, and phenytoin can decrease saquinavir levels. Delavirdine, ketoconazole, grapefruit juice, and other protease inhibitors may increase saquinavir levels. **Always carefully review patient's medication profile for other potential drug-drug interactions.**

Adolescent dosing: Patients in early puberty (Tanner I-II) should be dosed with pediatric regimens and those in late puberty (Tanner V) should be dosed with adult regimens. Adolescents who are at the midst of their growth spurt (Tanner III females and Tanner IV males) can be dosed by either pediatric or adult regimen with close monitoring of efficacy and toxicity.

Administer each dose with food or within 2 hr after a meal. Fortovase capsules are usually stored in the refrigerator; their stability will decrease to 3 mo once they are brought to room temperature. **Noncompliance can quickly promote resistant HIV strains.** When using in combination with ritonavir, doses > 400 mg PO BID for either ritonavir or saquinavir may be associated with risk for increased adverse effects.

SCOPOLAMINE HYDROBROMIDE

Hyoscine, Transderm Scop, Isopto
Anticholinergic agent

No   1   C

Inj: 0.3, 0.4, 0.86, 1 mg/mL
Transdermal: 1.5 mg/patch (4s); delivers 0.5 mg over 3 days
Ophthalmic solution: 0.25% (5, 15 mL)

Antiemetic (SC/IM/IV):
Children: 6 mcg/kg/dose Q6–8 hr PRN; **max. dose:** 300 mcg/dose
Adults: 0.32–0.65 mg/dose Q6–8 hr PRN

Continued

SCOPOLAMINE HYDROBROMIDE *continued*

Transdermal (≥12 yr): Apply patch behind the ear at least 4 hr prior to exposure to motion; remove after 72 hr.
Ophthalmic:
  Children, refraction: 1 drop BID for 2 days before procedure
  Children, iridocyclitis: 1 drop up to TID

Toxicities similar to atropine. **Contraindicated** in urinary or GI obstruction and glaucoma. May cause dry mouth, drowsiness, blurred vision. Transdermal route should **not** be used in children <12 yr. Drug withdrawal symptoms (nausea, vomiting, headache, and vertigo) have been reported following removal of transdermal patch in patients using the patch for >3 days. Systemic effects have been reported with both transdermal and ophthalmic preparations. Compress nasolacrimal ducts to minimize systemic effects when using ophthalmic preparations.

SELENIUM SULFIDE

Selsun, Exsel (Rx)
Topical antiseborrheic agent

No ? C

Lotion/shampoo: 1% (OTC), 2.5% (Rx and OTC)
Shampoo: 1% (OTC)

Seborrhea/dandruff: Massage 5–10 mL of 1% or 2.5% into wet scalp and leave on scalp × 2–3 min. Rinse thoroughly and repeat. Shampoo twice weekly × 2 weeks. Maintenance applications once every 1–4 weeks.
Tinea versicolor: Apply 2.5% to affected areas of skin. Allow to remain on skin × 30 min. Rinse thoroughly. Repeat QD × 7 days. Follow with monthly applications for 3 mo to prevent recurrences.

Rinse hands and body well after treatment. May cause local irritation, hair loss, and hair discoloration. **Avoid** eyes and genital area. Shampoo may be used for tinea capitis to reduce risk of transmission to others (does not eradicate tinea infection).
  For tinea versicolor, 15%-25% sodium hyposulfite or thiosulfate (Tinver lotion) applied to affected areas BID × 2–4 weeks is an alternative. Topical antifungals (e.g., clotrimazole, miconazole) may be used for small, focal infections.

SENNA

Senokot, Senna-Gen, and others
Laxative, stimulant

No 1 C

Granules (OTC): 326 mg/tsp
Rectal suppository (OTC): 652 mg
Syrup (OTC): 218 mg/5 mL (60 mL, 240 mL)

Continued

SENNA *continued*

Tabs (OTC): 187, 217, 374, 600 mg
Liquid (OTC): 33.3 mg/mL

Children:
    Oral: 10–20 mg/kg/dose PO QHS. **Max. doses** as shown below or
        1 mo–1 yr: 55–109 mg PO QHS to **max. dose:** 218 mg/24 hr
        1–5 yr: 109–218 mg PO QHS to **max. dose:** 436 mg/24 hr
        5–15 yrs: 218–436 mg PO QHS to **max. dose:** 872 mg/24 hr
    Rectal: Children >27 kg: 326 mg (½ suppository) PR QHS
Adults:
    Oral:
        Granules: 326 mg (1 tsp) at bedtime; **max. dose:** 652 mg (2 tsp) BID.
        Syrup: 436–654 mg (10–15 mL) at bedtime; **max. dose:** 654 mg (15 mL) BID.
        Tabs: 374 mg (2 tabs) at bedtime; **max. dose:** 748 mg (4 tabs) BID.
    Rectal: 652 mg (1 suppository) PR QHS; may repeat dose × 1 in 2 hr if needed.

Effects occur within 6–24 hr after oral administration. May cause nausea,
vomiting, diarrhea, and abdominal cramps. Active metabolite stimulates
Auerbach's plexus.

SERTRALINE HCl

Zoloft
Antidepressant (selective serotonin reuptake inhibitor [SSRI])   Yes   3   C

Tabs: 25, 50, 100 mg
Oral concentrate solution: 20 mg/mL (60 mL); contains 12% alcohol

Depression:
    Children 6–12 yr (data limited in this age group): Start at 25 mg PO QD.
        May increase dosage by 25 mg at 3-4 day intervals up to a **max. dose** of
    200 mg/24 hr.
    Children ≥13 yr and adults: Start at 50 mg PO QD. May increase dosage by 50 mg
    at 1-week intervals up to a **max. dose** of 200 mg/24 hr.
Obessessive compulsive disorder:
    Children 6–12 yr: Start at 25 mg PO QD. May increase dosage by 25 mg at 3–4
    day intervals or by 50 mg at 7-day intervals up to a **max. dose** of 200 mg/24 hr.
    Children ≥13 yr and adults: Start at 50 mg PO QD. May increase dosage by 50 mg
    at 1-week intervals up to **max. dose** of 200 mg/24 hr.

This drug should **not** be used in combination with an MAO inhibitor or within
14 days of discontinuing an MAO inhibitor. Use with **caution** in patients with
hepatic or renal impairment. Adverse effects include nausea, diarrhea, tremor,
and increased sweating. Hyponatremia and platelet dysfunction have been reported.

Continued

SERTRALINE HCl *continued*

Concurrent administration with warfarin may increase PT. Inhibits the CYP450 2D6 drug metabolizing enzyme.

Mix oral concentrate solution with 4 oz of water, ginger ale, lemon/lime soda, lemonade, or orange juice. After mixing, a slight haze may appear; this is normal. This dosage form should be used **cautiously** in patients with latex allergy because the dropper contains dry natural rubber.

SILVER SULFADIAZINE

No ? C

Silvadene, Thermazene, SSD Cream, SSD AF Cream
Topical antibiotic

Cream: 1% (20, 25, 50, 85, 400, 1000 g); contains methylparabens and propylene glycol

 Cover affected areas completely QD–BID. Apply cream to a thickness of ¹⁄₁₆ inch using sterile technique.

Contraindicated in premature infants and infants ≤2 mo due to concerns of kernicterus. Discard product if cream has darkened. Significant systemic absorption may occur in severe burns. Adverse effects include pruritus, rash, bone marrow suppression, hemolytic anemia, and interstitial nephritis. See p. 93 for more information.

SIMETHICONE

No ? C

Mylicon, Phazyme, Mylanta Gas, Gas-X, and others
Antiflatulent

Oral drops: 40 mg/0.6 mL (30 mL)
Caps: 125 mg
Tabs: 60, 95 mg
Chewable tabs: 40, 80, 125 mg

 Infants and children <2 yr: 20 mg PO QID PRN; **max. dose:** 240 mg/24 hr
2–12 yr: 40 mg PO QID PRN
>12 yr: 40–125 mg PO QPC and QHS PRN; **max. dose:** 500 mg/24 hr

 Efficacy has not been demonstrated for treating infant colic. Avoid carbonated beverages and gas-forming foods. Oral liquid may be mixed with water, infant formula, or other suitable liquids for ease of oral administration.

SODIUM BICARBONATE

Neut and others
Alkalinizing agent, electrolyte

Yes ? C

Inj: 4% (0.48 mEq/mL) (5 mL),4.2% (0.5 mEq/mL) (10 mL), 7.5% (0.89 mEq/mL), 8.4% (1 mEq/mL) (10, 50 mL)
Inj., premixed: 5% (0.6 mEq/mL) (500 mL)
Tabs: 300 mg (3.6 mEq), 325 mg (3.8 mEq), 520 mg (6.3 mEq), 600 mg (7.3 mEq), 650 mg (7.6 mEq)
Powder: 120, 480 g
Each 1 mEq bicarbonate provides 1 mEq Na^+

Cardiac arrest: See inside front cover.
Correction of metabolic acidosis: Calculate patient's dose with the following formulas.
Neonates, infants, and children:
   HCO_3^- (mEq) = 0.3 × weight (kg) × base deficit (mEq/L), OR
   HCO_3^- (mEq) = 0.5 × weight (kg) × [24 − serum HCO_3^- (mEq/L)]
Adults:
   HCO_3^- (mEq) = 0.2 × weight (kg) × base deficit (mEq/L), OR
   HCO_3^- (mEq) = 0.5 × weight (kg) × [24 − serum HCO_3^- (mEq/L)]
Urinary alkalinization (titrate dose accordingly to urine pH):
   Children: 84–840 mg (1–10 mEq)/kg/24 hr PO ÷ QID
   Adults: 4 g (48 mEq) × 1 followed by 1–2 g (12–24 mEq) PO Q4 hr. Doses up to 16 g (192 mEq)/24 hr have been used.

Contraindicated in respiratory alkalosis, hypochloremia, and inadequate ventilation during cardiac arrest. Use with **caution** in CHF, renal impairment, cirrhosis, hypocalcemia, hypertension, and concurrent corticosteroids. Maintain high urine output. Monitor acid-base balance and serum electrolytes. May cause hypernatremia (contains sodium), hypokalemia, hypomagnesemia, hypocalcemia, hyperreflexia, edema, and tissue necrosis (extravasation). Oral route of administration may cause GI discomfort and gastric rupture from gas production.
   For direct IV administration (cardiac arrest) in neonates and infants, use the 0.5 mEq/mL (4.2%) concentration or dilute the 1 mEq/mL (8.4%) concentration 1:1 with sterile water for injection and infuse at a rate no greater than 10 mEq/min. The 1 mEq/mL (8.4%) concentration may be used in children and adults for direct IV administration.
   For IV infusions (for all ages), dilute to a **maximum concentration** of 0.5 mEq/mL in dextrose or sterile water for injection and infuse over 2 hr using a **maximum rate** of 1 mEq/kg/hr.
   Sodium bicarbonate should not be mixed with or be in contact with calcium, norepinephrine, or dobutamine.

SODIUM PHOSPHATE

Fleet, Fleet Phospho-soda, Visicol
Laxative, enema/oral

Yes ? C

Enema (Fleet) (OTC): 6 g Na phos and 16 g Na biphosphate/100 mL
   Pediatric size: 67.5 mL
   Adult size: 133 mL
Oral solution (Fleet Phospho-soda) (OTC): 18 g Na phos and 48 g Na biphosphate/
100 mL (30, 45, 90, 237 mL); contains 96.4 mEq Na per 20 mL
Oral tabs (Visicol): 1.5 g

Not to be used for phosphorus supplementation. See *Phosphorus for
supplementation).*
   Enema:
  2–12 yr: 67.5 mL enema × 1. May repeat × 1
  >12 yr and adults: 133 mL enema × 1. May repeat × 1
Oral laxative (mix with equal volume of water):
  5–9 yr: 5 mL PO × 1
  10–12 yr: 10 mL PO × 1
  >12 yr: 20 to 30 mL PO × 1
Bowel preparation:
  Adult (Visicol): 4.5 g with 8 oz of liquid Q15 min. × 7 doses night prior to surgery
  and repeat 7 doses regimen 3–5 hr prior to procedure

Contraindicated in patients with severe renal failure, megacolon, bowel obstruction, and CHF. May cause hyperphosphatemia, hypernatremia, hypocalcemia,
hypotension, dehydration, and acidosis. Avoid retention of enema solution
and **do not exceed** recommended doses, because this may lead to severe electrolyte
disturbances due to enhanced systemic absorption. *Onset of action:* PO: 3–6 hr;
PR: 2–5 min.

SODIUM POLYSTYRENE SULFONATE

Kayexalate, SPS, Kionex
Potassium-removing resin

Yes ? C

Powder: 454, 480 g
Suspension: 15 g/60 mL (contains 21.5 mL sorbitol/60 mL and 0.1–0.3% alcohol)
(60, 120, 200, 500 mL)
Contains 4.1 mEq Na$^+$/g drug

Children:
  Usual dose: 1 g/kg/dose Q6 hr PO or Q2–6 hr PR

Continued

SODIUM POLYSTYRENE SULFONATE *continued*

Adults:
  PO: 15 g QD-QID
  PR: 30–50 g Q6 hr
NOTE: Suspension may be given PO or PR. Practical exchange ratio is 1 mEq K per 1 g resin. May calculate dose according to desired exchange.

1 mEq Na delivered for each mEq K removed. Use **cautiously** in presence of renal failure, CHF, hypertension, or severe edema. May cause hypokalemia, hypernatremia, hypomagnesemia, and hypocalcemia. Do **not** administer with antacids or laxatives containing Mg^{++} or Al^{+++}. Systemic alkalosis may result. Retain enema in colon for at least 30–60 min.

SPECTINOMYCIN
Trobicin
Antibiotic, aminoglycoside

Yes   ?   B

Inj: 2 g with 3.2 mL diluent, which contains 0.9% benzyl alcohol

Uncomplicated gonorrhea (in combination with a macrolide):
  Children <45 kg: 50 mg/kg IM × 1; **max. dose:** 2 g/dose
    ≥45 kg and ≥8 yr: 2 g IM × 1
Disseminated gonorrhea:
  ≥45 kg and ≥8 yr: 2 g IM Q12 hr × 7 days. Alternatively, may treat × 24–48 hr and switch to oral alternative.

Not effective for syphilis. Drug is primarily used to treat gonorrhea in patients who cannot tolerate cephalosporins or fluoroquinolones. **Not** recommended for treatment of pharyngeal infections. Vertigo, malaise, nausea, anorexia, chills, fever, and urticaria may occur. Repeat dosing will cause accumulation in renal failure. IM use only.

SPIRONOLACTONE
Aldactone
Diuretic, potassium sparing

Yes   1   D

Tabs: 25, 50, 100 mg
Suspension: 1, 2, 5, 25 mg/mL

Diuretic:
  Neonates: 1–3 mg/kg/24 hr ÷ QD–BID PO
  Children: 1–3.3 mg/kg/24 hr ÷ QD–QID PO

Continued

SPIRONOLACTONE *continued*

Adults: 25–200 mg/24 hr ÷ QD–QID PO (see remarks)
Max. dose: 200 mg/24 hr
Diagnosis of primary aldosteronism:
Children: 125–375 mg/m²/24 hr ÷ BID–QID PO
Adults: 400 mg QD PO × 4 days (short test) or 3–4 weeks (long test), then
100–400 mg QD maintenance.
Hirsutism in women:
Adults: 50–200 mg/24 hr ÷ QD–BID PO

Contraindicated in acute renal failure (see p. 951). May cause hyperkalemia,
GI distress, rash, and gynecomastia. May potentiate ganglionic blocking agents
and other antihypertensives. Monitor potassium levels and be aware of other
K^+ sources, K^+ sparing diuretics, and angiotensin-converting enzyme inhibitors (all
can increase K^+). May cause false elevation in serum digoxin levels measured by
radioimmunoassay.

Although TID–QID regimens have been recommended in adults, recent data suggest
QD–BID dosing is adequate.

STAVUDINE
Zerit, d4T
*Antiviral agent, nucleoside analogue reverse transcriptase
inhibitor*

Yes   3   C

Caps: 15, 20, 30, 40 mg
Oral solution: 1 mg/mL (200 mL)

Children:
<30 kg: 1 mg/kg/dose PO Q12 hr, do not exceed adult doses.
Adolescents and adults:
30–60 kg: 30 mg PO Q12 hr
>60 kg: 40 mg PO Q12 hr

Active against most AZT-resistant viral strains. Common side effects include
headache, GI discomfort, and rash. Peripheral neuropathy, pancreatitis, lactic
acidosis, severe hepatomegaly, and elevated liver enzymes have been reported.
Fatal lactic acidosis has been reported in pregnant women taking stavudine in
combination with didanosine. **Adjust dosage in renal impairment (see p. 944).**
Should **not** be given in combination with zidovudine (AZT) because of poor antiviral
effect.

Adolescent dosing: Patients in early puberty (Tanner I-II) should be dosed with
pediatric regimens and those in late puberty (Tanner V) should be dosed with adult
regimens. Adolescents who are at the midst of their growth spurt (Tanner III females
and Tanner IV males) can be dosed by either pediatric or adult regimen with close
monitoring of efficacy and toxicity.

Doses can be administered with food. *Oral solution:* Shake well before measuring
each dose and keep refrigerated (30-day stability after initial reconstitution).

For explanation of icons, see p. 572.

STREPTOKINASE

Kabikinase, Streptase
Thrombolytic enzyme

No   ?   C

Inj: 250,000; 600,000; 750,000; 1,500,000 IU

Thrombolytic: **Should be used in consultation with a hematologist.** Duration of therapy will depend on clinical response and generally does not exceed 3 days. *Children:* 3500–4000 U/kg over 30 min, followed by 1000–1500 U/kg/hr; **OR** 2000 U/kg load over 30 min followed by 2000 U/kg/hr. Duration of infusion is individualized based on response.

Pediatric safety and efficacy information is limited. **Contraindicated** with intra-cranial or intraspinal surgery, history of internal bleeding, recent streptococcal infection, or CVA within previous 2 mo. May cause hemorrhage, urticaria, itching, flushing, musculoskeletal pain, bronchospasm, and anaphylaxis. Monitor fibrinogen, thrombin clotting time, PT, and APTT when used as a thrombolytic.

Newborns have reduced plasminogen levels (~50% of adult values), which decrease the thrombolytic effects of streptokinase. Plasminogen supplementation may be necessary.

Not recommended in restoring patency of intravenous catheters. Hypotension, hypersensitivity reactions, apnea, and bleeding, some of which were life threatening, have been reported when used in this manner.

STREPTOMYCIN SULFATE

Antibiotic, aminoglycoside; antituberculous agent

Yes   1   D

Inj: 400 mg/mL (2.5 mL)
Powder for inj: 1 g

Tuberculosis (use as part of multi-drug regimen; see latest edition of AAP *Red Book):*
    Children:
Daily therapy: 20–40 mg/kg/24 hr IM QD
    Max. daily dose: 1 g/24 hr
    Twice weekly therapy: 20–40 mg/kg/dose IM twice weekly
    Max. daily dose: 1.5 g/24 hr
Adults:
    Daily therapy: 15 mg/kg/24 hr IM QD
    Max. daily dose: 1 g/24 hr
    Twice weekly therapy: 25–30 mg/kg/dose IM twice weekly
    Max. daily dose: 1.5 g/24 hr
Brucellosis, tularemia, plague, and rat bite fever: see latest edition of the *Red Book*.

Continued

STREPTOMYCIN SULFATE *continued*

Use with **caution** in preexisting vertigo, tinnitus, hearing loss, and neuromuscular disorders. Drug is administered via deep IM injection only. Follow auditory status. May cause CNS depression, other neurologic problems, myocarditis, or serum sickness.

Therapeutic levels: Peak 15–40 mg/L; trough: <5 mg/L. *Recommended serum sampling time at steady-state:* Trough within 30 min prior to the third consecutive dose and peak 30–60 min after the administration of the third consecutive dose. Therapeutic levels are not achieved in CSF.

Adjust dose in renal insufficiency (see p. 945).

SUCCIMER

Chemet, DMSA (dimercaptosuccinic acid)
Chelating agent

Yes ? C

Capsule: 100 mg

Lead chelation, children:
10 mg/kg/dose (or 350 mg/m^2/dose) PO Q8 hr × 5 days, then 10 mg/kg/dose (or 350 mg/m^2/dose) PO Q12 hr × 14 days.
Manufacturer recommends (see table below):

Wt (kg)	Dose (mg)
8–15	100
16–23	200
24–34	300
35–44	400
≥45	500

Give dose above every 8 hr for 5 days. Then give the same dose Q12 hr for an additional 14 days.

Use **caution** in patients with compromised renal function. Repeated courses may be necessary. Follow serum lead levels (see pp. 35–38). Allow minimum of 2 weeks between courses, unless blood levels require more aggressive management. Side effects include GI symptoms, increased LFTs (10%), rash, headaches, dizziness. **Co-administration with other chelating agents is not recommended.** Treatment of iron deficiency is recommended, as well as environmental remediation. Contents of capsule may be sprinkled on food for those who are unable to swallow capsule.

For explanation of icons, see p. 572.

SUCCINYLCHOLINE

Anectine, Quelicin, and others
Neuromuscular blocking agent

No   ?   C

Inj: 20 mg/mL (5, 10 mL), 50 mg/mL (10 mL), 100 mg/mL (5, 10 mL); may contain parabens and/or benzyl alcohol
Powder for inj: 100, 500, 1000 mg

Paralysis for intubation:
Infants and children:
  Initial:
  IV: 1–2 mg/kg/dose × 1
  IM: 3–4 mg/kg/dose × 1
  Max. dose: 150 mg/dose
  Maintenance: 0.3–0.6 mg/kg/dose IV Q5–10 min PRN.
  Continuous infusion not recommended.
Adults:
  Initial:
  IV: 0.3–1.1 mg/kg/dose × 1
  IM: 3–4 mg/kg/dose × 1
  Max. dose: 150 mg/dose
  Maintenance: 0.04–0.07 mg/kg/dose IV Q5–10 min PRN
Continuous infusion not recommended.

Pretreatment with atropine is recommended to reduce incidence of bradycardia. For rapid sequence intubation, see p. 5.

Cardiac arrest has been reported in children and adolescents primarily with skeletal muscle myopathies (e.g., Duchenne's muscular dystrophy). Identify developmental delays suggestive of a myopathy prior to use. Predose creatine kinase may be useful for identifying patients at risk. Monitoring of ECG for peaked T-waves may be useful in detecting early signs of this adverse effect.

May cause malignant hyperthermia (use dantrolene to treat), bradycardia, hypotension, arrhythmia, and hyperkalemia. Use with **caution** in patients with severe burns, paraplegia, or crush injuries and in patients with preexisting hyperkalemia. Beware of prolonged depression in patients with liver disease, malnutrition, pseudocholinesterase deficiency, hypothermia, and those receiving aminoglycosides, phenothiazines, quinidine, beta-blockers, amphotericin B, cyclophosphamide, diuretics, lithium, acetylcholine, and anticholinesterases. Diazepam may decrease neuromuscular blocking effects. *Duration of action:* 4–6 min IV, 10–30 min IM. Must be prepared to intubate within 1 min.

SUCRALFATE

Carafate and others
Oral antiulcer agent

Yes   ?   B

Tabs: 1 g
Suspension: 100 mg/mL (420 mL); contains sorbitol and parabens

Children: 40–80 mg/kg/24 hr ÷ Q6 hr PO
Adults: 1 g PO QID 1 hr AC and QHS

May cause vertigo, constipation, and dry mouth. Aluminum may accumulate in patients with renal failure. This may be augmented by the use of aluminum-containing antacids. Decreases absorption of phenytoin, digoxin, theophylline, cimetidine, fat-soluble vitamins, ketoconazole, omeprazole, quinolones, and oral anticoagulants. Administer these drugs at least 2 hr before or after sucralfate doses.

Drug requires an acidic environment to form a protective polymer coating for damaged GI tract mucosa. Doses as high as 1 g PO Q4 hr have been used in adults for stress ulcers.

SULFACETAMIDE SODIUM

Sulamyd and others
Ophthalmic antibiotic, sulfonamide derivative

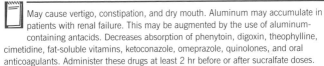

No   2   C

Ophthalmic solution: 10% (1, 2, 2.5, 5, 15 mL), 15% (2, 5, 15 mL), 30% (5, 15 mL)
Ophthalmic ointment: 10% (3.5 g)

>2 mo and adults:
Ophthalmic ointment: Apply ribbon QID and QHS (5 × 24 hr)
Drops: 1–2 drops Q2–3 hr to affected eye(s)

See *Sulfisoxazole.* 10% solution is used most frequently. May cause local irritation, stinging, burning, toxic epidermal necrolysis (rarely). Local irritation occurs more frequently with higher-strength preparations.

SULFADIAZINE

Various trade names
Antibiotic, sulfonamide derivative

Yes   2   B/D

Tabs: 500 mg
Suspension: 100 mg/mL

Continued

SULFADIAZINE *continued*

Congenital toxoplasmosis (administer with pyrimethamine and folinic acid)
(From Clin Infect Dis 18:38, 1994):
  Infants: 100 mg/kg/24 hr PO ÷ BID × 12 mo
Toxoplasmosis (administer with pyrimethamine and folinic acid):
  Children: 100–200 mg/kg/24 hr ÷ Q6 hr PO × 3–4 weeks
  Adults: 4–6 g/24 hr PO ÷ Q6 hr × 3–4 weeks
Rheumatic fever prophylaxis:
  ≤27 kg: 500 mg PO QD
  >27 kg: 1000 mg PO QD

Most cases of acquired toxoplasmosis do not require specific antimicrobial therapy. **Contraindicated** in porphyria and hypersensitivity to sulfonamides.
Use with **caution** in premature infants and infants <2 mo because of risk of hyperbilirubinemia, and in hepatic or renal dysfunction (30%-44% eliminated in urine). Maintain hydration. May cause increased effects of warfarin, methotrexate, and sulfonylureas due to drug displacement from protein binding sites. May cause fever, rash, hepatitis, SLE-like syndrome, vasculitis, bone marrow suppression, hemolysis (in patients with G6PD deficiency), and Stevens-Johnson syndrome. Pregnancy category changes from "B" to "D" if administered near term.

SULFAMETHOXAZOLE
Gantanol, Urobak
Antibiotic, sulfonamide derivative   Yes   2   B/D

Oral suspension: 500 mg/5 mL (480 mL)
Tabs: 500 mg

Children ≥2 mo: 50–60 mg/kg/dose PO × 1 followed by 50-60 mg/kg/24 hr PO ÷ Q12 hr; **max. dose:** 75 mg/kg/24 hr or 3000 mg/24 hr
Adults: 2 g PO × 1 followed by 1g PO BID–TID; **max. dose:** 3 g/24 hr

Contraindicated in porphyria, megaloblastic anemia due to folate deficiency, or near-term pregnancy. Use with **caution** in infants <2 mo, the presence of renal or liver disease, or G6PD deficiency. Maintain hydration. See sulfadiazine for toxicities and drug interactions.
Adjust dosage in renal impairment (see p. 945). Pregnancy category changes from "B" to "D" if administered near term. For combination with trimethoprim, see p. 664.

SULFASALAZINE

Salicylazo-sulfapyridine, SAS, Azulfidine, Azulfidine EN-tabs, and others
Antiinflammatory agent

Yes   2   B/D

Tabs: 500 mg
Enteric-coated tabs (Azulfidine EN-tabs): 500 mg

Ulcerative colitis:
  Children >6 yr:
    Initial dosing:
      Moderate/severe: 50–75 mg/kg/24 hr ÷ Q4–6 hr PO; **max. dose:** 6 g/24 hr
      Mild: 40–50 mg/kg/24 hr ÷ Q6 hr PO
    Maintenance: 30–50 mg/kg/24 hr ÷ Q4–8 hr PO; **max. dose:** 2 g/24 hr
  Adults:
    Initial: 3–4 g/24 hr ÷ Q4–6 hr PO
    Maintenance: 2 g/24 hr ÷ Q6–12 hr PO
    Max. dose: 6 g/24 hr
Juvenile rheumatoid arthritis:
  Children >6 yr: Start with 10 mg/kg/24 hr ÷ BID PO and increase by 10 mg/kg/24 hr Q7 days until planned maintenance dose is achieved. Usual maintenance dose is 30–50 mg/kg/24 hr ÷ BID PO up to a **maximum** of 2 g/24 hr.

Contraindicated in sulfa or salicylate hypersensitivity, porphyria, and GI or GU obstruction. Use with **caution** in renal impairment. Maintain hydration. May cause orange-yellow discoloration of urine and skin. May permanently stain contact lenses. May cause photosensitivity, hypersensitivity, blood dyscrasias, CNS changes, nausea, vomiting, anorexia, diarrhea, and renal damage. Hepatotoxicity has been reported. May cause hemolysis in patients with G6PD deficiency. Decreases folic acid absorption and reduces serum digoxin and cyclosporine levels. Slow acetylators may require lower dosage due to accumulation of active sulfapyridine metabolite. Pregnancy category changes to "D" if administered near term.

SULFISOXAZOLE

Gantrisin
Antibiotic, sulfonamide derivative

Yes   2   B/D

Tabs: 500 mg
Suspension: 500 mg/5 mL (480 mL); contains 0.3% alcohol and parabens
Syrup: 500 mg/5 mL (480 mL)
Ophthalmic solution: 4% (40 mg/mL) (15 mL)

Continued

SULFISOXAZOLE *continued*

Children ≥2 mo: 75 mg/kg/dose PO × 1 followed by 120–150 mg/kg/24 hr OR 4 g/m²/24 hr ÷ Q4–6 hr PO; **max. dose:** 6 g/24 hr

Adults: 2–4 g PO × 1 followed by 4–8 g/24 hr ÷ Q4–6 hr PO

Otitis media prophylaxis: 50 mg/kg/dose QHS PO

Rheumatic fever prophylaxis:

  <27 kg: 500 mg PO QD

  ≥27 kg: 1000 mg PO QD

Ophthalmic solution:

  Conjunctivitis or other superficial ocular infections: 1–2 drops Q1–4 hr; increase the time interval between doses as the condition improves.

  Trachoma (with systemic sulfonamide therapy): 2 drops Q2 hr.

Contraindicated in urinary obstruction or near-term pregnancy. Use with **caution** in infants <2 mo, the presence of renal or liver disease, or G6PD deficiency.

Maintain adequate fluid intake. See sulfadiazine for toxicities and drug interactions. Interferes with folate absorption. Usual duration of therapy for ophthalmic use is 7–10 days.

Adjust dose in renal impairment with systemic use (see p. 945). Pregnancy category changes to "D" if administered near term. For combination with erythromycin, see p. 682.

SUMATRIPTAN SUCCINATE

Imitrex

Antimigraine agent, selective serotonin agonist

Yes   1   C

Inj: 12 mg/mL (2 mL)

Unit use syringe: 6 mg/0.5mL syringe (2 syringes per box)

Tabs: 25, 50 mg

Oral suspension: 5 mg/mL ✂

Nasal spray (as a unit-dose spray device): 5 mg dose in 100 microliters (6 units per pack); 20 mg dose in 100 microliters (6 units per pack)

Adolescents and adults (see remarks):

  PO: 25 mg as soon as possible after onset of headache. If no relief in 2 hr, give 25–100 mg Q2 hr up to a **daily maximum** of 200 mg. **Max. single dose:** 100 mg/dose.

Max. daily dose: 200 mg/24 hr (with exclusive PO dosing or with an initial SC dose and subsequent PO dosing).

  SC: 6 mg × 1 as soon as possible after onset of headache. If no response, may give an additional dose of ≤6 mg 1 hr later. **Max. daily dose:** 12 mg/24 hr.

  Nasal: 5–20 mg/dose into one nostril or divided into each nostril. If headache returns, dose may be repeated in 2 hr up to a **maximum** of 40 mg/24 hr.

Continued

SUMATRIPTAN SUCCINATE *continued*

Contraindicated with concomitant administration of ergotamine derivatives, MAO inhibitors (and use within the past 2 weeks), or other vasoconstrictive drugs. Not for migraine prophylaxis. Use with **caution** in renal or hepatic impairment. A **max.** single dose of 50 mg has been recommended in adults with hepatic dysfunction. Acts as selective agonist for serotonin receptor. Induration and swelling at the injection site, flushing, dizziness, and chest, jaw, and neck tightness may occur with SC administration. Weakness, hyperreflexia, and incoordination have been reported with use in combination with SSRIs (e.g., fluoxetine, fluvoxamine, paroxetine, sertraline).

May cause coronary vasospasm if administered IV. **Use injectable form SC only!** *Onset of action:* 10–120 min SC, and 60–90 min PO. For nasal use, the safety of treating more than four headaches in a 30-day period has not been established.

Oral efficacy was not established in placebo-controlled trial in adolescents.

SURFACTANT, PULMONARY/ BERACTANT

Survanta   No
Bovine lung surfactant

Suspension: 25 mg/mL (4, 8 mL); contains 0.5–1.75 mg triglycerides, 1.4–3.5 mg free fatty acids, and <1 mg protein/1 mL drug

Prophylatic therapy: 4 mL/kg/dose intratracheally as soon as possible after delivery; up to four doses may be given at intervals no shorter than Q6 hr during the first 48 hr of life.
Rescue therapy: 4 mL/kg/dose intratracheally, immediately following the diagnosis of respiratory distress syndrome (RDS). May repeat dose as needed Q6 hr to maximum of four doses total.
Method of administration for above therapies: Each dose is divided into four 1 mL/kg aliquots; administer 1 mL/kg in each of four different positions (slight downward inclination with head turned to the right, head turned to the left; slight upward inclination with the head turned to the right, head turned to the left).

Transient bradycardia, O_2 desaturation, pallor, vasoconstriction, hypotension, endotracheal tube blockage, hypercarbia, hypercapnea, apnea, and hypertension may occur during the administration process. Other side effects may include pulmonary interstitial emphysema, pulmonary air leak, and posttreatment nosocomial sepsis. Monitor heart rate and transcutaneous O_2 saturation during dose administration, and arterial blood gases for postdose hyperoxia and hypocarbia.

All doses are administered intratracheally via a 5-French feeding catheter. If the suspension settles during storage, gently swirl the contents—**do not shake.** Drug is stored in the refrigerator, protected from light, and needs to be warmed by standing at room temperature for at least 20 min or warm in the hand for at least 8 min. Artificial warming methods should **not** be used.

For explanation of icons, see p. 572.

SURFACTANT, PULMONARY/ CALFACTANT

Infasurf

No

Bovine lung surfactant

Intratracheal suspension: 35 mg/mL (6 mL); contains 26 mg phosphatidylcholine and 0.26 mg surfactant protein B per 1 mL

Prophylactic therapy: 3 mL/kg/dose intratracheally as soon as possible after delivery; up to a total of three doses may be given Q12 hr.

Rescue therapy (see remarks): 3 mL/kg/dose intratracheally immediately after the diagnosis of respiratory distress syndrome (RDS). May repeat dose as needed Q12 hr to **maximum** of three doses total.

Method of administration for above therapies:

Manufacturer recommends administration through a side-port adapter into the endotracheal tube with two attendants (one to instill drug and another to monitor and position patient). Each dose is divided into two 1.5 mL/kg aliquots; administer 1.5 mL/kg in each of two different positions (infant positioned to the right or left-side dependent). Drug is administered while ventilation is continued over 20–30 breaths for each aliquot, with small bursts timed only during the inspiratory cycles. A pause followed by evaluation of respiratory status and repositioning should separate the two aliquots.

Common adverse effects include cyanosis, airway obstruction, bradycardia, reflux of surfactant into the endotracheal tube, requirement for manual ventilation, and reintubation. Monitor O_2 saturation and lung compliance after each dose such that oxygen therapy and ventilator pressure are adjusted as necessary.

All doses administered intratracheally via a 5-French feeding catheter. If suspension settles during storage, gently swirl the contents—**do not shake.** Drug is stored in the refrigerator, protected from light, and does not need to be warmed before administration. Unopened vials that have been warmed to room temperature (once only) may be refrigerated within 24 hr and stored for future use.

For rescue therapy, repeat doses may be administered as early as 6 hr after the previous dose, for a total of up to four doses if the infant is still intubated and requires at least 30% inspired oxygen to maintain a $PaO_2 \geq 80$ torr.

SURFACTANT, PULMONARY/ COLFOSCERIL PALMITATE

Exosurf Neonatal

No

Synthetic lung surfactant

Intratracheal suspension: 108 mg/10 mL (10 mL); contains 1.5 mg cetyl alcohol and 1 mg tyloxapol per 1 mL drug

Continued

FORMULARY

SURFACTANT, PULMONARY/COLFOSCERIL PALMITATE *continued*

Prophylactic therapy: 5 mL/kg intratracheally as soon as possible after delivery; give two additional doses at 12 and 24 hr if infant remains on ventilator support.

Rescue therapy: 5 mL/kg intratracheally as soon as the diagnosis of respiratory distress syndrome (RDS) is made. A second 5 mL/kg dose can be administered 12 hr later.

Method of administration for above therapies: Administer via a sideport on the special endotracheal tube adapter without interrupting mechanical ventilation. Each dose is divided into two 2.5 mL/kg aliquots; administer each 2.5 mL/kg dose over 1 to 2 min in small bursts timed with inspiration, with the infant's head in the midline position. Turn the infant's head and torso 45° to the right for 30 sec after the first aliquot, followed by turning the head and torso 45° to the left for 30 sec after the second aliquot.

Pulmonary hemorrhage, apnea, mucus plugging, and decrease in transcutaneous O_2 of >20% may occur. Monitor O_2 saturation, ECG, and blood pressure during dose administration, and arterial blood gases for postdose hyperoxia and hypocarbia after administration.

For intratracheal use only. Cetyl alcohol acts as a spreading agent, and tyloxapol is a nonionic surfactant that facilitates the dispersion of colfosceril and cetyl alcohol. Drug needs to be reconstituted with preservative-free sterile water for injection and is stable for 12 hr at room temperature after mixing. **Do not refrigerate.**

Suction infant prior to administration. Suction only if necessary until 2 hr after administration (unless signs of significant airway obstruction occur).

SURFACTANT, PULMONARY/ PORACTANT ALFA

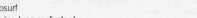

No

Curosurf
Porcine lung surfactant

Intratracheal suspension: 80 mg/mL (1.5, 3 mL): contains 0.3 mg surfactant protein B per 1 mL drug

Prophylactic therapy: 2.5 mL/kg/dose × 1 intratracheally as soon as possible after delivery; up to two subsequent 1.25 mL/kg/doses may be given at 12-hour intervals for a **max. total dose** of 5 mL/kg.

Rescue therapy: 2.5 mL/kg/dose × 1 intratracheally, immediately following the diagnosis of respiratory distress syndrome (RDS). May administer 1.25 mL/kg/dose Q12 hr × 2 doses as needed up to a **max. total dose** of 5 mL/kg.

Method of administration for above therapies: Each dose is divided into two aliquots, with each aliquot administered into one of the two main bronchi by positioning the infant with either the right or left side dependent. After the first aliquot is administered, remove the catheter from the ET tube and manually ventilate the infant with 100% oxygen at a rate of 40–60 breaths/min for 1 min. When the infant is stable, reposition the infant and administer the second dose. Then remove the catheter without flushing.

Continued

SURFACTANT, PULMONARY/PORACTANT ALFA *continued*

Transient episodes of bradycardia, decreased oxygen saturation, reflux of
surfactant into the endotracheal tube, and airway obstruction have occurred
during dose administration. Monitor O_2 saturation and lung compliance after
each dose, and adjust oxygen therapy and ventilator pressure as necessary.

All doses administered intratracheally via a 5-French feeding catheter. Suction infant
prior to administration and 1 hr after surfactant instillation (unless signs of significant
airway obstruction).

Drug is stored in the refrigerator and protected from light. Each vial of drug should
be slowly warmed to room temperature and gently turned upside-down for uniform
suspension **(do not shake)** before administration. Unopened vials that have been
warmed to room temperature (once only) may be refrigerated within 24 hr and stored
for future use.

TACROLIMUS
Prograf, FK506
Immunosuppressant

Yes   ?   C

Caps: 0.5, 1, 5 mg
Suspension: 0.5 mg/mL
Inj: 5 mg/mL (1 mL); contains alcohol and polyoxyl 60 hydrogenated castor oil
Topical ointment: 0.03%, 0.1% (30, 60 g)

Children:
  *Liver transplantation without preexisting renal or hepatic dysfunction (initial
    doses; titrate to therapeutic levels):*
    IV: 0.05–0.15 mg/kg/24 hr by continuous infusion
    PO: 0.15–0.3 mg/kg/24 hr ÷ Q12 hr
Adults (initial doses; titrate to therapeutic levels):
  IV: 0.05–0.1 mg/kg/24 hr by continuous infusion
  PO:
    Liver transplantation: 0.1–0.15 mg/kg/24 hr ÷ Q12 hr
    Kidney transplantation: 0.2 mg/kg/24 hr ÷ Q12 hr
*Atopic dermatitis (continue treatment for 1 week after clearing of signs and symp-
toms; see remarks):*
  Children ≥2 yr old: Apply a thin layer of the 0.03% ointment to the affected skin
  areas BID and rub in gently and completely.
  Adults: Apply a thin layer of the 0.03% or 0.1% ointment to the affected skin areas
  BID and rub in gently and completely.

IV dosage form **contraindicated** in patients allergic to polyoxyl 60 hydrogenated
castor oil. Experience in pediatric kidney transplantation is limited. Pediatric
patients have required higher mg/kg doses than adults. For BMT use (beginning
1 day before BMT), dose and therapeutic levels similar to those in liver transplantation
have been used.

Continued

TACROLIMUS *continued*

Major adverse events include tremor, headache, insomnia, diarrhea, constipation, hypertension, nausea, and renal dysfunction. Hypokalemia, hypomagnesemia, hyperglycemia, confusion, depression, infections, lymphoma, liver enzyme elevation, and coagulation disorders may also occur. Tacrolimus is a substrate of the CYP450 3A4 drug metabolizing enzyme. Calcium channel blockers, imidazole antifungals (ketoconazole, itraconazole, fluconazole, clotrimazole), macrolide antibiotics (erythromycin, clarithromycin, troleandomycin), cisapride, cimetidine, cyclosporine, danazol, methylprednisolone, and grapefruit juice can increase tacrolimus serum levels. In contrast, carbamazepine, phenobarbital, phenytoin, rifampin, and rifabutin may decrease levels. Reduce dose in renal or hepatic insufficiency.

Monitor trough levels (just prior to a dose at steady-state). Steady-state is generally achieved after 2–5 days of continuous dosing. Interpretation will vary based on treatment protocol and assay methodology (whole blood ELISA vs. MEIA vs. HPLC). Whole blood trough concentrations of 5–20 ng/mL have been recommended in liver transplantation. Trough levels of 7–20 ng/mL (whole blood) for the first 3 mo and 5–15 ng/mL after 3 mo have been recommended in renal transplantation.

Tacrolimus therapy generally should be initiated 6 hr or more after transplantation. PO is the preferred route of administration and should be administered on an empty stomach. IV infusions should be administered at concentrations between 0.004 and 0.02 mg/mL diluted in NS or D_5W.

TOPICAL USE: Do not use tacrolimus ointment with occlusive dressings; safety has not been evaluated. Skin burn sensation, pruritus, flu-like symptoms, allergic reaction, skin erythema, headache, and skin infection are the most common side effects.

TERBUTALINE

Brethine and others
Beta-2-adrenergic agonist

Yes   1   B

Tabs: 2.5, 5 mg
Suspension: 1 mg/mL
Inj: 1 mg/mL (1 mL)
Aerosol inhaler: 200 mcg/actuation (300 actuations per inhaler, 10.5 g)

PO: ≤12 yr: Initial: 0.05 mg/kg/dose TID, increase as required. **Max. dose:** 0.15 mg/kg/dose TID or total of 5 mg/24 hr.
  >12 yr and adults: 2.5–5 mg/dose PO TID
Max. dose:
    12–15 yr: 7.5 mg/24 hr
    >15 yr: 15 mg/24 hr
Nebulization:
  <2 yr: 0.5 mg in 2.5 mL NS Q4–6 hr PRN
  2–9 yr: 1 mg in 2.5 mL NS Q4–6 hr PRN
  >9 yr: 1.5–2.5 mg in 2.5 mL NS Q4–6 hr PRN

Continued

TERBUTALINE *continued*

SC: *≤12 yr:* 0.005–0.01 mg/kg/dose Q15–20 min × 2; **max. dose:** 0.4 mg/dose.
 >12 yr and adult: 0.25 mg/dose Q15–30 min PRN × 2; **max. dose:** 0.5 mg/4 hr
 period
Inhalations: 1–2 inhalations Q4–6 hr PRN
Continuous infusion, IV: 2–10 mcg/kg loading dose followed by infusion of 0.1–0.4
mcg/kg/min. May titrate in increments of 0.1–0.2 mcg/kg/min Q30 min, depending on
clinical response.
To prepare infusion: See inside front cover.

Nervousness, tremor, headache, nausea, tachycardia, arrhythmias, and palpitations may occur. Paradoxical bronchoconstriction may occur with excessive
use; if it occurs, discontinue drug immediately. Injectable product may be used
for nebulization. For acute asthma, nebulizations may be given more frequently than
Q4–6 hr. Use spacer device with inhaler to optimize drug delivery.

 Monitor heart rate, blood pressure, respiratory rate, and serum potassium when
using the continuous IV infusion route of administration. **Adjust dose in renal failure
(see p. 951).**

TETRACYCLINE HCl

Many brand names: Achromycin, Sumycin, Panmycin,
and others
Antibiotic

Yes   1   D

Tabs: 250, 500 mg
Caps: 250, 500 mg
Suspension: 125 mg/5 mL (60, 480 mL)
Ophthalmic ointment: 1% (3.5 g)
Ophthalmic drops: 1% (0.5, 1, 4 mL)
Topical ointment: 3% (14.2, 30 g)
Topical solution: 2.2 mg/mL (70 mL); contains 40% ethanol

Do not use in children <8 yr.
Children ≥8 yr: 25–50 mg/kg/24 hr PO ÷ Q6 hr.
 Max. dose: 3 g/24 hr
Adults: 1–2 g/24 hr PO ÷ Q6–12 hr
Ophthalmic:
 Neonatal prophylaxis: 1% ointment × 1 in both eyes.
 Solution: 2 drops into affected eye BID–QID
Acne vulgaris: Apply topical solution to affected areas BID

Not recommended in patients <8 yr due to tooth staining and decreased bone
growth. Also not recommended for use in pregnancy because these side effects
may occur in the fetus. The risk for these adverse effects is highest with long-
term use. May cause nausea, GI upset, hepatotoxicity, stomatitis, rash, fever, and
superinfection. Photosensitivity reaction may occur. Avoid prolonged exposure to

Continued

TETRACYCLINE HCl *continued*

sunlight. May decrease the effectiveness of oral contraceptives and may increase serum digoxin levels.

   Never use outdated tetracyclines because they may cause Fanconi-like syndrome. Do not give with dairy products or with any divalent cations (i.e., Fe^{++}, Ca^{++}, Mg^{++}). Give 1 hr before or 2 hr after meals.

   Adjust dose in renal failure (see p. 945).

   For topical use, pregnancy category is "B."

THEOPHYLLINE

TheoDur, Slo-bid Gyrocaps, Slo-Phyllin Gyrocaps, and many others

Bronchodilator, methylxanthine

No   1   C

Other dosage forms may exist

Immediate release:

   Tabs: 100, 125, 200, 250, 300 mg

   Caps: 100, 200 mg

   Elixir/solution/syrup: 80 mg/15 mL, 150 mg/15 mL. Some elixirs contain up to 20% alcohol. Some syrups and solutions are alcohol and dye free.

   Inj: 0.4, 0.8, 1.6, 2, 3.2, 4 mg/mL

Sustained release (see remarks):

   Tabs: 100, 200, 250, 300, 400, 450, 500, 600 mg

   Caps: 50, 60, 65, 75, 100, 125, 130, 200, 250, 260, 300, 400 mg

   Sustained release forms should not be chewed or crushed. Capsules may be opened and contents may be sprinkled on food.

   Dosing intervals are for immediate-release preparations.
   For sustained-release preparations divide daily dose QD-TID based on product (see table on p. 862).

Neonatal apnea:

   Load: 5 mg/kg/dose PO × 1

   Maintenance: 3–6 mg/kg/24 hr PO ÷ Q6–8 hr

Bronchospasm; PO:

   Loading dose: 1 mg/kg/dose for each 2 mg/L desired increase in serum theophylline level.

   Maintenance, infants (<1 yr):

      Preterm:

         <24 days old (postnatal): 1 mg/kg/dose PO Q12 hr

         ≥24 days old (postnatal): 1.5 mg/kg/dose PO Q12 hr

      Full-term up to 1 yr: Total daily dose (mg) = [(0.2 × age in weeks) + 5] × (kg body weight)

         ≤6 mo: Divide daily dose Q8 hr

         >6 mo: Divide daily dose Q6 hr

Continued

THEOPHYLLINE *continued*

Maintenance, children >1 yr and adults without risk factors for altered clearance (see remarks):

<45 kg: Begin therapy at 12–14 mg/kg/24 hr ÷ Q4–6 hr up to a **max. dose** of 300 mg/24 hr. If needed based on serum levels, gradually increase to 16–20 mg/kg/24 hr ÷ Q4–6 hr. **Max. dose:** 600 mg/24 hr

≥45 kg: Begin therapy with 300 mg/24 hr ÷ Q6–8 hr. If needed based on serum levels, gradually increase to 400–600 mg/24 hr ÷ Q6–8 hr.

Drug metabolism varies widely with age, drug formulation, and route of administration. Most common side effects and toxicities are nausea, vomiting, anorexia, abdominal pain, gastroesophageal reflux, nervousness, tachycardia, seizures, and arrhythmias.

Serum levels should be monitored. Therapeutic levels: bronchospasm: 10–20 mg/L; apnea: 7–13 mg/L. Half-life is age-dependent: 30 hr (newborns); 6.9 hr (infants); 3.4 hr (children); 8.1 hr (adults). See aminophylline for guidelines for serum level determinations. Theophylline is a substrate for CYP 450 1A2. Levels are increased with allopurinol, alcohol, ciprofloxacin, cimetidine, clarithromycin, disulfiram, erythromycin, estrogen, isoniazid, propranolol, thiabendazole, and verapamil. Levels are decreased with carbamazepine, isoproterenol, phenobarbital, phenytoin, and rifampin.

Use ideal body weight in obese patients when calculating dosage because of poor distribution into body fat. Risk factors for increased clearance include: smoking, cystic fibrosis, hyperthyroidism, and high protein carbohydrate diet. Factors for decreased clearance include CHF, correction of hyperthyroidism, fever, viral illness, and sepsis.

Suggested dosage intervals for sustained-release products (see table below):

THEOPHYLLINE SUSTAINED-RELEASE PRODUCTS

Trade Name	Available Strengths	Dosage Interval
CAPSULES		
Aerolate	65, 130, 260 mg	Q8–12 hr
Slo-bid Gyrocaps	50, 75, 100, 125, 200, 300 mg	Q8–12 hr
Slo-Phyllin Gyrocaps	60, 125, 250 mg	Q8–12 hr
Theo 24	100, 200, 300, 400 mg	Q24 hr
Theobid Duracaps	260 mg	Q12 hr
Theoclear-LA or Theospan-SR	130, 260 mg	Q12 hr
Theovent	125, 250 mg	Q12 hr
TABLETS		
Theophylline SR	100, 200, 300 mg	Q12–24 hr
Quibron-T/SR Dividose	300 mg	Q8–12 hr
Respbid	250, 500 mg	Q8–12 hr
Sustaire	100, 300 mg	Q8–12 hr
Theo Dur	100, 200, 300, 450 mg	Q8–24 hr
Theocron	100, 200, 300 mg	Q12–24 hr
Theolair SR	200, 250, 300, 500 mg	Q8–12 hr
Theo-Sav	100, 200, 300 mg	Q8–24 hr
Theo X	100, 200, 300 mg	Q12–24 hr
T-phyl	200 mg	Q8–12 hr
Uni-Dur or Uniphyl	400, 600 mg	Q24 hr

THIABENDAZOLE

Mintezol
Anthelmintic

Yes   ?   C

Suspension: 500 mg/5 mL
Chew tabs: 500 mg; contains saccharin
Topical suspension: 10–15%
Topical ointment: 10% in white petrolatum

Children and adults: 50 mg/kg/24 hr PO ÷ BID; **max. dose:** 3 g/24 hr
Duration of therapy (consecutive days):
  Strongyloides: × 2 days (5 days for disseminated disease)
  Cutaneous larva migrans: × 2–5 days
  Visceral larva migrans: × 5–7 days
  Trichinosis: × 2–4 days
Angiostrongylosis: 75 mg/kg/24 hr PO ÷ TID × 3 days; **max. dose:** 3 g/24 hr
Topical therapy for cutaneous larva migrans: Apply sparingly to all lesions 4–6 ×/24 hr
until lesions are inactivated. See Arch Dermatol 129:588;1993 for additional
information.

Use with **caution** in renal or hepatic impairment. Nausea, vomiting, and vertigo
are frequent side effects. May cause abnormal sensation in eyes, xanthopsia,
blurred vision, dry mucous membranes, rash, hypersensitivity, erythema
multiforme, leukopenia, and hallucinations. May increase serum levels of theophylline
or caffeine. Clinical experience in children weighing <13.6 kg (30 lb) is limited.

THIAMINE/VITAMIN B$_1$

VITAMIN B$_1$, Thiamilate, and others
Water-soluble vitamin

No   1   A/C

Tabs: 25, 50, 100, 250, 500 mg
Enteric coated tabs: 20 mg
Inj: 100 mg/mL, 200 mg/mL; may contain benzyl alcohol

For US RDA, see pp. 460–461.
Beriberi (thiamine deficiency):
  Children: 10–25 mg/dose IM/IV QD (if critically ill) or 10–50 mg/dose PO QD ×
  2 weeks, followed by 5–10 mg/dose QD × 1 mo.
  Adults: 5–30 mg/dose IM/IV TID × 2 weeks, followed by 5–30 mg/24 hr PO ÷ QD
  = TID × 1 mo.
Wernicke's encephalopathy syndrome: 100 mg IV × 1, then 50–100 mg IM/IV QD
until patient resumes a normal diet. (Administer thiamine before starting glucose
infusion.)

Continued

For explanation of icons, see p. 572.

THIAMINE/VITAMIN B$_1$ *continued*

Multivitamin preparations contain amounts meeting RDA requirements. Allergic reactions and anaphylaxis may occur, primarily with IV administration. *Therapeutic range:* 1.6–4 mg/dL. High-carbohydrate diets or IV dextrose solutions may increase thiamine requirements. Large doses may interfere with serum theophylline assay. Pregnancy category changes to "C" if used in doses above the RDA.

THIOPENTAL SODIUM

Pentothal and others
Barbiturate

Yes   1   C

Inj: 250, 400, 500 mg, 1, 2.5, 5 g (reconstituted to 20 mg/mL or 25 mg/mL)
Rectal suspension: 400 mg/g (2 g)

Cerebral edema: 1.5–5 mg/kg/dose IV. Repeat PRN for increased ICP.
Anesthesia induction, children and adults:
    IV: 2–6 mg/kg: Use lower doses in patients with hemodynamic instability. See pp. 4–6, for rapid sequence intubation.
Deep sedation:
    Children: 30 mg/kg PR × 1; **max. dose:** 1 g/dose

Contraindicated in acute intermittent porphyria. May cause respiratory depression, hypotension, anaphylaxis, and decreased cardiac output.
Onset of action: 30–60 sec for IV; 7–10 min for PR. *Duration of action:* 5–30 min for IV; 90 min for PR.
Adjust dose in renal failure (see p. 951).

THIORIDAZINE

Mellaril and others
Antipsychotic, phenothiazine derivative

No   ?   C

Tabs: 10, 15, 25, 50, 100, 150, 200 mg
Oral concentration: 30, 100 mg/mL (120 mL); may contain alcohol
Suspension: 25 mg/5 mL, 100 mg/5 mL (480 mL)

Children 2–12 yr: 0.5–3 mg/kg/24 hr PO ÷ BID-TID. **Max. dose:** 3 mg/kg/24 hr
>12 yr and adults: Start with 75–300 mg/24 hr PO ÷ TID. Then gradually increase PRN to **max. dose** of 800 mg/24 hr ÷ BID–QID

Continued

THIORIDAZINE *continued*

Indicated for schizophrenia unresponsive to standard therapy. **Contraindicated** in severe CNS depression, brain damage, narrow-angle glaucoma, blood dyscrasias, and severe liver or cardiovascular disease. **DO NOT** co-administer with drugs that may inhibit the CYP 450 2D6 isoenzymes (e.g., SSRIs such as fluoxetine, fluvoxamine, paroxetine; and beta-blockers such as propranolol and pindolol); drugs that may widen the QTc interval (e.g., disopyramide, procainamide, quinidine); and in patients with known reduced activity of CYP 450 2D6.

May cause drowsiness, extrapyramidal reactions, autonomic symptoms, ECG changes (QTc prolongation in a dose-dependent manner), arrhythmias, paradoxical reactions, and endocrine disturbances. Long-term use may cause tardive dyskinesia. Pigmentary retinopathy may occur with higher doses; a periodic eye examination is recommended. More autonomic symptoms and less extrapyramidal effects than chlorpromazine. Concurrent use with epinephrine can cause hypotension. Increased cardiac arrhythmias may occur with tricyclic antidepressants. Do not simultaneously administer oral liquid dosage form with carbamazepine oral suspension because an orange rubbery precipitate may form.

In an overdose situation, monitor ECG and avoid drugs that can widen QTc interval.

TIAGABINE

Gabitril
Anticonvulsant

No   ?   C

Tabs: 2, 4, 12, 16, 20 mg

Adjunctive therapy for partial seizures:
≥12 yr and adults: Start at 4 mg PO QD × 7 days. If needed, increase dose to 8 mg/24 hr PO ÷ BID. Dosage may be increased further by 4–8 mg/24 hr at weekly intervals (daily doses may be divided BID-QID) until a clinical response is achieved or up to specified **maximum dose.**

Max. dose:
12–18 yr: 32 mg/24 hr
Adults: 56 mg/24 hr

Use with **caution** in hepatic insufficiency (may need to reduce dose and/or increase dosing interval). Most common side effects include dizziness, asthenia, nausea, nervousness, tremor, abdominal pain, confusion, and difficulty in concentrating. Cognitive/neuropsychiatric symptoms resulting in nonconvulsive status epilepticus requiring subsequent dose reduction or drug discontinuation have been reported.

Tiagabine's clearance is increased by concurrent hepatic enzyme-inducing anti-epileptic drugs (e.g., phenytoin, carbamazepine, and barbiturates). Lower doses or a slower titration for clinical response may be necessary for patients receiving non-enzyme–inducing drugs (e.g., valproate, gabapentin, and lamotrigine). Avoid abrupt discontinuation of drug.

TID dosing schedule may be preferred because BID schedule may not be well tolerated. Doses should be administered with food.

For explanation of icons, see p. 572.

TICARCILLIN

Ticar
Antibiotic, penicillin (extended spectrum)

Yes 1 B

Inj: 1, 3, 6, 20, 30 g
Each g contains 5.2–6.5 mEq Na

Neonates, IM/IV:
  ≤7 days:
    <2 kg: 150 mg/kg/24 hr ÷ Q12 hr
    ≥2 kg: 225 mg/kg/24 hr ÷ Q8 hr
  >7 days:
    <1.2 kg: 150 mg/kg/24 hr ÷ Q12 hr
    1.2–2 kg: 225 mg/kg/24 hr ÷ Q8 hr
    >2 kg: 300 mg/kg/24 hr ÷ Q6–8 hr
Infants and children (IM/IV): 200–300 mg/kg/24 hr ÷ Q4–6 hr. **Max. dose:** 24 g/24 hr
Cystic fibrosis (IM/IV): 300–600 mg/kg/24 hr ÷ Q4–6 hr. **Max. dose:** 24 g/24 hr
Adults (IM/IV): 1–4 g/dose Q4–6 hr; **max. dose:** 24 g/24 hr

May cause decreased platelet aggregation, bleeding diathesis, hypernatermia, hematuria, hypokalemia, hypocalcemia, allergy, rash, and increased AST. Like other penicillins, CSF penetration occurs only with inflamed meninges. Do not mix with aminoglycoside in same solution. May cause false-positive tests for urine protein and serum Coombs'.
Adjust dose in renal failure (see p. 945).

TICARCILLIN/CLAVULANATE

Timentin
Antibiotic, penicillin (extended spectrum with beta-lactamase inhibitor)

Yes 1 B

Inj: 3.1 g (3 g ticarcillin and 0.1 g clavulanate); contains 4.75 mEq Na$^+$ and 0.15 mEq K$^+$ per 1 g drug

Doses should be based on ticarcillin component; see *Ticarcillin*.
Max. dose: 18–24 g/24 hr

Activity similar to ticarcillin except that beta-lactamase inhibitor broadens spectrum to include *S. aureus* and *H. influenzae*. See *Ticarcillin* for side effects. Like other penicillins, CSF penetration occurs only with inflamed meninges. May cause false-positive tests for urine protein and serum Coombs'.
Adjust dosage in renal impairment (see p. 945).

TOBRAMYCIN

Nebcin, Tobrex, TOBI, and others
Antibiotic, aminoglycoside

Yes   ?   D

Inj: 10, 40 mg/mL; may contain phenol and bisulfites
Powder for inj: 1.2 g
Ophthalmic ointment: 0.3% (3.5 g)
Ophthalmic solution: 0.3% (5 mL)
Nebulizer solution (TOBI): 300 mg/5 mL (preservative free) (56s)

Neonates, IM/IV (see table below):

Postconceptional Age (weeks)	Postnatal Age (days)	Dose (mg/kg/ dose)	Interval (hr)
≤29*	0–28	2.5	24
	>28	3	24
30–36	0–14	3	24
	>14	2.5	12
≥37	0–7	2.5	12
	>7	2.5	8

*Or significant asphyxia.

Child: 6–7.5 mg/kg/24 hr ÷ Q8 hr IV/IM
Cystic fibrosis: 7.5–10 mg/kg/24 hr ÷ Q8 hr IV
Adults: 3–6 mg/kg/24 hr ÷ Q8 hr IV/IM
Ophthalmic:
    Children and adults: Apply thin ribbon of ointment to affected eye BID-TID; or 1–2
    drops of solution to affected eye Q4 hr
Inhalation:
    Cystic fibrosis prophylaxis therapy (TOBI):
        ≥6 yr and adults: 300 mg Q12 hr administered in repeated cycles of 28 days on
        drug followed by 28 days off drug

Use with **caution** in patients receiving anesthetics or neuromuscular blocking
agents, and in patients with neuromuscular disorders. May cause ototoxicity,
nephrotoxicity, and myelotoxicity. Serious allergic reactions including anaphylaxis, and dermatologic reactions including exfoliative dermatitis, toxic epidermal
necrolysis, erythema multiforme, and Stevens Johnson syndrome have been reported
rarely. **Ototoxic effects synergistic with furosemide.**

Higher doses are recommended in patients with cystic fibrosis, neutropenia, or
burns. **Adjust dose in renal failure (see p. 945).** Monitor peak and trough levels.
    Therapeutic peak levels:
        6–10 mg/L in general
        8–10 mg/L in pulmonary infections, neutropenia, and severe sepsis

Continued

TOBRAMYCIN *continued*

Therapeutic trough levels: <2 mg/L. *Recommended serum sampling time at steady-state:* Trough within 30 min prior to the third consecutive dose and peak 30–60 min after the administration of the third consecutive dose.

For inhalation use with other medications in cystic fibrosis, use the following order of administration: bronchodilator first, chest physiotherapy, other inhaled medications (if indicated), and tobramycin last.

TOLMETIN SODIUM

Tolectin
Nonsteroidal antiinflammatory agent

No   1   C/D

Tabs: 200, 600 mg
Capsules: 400 mg
Contains 0.8 mEq Na per 200 mg drug

Children ≥2 yr:
Antiinflammatory:
   Initial: 20 mg/kg/24 hr ÷ TID-QID PO. May increase in increments of 5 mg/kg/24 hr to **max. dose** of 30 mg/kg/24 hr or 2 g/24 hr
   Analgesic: 5–7 mg/kg/dose PO Q6–8 hr. **Max. dose:** 30 mg/kg/24 hr or 2 g/24 hr
Adults:
   Initial: 400 mg TID PO
   Maintenance: Titrate to desired effect. Usually, 600–1800 mg/24 hr ÷ TID PO.
   Max. dose: 2 g/24 hr

May cause GI irritation or bleeding, CNS symptoms, platelet dysfunction, or false-positive proteinuria. May increase the effects of warfarin and methotrexate.
Pregnancy category changes to "D" if used in third trimester or near delivery.
Take with food or milk.

TOLNAFTATE

Tinactin, Aftate, and many others
Antifungal agent

No   ?   C

Topical aerosol liquid (OTC): 1% (60, 120 mL)
Aerosol powder (OTC): 1% (100, 150 g)
Cream (OTC): 1% (15, 30 g)
Gel (OTC): 1% (15 g)
Topical powder (OTC): 1% (45, 90 g)
Topical solution (OTC): 1% (10, 60 mL)

Continued

TOLNAFTATE *continued*

Topical:
Apply 1–2 drops of solution or small amount of gel, liquid, cream, or powder to affected areas BID for 2–4 weeks.

May cause mild irritation and sensitivity. Avoid eye contact. **Do not use** for nail or scalp infections.

TOPIRAMATE

Topamax
Anticonvulsant

Yes ? C

Sprinkle caps: 15, 25 mg
Tabs: 25, 100, 200 mg

Children 2–16 yr: Start with 1–3 mg/kg/dose (**max. dose:** 25 mg/dose) PO QHS × 7 days, then increase by 1–3 mg/kg/24-hr increments at 1- to 2-week intervals (divide daily dose BID) to response. Usual maintenance dose is 5–9 mg/kg/24 hr PO ÷ BID.

≥*17 yr and adults:* Start with 25–50 mg PO QHS × 7 days, then increase by 25–50 mg/24-hr increments at 1-week intervals until adequate response. Doses >50 mg should be divided BID. Consult with neurologist.
Usual maintenance dose: 400 mg/24 hr.
Doses above 1600 mg/24 hr have not been studied.

Used as adjunctive therapy for primary generalized tonic-clonic or partial seizures, and Lennox-Gastaut syndrome. Use with **caution** in renal and hepatic dysfunction (decreased clearance) and sulfa hypersensitivity. **Reduce dose by 50% when creatinine clearance is <70 mL/min.** Common side effects (incidence lower in children) include ataxia, cognitive dysfunction, dizziness, nystagmus, paresthesia, sedation, visual disturbances, nausea, dyspepsia, and kidney stones. Secondary angle-closure glaucoma characterized by ocular pain, acute myopia, and increased intraocular pressure has been reported and may lead to blindness if left untreated. Patients should be instructed to seek immediate medical attention if they experience blurred vision or periorbital pain.

Drug is metabolized by and inhibits the cytochrome P 450 2C19 isoenzyme. Phenytoin, valproic acid, and carbamazepine may decrease topiramate levels. Topiramate may decrease valproic acid, digoxin, and ethinyl estradiol (to decrease oral contraceptive efficacy), but may increase phenytoin levels. Alcohol and CNS depressants may increase CNS side effects. Carbonic anhydrase inhibitors (e.g., acetazolamide) may increase risk of nephrolithiasis or paresthesia.

Doses may be administered with or without food. Sprinkle capsule may be opened and sprinkled on small amount of food (e.g., 1 teaspoonful of applesauce) and swallowed whole (do not chew). Maintain adequate hydration to prevent kidney stone formation.

For explanation of icons, see p. 572.

TRAZODONE

Desyrel and many others
Antidepressant, triazolopyridine-derivative

No   3   C

Tabs: 50, 100, 150, 300 mg

Depression (titrate to lowest effective dose):
Children (6–18 yr): Start at 1.5–2 mg/kg/24 hr PO ÷ BID–TID; if needed,
   gradually increase dose Q3–4 days up to a **maximum** of 6 mg/kg/24 hr ÷ TID
Adults: Start at 150 mg/24 hr PO ÷ TID; if needed, increase by 50 mg/24 hr Q3–4
days up to a **maximum** of 600 mg/24 hr for hospitalized patients (400 mg/24 hr for
ambulatory patients).

Use with **caution** in preexisting cardiac disease, initial recovery phase of MI, and
electroconvulsive therapy. Common side effects include dizziness, drowsiness,
dry mouth, and diarrhea. Seizures, tardive dyskinesia, EPS, arrhythmias,
priapism, blurred vision, neuromuscular weakness, anemia, orthostatic hypotension,
and rash have been reported. Trazodone may increase digoxin levels and increase CNS
effects of alcohol, barbiturates, and other CNS depressants. Maximum antidepressant
effect is seen at 2–6 weeks.

TRETINOIN

Retin-A, Retin-A Micro, Avita, Renova
Retinoic acid derivative, topical acne product

No   ?   C

Cream: 0.02% (40 g), 0.025% (20, 45 g), 0.05% (20, 40, 45, 60 g), 0.1%
(20, 45 g)
Topical gel: 0.01%, 0.025%; may contain 90% alcohol (15, 45 g)
Topical gel (Retin-A Micro): 0.1%; contains glycerin, propylene glycol, benzyl alcohol
(20, 45 g)
Topical liquid: 0.05%; contains 55% alcohol (28 mL)

Topical:
Children >12 yr and adults: Gently wash face with a mild soap, pat the skin dry,
   and wait 20 to 30 min before use. Initiate therapy with either 0.025% cream
   or 0.01% gel and apply a small "pea-sized" amount to the affected areas of the
face QHS.

Contraindicated in sunburns. **Avoid** excessive sun exposure. If stinging or
irritation occurs, decrease frequency of administration to QOD. **Avoid** contact
with eyes, ears, nostrils, mouth, or open wounds. Local adverse effects include
irritation, erythema, excessive dryness, blistering, crusting, hyperpigmentation or
hypopigmentation, and acne flare-ups. Concomitant use of other topical acne products
may lead to significant skin irritation. Onset of therapeutic benefits may be experienced
within 2–3 weeks with optimal effects in 6 weeks.

TRIAMCINOLONE

Azmacort, Nasacort, Tri-Nasal, Nasacort AQ, Kenalog, Aristocort, and others

Corticosteroid

No   ?   C

Nasal inhaler (Nasacort): 55 mcg/actuation (100 actuations per 10 g)
Nasal spray:
 Tri-Nasal: 50 mcg/actuation (120 actuations per 15 mL)
 Nasacort AQ: 55 mcg/actuation (30 actuations per 6.5 g, 120 actuations per 16.5 g)
Oral inhaler: 100 mcg/actuation (240 actuations per 20 g)
Tabs: 1, 2, 4, 8 mg
Oral syrup: 4 mg/5 mL (120 mL)
Cream: 0.025%, 0.1%, 0.5%
Ointment: 0.025%, 0.1%, 0.5%
Lotion: 0.025%, 0.1% (60 mL)
Topical aerosol: 0.2 mg/2-second spray (23, 63 g); contains 10.3% alcohol
Dental paste: 0.1% (5 g)
See pp. 908–909 for potency rankings and sizes of topical preparations.
Inj as acetonide: 3, 10, 40 mg/mL; contains benzyl alcohol
Inj as diacetate: 25, 40 mg/mL; contains polyethylene glycol and benzyl alcohol; for IM injection use only
Inj as hexacetonide: 5, 20 mg/mL; contains benzyl alcohol

Oral inhalation:
 Children 6–12 yr: 1–2 puffs TID–QID or 2–4 puffs BID; **max. dose:** 12 puffs/ 24 hr
 ≥12 yr and adults: 2 puffs TID–QID or 4 puffs BID; **max. dose:** 16 puffs/24 hr
 NIH-National Heart Lung and Blood Institute recommendations (divide daily doses BID–QID): See pp. 911–912.
Intranasal (always titrate to lowest effective dose after symptoms are controlled):
 Nasacort:
  Children 6–11 yr: 2 sprays in each nostril QD
  ≥12 yr and adults: 2 sprays in each nostril QD; may increase to 4 sprays/ nostril/24 hr ÷ QD–QID
 Nasacort AQ:
  Children 6–11 yr: Start with 1 spray in each nostril QD. If no benefit in 1 week, dose may be increased to 2 sprays in each nostril QD.
  ≥12 yr and adults: 2 sprays in each nostril QD
Topical: Apply to affected areas QD–TID
Systemic use: Use ⅙ of Cortisone dose. See p. 913.
Intralesional, ≥12 yr and adults (as diacetate or acetonide): 1 mg/site at intervals of 1 week or more. May give separate doses in sites >1 cm apart, not to exceed 30 mg.

Rinse mouth thoroughly with water after each use of the oral inhalation dosage form. Nasal preparations may cause epistaxis, cough, fever, nausea, throat irritation, and dyspepsia. Topical preparations may cause dermal atrophy,

Continued

TRIAMCINOLONE *continued*

telangiectasias, and hypopigmentation. Topical steroids should be used with **caution** on the face and in intertriginous areas. See p. 183.

Dosage adjustment for hepatic failure with systemic use may be necessary.

TRIAMTERENE

Dyrenium
Diuretic, potassium sparing

Yes ? B

Caps: 50, 100 mg

Children: 2–4 mg/kg/24 hr ÷ QD–BID PO. May increase up to a **maximum** of 6 mg/kg/24 hr or 300 mg/24 hr.
Adults: 50-100 mg/24 hr ÷ QD–BID PO; **max. dose:** 300 mg/24 hr

Do not use if GFR <10 mL/hr. **Adjust dose in renal impairment (see p. 951).** Monitor serum electrolytes. May cause hyperkalemia, hyponatremia, hypomagnesemia, and metabolic acidosis. Interstitial nephritis, thrombocytopenia, and anaphylaxis have been reported.

Concurrent use of ACE inhibitors may increase serum potassium. Use with **caution** when administering medications with high potassium load (e.g., some penicillins), and in patients with hepatic impairment or on high-potassium diets. Cimetidine may increase effects. This drug is also available as a combination product with hydrochlorothiazide. Administer doses with food to minimize GI upset.

TRIETHANOLAMINE POLYPEPTIDE OLEATE

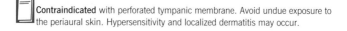

Cerumenex
Otic cerumenolytic

No ? C

Solution: 10% (6, 12 mL)

Children and adults: Fill ear canal and insert cotton plug. After 15–30 min, flush ear with warm water. May repeat dose in the presence of unusually hard impactions.

Contraindicated with perforated tympanic membrane. Avoid undue exposure to the periaural skin. Hypersensitivity and localized dermatitis may occur.

TRIMETHOBENZAMIDE HCl

Tigan and others
Antiemetic

No   ?   C

Caps: 100, 250 mg
Suppository: 100 mg (10s), 200 mg (10s, 50s); contains 2% benzocaine
Inj: 100 mg/mL (2, 20 mL); may contain phenol or parabens

Children:
<13.6 kg (excluding premature and newborn infants):
  PR: 100 mg/dose TID-QID.
13.6–40.9 kg:
  PO/PR: 100–200 mg/dose TID-QID
Adults:
  PO: 250 mg/dose TID-QID
  PR/IM: 200 mg/dose TID-QID

Do not use in premature or newborn infants. Avoid use in patients with hepatotoxicity, acute vomiting, or allergic reaction. CNS disturbances are common in children (extrapyramidal symptoms, drowsiness, confusion, dizziness). Hypotension, especially with IM use, may occur. Suppository contains 2% benzocaine. **IM not recommended in children.**

TRIMETHOPRIM-SULFAMETHOXAZOLE

See Co-Trimoxazole

UROKINASE

Abbokinase, Abbokinase Open Cath
Thrombolytic enzyme

No   ?   B

Inj: 5000 U/mL (Abbokinase Open Cath); 250,000 U (both products are preservative free)

Deep vein thromboses and pulmonary emboli: **Should be used in consultation with a hematologist.** 4400 U/kg over 10 min, followed by 4400 U/kg/hr for 6–12 hr; some patients may require 12–72 hr of therapy. Titrate to effect.

Continued

UROKINASE *continued*

Occluded IV catheter:

  Aspiration method: Use 5000 U/mL concentrate. Instill into catheter a volume equal to the internal volume of catheter over 1–2 min, leave in place for 1–4 hr, then aspirate. May repeat with 10,000 U/mL in each lumen if no response. **DO NOT** infuse into patient.

  IV infusion method: 150–200 U/kg/hr in each lumen for 8–48 hr at a rate of at least 20 mL/hr.

  For dialysis patients: 5000 U in each lumen administered over 1–2 min; leave drug in for 1–2 days, then aspirate

Contraindicated for patients with active internal bleeding, bacterial endocarditis, intracranial neoplasm, arteriovenous malformation, aneurysm, bleeding diathesis, DIC, history of CVA within the past 2 mo, or recent trauma/surgery. Monitor fibrinogen, thrombin clotting time, PT, and APTT when used as a thrombolytic (before and during continuous infusion therapy).

Discontinue administration if signs of bleeding occur. Side effects include allergic reactions, fever, rash, and bronchospasm.

Newborns have reduced plasminogen levels (~50% of adult values), which decrease the thrombolytic effects of urokinase. Plasminogen supplementation may be necessary.

Product may not be available due to FDA concerns with manufacturing deficiencies. The FDA recommends that urokinase be reserved for only those situations in which there are no alternatives and the use of the drug is deemed critical to the care of the patient.

URSODIOL

Actigall, Urso
Gallstone solubilizing agent, cholelitholytic agent

No   ?   B

Suspension: 60 mg/mL
Caps (Actigall): 300 mg
Tabs (Urso): 250 mg

Children: 10–15 mg/kg/24 hr QD PO
Adults: 8–10 mg/kg/24 hr ÷ BID–TID PO
  Cystic fibrosis (to improve fatty acid metabolism in liver disease): 15–30 mg/kg/24 hr ÷ QD–TID PO

Contraindicated in calcified cholesterol stones, radiopaque stones, bile pigment stones, or stones >20 mm in diameter. May cause GI disturbance, rash, arthralgias, anxiety, headache, and elevated liver enzymes. Aluminum-containing antacids, cholestyramine, and oral contraceptives decrease ursodiol effectiveness. Dissolution of stones may take several months. Stone recurrence occurs in 30%–50% of patients within 5 yr.

Limited data for use in TPN-induced cholestasis at 30 mg/kg/24 hr ÷ TID PO (Gastroenterology 111(3):716-9;1996).

VALACYCLOVIR

Valtrex
Antiviral agent

Yes   1   B

Tabs: 500, 1000 mg

Herpes zoster (see remarks):
  Adults (immunocompetent): 1 g/dose PO TID × 7 days within 48–72 hr of onset
    of rash.
Genital herpes:
  Adolescents and adults:
    Initial episodes: 1 g/dose PO BID × 10 days.
    Recurrent episodes: 500 mg/dose PO BID × 3 days.
    Suppressive therapy: 500–1000 mg/dose PO QD × 1 yr, then reassess for
      recurrences

This pro-drug is metabolized to acyclovir and L-valine with better oral absorption
than acyclovir. Use with **caution** in hepatic or renal insufficiency. **Adjust dose in
renal insufficiency (see p. 96).** Thrombotic thrombocytopenic purpura/hemolytic
uremic syndrome (TTP/HUS) has been reported in patients with advanced HIV
infection and in bone marrow and renal transplant recipients. Probenecid or cimetidine
can reduce the rate of conversion to acyclovir. See acyclovir for additional drug
interactions and adverse effects.

For initial episodes of genital herpes, therapy is most effective when initiated within
48 hr of symptom onset. Therapy should be initiated immediately after the onset of
symptoms in recurrent episodes (no efficacy data when initiating therapy >24 hr after
onset of symptoms). Data are not available for use as suppressive therapy for periods
>1 yr.

Valacyclovir **CANNOT** be substituted for acyclovir on a one-to-one basis. Doses may
be administered with or without food.

VALGANCICLOVIR

Valcyte
Antiviral agent

Yes   ?   C

Tabs: 450 mg

CMV retinitis:
  Adults:
    Induction therapy: 900 mg PO BID × 21 days with food
    Maintenance therapy: 900 mg PO QD with food

Continued

VALGANCICLOVIR *continued*

This pro-drug is metabolized to ganciclovir with better oral absorption than ganciclovir. Use with **caution** in renal insufficiency. **Adjust dose in renal insufficiency (see p. 946).** May cause headache, insomnia, peripheral neuropathy, diarrhea, vomiting, neutropenia, anemia, and thrombocytopenia. See *Ganciclovir* for drug interactions and additional adverse effects.

Valganciclovir **CANNOT** be substituted for ganciclovir on a one-to-one basis. All doses are administered with food.

VALPROIC ACID

Depakene, Depacon, and others
(Depakote—*See Divalproex sodium*)
Anticonvulsant

No   1   D

Caps: 250 mg
Syrup: 250 mg/5 mL (473 mL); may contain parabens
Inj (Depacon): 100 mg/mL (5 mL)

Oral:
  Initial: 10–15 mg/kg/24 hr ÷ QD–TID
    Increment: 5–10 mg/kg/24 hr at weekly intervals to **max. dose** of 60 mg/kg/24 hr
  Maintenance: 30–60 mg/kg/24 hr ÷ BID–TID. Due to drug interactions, higher doses may be required in children on other anticonvulsants.
Intravenous (use only when PO is not possible):
  Use same PO daily dose ÷ Q6 hr. Convert back to PO as soon as possible.
Rectal (use syrup, diluted 1:1 with water, given PR as a retention enema):
  Load: 20 mg/kg/dose
  Maintenance: 10–15 mg/kg/dose Q8 hr
Migrane prophylaxis:
  Children: 15–30 mg/kg/24 hr PO ÷ BID
  Adult: Start with 500 mg/24 hr ÷ PO BID. Dose may be increased to a **maximum** of 1000 mg/24 hr ÷ PO BID. If using divalproex sodium extended-release tablets, administer daily dose QD.

Contraindicated in hepatic disease. May cause GI, liver, blood, and CNS toxicity; weight gain; transient alopecia; pancreatitis (potentially life-threatening); nausea; sedation; vomiting; headache; thrombocytopenia; platelet dysfunction; rash; and hyperammonemia. Hepatic failure has occurred, especially in children <2 yr. Idiosyncratic life-threatening pancreatitis has been reported in children and adults.

Valproic acid is a substrate for CYP 450 2C19 isoenzyme and an inhibitor of CYP 450 2C9, 2D6 and 3A3/4 (weak). It increases amitriptyline/nortriptyline, phenytoin, diazepam, and phenobarbital levels. Concomitant phenytoin, phenobarbital, topiramate, meropenem, and carbamazepine may decrease valproic acid levels. Amitriptyline or nortriptyline may increase valproic acid levels. May interfere with urine ketone and thyroid tests.

Continued

VALPROIC ACID continued

Do not give syrup with carbonated beverages. Use of IV route has not been evaluated for >14 days of continuous use. Infuse IV over 1 hr up to a **max. rate** of 20 mg/min.

Therapeutic levels: 50–100 mg/L. *Recommendations for serum sampling at steady-state:* Obtain trough level within 30 min prior to the next scheduled dose after 2–3 days of continuous dosing. Monitor CBC and LFTs prior to and during therapy.

VANCOMYCIN

Vancocin and others
Antibiotic

Yes   ?   C/B

Inj: 0.5, 1, 5, 10 g
Caps: 125, 250 mg
Solution: 1 g (reconstitute to 250 mg/5 mL), 10 g (reconstitute to 500 mg/6 mL)

 Neonates, IV (see table below):

	Postnatal Age	
Weight	<7 Days	≥7 Days
<1.2 kg	15 mg/kg/dose Q24 hr	15 mg/kg/dose Q24 hr
1.2–2 kg	10–15 mg/kg/dose Q12–18 hr	10–15 mg/kg/dose Q8–12 hr
>2 kg	10–15 mg/kg/dose Q8–12 hr	15–20 mg/kg/dose Q8 hr

Infants and children, IV:
  CNS infection: 60 mg/kg/24 hr ÷ Q6 hr
  Other infections: 40 mg/kg/24 hr ÷ Q6–8 hr
  Max. dose: 1 g/dose
Adults: 2 g/24 hr ÷ Q6–12 hr IV; **max. dose:** 4 g/24 hr
C. difficile colitis:
  Children: 40–50 mg/kg/24 hr ÷ Q6 hr PO × 7–10 days
    Max. dose: 500 mg/24 hr
  Adults: 125 mg/dose PO Q6 hr × 7–10 days
Endocarditis prophylaxis: pp. 159–160.

Ototoxicity and nephrotoxicity may occur and may be exacerbated with concurrent aminoglycoside use. **Adjust dose in renal failure (see p. 886).** Low concentrations of the drug may appear in CSF with inflamed meninges. "Red man syndrome" associated with rapid IV infusion may occur. Infuse over 60 min (may infuse over 120 min if 60-min infusion is not tolerated). **Note:** Diphenhydramine is used to reverse "red man syndrome." Allergic reactions have been reported.

Although the monitoring of serum levels is controversial, the following guidelines are recommended. *Therapeutic levels:* Peak: 25–40 mg/L; trough: <10 mg/L. *Recommended serum sampling time at steady-state:* Trough within 30 min prior to the third consecutive dose and peak 60 min after the administration of the third consecutive dose.

Continued

VANCOMYCIN *continued*

Metronidazole (PO) is the drug of choice for *C. difficile* colitis; vancomycin should be avoided due to the emergence of vancomycin-resistant enterococcus. Pregnancy category "B" is assigned with the oral route of administration.

VARICELLA-ZOSTER IMMUNE GLOBULIN (HUMAN)
VZIG
Hyperimmune globulin

No   ?   C

1 vial = 125 U (~1.25 mL), 625 U (~6.25 mL); contains 10%–18% globulin

≤10 kg: 125 U IM
  10.1–20 kg: 250 U IM
    20.1–30 kg: 375 U IM
30.1–40 kg: 500 U IM
>40 kg: 625 U IM (**maximum** 2.5 mL per injection site)
Max. dose: 625 U/dose

Contraindicated in severe thrombocytopenia because of IM injection. See pp. 339–341 for indications. Doses ideally should be given within 48 hr of exposure and no later than 96 hr postexposure. Local discomfort, redness, and swelling at the injection site may occur. **May induce anaphylactic reactions in immunoglobulin A–deficient individuals.** Interferes with immune response to live virus vaccines such as measles, mumps, and rubella; defer administration of live vaccines 5 mo or longer after VZIG dose.

VASOPRESSIN
Pitressin and others
Antidiuretic hormone analog

No   ?   B

Inj: 20 U/mL (aqueous) (0.5, 1, 10 mL)

Diabetes insipidus: Titrate dose to effect
SC/IM:
  Children: 2.5–10 U BID–QID
  Adults: 5–10 U BID–QID
Continuous infusion (adults and children): Start at 0.5 milliunit/kg/hr (0.0005 U/kg/hr). Double dosage every 30 min PRN up to **max. dose** of 10 milliunit/kg/hr (0.01 U/kg/hr)

Continued

VASOPRESSIN *continued*

Growth hormone and corticotropin provocative tests:
    Children: 0.3 U/kg IM; **max. dose:** 10 U
    Adult: 10 U IM
GI hemorrhage (IV):
    Children: Start at 0.002–0.005 U/kg/min. Increase dose as needed to **max. dose** of
    0.01 U/kg/min.
    Adults: Start at 0.2–0.4 U/min. Increase dose as needed to **max. dose** of
    0.9 U/min.
Cardiac arrest, ventricular fibrillation, and pulseless ventricular tachycardia:
    Adults: 40 U IV × 1

Use with **caution** in seizures, migraine, asthma, and vascular disease. Side effects include tremor, sweating, vertigo, abdominal discomfort, nausea, vomiting, urticaria, anaphylaxis, hypertension, and bradycardia. May cause vasoconstriction, water intoxication, and bronchoconstriction. *Drug interactions:* Lithium, demeclocycline, heparin and alcohol reduce activity; carbamazepine, tricyclic antidepressants, fludrocortisone, and chlorpropamide increase activity.

Do not abruptly discontinue IV infusion (taper dose). Patients with variceal hemorrhage and hepatic insufficiency may respond to lower dosages. Monitor fluid intake and output, urine specific gravity, urine and serum osmolality, and sodium.

VECURONIUM BROMIDE

Norcuron
Nondepolarizing neuromuscular blocking agent

Yes ? C

Inj: 10, 20 mg; may contain benzyl alcohol

Neonates:
    Initial: 0.1 mg/kg/dose IV
    Maintenance: 0.03–0.15 mg/kg/dose IV Q1–2 hr PRN
>7 week–1 yr:
    Initial: 0.08–0.1 mg/kg/dose IV
    Maintenance: 0.05–0.1 mg/kg/dose IV Q1 hr PRN;
    >1 yr–adults:
    Initial: 0.08–0.1 mg/kg/dose IV
    Maintenance: 0.05–0.1 mg/kg/dose IV Q1 hr PRN; may administer via continuous
    infusion at 0.05–0.07 mg/kg/hr IV

Use with **caution** in patients with renal or hepatic impairment, and neuromuscular disease. Infants from 7 weeks to 1 yr are more sensitive to the drug and may have a longer recovery time. Children (1–10 yr) may require higher doses and more frequent supplementation than adults. Enflurane, isoflurane, aminoglycosides, beta-blockers, calcium channel blockers, clindamycin, furosemide, magnesium salts, quinidine, procainamide, and cyclosporine may increase the potency and duration

Continued

For explanation of icons, see p. 572.

VECURONIUM BROMIDE *continued*

of neuromuscular blockade. Calcium, caffeine, carbamazepine, phenytoin, steroids (chronic use), acetylcholinesterases, and azathioprine may decrease effects. May cause arrhythmias, rash, and bronchospasm.

Neostigmine, pyridostigmine, or edrophonium are antidotes. Onset of action within 1–3 min. Duration is 30–40 min. See p. 5, for rapid sequence intubation.

VERAPAMIL

Isoptin, Calan, Verelan, and others
Calcium channel blocker

Yes   1   C

Tabs: 40, 80, 120 mg
Extended/sustained-release tabs: 120, 180, 240 mg
Extended/sustained-release caps: 100, 120, 180, 200, 240, 300, 360 mg
Inj: 2.5 mg/mL
Suspension: 50 mg/mL

IV for dysrhythmias: Give over 2–3 min. May repeat once after 30 min.
1–15 yr, for PSVT: 0.1–0.3 mg/kg; **max. dose:** 5 mg first dose, 10 mg second dose.
Adults, for SVT: 5–10 mg (0.075–0.15 mg/kg), 10 mg second dose.
PO for hypertension:
Children: 4–8 mg/kg/24 hr ÷ TID
Adults: 240–480 mg/24 hr ÷ TID-QID
Divide QD-BID for extended sustained-release preparations.
Adult antianginal dose: 80 mg/dose Q6–8 hr PO; **max. dose:** 480 mg/24 hr

Contraindications include hypersensitivity, cardiogenic shock, severe CHF, sick-sinus syndrome, or AV block. **Due to negative inotropic effects, verapamil should not be used to treat SVT in an emergency setting in infants. Avoid IV use** in neonates and young infants due to apnea, bradycardia, and hypotension. Monitor ECG. **Have calcium and isoproterenol available to reverse myocardial depression.** May decrease neuromuscular transmission in patients with Duchenne's muscular dystrophy and worsen myasthenia gravis.

Drug is a substrate of CYP 450 1A2, and 3A3/4; and an inhibitor of CYP 3A4. Barbiturates, sulfinpyrazone, phenytoin, vitamin D, and rifampin may decrease serum levels/effects of verapamil; quinidine may increase serum levels/effects. Verapamil may increase effects of beta-blockers (severe myocardial depression), carbamazepine, cyclosporine, digoxin, ethanol, fentanyl, lithium, nondepolarizing muscle relaxants, and prazosin. **Reduce dose in renal insufficiency (see p. 951).**

VIDARABINE

Adenine arabinoside, ara-A, Vira-A
Antiviral agent

No   ?   C

Ophthalmic ointment: 3% monohydrate (2.8% vidarabine base) (3.5 g)

Keratoconjunctivitis (HSV, VZV): Apply ½-inch ribbon of ointment to lower conjunctival sac Q3 hr, 5 × /24 hr until complete reepithelialization has occurred, then decrease dose to BID for an additional 7 days.
If there are no signs of improvement after 7 days, or if complete reepithelialization has not occurred in 21 days, consider other forms of therapy.

Ophthalmic product may cause burning, lacrimation, keratitis, photophobia, and blurred vision. Ophthalmic steroids are **contraindicated** in suspected herpetic keratoconjunctivitis.

VITAMIN A

Aquasol A and others
Vitamin, fat soluble

No   ?   A/X

Drops (water miscible): 5000 IU/0.1 mL (30 mL)
Caps: 5000 IU (OTC), 10,000 IU (OTC), 15,000 IU (OTC), 25,000 IU, 50,000 IU
Tabs: 5000 IU (OTC), 10,000 IU (OTC), 15,000 IU
Inj: 50,000 IU/mL (2 mL)

US RDA: See pp. 460–461.
Supplementation in measles (6 mo to 2 yr)
 6 mo–1 yr: 100,000 IU/dose QD PO × 2 days. Repeat 1 dose at 4 weeks.
 1–2 yr: 200,000 IU/dose QD PO × 2 days. Repeat 1 dose at 4 weeks.
Malabsorption syndrome prophylaxis:
 Children >8 yr and adults: 10,000–50,000 IU/dose QD PO of water-miscible product.

High doses above the US RDA are teratogenic (category X). The use of vitamin A in measles is recommended in children 6 mo to 2 yr who are either hospitalized or who have any of the following risk factors: immunodeficiency, ophthalmologic evidence of vitamin A deficiency, impaired GI absorption, moderate to severe malnutrition, and recent immigration from areas with high measles mortality. May cause GI disturbance, rash, headache, increased ICP (pseudotumor cerebri), papilledema, and irritability. Mineral oil, cholestyramine, and neomycin will reduce vitamin A absorption. See pp. 463–465 for multivitamin preparations.

FORMULARY

VITAMIN B₁
See Thiamine

VITAMIN B₂
See Riboflavin

VITAMIN B₃
See Niacin

VITAMIN B₆
See Pyridoxine

VITAMIN B₁₂
See Cyanocobalamin

VITAMIN C
See Ascorbic acid

VITAMIN D₂
See Ergocalciferol

VITAMIN E/ALPHA-TOCOPHEROL
Aquasol E, Liqui-E, and others
Vitamin, fat soluble

Yes ? A/C

Tabs (OTC): 100, 200, 400, 500, 800 IU
Caps (OTC): 100, 200, 400, 500, 600, 800, 1000 IU
Caps, water miscible: 73.5, 147, 165, 330 mg; 100, 200, 400 IU
Drops: 50 IU/mL (water miscible)
Liquid: 400 IU/15 mL (water miscible)

 US RDA: See pp. 460–461.
Vitamin E deficiency, PO: Follow levels
  Use water-miscible form with malabsorption

Continued

VITAMIN E/ALPHA-TOCOPHEROL *continued*

Neonates: 25–50 IU/24 hr
Children: 1 IU/kg/24 hr
Adults: 60–75 IU/24 hr
Cystic fibrosis (use water-miscible form): 5–10 IU/kg/24 hr PO QD; **max. dose:** 400 IU/24 hr

Adverse reactions include GI distress, rash, headache, gonadal dysfunction, decreased serum thyroxine and triiodothyronine, and blurred vision. Necrotizing enterocolitis has been associated with large doses (>200 U/24 hr). May increase hypoprothrombinemic response of oral anticoagulants (e.g., warfarin), especially in doses >400 IU/24 hr.

One unit of vitamin E = 1 mg of ᴅʟ-alpha-tocopherol acetate. In malabsorption, water-miscible preparations are better absorbed. *Therapeutic levels:* 6–14 mg/L.

Pregnancy category changes to "C" if used in doses above the RDA. See pp. 463–465 for multivitamin preparations.

VITAMIN K
See Phytonodione

WARFARIN
Coumadin, Sofarin
Anticoagulant

Yes   1   D

Tabs: 1, 2, 2.5, 3, 4, 5, 6, 7.5, 10 mg
Inj: 5 mg

Infants and children:
Loading dose:
Baseline INR 1–1.3: 0.1–0.2 mg/kg/dose PO QD × 2 days; **max. dose:** 10 mg/dose
Liver dysfunction: 0.1 mg/kg/dose PO QD × 2 days; **max. dose:** 5 mg/dose
Maintenance dose: 0.1 mg/kg/24 hr PO QD. Adjust dose to achieve the desired INR or PT. *Maintenance dose range:* 0.05–0.34 mg/kg/24 hr PO QD. See remarks.
Adults: 5–15 mg PO QD × 2–5 days. Adjust dose to achieve the desired INR or PT. *Maintenance dose range:* 2–10 mg/24 hr PO QD.

Contraindicated in severe liver or kidney disease, uncontrolled bleeding, GI ulcers, and malignant hypertension. Acts on vitamin K–dependent coagulation factors II, VII, IX, and X. Side effects include fever, skin lesions, skin necrosis

Continued

WARFARIN continued

(especially in protein C deficiency), anorexia, nausea, vomiting, diarrhea, hemorrhage, and hemoptysis.

Warfarin is a substrate for CYP 450 1A2, 2C8, 2C9, 2C18, 2C19, and 3A3/4, and inhibits CYP 2C9. Chloramphenicol, chloral hydrate, cimetidine, delavirdine, fluconazole, fluoxetine, metronidazole, indomethacin, nonsteroidal antiinflammatory agents, omeprazole, quinidine, salicylates, sulfonamides, zafirlukast, and zileuton may increase warfarin's effect. Ascorbic acid, barbituates, carbamazepine, cholestyramine, dicloxacillin, griseofulvin, oral contraceptives, rifampin, spironolactone, sucralfate, and vitamin K (including foods with high content) may decrease warfarin's effect.

Younger children generally require higher doses to achieve desired effect. A cohort study of 262 children found that infants <1 yr required an average daily dose of 0.32 mg/kg and teenagers 11–18 yr required 0.09 mg/kg to maintain a target INR of 2–3. Children receiving Fontan cardiac surgery may require smaller doses than children with either congenital heart disease (without Fontan) or no congenital heart disease. See Chest 2001; 119:344-370S and Blood 1999; 94(9):3007-3014 for additional information.

The INR (international ratio) is the recommended test to monitor warfarin anticoagulant effect. Monitor INR after 5–7 days of new dosage. The particular INR desired is based on the indication. An INR of 2–3 has been recommended for prophylaxis and treatment of DVT, pulmonary emboli, and bioprosthetic heart valves. An INR of 2.5–3.5 has been recommended for mechanical prosthetic heart valves and the prevention of recurrent systemic emboli. If PT is monitored, it should be 1.5–2 times the control.

Onset of action occurs within 36–72 hr and peak effects occur within 5–7 days. **The antidote is vitamin K and/or fresh frozen plasma.**

ZAFIRLUKAST

Accolate
Antiasthmatic, leukotriene receptor antagonist

No   3   B

Tabs: 10, 20 mg

Asthma:
Children 5–11 yr: 10 mg PO BID
Children ≥12 yr and adults: 20 mg PO BID

Use with **caution** in hepatic insufficiency; **50%–60% reduction in clearance occurs in alcoholic cirrhosis.** May cause headache, dizziness, nausea, diarrhea, abdominal pain, vomiting, generalized pain, asthenia, myalgia, fever, LFT elevation, and dyspepsia. Eosinophilia, vasculitic rash, worsening pulmonary symptoms, cardiac complications, and/or neuropathy have been reported primarily in patients with oral steroid dose reduction. Hepatitis, hyperbilirubinemia, and hypersensitivity reactions (e.g., urticaria, angioedema, and rashes) have also been reported.

Drug is a substrate for CYP 450 2C9 and inhibits CYP 450 2C9 and 3A3/4 isoenzymes. Erythromycin, terfenadine, and theophylline decrease zafirlukast levels,

Continued

ZAFIRLUKAST *continued*

whereas aspirin increases levels. Zafirlukast may increase the effects of warfarin. Administer doses on an empty stomach, at least 1 hr prior or 2 hr after eating.

ZALCITABINE

Hivid, dideoxycytidine, ddC
Antiviral agent, nucleoside analogue reverse transcriptase inhibitor

Yes   3   C

Tabs: 0.375, 0.75 mg
Syrup (available only by compassionate use program via Roche Pharmaceuticals): 0.1 mg/mL

Children: 0.01 mg/kg/dose PO TID
Adolescents and adults: 0.75 mg PO TID

Use with **caution** in patients with liver disease, pancreatitis, or severe myelosuppression. Peripheral neuropathy, headaches, GI disturbances, and malaise are common side effects. Other side effects include bone marrow suppression, hepatitis, pancreatitis, hypertension, rash, oral and esophageal ulcers, myalgias, and fatigue. Lactic acidosis and severe hepatomegaly with steatosis, including fatal cases, have been reported.

Amphotericin, cimetidine, foscarnet, and aminoglycosides may reduce clearance and increase chances of peripheral neuropathy. In addition, drugs that cause peripheral neuropathy (e.g., ddI) should **not** be used in combination with ddC. Concurrent use of IV pentamidine can increase risk of pancreatitis.

Adolescent dosing: Patients in early puberty (Tanner I-II) should be dosed with pediatric regimens and those in late puberty (Tanner V) should be dosed with adult regimens. Adolescents who are at the midst of their growth spurt (Tanner III females and Tanner IV males) can be dosed by either pediatric or adult regimen with close monitoring of efficacy and toxicity.

Antacids can decrease absorption. **Reduce dose in renal dysfunction (see p. 946).** Administer doses on an empty stomach; 1 hr before or 2 hr after meals.

ZANAMIVIR

Relenza
Antiviral

No   ?   C

Powder for inhalation: 5 mg/inhalation (5 rotadisks [4 inhalations/rotadisk] with diskhaler)

Continued

Treatment of uncomplicated influenza (initiate therapy within 2 days of onset of symptoms):

  ≥7 yrs and adults:

  Day 1: 10 mg inhaled (as two 50-mg inhalations) BID (2–12 hr between the two doses) × 2 doses

  Day 2–5: 10 mg inhaled (as two 50-mg inhalations) Q12 hr × 4 days

Currently indicated for the treatment of influenza A and B strains. **Not recommended** for patients with underlying respiratory diseases (e.g., asthma) because bronchospasm may occur and efficacy could not be demonstrated. May cause nasal discomfort, cough, and throat/tonsil discomfort and pain. Allergic reactions involving oropharyngeal edema and serious skin rashes have been reported; discontinue therapy if this occurs.

See package insert for specific instructions for using the rotadisk/diskhaler system. If patient is concurrently using an inhaled bronchodilator, use the bronchodilator before taking zanamivir.

ZIDOVUDINE

Retrovir, AZT

Antiviral agent, nucleoside analogue reverse transcriptase inhibitor

Yes 3 C

Caps: 100 mg
Tabs: 300 mg
Liquid: 50 mg/5 mL
Inj: 10 mg/mL
In combination with lamivudine (3TC) as Combivir:
  Tabs: 300 mg zidovudine + 150 mg lamivudine
In combination with abacavir and lamivudine (3TC) as Trizivir:
  Tabs: 300 mg zidovudine + 300 mg abacavir + 150 mg lamivudine

See pp. 366–370 for indications. See also latest edition of AAP *Red Book.* Dosages may differ in separate protocols.

  Children 3 mo–12 yr:

PO: 160 mg/m^2/dose Q8 hr. Dose can range from 90–180 mg/m^2/dose Q6–8 hr.

  Intermittent IV: 120 mg/m^2/dose Q6 hr

  Continuous IV infusion: 20 mg/m^2/hr

≥12 yr and adults:

  PO: 200 mg/dose TID, or 300 mg/dose BID; **max. dose:** 600 mg/24 hr.

    Combivir: 1 tablet PO BID

    Trizivir (≥40 kg): 1 tablet PO BID

  IV: 1 mg/kg/dose Q4 hr

Continued

ZIDOVUDINE *continued*

Prevention of vertical transmission:
> *14–34 weeks of pregnancy:*
> > *Until labor:* 100 mg PO 5 × /24 hr or 600 mg/24 hr PO ÷ BID-TID
> > *During labor:* 2 mg/kg/dose IV over 1 hr followed by 1 mg/kg/hr IV infusion until umbilical cord is clamped.
>
> *Neonate:* 2 mg/kg/dose Q6 hr PO or 1.5 mg/kg/dose Q6 hr IV over 60 min. Begin within 12 hr of birth and continue until 6 weeks of age.
> *Premature infant (from ACTG 331 initiate therapy within 12 hr of birth and continue for 6 weeks):*
> > *<30 weeks gestation:* 2 mg/kg/dose PO Q12 hr or 1.5 mg/kg/dose IV Q12 hr for first 4 weeks of life, then reduce dosing interval to Q8 hr thereafter.
> > *≥30 weeks gestation:* 2 mg/kg/dose PO Q12 hr or 1.5 mg/kg/dose IV Q12 hr for first 2 weeks of life, then reduce dosing interval to Q8 hr thereafter. Dosage interval may be further reduced to Q6 hr when the child reaches full term (40 weeks postconceptional age [PCA]).

Needle-stick prophylaxis: 200 mg/dose PO TID or 300 mg/dose PO BID × 28 days. Use in combination with lamivudine 150 mg/dose PO BID, and indinavir 800 mg/dose PO TID × 28 days.

Use with **caution** in patients with impaired renal or hepatic function. Dosage reduction is recommended in severe renal impairment and may be necessary in hepatic dysfunction. Drug penetrates well into the CNS. Most common side effects include anemia, granulocytopenia, nausea, and headache (dosage reduction, erythropoietin, filgrastim/GCSF, or discontinuation may be required depending on event). Seizures, confusion, rash, myositis, myopathy (use >1 yr), hepatitis, and elevated liver enzymes have been reported. Macrocytosis is noted after 4 weeks of therapy and can be used as an indicator of compliance. Lactic acidosis and severe hepatomegaly with steatosis, including fatal cases, have been reported.

Do not use in combination with stavudine because of poor antiretroviral effect. Effects of interacting drugs include increased toxicity (acyclovir, trimethoprim-sulfamethoxazole), increased hematological toxicity (ganciclovir, interferon-alpha, marrow suppressive drugs), and granulocytopenia (drugs that affect glucuronidation). Methadone, atovaquone, cimetidine, valproic acid, probenecid, and fluconazole may increase levels of zidovudine, whereas rifampin, rifabutin, and clarithromycin may decrease levels.

Some NIH Pediatric HIV Working Group participants use 180 mg/m^2/dose Q12 hr PO when using other antiretroviral combinations in children 3 mo–12 yr (data are limited).

Adolescent dosing: Patients in early puberty (Tanner I-II) should be dosed with pediatric regimens and those in late puberty (Tanner V) should be dosed with adult regimens. Adolescents who are at the midst of their growth spurt (Tanner III females and Tanner IV males) can be dosed by either pediatric or adult regimen with close monitoring of efficacy and toxicity.

Do not administer IM. IV form is incompatible with blood product infusions and should be infused over 1 hr (intermittent IV dosing). Despite manufacturer recommendations of administering oral doses 30 min prior to or 1 hr after meals, doses may be administered with food.

ZILEUTON

Zyflo

Antiasthmatic, 5-lipoxygenase inhibitor

No   ?   C

Tabs: 600 mg

Asthma:
Children ≥12 yr and adults: 600 mg PO QID (with meals and at bedtime)

Contraindicated in active liver disease or transaminase elevations ≥3 times the upper limit of normal. Major adverse effects include headache, dyspepsia, nausea, abdominal pain, and elevated transaminase levels. Fatigue, dizziness, insomnia, paresthesia, and rash have also been reported.

Zileuton is a substrate for CYP 450 1A2, 2C9, and 3A3/4 isoenzymes and inhbits CYP 450 1A2 and 3A3/4. May increase the effects and/or toxicity of alprazolam, astemizole **(contraindicated),** clozapine, digoxin, propranolol, terfenadine **(contraindicated),** theophylline, and warfarin. Doses may be administered with or without food.

ZINC SALTS

Trace mineral

No   ?   C

Tabs as sulfate (OTC), 23% elemental: 66, 110, 200 mg
Caps as sulfate, 23% elemental: 220 mg
Tabs as gluconate, 14.3% elemental (OTC): 10, 15, 50 mg
Liquid as sulfate: 2.27 mg elemental Zn/mL
Inj as sulfate: 1 mg, 5 mg elemental Zn/mL; may contain benzyl alcohol
Inj as chloride: 1 mg elemental Zn/mL

Zinc deficiency:
Infants and children: 0.5–1 mg elemental Zn/kg/24 hr PO ÷ QD-TID.
    Adults: 25-50 mg elemental Zn/dose (100–220 mg Zn sulfate/dose) PO TID
US RDA: See p. 462.
For supplementation in parenteral nutrition, see p. 502.

Nausea, vomiting, GI disturbances, leukopenia, and diaphoresis may occur. Gastric ulcers, hypotension, and tachycardia may occur at high doses. Patients with excessive losses (burns) or impaired absorption require higher doses.
Therapeutic levels: 70–130 mcg/dL. May decrease the absorption of penicillamine, tetracycline, and fluoroquinolones (e.g., ciprofloxacin). Drugs that increase gastric pH (e.g., H_2 antagonists and proton pump inhibitors) can reduce the absorption of zinc.

Approximately 20%–30% of oral dose is absorbed. Oral doses may be administered with food if GI upset occurs.

BIBLIOGRAPHY

1. Package inserts of medications.
2. Committee on Drugs. The transfer of drugs and other chemicals into human milk. Pediatrics 2001; 108(3):776-789.
3. Briggs GG, Freeman RK, Yaffe SJ. A reference guide to fetal and neonatal risk: drugs in pregnancy and lactation, 5th ed. Baltimore, Md: Williams & Wilkins; 1998.
4. Pickering LK et al. 2000 Red Book: Report of the Committee on Infectious Diseases, 25th ed. Elk Grove Village, Ill: American Academy of Pediatrics; 2000.
5. Gilbert DN, Moellering RE, Sande MA. The Sanford guide to antimicrobial therapy, 31st ed. Vienna, Va: Antimicrobial Therapy, Inc; 2001.
6. Nelson JD, Bradley, JS. 2000-2001 Nelson's pocket book of pediatric antimicrobial therapy, 14th ed. Philadelphia: Lippincott, Williams & Wilkins; 2000.
7. Bartlett JG, Gallant JE. 2001-2002 medical management of HIV infection. Timonium, Md: H & N Printing & Graphics; 2001.
8. Young TE, Mangum OB. Neofax: a manual of drugs used in neonatal care, 14th ed. Raleigh, NC: Acorn Publishing; 2001.
9. McEvoy GK et al. AHFS 2001 drug information. Bethesda, Md: American Society of Health-System Pharmacists; 2001.
10. Facts and Comparisons: E Facts, online drug information service, www.efacts.com, Philadelphia: JB Lippincott.
11. Micromedex Inc. Micromedex healthcare series, vol 111, expires 3/2002.
12. Takemoto CK, Hodding JH, Kraus DM. Pediatric dosage handbook, 8th ed. Hudson, Ohio: Lexi-Comp Inc; 2001.
13. Ellsworth AJ et al. 2001-2002 Mosby's medical drug reference. St. Louis: Mosby; 2001.
14. National Library of Medicine. The HIV/AIDS treatment information service (ATIS). www.hivatis.org.
15. National Institutes of Health: National Heart, Lung and Blood Institute–Expert Panel Report 2. Clinical practice guidelines: guidelines for the diagnosis and management of asthma. NIH Pub. No. 97-4051; April 1997.
16. Hazinski MF, Cummins RO, Field JM. 2000 handbook of emergency cardiovascular care for healthcare providers. American Heart Association; 2000.
17. Monagle P et al. Antithrombotic therapy in children: sixth ACCP Consensus Conference on Antithrombotic Therapy. Chest 2001; 119:344-370S.
18. American Thoracic Society. Targeted tuberculin testing and treatment of latent tuberculosis infection. Am J Respir Crit Care Med 2000; 161:1376-1395.
19. Burg FD et al. Gellis & Kagan's current pediatric therapy. 16th ed. Philadelphia: WB Saunders; 1999.
20. Prescribing reference for pediatricians, vol 12. New York: Prescribing Reference Inc; 2001.
21. Food and Drug Administration: Safety Information and Adverse Event Reporting Program. http://www.fda.gov/medwatch/.

26

DRUG DOSES

ANALGESIA AND SEDATION

Javier Tejedor-Sojo, MD

I. ASSESSMENT OF PAIN

A. INFANT[1]

1. **Physiologic response:** Seen primarily in early onset of acute pain; subsides with continuing or chronic pain. Increases in blood pressure, heart rate, and respiratory rate; oxygen desaturation; crying; diaphoresis; flushing; pallor.
2. **Behavioral response:** Observe characteristics and duration of cry, facial expressions, visual tracking, body movements, and response to stimuli.

B. PRESCHOOLER

In addition to physiologic and behavioral responses, use the "FACES" pain rating scale to assess the intensity of the pain (Fig. 27-1).

C. SCHOOL-AGE AND ADOLESCENT

Evaluate physiologic and behavioral responses, and ask about description, location, and character of pain. Use a pain rating scale in which 0 is no pain and 10 is the worst pain ever experienced by the patient.

II. ANALGESICS[2,3]

A. NONNARCOTIC ANALGESICS

Nonnarcotic analgesics are commonly used in the management of mild to moderate pain of nonvisceral origin. They can be administered alone or in combination with opiates (Table 27-1).

1. **Acetaminophen:** Weak analgesic with antipyretic activity.
2. **Nonsteroidal antiinflammatory drugs (NSAIDs):** Especially useful for sickle cell, bony, rheumatic, and inflammatory pain. Recommend H_2-receptor blocker, or switching to cyclooxygenase-2 inhibitor (COX-2) for prolonged use.

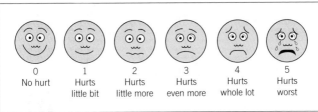

FIG. 27-1

FACES pain rating scale. *(From Wong DL. Whaley and Wong's essentials of pediatric nursing, 5th ed. St Louis: Mosby, 1995.)*

TABLE 27-1
NONNARCOTIC ANALGESICS

Drug	Dose	Route	Interval	GI Irritation	Platelet Inhibition
Acetaminophen*	10-15 mg/kg/dose, max. 75 mg/kg/day, adult dose 325-650 mg/dose, max. 4 g/day	PO/PR	Q4-6hr	No	No
Aspirin†	10-15 mg/kg/dose, max. 4 g/day	PO/PR	Q4hr	Yes	Yes
Celecoxib‡	100-200 mg/day (adults)	PO	Q12-24hr	Yes	Yes
Choline MG trisalicylate†	7.5-15 mg/kg/dose, adult dose 500 mg-1.5 g (dose based on salicylate content)	PO	Q6-8hr (pediatric) Q8-24hr (adult)	Yes	No
Ibuprofen	5-10 mg/kg/dose, max. 40 mg/kg/day, adult dose 200-800 mg/dose, max. 3.2 g/day	PO	Q6-8hr	Yes	Yes
Ketorolac	0.5 mg/kg/dose, max. dose 30 mg Q6hr or 120 mg/day (max. 3-5 day use) Children >50 kg and adults: 10 mg/dose, max. dose 40 mg/day	IV/IM PO	Q6hr Q6hr	Yes Yes	Yes Yes
Naproxen	5-10 mg/kg/dose, adult dose 250-500 mg, max. 1250 mg/day	PO	Q8-12hr	Yes	Yes
Rofecoxib‡	12.5-50 mg/day (adults)	PO	Q24hr	Yes	Yes

Celecoxib information from Celecoxib for arthritis. The medical letter on drugs and therapeutics 1999; 41(1045):11-12.
PO, by mouth; PR, by rectum.
*Does not have antiinflammatory properties. Initial rectal dose: 25-40 mg/kg.
†Contraindicated in patients <16 years of age with varicella or influenza because there is an association with Reye syndrome. May be used for the treatment of rheumatic pain.
‡Dosing not studied in children.

B. OPIATES (Table 27-2)

C. LOCAL ANESTHETICS

Local anesthetics are used primarily to anesthetize areas for minor procedures. They are administered topically, subcutaneously, into peripheral nerves, or centrally (epidural/spinal).

1. **Injectable local anesthetics** (Table 27-3)

a. Infiltration of the skin at the site; used for painful procedures such as wound closure, blood drawing, intravenous (IV) line placement, or lumbar puncture. To reduce stinging from injection, alkalinize the anesthetic; add 1 mL (or 1 mEq) sodium bicarbonate to 9 mL lidocaine, or 1 mL sodium bicarbonate to 29 mL bupivacaine. To enhance efficacy and duration, use local anesthetics with epinephrine. Never use local anesthetics with epinephrine in areas supplied by end-arteries (e.g., pinna, digits, nasal tip, and penis).

b. Peripheral nerve blocks

   (1) *Digital nerve block:* Indicated in finger or toe laceration repair, setting a fracture, paronychia drainage, or nail removal.

   Technique: Cleanse the skin. Insert a 25-gauge needle at the metacarpophalangeal (MCP) junction on either side of the digit. Keep the needle perpendicular to the plane of the hand and foot and advance from the dorsal to palmar surface while injecting slowly. Use 1 to 3 mL of epinephrine-free anesthetic. This block should not be performed if there is uncertainty regarding the blood supply to the digit (Fig. 27-2).

   (2) *Penile nerve block:* Indicated in circumcision, meatotomy, and hypospadias repair.

   Technique: Cleanse the skin. The nondominant hand holds the penis forward and down. A 25-gauge needle is inserted at the 11 and 1 o'clock positions at the base of the penis. Inject 0.5 to 3 mL of epinephrine-free anesthetic in Buck's fascia, 3 to 5 mm below the surface of the skin (Fig. 27-3).

   (3) *Hematoma block:* Used for reduction of closed fractures.

   Technique: Provide systemic sedation, anxiolysis, and analgesia as indicated (see Section IV). Using sterile technique, aspirate fracture hematoma with 20- to 22-gauge needle and inject 1% lidocaine (epinephrine-free). After 5 to 10 minutes, reduce fracture.

2. **Topical local anesthetics**

a. EMLA (Eutectic Mixture of Local Anesthetics): Topical emulsion of lidocaine (2.5%) and prilocaine (2.5%) applied to intact skin to produce anesthesia. Applied, then covered with an occlusive dressing; onset of complete anesthesia in 60 to 90 minutes. Indicated for procedures in which intact skin is punctured, such as venipuncture, circumcision, lumbar puncture, and bone marrow aspiration. EMLA should not be used in patients with congenital/idiopathic methemoglobinemia or in infants <12 months of age receiving treatment with other methemoglobin-inducing agents.

TABLE 27-2
COMMONLY USED OPIATES

Drug	Equianalgesic Doses (mg/kg/dose)	Route	Onset (min)	Duration (hr)	Side Effects	Comments
Codeine	1.2	PO	30-60	3-4	Nausea/vomiting	Use with acetaminophen for synergy.
Fentanyl	0.001	IV	1-2	0.5-1	Bradycardia, chest wall rigidity with high boluses (>5 mcg/kg but can occur with low doses)	Levels of unbound drug are higher in newborns than older patients.
	0.001	Transdermal	12	2-3		
	0.01	Transmucosal	15			
Hydromorphone	0.015	IV/SC	5-10 (IV)	3-4	May cause nausea, sedation, pruritus	Less sedation, nausea, pruritus than morphine.
	0.02-0.1	PO	30-60			
Meperidine	1.0	IV	5-10	3-4	Tachycardia, catastrophic interaction with MAO inhibitors, metabolite can cause seizures, can induce asthma attacks (from Na bisulfite)	Euphoric effects are greater than with morphine. Low doses stop shivering (0.1-0.25 mg/kg)
	1.5-2.0	PO	30-60	2-4		
Methadone*	0.1	IV	5-10	4-24	Nausea, sedation	Intial dose may produce analgesia for 3-4 hr; duration of action is increased with repeated dosing.
	0.1	PO	30-60	4-24		
Morphine	0.1	IV	5-10	3-4	Nausea, sedation, pruritus, constipation, seizures in neonates	Available in sustained release form for chronic pain.
	0.1-0.2	IM/SC	10-30	4-5		
	0.3-0.5	PO	30-60	4-5		
Oxycodone	0.1	PO	30-60	3-4	May contain Na metabisulfite, which can precipitate anaphylaxis	Much less nauseating than codeine. Available in sustained release form for chronic pain.

From Yaster M et al. Pediatric pain management and sedation handbook. St. Louis: Mosby; 1997.
*When converting to methadone as part of an opioid taper, give 30% of the total converted dose initially and assess the need for a higher dose at subsequent intervals.

ANALGESIA AND SEDATION 27

TABLE 27-3
COMMONLY USED INJECTABLE LOCAL ANESTHETICS*

Agent	Concentration (%)	Max Dose without Epinephrine (mg/kg)	Max Dose with Epinephrine (mg/kg)	Onset (min)	Duration Alone (hr)	Duration with Epinephrine (hr)
Lidocaine	0.5-2	5	7	3	0.5-2	1-3
Bupivacaine	0.25	2.5	3	15	2-4	4-8

Modified from St. Germaine Brent A. Pediatr Clin North Am 2000; 47(3):651-679 and Yaster M et al. Pediatric pain management and sedation handbook. St. Louis: Mosby; 1997.
*1% concentration of any local anesthetic = 10 mg/ml.

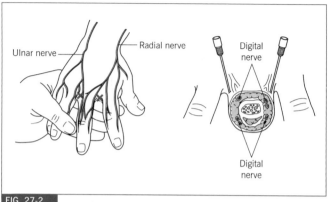

FIG. 27-2

Digital nerve block. *(From Yaster M et al. Pediatric pain management and sedation handbook. St Louis: Mosby; 1997.)*

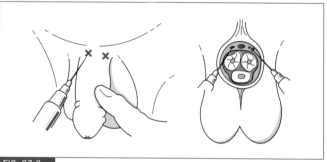

FIG. 27-3

Penile nerve block. *(From Yaster M, Maxwell LG. Pediatric regional anesthesia. Anesthesiology 1989; 70:324-338.)*

b. Viscous lidocaine: Often combined with diphenhydramine and Maalox for mucosal analgesia (mucositis, stomatitis). Not recommended in young children who cannot expectorate. Systemic toxicity can occur with mucosal absorption. Maximum dose is 3 mg/kg/dose every 2 hours as needed.

c. Lidocaine jelly: Useful for decreasing pain with nasogastric tube placement or urethral catheterization.

d. LET (Lidocaine, Epinephrine, Tetracaine): Provides topical local anesthesia for dermal lacerations. It is applied to an open wound either

TABLE 27-4

ORDERS FOR PCA

Drug	Basal Rate (mcg/kg/hr)	Bolus Dose (mcg/kg)	Lockout Period (min)	Boluses/hr	Max. Dose/hr (mcg/kg)
Morphine	10-30	10-30	6-10	4-6	100-150
Hydromorphone	3-5	3-5	6-10	4-6	15-20
Fentanyl	0.5-1	0.5-1	6-10	2-3	2-4

Modified from Yaster M et al. Pediatric pain management and sedation handbook. St. Louis: Mosby; 1997.

27

ANALGESIA AND SEDATION

in a gel or liquid form. 1 to 3 mL is applied with a cotton-tipped applicator/cotton ball and held in place for 20 to 30 minutes. Contraindicated in areas supplied by end-arteries (e.g., pinna, nose, penis, and digits). Maximum dose for topical lidocaine is 3 mg/kg/dose.[2]

e. TAC (Tetracaine, Adrenaline [epinephrine], Cocaine): 1 to 3 mL provides topical local anesthesia for dermal lacerations; applied to open wound in either a gel or liquid form. A few drops are applied directly to the wound, and the remainder of the 3 mL is applied by cotton-tipped applicator/cotton ball and held in place with firm pressure for 10 minutes. Contraindicated in areas supplied by end-arteries, on mucous membranes, on areas adjacent to mucous membranes, and in patients taking monoamine oxidase (MAO) inhibitors. Reapplication is contraindicated because of risk of toxicity. Seizures have been reported even with appropriate dosing. Maximum dose for cocaine is 3 mg/kg.

III. PATIENT-CONTROLLED ANALGESIA (PCA)

A. DEFINITION

PCA is a device that enables a patient to self-administer small doses of analgesics. A family member, caregiver, or nurse may administer doses also, especially in young children.

B. INDICATIONS

Acute/chronic pain secondary to sickle cell disease, surgery, burns, trauma, and cancer. Also for preemptive pain management (e.g., to facilitate dressing changes).

C. ROUTES OF ADMINISTRATION

IV, subcutaneous (SC), or epidural/spinal.

D. AGENTS (Table 27-4)

IV. SEDATION[2,4,5]

A. DEFINITIONS

1. **Moderate sedation:** Controlled state of depressed consciousness during which the child retains airway reflexes and a patent airway, responds to age-appropriate commands, and tolerates a noxious procedure.

2. **Deep sedation:** Controlled state of depressed consciousness during which airway reflexes and a patent airway may not be retained and the child is unable to respond to physical or verbal stimuli. Moderate sedation can easily progress to deep sedation, and most procedures performed on children under 5 years of age require deep sedation.

B. PRINCIPLES

Principles for providing sedation include the following:

1. Safety.
2. Minimize pain and discomfort, produce amnesia, control behavior, and immobilize.
3. Ensure rapid return of consciousness and airway control.
4. Ability to rescue patient because complications can easily occur.

C. PREPARATION

1. **Patient must be NPO for solids and clear liquids.** Classification of breast milk as a clear liquid versus solid remains controversial (Table 27-5).
2. Obtain written informed consent.
3. Obtain a focused patient history regarding asthma, apnea, organ dysfunction (cardiac, renal, liver), prematurity, co-morbidities, and adverse reactions to sedatives/anesthesia. Physical examination with specific attention to HEENT, lungs, and cardiac examination. If risk of conscious sedation is too high, consider obtaining an anesthesia consultation, or perform the procedure in the operating room under general anesthesia.
4. **Have an emergency plan ready.** Make sure qualified back-up personnel are close by.
5. Intravenous access.
6. Airway equipment:
   a. Suction.
   b. Oxygen.
   c. Airway equipment: Oral/nasal airway, laryngoscope and appropriate-sized blades, appropriate-sized endotracheal tubes (ETT) with stylet, tape, bag-valve with appropriate-sized mask.
   d. Pharmacy.
      (1) Intubation medications: Atropine, anesthetic, sedative/hypnotic, paralytic

TABLE 27-5		
FASTING RECOMMENDATIONS (HOURS)		
Age	Milk/Solids	Clear Liquids
<6 mo	4	2
6-36 mo	6	2-3
>36 mo	6-8	2-3

From Yaster M et al. Pediatric pain management and sedation handbook. St Louis: Mosby; 1997.

    (2) Emergency medications: Epinephrine, atropine, lidocaine, glucose.

    (3) Reversal agents: Naloxone, flumazenil.

D. MONITORING

1. **Baseline vital signs (including pulse oximetry) should be obtained initially; heart rate and oxygen saturation should be monitored continuously.** Blood pressure and respiratory rate should be monitored intermittently. Vital signs should be recorded at 5-minute intervals.

2. **Airway:** Airway patency and adequacy of ventilation through capnography, auscultation, or direct visualization should be assessed frequently.

E. PHARMACOLOGIC AGENTS (Table 27-6)

Central nervous system (CNS), cardiovascular, and respiratory depression are potentiated by combining sedative drugs and/or opioids and by rapid drug infusion. Titrate to effect (Fig. 27-4).

1. **Benzodiazepines:** Table 27-7.

2. **Opiates:** See Table 27-2.

3. **Barbiturates:** Table 27-8.

4. **Ketamine:** A nonbarbiturate that causes potent dissociative anesthesia and analgesia. An antisialagogue such as atropine or glycopyrrolate can be given concomitantly to counteract the increased mucous/salivary gland secretory effects of ketamine. A benzodiazepine may also be given with ketamine to ameliorate the hallucinogenic effects of the latter; however, there is also evidence that disputes the benefits of benzodiazepines in preventing emergence phenomena after ketamine administration (Table 27-9).

5. **Sedating antihistamines (diphenhydramine, hydroxyzine):** Mild sedative hypnotics used for preprocedure sedation and treatment of opiate-induced pruritus. See Formulary for dosing.

6. Reversal agents

a. Naloxone: Opioid antagonist.

    (1) Indications: Opioid overdose, respiratory depression, newborn with acute maternal opiate exposure **(Caution: can precipitate withdrawal),** pruritus, urinary retention, biliary spasm.

    (2) See Formulary for dosing. In the nonarrest situation, use the lowest effective dose (start at 0.001 mg/kg) to reverse respiratory depression and not analgesia.[5]

    (3) Onset and duration: Onset 1 to 2 minutes when administered IV, 2 to 5 minutes by other routes. Duration is 45 minutes, which may be shorter than the duration of action of the opiate. Patients may require repeated doses. Monitor for the return of respiratory depression.

b. Flumazenil: Benzodiazepine antagonist.

    (1) See Formulary for dosing.

    (2) Onset and duration: Onset is usually within 1 to 3 minutes. Duration

27

ANALGESIA AND SEDATION

TABLE 27-6

PROPERTIES OF COMMON SEDATIVE AGENTS

	Anxiolysis	Analgesia	Sedation/Hypnosis	Reversible	Indications/Comments
Benzodiazepines (see Table 27-7)	Yes	No	Yes	Yes	Amnesia/anxiolysis for nonpainful procedures May use in combination with opiates/ketamine for painful procedures
Opiates (see Table 27-2)	No	Yes	Yes	Yes	Sedation/analgesia for painful procedures
Ketamine (see Table 27-9)	Yes	Yes	Yes	No	Dissociative anesthesia/analgesia for painful procedures (fractures, bone marrow aspiration) Administer benzodiazepine + antisialagogue (atropine or glycopyrrolate) concomitantly
Barbiturates (see Table 27-8)	No	No	Yes	No	Immobility for nonpainful procedures (CT, MRI) Titrate IV dosage slowly to effect
Chloral Hydrate*	No	No	Yes	No	Fails to provide adequate immobility 30%-40% of time Avoid in pre-term and term infants

*The high rate of failure of chloral hydrate combined with its adverse effects increase the risk/benefit profile of this agent. It is our recommendation to consider alternative sedatives whenever possible. See Formulary for dosing recommendations.

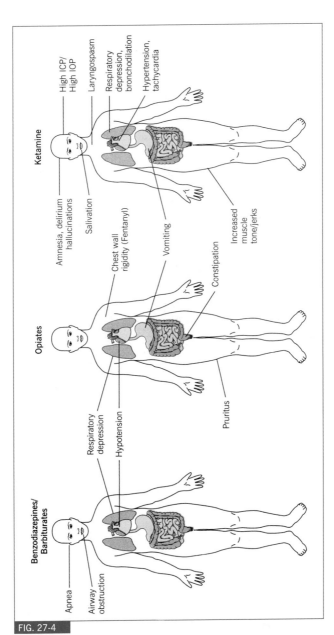

FIG. 27-4

Common side effects of sedatives/analgesics.

27

ANALGESIA AND SEDATION

TABLE 27-7
COMMONLY USED BENZODIAZEPINES*

Action	Drug	Routes	Onset (min)	Dose (mg/kg/dose)	Duration (hr)
Short	Midazolam (Versed)	IV/IM/PO/PR/IN	IV 1-3	IV 0.05-0.1 titrated to effect (max. dose 0.4 mg/kg)	1-2
			IM 5-10	IM 0.1-0.2 (max. dose 10 mg)	1-2
			PO[a] 10-30	PO 0.5 (max. dose 20 mg)	1-2
			PR[a] 10	PR 0.5 (max. dose 20 mg)	1-2
			IN[a] 5-10	IN 0.2-0.5 (max. dose 7.5 mg)	1-2
Medium	Diazepam (Valium)	IV/PO/PR	IV 1-3	IV 0.05-0.2	0.25-1
			PO 30-60	PO 0.2-0.5	2-3
			PR 7-15	PR 0.2-0.5	2-3
Long	Lorazepam (Ativan)	IV/IM/PO/PR	IV 1-5	IV 0.05 (max. single dose 2 mg)	3-4
			IM 10-20	IM 0.05 (max. single dose 4 mg)	3-6
			PO 30-60	PO 0.05 (max. single dose 4 mg)	3-6

From Yaster M et al. Pediatric pain management and sedation handbook. St. Louis: Mosby; 1997 and St. Germaine Brent A. Pediatr Clin North Am 2000; 47(3):651-679.
IN, intranasal; *PR*, rectal.
*Use IV solution for PO, PR, and IN administration. Rectal diazepam gel (Diastat) is available.

TABLE 27-8

PHARMACOKINETICS OF COMMON BARBITURATES

Drug	Route	Onset (min)	Duration (hr)	Dose
Methohexital	PR	5-10	1-1.5	Initial dose: 20-30 mg/kg Max. dose: 1 g
Pentobarbital	IV	1-10	1-4	Initial dose: 1-3 mg/kg Titrate to max. dose of 6 mg/kg or 150-200 mg
	IM	5-15	2-4	Initial dose: 2-6 mg/kg Max. dose: 6 mg/kg or 150 mg
	PO/PR	15-60	2-4	Initial dose: 2-6 mg/kg Max. dose: 6 mg/kg or 200 mg PO, 150 mg (PR)
Thiopental	PR	5-10	1-1.5	Initial dose: 20-30 mg/kg Max. dose: 1 g

Modified from Yaster M et al. Pediatric pain management and sedation handbook. St. Louis: Mosby; 1997 and St. Germaine Brent A. Pediatr Clin North Am 2000; 47(3):651-679 and Cote CJ et al. A practice of anesthesia for infants and children. Philadelphia: WB Saunders; 2001.

is 45 to 60 minutes, which may be shorter than the duration of benzodiazepine. Monitor for the return of respiratory depression for at least 2 hours.

   (3) **Caution: May precipitate seizures, particularly in patients with an underlying seizure disorder, or in those with tricyclic antidepressant overdose.**
F. **EXAMPLES OF SEDATION PROTOCOLS** (Table 27-10)

V. OPIOID/SEDATIVE TAPERING[2]

1. Patients should receive a tapering schedule if they have received frequent opioid analgesics/sedatives for more than 5 to 10 days.
2. Convert all drugs that the patient is receiving to a single equianalgesic member of that group (Table 27-11).
3. Change drug dosing from continuous infusion to intermittent IV/oral (PO) bolus therapy around the clock.
4. Start weaning baseline dose by 10% to 20% of the *original daily dose* every 1 to 2 days (e.g., to start tapering from a morphine dose of 40 mg/day, decrease the daily dose by 4 to 8 mg every 1 to 2 days).
5. If not done previously, convert IV dosing to equivalent PO administration 1 to 2 days before discharge and continue titration as outlined above.

27

ANALGESIA AND SEDATION

TABLE 27-9

KETAMINE DOSING AND PHARMACOKINETICS*

Dose (mg/kg)	Onset (min)	Duration (min)	CNS Effects	Cardiovascular Effects	Respiratory Effects	Other Effects
SEDATION						
IM 2-3	5-15	30-90	Increased intracranial pressure Emergence delirium Potent hallucinogen	Increased heart rate, blood pressure, cardiac output, systemic and pulmonary vascular resistance (can reverse right to left shunt particularly during 'Tet' spells in patients with tetralogy of Fallot) Direct myocardial depressant	Apnea with rapid IV infusion Bronchodilation Increased secretions Laryngospasm and coughing secondary to increased secretions	Increased muscle tone, jerking movements Increased intraocular pressure Nausea and emesis
PO/PR 4-6	20-45	60-120+				

Modified from Yaster M et al. Pediatric pain management and sedation handbook. St. Louis: Mosby; 1997 and St. Germaine Brent A. Pediatr Clin North Am 2000; 47(3):651-679 and Cote CJ et al. A practice of anesthesia for infants and children. Philadelphia: WB Saunders; 2001.

*These effects apply regardless of the route of administration. The presence of vocalization does not represent failure. Similarly some movement can be seen with adequate analgesia/anesthesia. Nystagmus indicates likely therapeutic effect.

TABLE 27-10

EXAMPLES OF SEDATION PROTOCOLS

	Dosage	Comments
Midazolam +	0.1 mg/kg IV × 3 doses prn	High likelihood of respiratory depression
Fentanyl	1 mcg/kg IV × 3 doses prn	Infuse fentanyl no faster than at 3-minute intervals
Midazolam +	0.1 mg/kg IV × 3 doses prn	
Atropine +	0.01 mg/kg IV × 1 dose (min 0.1 mg/dose; max 0.4 mg/dose)	Give atropine and midazolam before administering ketamine
Ketamine	3 mg/kg IM × 1 dose or 4 mg/kg PO × 1 dose*	

NOTE:
1. Use airway opening maneuvers, verbal/physical stimuli, oxygen mask, positive pressure ventilation, and reversal agents as indicated if there is concern of oversedation.
2. Recovery after above sedation protocols varies but typically ranges from 60-120 minutes.
3. These examples reflect commonly used current protocols at the Johns Hopkins Children's Center; variations of the above are common at other institutions.

*Ketamine can be given IV but the risk of inducing general anesthesia is very high; this should only be used by providers highly skilled in airway management.

TABLE 27-11

RELATIVE POTENCIES AND EQUIVALENCE OF OPIOIDS

	IV Dose (mg/kg)	Equivalent PO Dose (mg/kg)	Ratio of Morphine Equivalence
Morphine	0.1	0.3-0.5	1
Fentanyl	0.001	0.001 (Transdermal) 0.01-0.015 (Transmucosal)	50-100
Hydromorphone	0.015	0.02-0.1	5-7
Meperidine	1	1.5-2	0.1
Methadone	0.1	0.1	0.25

From Yaster M et al. Pediatric pain management and sedation handbook. St Louis: Mosby; 1997.

27

ANALGESIA AND SEDATION

REFERENCES

1. Wong DL. Whaley and Wong's essentials of pediatric nursing, 5th ed. St Louis: Mosby, 1995.
2. Yaster M et al. Pediatric pain management and sedation handbook. St Louis: Mosby; 1997.
3. Yaster M, Maxwell LG. Pediatric regional anesthesia. Anesthesiology 1989; 70:324-338.
4. St. Germaine Brent A. The management of pain in the emergency department. Pediatr Clin North Am 2000; 47(3):651-679.
5. Cote CJ et al. A practice of anesthesia for infants and children. Philadelphia: WB Saunders, 2001.

FORMULARY ADJUNCT

Shalloo Sachdev, MD

I. TOPICAL CORTICOSTEROIDS

a. Table 28-1 provides a listing of topical steroids from the most potent (group I) to the least potent (group VII). Use intermediate- and low-potency steroids (groups IV-VII) for pediatric patients. Topical steroid use is contraindicated in the treatment of varicella.

b. Occlusive dressings (including waterproof diapers) increase systemic absorption of topical steroids and should not be used with high-potency preparations. Topical steroids should be used with caution in intertriginous areas and on the face.

c. Apply once or twice daily. Penetration of the skin is greatest with ointments, with decreasing effectiveness in gels, creams, and lotions. Prolonged use may result in cutaneous and systemic side effects.

d. A gram of topical cream or ointment should cover a 10×10 cm area. A 30- to 60-g tube will cover the entire body of an adult once.

28

II. COMMON INDICATIONS AND DOSES OF SYSTEMIC CORTICOSTEROIDS

A. ENDOCRINE[1]

1. Physiologic replacement

a. Cortisone acetate: PO: 24-36 mg/m^2/24hr ÷ Q8hr; IM/IV: 12-18 mg/m^2/dose QD.

b. Hydrocortisone: PO: 18-30 mg/m^2/24hr ÷ Q8hr; IM/IV: 9-12 mg/m^2/dose.

c. Prednisolone/prednisone: PO: 4-6 mg/m^2/24hr ÷ Q12hr.

d. Dexamethasone: PO/IM/IV: 0.5-0.75 mg/m^2/24hr ÷ Q6-12hr.

2. Stress dosing: Consider for patients on glucocorticoid therapy >1 month.

a. PO/IM: 2 to 4 times the physiologic replacement dose. Give preoperatively and postoperatively, with gradual decrease to a maintenance dose.

b. IV: Hydrocortisone sodium succinate (Solu-Cortef): 25-100 mg/m^2/24hr (give as a continuous infusion). If IV access is not available, administer 25 mg/m^2/dose IM Q8hr.

3. Adrenal insufficiency

a. Chronic: See "Physiologic replacement" above.

b. Acute

    (1) Fluids: Start hydration with 20 mL/kg D$_5$ NS, then 60 mL/kg D$_5$ NS administered over 24 hours.

    (2) Steroids: Hydrocortisone sodium succinate (Solu-Cortef) 50 mg/m^2 IV bolus, then begin continuous infusion over 24 hours as per "stress dosing" protocol above.

TABLE 28-1

TOPICAL STEROID POTENCY RANKING

Group	Brand	Generic Name	Sizes (in grams unless otherwise specified)
I (MOST POTENT)	Temovate cr, ot 0.05%	Clobetasol propionate	15, 30, 45
	Diprolene ot 0.05%, cr 0.05%	Betamethasone dipropionate	15, 45
	Diprolene AF		15, 45
	Psorcon ot 0.05%	Diflorasone diacetate	15, 30, 60
	Ultravate cr, ot 0.05%	Halobetasol dipropionate	15, 45
II	Cyclocort ot 0.1%	Amcinonide	15, 30, 60
	Diprosone ot 0.05%	Betamethasone dipropionate	15, 45
	Elocon ot 0.1%	Mometasone furoate	15, 45
	Florone ot 0.05%	Diflorasone diacetate	15, 30, 60
	Halog cr, ot, sl 0.1%	Halcinonide	15, 30, 60, 240 sl: 20, 60 mL
	Lidex cr, gl, ot, sl 0.05%	Fluocinonide	15, 30, 60, 120 sl: 20, 60 mL
	Maxiflor ot 0.05%	Diflorasone diacetate	15, 30, 60
	Maxivate cr, ot 0.05%	Betamethasone dipropionate	15, 45
	Topicort cr, ot 0.25%	Desoximetasone	15, 60, 120
	Topicort gl 0.05%		15, 60
III	Aristocort A ot 0.1%	Triamcinolone acetonide	15, 60
	Cyclocort cr, lt 0.1%	Amcinonide	15, 30, 60 lt: 20, 60 mL
	Diprosone cr 0.05%	Betamethasone dipropionate	15, 45
	Florone cr 0.05%	Diflorasone diacetate	15, 30, 60
	Lidex E cr 0.05%	Fluocinonide	15, 30, 60, 120
	Maxiflor cr 0.05%	Diflorasone diacetate	15, 30, 60
	Maxivate lt 0.05%	Betamethasone dipropionate	60 mL
	Valisone ot 0.1%	Betamethasone valerate	14, 45
IV	Aristocort ot 0.1%	Triamcinolone acetonide	15, 60, 240, 454
	Cordran ot 0.05%	Flurandrenolide	15, 30, 60, 225
	Elocon cr, lt 0.1%	Mometasone furoate	15, 45 lt: 30, 60 mL

From Ferndale Laboratories, Ferndale, MI.

cr, Cream; *gl,* gel; *lt,* lotion; *ot,* ointment; *sl,* solution.

NOTE: There are other topical steroid preparations containing dexamethasone, flumethasone, prednisolone, and methylprednisolone.

TABLE 28-1			

TOPICAL STEROID POTENCY RANKING—cont'd

Group	Brand	Generic Name	Sizes (in grams unless otherwise specified)
IV (cont'd)			
	Kenalog cr, ot 0.1%	Triamcinolone acetonide	15, 60, 80, 240
	Kenalog aerosol 0.2%	Triamcinolone acetonide	63
	Dermatop cr, ot 0.1%	Prednicarbate	15, 60
	Synalar ot 0.025%	Fluocinolone acetonide	15, 30, 60, 120, 425
	Topicort LP cr 0.05%	Desoximetasone	15, 60
V	Cordran cr 0.05%	Flurandrenolide	15, 30, 60, 225
	Kenalog lt 0.1%	Triamcinolone acetonide	15, 60 mL
	Kenalog ot 0.025%		15, 60, 80, 240
	Locoid cr, ot 0.1%	Hydrocortisone butyrate	15, 45
	Synalar cr 0.025%	Fluocinolone acetonide	15, 30, 60, 425
	Tridesilon ot 0.05%	Desonide	15, 60
	Valisone cr, lt 0.1%	Betamethasone valerate	15, 45, 110, 430 lt: 20, 60 mL
	Westcort cr, ot 0.2%	Hydrocortisone valerate	15, 45, 60 cr only: 120
VI	Aclovate cr, ot 0.05%	Alclometasone dipropionate	15, 45
	Aristocort cr 0.1%	Triamcinolone acetonide	15, 60, 240, 2520
	Kenalog cr, lt 0.025%	Triamcinolone acetonide	15, 60, 80, 240, 2520 lt: 60 mL
	Locoid sl 0.1%	Hydrocortisone butyrate	20, 60 mL
	Locorten cr 0.03%	Flumethasone pivalate	15, 60
	Synalar cr, sl 0.01%	Fluocinolone	15, 45, 60, 425 sl: 20, 60 mL
	Tridesilon cr 0.05%	Desonide	15, 60
VII (LEAST POTENT)	Hytone cr, ot, lt 1%	Hydrocortisone	cr, ot: 30 cr, lt: 120 mL
	Hytone cr, ot, lt 2.5%		cr, ot: 30 cr, lt: 60 mL

4. Congenital adrenal hyperplasia

a. Non-salt losing: See "Physiologic replacement" on p. 907.

b. Salt losing: Fludrocortisone acetate (Florinef): PO: Usually 0.1 mg/m^2/24 hours, with a range of 0.05-0.3 mg/24 hours in addition to physiologic glucocorticoid replacement. Dose is adjusted for blood pressure and plasma rennin activity.[1,2]

B. PULMONARY

1. Airway edema

a. Dexamethasone: PO/IV/IM: 0.5-2 mg/kg/24hr ÷ Q6hr. Begin 24 hours before extubation and continue for 4 to 6 doses after extubation.

b. Croup: Dexamethasone 0.6 mg/kg/dose IM/IV × 1. Dexamethasone 0.15 mg/kg PO may be used for outpatient therapy for mild croup.[3,4] Inhaled budesonide 2 mg Q12hr (maximum: four doses).[5]

2. Acute asthma

a. Prednisone/prednisolone
   (1) PO: 2 mg/kg/24hr ÷ Q12-24hr × 3 to 7 days.
   (2) Maximum dose: 80 mg/24hr.

b. Methylprednisolone
   (1) IV/IM: Load (optional) 2 mg/kg/dose × 1.
   (2) Maintenance: 2 mg/kg/24hr ÷ Q6-8hr.

c. Hydrocortisone
   (1) IV: Load (optional) 4-8 mg/kg/dose; maximum dose: 250 mg.
   (2) Maintenance: 8 mg/kg/24hr ÷ Q6hr.

C. MISCELLANEOUS

1. Antiemetic (chemotherapy induced): Dexamethasone

a. IV: Initial: 10 mg/m^2/dose (maximum dose: 20 mg).

b. Subsequent: 5 mg/m^2/dose Q6hr.

2. Cerebral edema: Dexamethasone

a. PO/IM/IV: Loading dose: 1-2mg/kg/dose × 1.

b. Maintenance: 1-1.5 mg/kg/24hr ÷ Q4-6hr (maximum dose: 16 mg/24 hours).

3. Spinal cord injury: Methylprednisolone

a. 30 mg/kg bolus dose over 15 minutes, followed 45 minutes later by a continuous infusion of 5.4 mg/kg/hr × 23 hours.[6,7] Should be administered within 8 hours of injury for efficacy.

b. Methylprednisolone does not appear to be of benefit in acute head injury.

4. Bacterial meningitis[8]

a. Indications
   (1) Dexamethasone is recommended for children >6 weeks old with Hib meningitis.
   (2) Dexamethasone could be considered for children >6 weeks old with pneumococcal meningitis, but this is still controversial.

b. Dose: Dexamethasone—0.15 mg/kg/dose IV Q6hr × 48 hours. Ideally given with or just before first parenteral antibiotic dose. Initiation >4 hours after parenteral antibiotics is unlikely to be effective. Do not delay antibiotic therapy because of steroid administration.

5. **Idiopathic thrombocytic purpura**[9]
a. Indications: Clinical bleeding.
b. Dose: Pulse steroid therapy with dexamethasone 20-25 mg/m^2 IV × 4 days.[9]

6. **Transfusion reactions:** Methylprednisolone
a. IV: 0.5-1 mg/kg before initiation of blood product transfusion in patients with known transfusion reaction.[10]
b. If hives and/or itching present during transfusion, curtail transfusion and administer methylprednisolone.

III. INHALED CORTICOSTEROIDS FOR AIRWAY INFLAMMATION
(Table 28-2)

28

FORMULARY ADJUNCT

TABLE 28-2
ESTIMATED COMPARATIVE DAILY DOSAGES FOR INHALED CORTICOSTEROIDS

Drug	Low Dose	Medium Dose	High Dose
CHILDREN			
Beclomethasone dipropionate	84-336 mcg	336-672 mcg	>672 mcg
42 mcg/puff	(2-8 puffs)	(8-16 puffs)	(>16 puffs)
84 mcg/puff	(1-4 puffs)	(4-8 puffs)	(>8 puffs)
Budesonide DPI:	100-200 mcg	200-400 mcg	>400 mcg
200 mcg/dose		(1-2 inhalations)	(>2 inhalations)
Respules:	0.25 mg	0.5 mg	1 mg
0.25 mg/2 mL, 0.5 mg/2 mL			
Flunisolide	500-750 mcg	1000-1250 mcg	>1250 mcg
250 mcg/puff	(2-3 puffs)	(4-5 puffs)	(>5 puffs)

From Expert Panel Report II. Guidelines for the diagnosis and management of asthma. National Institutes of Health Pub. No. 97-4051. Bethesda, Md: National Asthma Education and Prevention Program; 1997.

NOTE: The most important determinant of appropriate dosing is the clinician's judgment of the patient's response to therapy. The clinician must monitor the patient's response on several clinical parameters and adjust the dose accordingly. The stepwise approach to therapy emphasizes that once control of asthma is achieved, the dose of medication should be carefully titrated to the minimum dose required to maintain control, thus reducing the potential for adverse effect. The reference point for the range of doses in children is data on the safety of inhaled corticosteroids in children, which in general, suggest that the dose ranges are equivalent to those of beclomethasone dipropionate 200-400 mcg/day (low dose), 400-800 mcg/day (medium dose), and >800 mcg/day (high dose). Metered-dose inhaler (MDI) dosages are expressed as the activator dose (the amount of drug leaving the activator and delivered to the patient), which is the labeling required in the United States. Dry-powder inhaler (DPI) doses are expressed as the amount of drug in the inhaler after activation.

cont'd

TABLE 28-2

ESTIMATED COMPARATIVE DAILY DOSAGES FOR INHALED CORTICOSTEROIDS—cont'd

Drug	Low Dose	Medium Dose	High Dose
Fluticasone	88-176 mcg	176-440 mcg	>440 mcg
MDI:	(2-4 puffs)	(4-10 puffs)	—
44 mcg/puff			
110 mcg/puff	—	(2-4 puffs)	(>4 puffs)
220 mcg/puff	—	(1-2 puffs)	(>2 puffs)
DPI (Rotadisk):	(2-4 inhalations,	(2-4 inhalations,	(>4 inhalations,
50, 100, 250 mcg/	50 mcg)	100 mcg)	100 mcg)
dose			(>2 inhalations,
			250 mcg)
Triamcinolone acetonide	400-800 mcg	800-1200 mcg	>1200 mcg
100 mcg/puff	(4-8 puffs)	(8-12 puffs)	(>12 puffs)
ADULTS			
Beclomethasone	168-504 mcg	504-840 mcg	>840 mcg
dipropionate			
42 mcg/puff	(4-12 puffs)	(12-20 puffs)	(>20 puffs)
84 mcg/puff	(2-6 puffs)	(6-10 puffs)	(>10 puffs)
Budesonide	200-400 mcg	400-600 mcg	>600 mcg
DPI:	(1-2 inhalations)	(2-3 inhalations)	(>3 inhalations)
200 mcg/dose			
Respules:	0.25 mg	0.5 mg	1 mg
0.25 mg/2 mL,			
0.5 mg/2 mL			
Flunisolide	500-1000 mcg	1000-2000 mcg	>2000 mcg
250 mcg/puff	(2-4 puffs)	(4-8 puffs)	(>8 puffs)
Fluticasone	—	264-660 mcg	>660 mcg
MDI:	(2-6 puffs)	—	—
44 mcg/puff			
110 mcg/puff	(2 puffs)	(2-6 puffs)	(>6 puffs)
220 mcg/puff	—	—	(>3 puffs)
DPI (Rotadisk):	(2-6 inhalations,	(3-6 inhalations,	(>6 inhalations,
50, 100, 250 mcg/	50 mcg)	100 mcg)	100 mcg; or
dose			>2 inhala-
			tions, 250
			mcg)
Triamcinolone acetonide	400-1000 mcg	1000-2000 mcg	>2000 mcg
100 mcg/puff	(4-10 puffs)	(10-20 puffs)	(>20 puffs)

IV. DOSE EQUIVALENCE OF COMMONLY USED STEROIDS
(Table 28-3)

V. INSULIN (Table 28-4)

All preparations except Lantus are available as human, purified pork, pork/beef, and beef. The human and more purified preparations produce less subcutaneous atrophy and less insulin resistance. For the management of diabetic ketoacidosis, see p. 213.

TABLE 28-3
DOSE EQUIVALENCE OF COMMONLY USED STEROIDS*

Drug	Glucocorticoid Effect Equivalent to 100 mg Cortisol PO	Mineralocorticoid (mg): Na Retention Effect Equivalent to 0.1 mg Florinef†
Cortisone	125	20
Cortisol (hydrocortisone)	100	20
Prednisone	25	50
Prednisolone	20-25	50
Methylprednisolone	15-20	No effect
Triamcinolone	10-20	No effect
9α-Fluorocortisol	6.5	0.1
Dexamethasone	1.5-3.75	No effect

Modified from Kappy MS, Blizzard RM, Migeon CJ, editors. The Diagnosis and treatment of endocrine disorders in childhood and adolescence, 4th ed. Springfield, Ill: Charles C Thomas; 1994.
*The doses give approximately equivalent clinical effects. When using this table, select equipotent doses based on glucocorticoid or mineralocorticoid effect, because this is different for each drug.
†Total physiologic replacement for salt retention is usually 0.1 mg Florinef, regardless of size.

TABLE 28-4
PHARMACOKINETICS OF INSULINS

Insulin	Onset (hr)	Peak (hr)	Effective Duration (hr)	Maximum Duration (hr)
ANIMAL				
Regular	0.5-2	3-4	4-6	6-8
Semi-Lente	1-1.5	5-10	12-16	
NPH*	4-6	8-14	16-20	20-24
Lente	4-6	8-14	16-20	20-24
Ultralente	8-14	Minimal	24-36	24-36
HUMAN				
Lispro†	0.15-0.25	0.5-1.5	3	4
Regular	0.5-1	2-3	3-6	4-6
NPH*	2-4	4-10	10-16	14-18
Lente	3-4	4-12	12-18	16-20
OTHER				
Insulin glargine (Lantus)‡			24	24

Modified from American Diabetes Association. The diabetes desk professional edition: how to control and manage diabetes mellitus. The Association; 2001.
NOTE: All preparations are available as U-100 (100 U/mL) except for those that follow. Dilutions may be necessary to accurately deliver small doses.
U-500 (purified pork): 50 U regular/mL.
U-70/30 (human or purified pork): 70 U/mL NPH, 30 U/mL regular.
U-50/50 (human): 50 U/mL NPH, 50 U/mL regular.
*Human neutral protamine Hagedorn (NPH) may have a slightly decreased duration of action compared with pork-derived NPH. Therefore the dose conversion may not be 1:1.
†Give 15 minutes before a meal and use in conjunction with a longer-acting form of insulin.
‡rDNA origin. After injection into the subcutaneous tissue, the acidic solution is neutralized, leading to microprecipitates from which small amounts of insulin glargine are slowly released, resulting in relatively constant concentration over 24 hours without a pronounced peak. Usually given at bedtime. Cannot be mixed in a syringe with other insulins. From Micromedex, July 2001.

28

FORMULARY ADJUNCT

VI. PANCREATIC ENZYME SUPPLEMENTS (Table 28-5)

TABLE 28-5

PANCRELIPASE*

Product	Dosage Form	Lipase (USP) Units	Amylase (USP) Units	Protease (USP) Units
Cotazym	Capsule	8000	30,000	30,000
Cotazym-S	Capsule, enteric-coated sphere	5000	20,000	20,000
Creon 5	Capsule, delayed release with enteric-coated microsphere	5000	16,600	18,750
Creon 10	Same as Creon 5	10,000	33,200	37,500
Creon 20	Same as Creon 5	20,000	66,400	75,000
Pancrease	Capsule, delayed release	4500	20,000	25,000
Pancrease MT	Capsule, enteric-coated microtabs			
4		4000	12,000	12,000
10		10,000	30,000	30,000
16		16,000	48,000	48,000
20		20,000	56,000	44,000
Pancreacarb MS 8	Delayed-release capsule, enteric-coated, microsphere	8000	40,000	45,000
Ultrase	Capsule, enteric-coated, microsphere	4500	20,000	25,000
Ultrase MT	Capsule, enteric-coated minitab			
6		6000	19,500	19,500
12		12,000	39,000	39,000
18		18,000	58,500	58,500
20		20,000	65,000	65,000
Viokase	Powder 1/4 tsp = 0.7 g	16,800/0.7 g	70,000/0.7 g	70,000/0.7 g
	Tablet	8000	30,000	30,000
Zymase	Capsule	12,000	24,000	24,000

Modified from Taketomo CK, Hodding JH, Kraus DM. American Pharmaceutical Association pediatric dosage handbook. Hudson, Ohio: Lexi-Comp; 1998 and Solvay Pharmaceuticals, Inc. 1994; Fact and Comparisons: September, 1998; Scandipharm Product Information: July 1994 and May 1995.
*See Formulary for side effects associated with administration.

VII. COMMON INDUCERS AND INHIBITORS OF THE CYTOCHROME P450 SYSTEM (Table 28-6)

TABLE 28-6
INDUCERS AND INHIBITORS OF THE CYTOCHROME P450 SYSTEM

Isoenzyme	Substrate (drug metabolized by isoenzyme)	Inhibitors	Inducers
CYP1A2	Caffeine, tacrine, theophylline, lidocaine, R-warfarin	Cimetidine, ciprofloxacin, erythromycin, tacrine	Omeprazole, smoking, phenobarbital
CYP2B6	Cocaine, ifosphamide, cyclophosphamide	Chloramphenicol	Phenobarbital
CYP2C9/10	S-Warfarin, phenytoin, tolbutamide, diclofenac, piroxicam	Amiodarone, fluconazole, lovastatin	Rifampin, phenobarbital
CYP2C19	Diazepam, omeprazole, mephenytoin	Fluvoxamine, fluoxetine, omeprazole, felbamate	Rifampin, phenobarbital
CYP2D6	Codeine, haloperidol, dextromethorphan, tricyclic antidepressants, phenothiazines, metoprolol, propranolol (4-OH), venlafaxine, risperidone, encainide, paroxetine, sertraline	Quinidine, fluoxetine, sertraline, amiodarone, propoxyphene	None known
CYP2E1	Acetaminophen, alcohol	Disulfiram	Isoniazid, alcohol
CYP3A3/4	Nifedipine, verapamil, cyclosporine, carbamazepine, terfenadine, cisapride, astemizole, tacrolimus, midazolam, alfentanil, diazepam, loratadine, ifosphamide, cyclophosphamide, ritonavir, indinavir	Erythromycin, cimetidine, clarithromycin, fluvoxamine, fluoxetine, ketoconazole, itraconazole, grapefruit juice, metronidazole, ritonavir, indinavir, mibefradil	Rifampin, phenytoin, phenobarbital, carbamazepine

Modified from Hansten PD, Horn JR. Hansten and Horn's drug interaction analysis and management. Vancouver, BC, Canada: Applied Therapeutics; 1997.
CYP, Cytochrome P450.
Note: The cytochrome P450 enzyme system is composed of different isoenzymes. Each isoenzyme metabolizes a unique group of drugs or substrates. When an *inhibitor* of a particular isoenzyme is introduced, the serum concentration of any drug or *substrate* metabolized by that particular isoenzyme will *increase.* When an *inducer* of a particular isoenzyme is introduced, the serum concentration of drugs or *substrates* metabolized by that particular isoenzyme will *decrease.*

28

FORMULARY ADJUNCT

VIII. OPHTHALMIC DRUGS (Table 28-7)

TABLE 28-7

OPHTHALMIC DRUGS

Brand Name	Ingredient	Indication	Dose
Bleph-10 (> 2 mo) (Soln: 2.5 mL, 5 mL, 15 mL; Oint 3.5 g)	Sulfacetamide sodium 10% Oph soln contains benzalkonium chloride Oph oint contains phenylmercuric acetate	Conjunctivitis Oph soln used as adjunct in trachoma	1-2 gtt Q2-3hr or small amount of oint Q3-4hr for 7-10 days Trachoma: 2 gtt Q2hr with systemic therapy
Garamycin Oph Soln and Oint (Soln: 5 mL; Oint: 35 g)	Gentamicin as sulfate	Conjunctivitis	Severe infections: 2 gtt Q1hr. Mild-moderate infections: 1-2 gtt Q4hr, or oint: bid-tid
Ilotycin (Oint: ⅛ oz)	Erythromycin (5 mg/g)	Conjunctivitis Prophylaxis of ophthalmia neonatorum	Small amount of oint ≥qd 0.5-1 cm to each conjunctival sac
Neosporin (Oint: 3.75 g; Soln: 10 mL)	Oint (per g): Polymyxin B sulfate (10,000 units), bacitracin Zn (400 units), neomycin sulfate (3.5 mg) Soln (per mL): Polymyxin B sulfate (10,000 U), neomycin sulfate (1.75 mg), gramicidin (0.025 mg), 0.5% alcohol	Conjunctivitis	1-2 gtt or small amount of oint 2-4 times daily for 7-10 days For acute infections, use 1-2 gtt 2-4 times Q1hr initially
Ocuflox (>1 yr) (Soln: 5 mL, 10 mL)	Ofloxacin 0.3%, benzalkonium chloride	Conjunctivitis Corneal ulcer	1-2 gtt Q2-4hr × 2 days, then qid × 5 days 1-2 gtt Q30 min while awake; at 4 hr and 6 hr during sleep × 2 days; then 1-2 gtt Q1hr while awake for 5-7 days, then qid until treatment completion

Polysporin (Oint: 3.75 g)	Polymyxin B sulfate (10,000 U), bacitracin zinc (500 U) per g of oint	Conjunctivitis	Q3-4hr; do not use >7 days
Polytrim (> 2 mo) (Soln: 10 mL)	Trimethoprim sulfate (1 mg), polymyxin B sulfate (10,000 U/mL), benzalkonium chloride	Conjunctivitis	1 gtt Q3hr × 7-10 days
Tobrex (Soln: 5 mL; Oint: 3.5 g)	Soln: Tobramycin 0.3%, benzalkonium chloride Oint: Tobramycin 0.3%, chlorobutanol	Conjunctivitis	Severe infections: 2 gtt Q1hr or 0.5 inch of ointment Q3-4hr Mild-moderate infections: 1-2 gtt Q4hr or 0.5 inch of oint BID-TID
Vira-A (> 2 yr) (Oint; 3.5 g)	Vidarabine 3%	Acute keratoconjunctivitis, recurrent epithelial keratitis caused by HSV 1 and 2	0.5 inch in lower conjunctival sac five times daily (Q3hr); continue for 7 more days (BID) after re-epithelialization
Viroptic (> 6yr) (Soln: 7.5 mL)	Trifluridine 1%, contains thimerosal	Primary keratoconjunctivitis, recurrent epithelial keratitis caused by HSV 1 and 2	1 gtt Q2hr while awake (maximum 9 gtt/day) 1gtt Q4hr × 7days after re-epithelialization (maximum 21 days)
Alocril (≥ 3 yr) (Soln: 5 mL)	Nedocromil sodium 2% (mast cell stabilizer), benzalkonium chloride	Allergic conjunctivitis	1-2 gtt several times a day; remove contact lenses during therapy
Alomide (> 2 yr) (Soln: 10 mL)	Lodoxamide tromethamine 0.1% (mast cell stabilizer)	Vernal conjunctivitis and keratitis, keratoconjunctivitis	1-2 gtt QID up to 3 mo

From Prescribing reference for pediatricians. Spring-Summer 2001.

cont'd

28

FORMULARY ADJUNCT

TABLE 28-7

OPHTHALMIC DRUGS—cont'd

Brand Name	Ingredient	Indication	Dose
Corticosporin (Oph Susp: 7.5 mL; Oph oint: 3.5 g)	Susp (per mL): Polymyxin B sulfate (10,000 U), neomycin sulfate (0.35%), hydrocortisone (1%). Oint (per g): Polymyxin B sulfate (10,000 U), neomycin sulfate (0.35%), bacitracin zinc (400 U), hydrocortisone (1%)	Ocular inflammation associated with infection **Contraindicated in fungal, viral, or mycobacterial infection** Use with caution in glaucoma, corneal or scleral thinning	1-2 gtt or small amount of oint 3-4 times daily
Poly-Pred (Susp: 5 mL, 10 mL)	Susp (per mL): Prednisolone acetate (0.5%), neomycin sulfate (0.35%), polymyxin B sulfate (10,000 U)	Ocular inflammation associated with infection **Contraindicated in fungal, viral, or mycobacterial infections** Use with caution in glaucoma, corneal or scleral thinning	1-2 gtt Q3-4hr

From Prescribing reference for pediatricians. Spring-Summer 2001.

IX. OXIDIZING AGENTS AND GLUCOSE-6-PHOSPHATE DEHYDROGENASE (G6PD) DEFICIENCY (Box 28-1)

BOX 28-1

OXIDIZING AGENTS AND G6PD DEFICIENCY

p-Aminosalicylic acid
Acetaminophen (Phenacetin)*
Acetylsalicylic acid
Aniline dyes
Antipyrine
Ascorbic acid†
Chloramphenicol‡
Dapsone (diaminodiphenylsulfone)
Fava beans
Furazolidone (Furoxone)
Henna
Methylene blue*
Naphthalene*
Nitrofurantoin (Furadantin)
Primaquine
Probenecid
Salicylazosulfapyridine (Azulfidine)
Sulfacetamide (Sulamyd)
Sulfanilamide
Sulfisoxazole (Gantrisin)*
Sulfoxone*
Trisulfapyrimidine (Sultrin)
Vitamin K, water-soluble analogs only

NOTE: These drugs and chemicals may cause hemolysis of "reacting" (primaquine-sensitive) red blood cells (e.g., in patients with G6PD deficiency).
*Only slightly hemolytic to G6PD A patients in very large doses.
†Hemolytic in G6PD Mediterranean but not in G6PD A or Canton.
‡In massive doses.

X. HERBAL MEDICINES IN PEDIATRICS AND ADOLESCENCE (Table 28-8)

XI. PSYCHIATRY DRUG FORMULARY (Table 28-9)

XII. CHEMOTHERAPEUTIC AGENTS (Table 28-10)

28

FORMULARY ADJUNCT

TABLE 28-8

HERBAL MEDICINES IN PEDIATRICS AND ADOLESCENCE

Herb	Compound	Use	Evidence for Efficacy	Precautions and Adverse Reactions
Aloe	Anthraquinone	Constipation		Long-term use leads to electrolyte losses, especially potassium Should not be used in children <12
Blood root	Berberine	Antiplaque agent for gingivitis, antimicrobial, antiinflammatory	No proven evidence	Emetic effect in doses above 0.03 g
Chickweed	Saponin	Internally: Rheumatism, gout, stiffness of joints, tuberculosis Externally: inflammation of eyes, eczema	No proven evidence	No known health hazards
Colt's foot	Pyrrolizidine alkaloid	Cough, bronchitis, inflammation of mouth and pharynx	No proven evidence	May cause hepatotoxicity, carcinogenic/mutagenic effects when consumed internally
Comfrey	Pyrrolizidine alkaloid	Antiinflammatory, demulcent, hypotensive effects	Approved by Commission E for blunt injuries, bruises, sprains	May cause hepatotoxicity, carcinogenic/mutagenic effects when consumed internally
Fever few	Volatile oil	Migraine, arthritis, rheumatic diseases, allergies	Animal experiments show that fever few slows down platelet aggregation, prostaglandin synthesis, and histamine release	May interact with antithrombotic medications such as aspirin and warfarin

Golden seal	Berberine	Eye infections, chlamydia trachomatis, acute diarrhea	No proven evidence	Long-term use can lead to digestive disorders, constipation, excitatory states, hallucinations. High doses can lead to breathing difficulty, bradycardia, spasms, and central paralysis
Lily-of-the-Valley	Cardioactive steroid glycoside	Positive inotropic effect, for arrhythmia	Only older studies available	Nausea, vomiting, headache, stupor, cardiac arrhythmias. **Not to be used without consultation with a cardiologist**
Uva Ursi	Anthraquinone	Infections of the urinary tract	In vitro antimicrobial effect	Liver damage can occur with extended use. Overdosage can lead to inflammation and irritation of the bladder and urinary tract mucous membranes. Contraindicated in children <12
Witch hazel	Tannin	Hemorrhoids, inflammation of the skin, mouth and pharynx, wounds, burns		If taken internally can lead to digestive complaints

Modified from Physician's drug reference for herbal medicines, 2nd ed. Montvale, NJ: Medical Economics; 2000 and Gardiner P, Kemper KJ. Herbs in pediatric and adolescent medicine. Peds Rev 2000; 21(2):44-57.

This is not a comprehensive list. Please refer to Physician's drug reference for herbal medicines, 2nd ed. Montvale, NJ: Medical Economics; 2000, for more complete review.

28

FORMULARY ADJUNCT

TABLE 28-9

PSYCHIATRY DRUG FORMULARY

STIMULANTS (ADHD TREATMENT)

Agent	Suggested Dose	Kinetics	Side Effects/Comments
Methylphenidate (Ritalin) 5 mg, 10 mg, 20 mg tabs	Starting dose 5 mg bid (breakfast/lunch) or 0.3 mg/kg/dose Increase 2.5-5 mg Qwk as needed Max dose: 80 mg/day + BID-QID	Onset: Within 30 min Peak action: 1.9 hr Duration: 4-6 hr	Nervousness, insomnia, anorexia, unveiling of tics, stomach aches, headaches, dysphoria. Use with caution in children with seizure disorder. Contraindicated with MAOIs. Monitor height, weight, and blood pressure. Avoid caffeine and decongestants.
Methylphenidate Sustained Release (Ritalin SR) 20 mg tabs	Starting dose: 20 mg QD Max dose: 80 mg/day	Onset: 60-90 min Peak action: 4.7 hr Duration: 8 hr	Do not crush or chew tablets. See comments for methylphenidate.
Methylphenidate Extended Release (Concerta) 18 mg, 36 mg, 54 mg tabs Also available: (Metadate ER) 10, 20 mg tabs (Methylin ER) 10, 20 mg tabs	Starting dose: 18 mg QD Max dose: 54 mg/day	Peak action: 6-8 hr Duration: 12 hr	See comments for methylphenidate.

Dextroamphetamine Short-Acting (Dexedrine) 5 mg tabs	Starting dose 3-5 yr: 2.5 mg BID or 0.15 mg/kg/dose Adjust by 2.5-5 mg Qwk Starting dose ≥6 yr: 5 mg QD or BID Increase by 5 mg Qwk Max dose: 40 mg/day + QD–TID	Onset: 20-60 min Peak action: 2 hr Duration: 4-6 hr	See comments for methylphenidate.
Dextroamphetamine Long-Acting (Dexedrine Spansule) 5 mg, 10 mg, 15 mg capsules	Starting dose 5-8 yr: 10 mg QD Increase by 5 mg Qwk Max dose: 15 mg QD Starting dose ≥9 yr: 15 mg QD Increase by 5 mg Qwk Max dose: 30 mg QD	Onset: 60-90 min Peak action: 8-10 hr	See comments for methylphenidate.
Mixed Amphetamine Salts (Adderall) 5 mg, 10 mg, 20 mg, 30 mg tabs	Starting dose 3-5 yr: 2.5 mg Qam Increase by 2.5-5 mg Qwk Starting dose ≥6 yr: 5 mg QD Increase by 5 mg Qwk	Onset: Estimated at 30 min Duration: Estimated at 5-7 hr	See comments for methylphenidate.

From Physician's desk reference, 54th ed. Montvale, NJ: Medical Economics; 2000; Riddle MA et al. J Am Acad Child Adolesc Psychiatry. 1999; 38:546-556; Findling RL, Blumer JL, editors. Child and adolescent psychopharmacology. Pediatr Clin North Am. 1998; 45(5); Shoaf TL, Emslie GJ, Mayes TL. Pediatr Ann 2001; 30(3):130-171; Emslie GJ, Mayes TL, Hughes CW. Updates in the pharmacologic treatment of childhood depression. In: Dunner DL, Rosenbaum JF, editors. The Psychiatric Clinics of North America annual of drug therapy. Philadelphia: W.B. Saunders; 2000; 235-256; and Velosa JF, Riddle MA. Child Adolesc Psychiatr Clin N Am 2000; 9:119-133.

MAOIs, Monoamine oxidase inhibitors.

Note: Additional information for many of these drugs can be found in the Formulary.

Most of these drugs have not been FDA approved for pediatric use. They are listed here based on material presented in Findling RL, Blumer JL as a reference guide. It should be noted that most that have not undergone rigorous extensive safety or efficacy testing in the pediatric age group.

cont'd

28

FORMULARY ADJUNCT

TABLE 28-9

PSYCHIATRY DRUG FORMULARY—cont'd

Agent	Suggested Dose	Kinetics	Side Effects/Comments
NONPSYCHOSTIMULANTS (ADHD TREATMENT)			
Clonidine (Catapres)	Starting dose: 0.05 mg QID Titrate nightly dose by increments of 0.05 mg as needed to a maximum of 0.4 mg	Peak response: 2-4 hr	Dry mouth, dizziness, drowsiness, fatigue, constipation, arrhythmias, anorexia. Monitor ECG, blood pressure, heart rate. Slow taper because sudden withdrawal can cause rebound hypertension.
Guanfacine (Tenex)	Starting dose: 0.5 mg Qam, 3 pm, plus 1 mg QHS	Peak response: 1-4 hr	Monitor ECG, blood pressure, heart rate. See comments on clonidine.
ANTIPSYCHOTICS			
Clozapine (Clozaril)	Starting dose: 6.25 mg/day Titrate upward by 6.25 mg/wk in divided doses Max dose: Prepubescent: 300 mg/day Adolescent: 400 mg/day		Obtain baseline EEG. Repeat EEG prn for sudden behavioral deterioration. Monitor CBC. Because of potentially lethal hematologic changes, use is reserved for patients resistant to treatment.
Haloperidol (Haldol)	See Formulary		Obtain baseline ECG, HR, BP, LFTs. Check Q3 mo, with dose changes. In general, anticholinergic effects include orthostatic hypotension, sedation, weight gain, dystonic reactions; tardive dyskinesia, akathisia, neuroleptic malignant syndrome.

Olanzapine (Zyprexa)	Prepubescent: 2.5 mg QD Adolescent: 5 mg QD Increase Q3-4 days to maximum of 20 mg/day	See comments for haloperidol.
Risperidone (Risperdal)	Prepubescent: 2.5 mg QD Adolescent: 0.5 mg/day QD-BID Adult: 1 mg BID Increase Q wk 1mg BID as needed Max dose: 3 mg BID	Renal/hepatic dosing. See comments for haloperidol; hyperprolactinemia, amenorrhea, galactorrhea.
Quetiapine (Seroquel)	Prepubescent: 12.5-750 mg/day Adolescent: 25-750 mg/day Adults: 150-750 mg/day	See comments for haloperidol. Baseline and semiannual ophthalmologic examination recommended because cataracts occurred in drug studies in canines.
Ziprasidone	120 mg/day	Dyspepsia, constipation, nausea, abdominal pain. Low incidence of extrapyramidal side effects.
ANXIOLYTICS		
Buspirone (BuSpar) Please see SSRI and venlafaxine	Prepubescent: 2.5-5 mg/day Increase by 2.5 mg/day Q3-4 days Max dose: 20 mg/day ÷ Q12hr Adolescent: 5-10 mg/day Increase by 5 mg/day Q3-4 days Max dose: 60 mg/day ÷ Q12hr	Tachycardia, central nervous system (CNS) effects (headache, insomnia, confusion, dizziness); gastrointestinal (GI) effects.

From Physician's desk reference, 54th ed. Montvale, NJ: Medical Economics; 2000; Riddle MA et al. J Am Acad Child Adolesc Psychiatry, 1999; 38:546-556; Findling RL, Blumer JL, editors. Child and adolescent psychopharmacology. Pediatr Clin North Am. 1998; 45(5); Shoaf TL, Emslie GJ, Mayes TL. Pediatr Ann 2001; 30(3):130-171; Emslie GJ, Mayes TL, Hughes CW. Updates in the pharmacologic treatment of childhood depression. In: Dunner DL, Rosenbaum JF, editors. The Psychiatric Clinics of North America annual of drug therapy. Philadelphia: W.B. Saunders; 2000; 235-256; and Velosa JF, Riddle MA. Child Adolesc Psychiatr Clin N Am 2000; 9:119-133.

cont'd

28

FORMULARY ADJUNCT

TABLE 28-9

PSYCHIATRY DRUG FORMULARY—cont'd

Agent	Suggested Dose	Kinetics	Side Effects/Comments
MOOD STABILIZERS			
Lithium	See Formulary Therapeutic level: 0.6-1.5 mEq/L.		Obtain levels Qwk until stable. Check baseline renal, hepatic, thyroid panels, calcium, CBC, ECG.
Divalproex sodium (Depakote)	15 mg/kg/day ÷ bid-tid Max: 60 mg/kg Therapeutic level: 50-60 mEq/L		Obtain β-HCG, CBC, LFTs before therapy. LFT, CBC Q6 mo. Can cause pancreatitis, polycystic ovarian syndrome.
Carbamazepine (Tegretol)	See Formulary		Obtain CBC, LFTs, β-HCG before therapy.
ANTIDEPRESSANTS/ANXIOLYTICS			
Selective Serotonin Reuptake Inhibitors (SSRIs)			
Fluoxetine (Prozac)	Starting dose < 12 yr: 5-10 mg/day Maintenance: 10-30 mg/day Starting dose ≥12 yr: 10 mg/day Maintenance: 20-40 mg/day Max dose: 60 mg/day		Do not use if MAOIs have been used in previous 14 days. Can cause GI upset, CNS side effects (headaches, nervousness, sedation), activate bipolar switchbacks.
Fluvoxamine (Luvox)	Starting dose <12 yr: 25 mg QHS Maintenance: 100-200 mg/day Starting dose ≥12 yr: 25-50 mg QHS Maintenance: 150-300 mg/day		Contraindications: MAOIs, cisapride, terfenadine, astemizole. Smoking increases levels.
Paroxetine (Paxil)	Starting dose <12 yr: 5-10 mg/day Maintenance: 10-20 mg/day Starting dose ≥12 yr: 10-20 mg/day Maintenance: 20-40 mg/day		Purpura, hyponatremia, cytochrome p450 system (multiple drug interactions). Also see comments for fluoxetine.

Drug	Dose	Comments
Sertraline (Zoloft)	Starting dose <12 yr: 25 mg/day Maintenance: 100-150 mg/day Starting dose ≥12 yr: 25-50 mg/day Maintenance: 150-200 mg/day	See comments for fluoxetine.
Citalopram (Celexa)	<12 yr: 10-20 mg/day ≥12 yr: 10-40 mg/day	See comments for fluoxetine; multiple drug interactions.
Tricyclics (TCAs)		
Nortriptyline (Pamelor)	See Formulary	Obtain baseline CBC, LFTs, BP, ECG. Recheck with every dose increase and Q1mo × 6 mo. Check TCA level with each ECG. Side effects include anticholinergic effects (dry mouth, weight gain, sedation). Slow taper recommended.
Imipramine (Tofranil)	See Formulary	See comments for nortriptyline.
Desipramine (Norpramin)	Prepubescent: 1-3 mg/kg/day (QHS or + bid) Adolescent: 25-50 mg/day	Blood dyscrasia, GI side effects, photosensitivity, arrhythmias. See comments for nortriptyline. Does not cause weight gain. Therapeutic level: 150-250 mcg/mL.
Anafranil (Clomipramine)	>10 yr: With food, 25 mg/day Increase over 2 wk to 100 mg/day or 3 mg/kg/day in divided doses	Seizures, anticholinergic effect, nausea, anorexia, weight gain.

From Physician's desk reference, 54th ed. Montvale, NJ: Medical Economics; 2000; Riddle MA et al. J Am Acad Child Adolesc Psychiatry. 1999; 38:546-556; Findling RL, Blumer JL, editors. Child and adolescent psychopharmacology. Pediatr Clin North Am. 1998; 45(5); Shoaf TL, Emslie GJ, Mayes TL. Pediatr Ann 2001; 30(3):130-171; Emslie GJ, Mayes TL, Hughes CW. Updates in the pharmacologic treatment of childhood depression. In: Dunner DL, Rosenbaum JF, editors. The Psychiatric Clinics of North America annual of drug therapy. Philadelphia: W.B. Saunders; 2000; 235-256; and Velosa JF, Riddle MA. Child Adolesc Psychiatr Clin N Am 2000; 9:119-133.

cont'd

FORMULARY ADJUNCT **28**

TABLE 28-9

PSYCHIATRY DRUG FORMULARY—cont'd

Agent	Suggested Dose	Kinetics	Side Effects/Comments
ANTIDEPRESSANTS/ANXIOLYTICS—cont'd			
Serotonin Norepinephrine Reuptake Inhibitors			
Venlafaxine (Effexor)	Starting dose prepubescent: 37.5 mg/day Maintenance: 75-150 mg/day Starting dose adolescent: 37.5-75 mg/day Maintenance: 150-300 mg/day		Nausea, dizziness, somnolence, constipation, xerostomia.
5-HT Blockers			
Nefazodone (Serzone)	Start 50 mg bid. Titrate to effectiveness by 50 mg Q3 days Max dose Children: 300 mg/day >12 yr: 600 mg/day		Nausea, dizziness, priapism, agitation, dry mouth, vision changes. Contraindications: MAOIs, astemizole, cisapride, terfenadine.

Other		
Bupropion Sustained Release (Wellbutrin SR)	≥18 yr: 100 mg bid × 3 days If tolerated, increase by 100 mg TID (minimum Q6hr) Max dose: 450 mg/day, 150 mg/dose/hr	CNS stimulation, weight change, dry mouth, headache, GI effects, insomnia. Contraindications: seizures, eating disorders, MAOIs.
Mirtazapine (Remeron)	≥18 yr: Initially 15 mg QHS Increase Q1-2 wk	Obtain baseline CBC, LFTs, and monitor periodically. Side effects: Increased appetite, weight gain, dizziness, nausea dry mouth, constipation, CNS effects (somnolence), hypotension/hypertension, elevated triglycerides, cholesterol.

From Physician's desk reference, 54th ed. Montvale, NJ: Medical Economics; 2000; Riddle MA et al. J Am Acad Child Adolesc Psychiatry, 1999; 38:546-556; Findling RL, Blumer JL, editors. Child and adolescent psychopharmacology. Pediatr Clin North Am. 1998; 45(5); Shoaf TL, Emslie GJ, Mayes TL. Pediatr Ann 2001; 30(3):130-171; Emslie GJ, Mayes TL, Hughes CW. Updates in the pharmacologic treatment of childhood depression. In: Dunner DL, Rosenbaum JF, editors. The Psychiatric Clinics of North America annual of drug therapy. Philadelphia: W.B. Saunders; 2000; 235-256; and Velosa JF, Riddle MA. Child Adolesc Psychiatr Clin N Am 2000; 9:119-133.

FORMULARY ADJUNCT

TABLE 28-10

CHARACTERISTICS OF CHEMOTHERAPEUTIC AGENTS

Drug Name (drug class in italics)	Acute Toxicity (DLT*)	Long-term Toxicity
Asparaginase (L-ASP, Elspar, PEG-ASP) *Enzyme*	DLT: Pancreatitis, seizures, hypersensitivity reactions (both acute and delayed; less with PEG modified), encephalopathy Other: Nausea, pancreatitis, hyperglycemia, azotemia, fever, coagulopathy, sagittal sinus thrombosis and other venous thromboses, hyperammonemia	Neurologic deficits secondary to stroke
Bleomycin (Blenoxane) *DNA strand breaker*	DLT†: Anaphylaxis, pneumonitis Other: Pain, fever, chills, mucositis, skin reactions	Pulmonary fibrosis related to cumulative dose
Busulfan (Myleran) *Alkylator*	DLT: Myelosuppression, mucositis, seizures, hepatic venoocclusive disease Other: Hyperpigmentation, hypotension	Infertility, endocardial fibrosis, secondary malignancy
Carboplatin (CBDCA, Paraplatin) *DNA cross-linker*	DLT†: Thrombocytopenia, nephrotoxicity Other: Severe emesis, ototoxicity, peripheral neuropathy, optic neuritis (rare)	Renal insufficiency (less than cisplatin), hearing loss
Carmustine (bis-chloronitrosourea, BCNU, BiCNU) *Alkylator*	DLT: Myelosuppression (prolonged cumulative) Other: Vesicant, brownish discoloration of skin, hepatic and renal toxicity, severe emesis	Pulmonary fibrosis, infertility, secondary malignancy
Cisplatin (Platinol, cis-platinum, CDDP) *DNA cross-linker*	DLT†: Tubular and glomerular nephrotoxicity (related to cumulative dose), peripheral neuropathy Other: Severe emesis, myelosuppression, ototoxicity, SIADH (rare), papilledema and retrobulbar neuritis (rare)	Renal insufficiency, hearing loss, peripheral neuropathy
Cladribine (2-CdA, Leustatin) *Antimetabolite or nucleotide analog*	Myelosuppression, nausea and vomiting, headache, fever, chills, fatigue	
Cyclophosphamide (CTX, Cytoxan) *Alkylator prodrug*	DLT: Leukopenia, cardiomyopathy Other: Hemorrhagic cystitis (improved by mesna), emesis, direct ADH effect	Infertility, cardiomyopathy, secondary malignancy, leukoencephalopathy

Cytarabine (Ara-C) *Antimetabolite or nucleotide analog*	DLT†: Myelosuppression, cerebellar toxicity Other: Nausea and vomiting, anorexia, diarrhea, metallic taste, severe gastrointestinal ulceration, conjunctivitis, lethargy, ataxia, nystagmus, slurred speech, respiratory distress rapidly progressing to pulmonary edema, influenza-like syndrome, fever	Leukoencephalopathy
Dacarbazine (DIC, DTIC, imidazole carboxamide) *Alkylator*	DLT: Myelosuppression Other: Severe emesis, transaminitis, facial paresthesias (rare), rash	Infertility
Dactinomycin (actinomycin-D) *Antibiotic*	DLT: Myelosuppression, severe diarrhea Other: Vesicant, nausea, acne, erythema, radiation recall, hepatic venoocclusive disease	Secondary malignancy
Daunorubicin (daunomycin) *Anthracycline*	DLT‡: Leukopenia, arrhythmia, congestive heart failure (related to cumulative dose) Other: Stomatitis, emesis, vesicant, red urine, radiation recall	Cardiomyopathy
Doxorubicin (Adriamycin) *Anthracycline*	Refer to daunorubicin	Cardiomyopathy
Etoposide (VP-16, VePesid) *Topoisomerase inhibitor*	DLT: Leukopenia, anaphylaxis (rare), transient cortical blindness Other: Hyperbilirubinemia transaminitis, peripheral neuropathy (rare), hypotension	Secondary malignancy (AML)

ADH, Antidiuretic hormone; *AML,* acute myeloid leukemia; *MAOI,* monoamine oxidase inhibitors; *SGOT,* serum glutamic-oxaloacetic transaminase; *SIADH,* syndrome of inappropriate antidiuretic hormone.

*The dose-limiting toxicity (DLT) is the toxicity most likely to require adjustment or withholding of drug.

†Dose must be adjusted in renal insufficiency.

‡Dose must be adjusted in hyperbilirubinemia.

§Dose must be adjusted in renal insufficiency and in patients with third spacing.

cont'd

FORMULARY ADJUNCT **28**

TABLE 28-10
CHARACTERISTICS OF CHEMOTHERAPEUTIC AGENTS—cont'd

Drug Name (drug class in italics)	Acute Toxicity (DLT*)	Long-term Toxicity
Fludarabine (Fludara) *Purine antimetabolite or nucleotide analog*	Myelosuppression†, anorexia, increased SGOT, somnolence, fatigue	Peripheral neuropathy, immune suppression
Fluorouracil (5-FU, Adrucil) *Nucleotide analog*	DLT: Myelosuppression (reversible with uridine), mucositis, severe diarrhea Other: Hand-foot syndrome, tear duct stenosis, hyperpigmentation, loss of nails; cerebellar syndrome (rare), and anaphylaxis	—
Hydroxyurea (Hydrea) *Ribonucleotide reductase inhibitor*	DLT: Leukopenia, pulmonary edema (rare) Other: Megaloblastic erythropoiesis, hyperpigmentation, azotemia, transaminitis, radiation recall	—
Idarubicin (Idamycin) *Anthracycline*	DLT: Arrhythmia, cardiomyopathy (cumulative) Other: Vesicant, diarrhea, mucositis, enterocolitis	Cardiomyopathy
Ifosfamide (isophosphamide, Ifex) *Alkylator prodrug*	DLT†: Myelosuppression, encephalopathy (rarely progressing to death), renal tubular damage Other: Emesis, hemorrhagic cystitis (improved with Mesna), direct ADH effect	Secondary malignancy, infertility
Liposomal doxorubicin (Doxil) *Anthracycline*	Refer to Daunorubicin	Refer to Daunorubicin
Lomustine (CCNU) *Alkylating agent*	Myelosuppression, nausea and vomiting, disorientation, fatigue	Secondary malignancy (leukemia)
Mechlorethamine (nitrogen mustard, HN₂ [mustine], Mustargen) *Alkylator*	DLT: Leukopenia, thrombocytopenia Other: Severe emesis, vesicant (antidote sodium thiosulfate), peptic ulcer (rare)	Secondary malignancy, infertility

Drug	Toxicity
Melphalan (L-PAM, Alkeran) *Alkylator*	DLT: Prolonged leukopenia (6-8 wk), mucositis, diarrhea Other: Pruritus, emesis	Pulmonary fibrosis, secondary malignancy, infertility, cataracts
Mercaptopurine (6-MP) *Nucleotide analog*	DLT: Hepatic necrosis and encephalopathy (especially doses >2.5 mg/kg/day) Other: Vesicant, headache, diarrhea, nausea	Cirrhosis
Methotrexate (MTX, Folex, Mexate, amethopterin) *Folate antagonist*	DLTs: Stomatitis, diarrhea, renal dysfunction, encephalopathy, cortical blindness, ventriculitis (intrathecal) Other: Photosensitivity, erythema, excessive lacrimation, transaminitis	Leukoencephalopathy, cirrhosis, pulmonary fibrosis, aseptic necrosis of bone, osteoporosis
Mitoxantrone (Novantrone, DHAD, DHAQ, dihydroxyanthracenedione) *DNA intercalator*	DLT: Myelosuppression, cumulative cardiomyopathy Other: Stomatitis, blue-green urine and serum	Cardiomyopathy
Paclitaxel (Taxol) *Tubulin inhibitor*	DLT: Neutropenia, anaphylaxis, ventricular tachycardia and myocardial infarction (rare) Other: Mucositis, peripheral neuropathy, bradycardia, hypertriglyceridemia	Too soon to know
Procarbazine (Matulane) *Alkylator*	DLT: Encephalopathy; pancytopenia, especially thrombocytopenia Other: Emesis, paresthesias, dizziness, ataxia, hypotension; adverse effects with tyramine-rich foods, ethanol, MAOIs, meperidine, and many other drugs	Secondary malignancy, infertility
Teniposide (VM-26) *Topoisomerase inhibitor*	DLT: Leukopenia, anaphylaxis (rare) Other: Hyperbilirubinemia, transaminitis	Secondary malignancy (AML)
Thioguanine (6-TG, 6-thioguanine) *Nucleotide analog*	DLT: Myelosuppression, bronchospasm and shock with rapid IV infusion, stomatitis, diarrhea Other: Hyperbilirubinemia, transaminitis, decreased vibratory sensation, ataxia, dermatitis	—

cont'd

28

FORMULARY ADJUNCT

TABLE 28-10
CHARACTERISTICS OF CHEMOTHERAPEUTIC AGENTS—cont'd

Drug Name (drug class in italics)	Acute Toxicity (DLT*)	Long-term Toxicity
Thiotepa *Alkylating agent*	DLT: Cognitive impairment, leukopenia Other: Increased SGOT, headache, dizziness, rash, desquamation	Secondary malignancy (leukemia) impaired fertility, weakness of lower extremities
Topotecan (Hycamptamine) *Topoisomerase inhibitor*	DLT: Leukopenia, peripheral neuropathy (rare), Horner's syndrome Other: Nausea, diarrhea, transaminitis, headache	Too soon to know
Vinblastine (Velban, VBL, vincaleukoblastine) *Microtubule inhibitor*	DLT‡: Leukopenia Other: Vesicant (improved by hyaluronidase and applied heat), constipation, bone pain (especially in the jaw), peripheral and autonomic neuropathy, rarely SIADH	—
Vincristine (VCR, Oncovin) *Microtubule inhibitor*	DLT‡: Peripheral and autonomic neuropathy, encephalopathy Other: Vesicant, bone pain, constipation, SIADH (rare)	—

ADJUNCTS TO CHEMOTHERAPY

Drug	Role	Toxicity
Amifostine	Reduces the toxicity of radiation and alkylating agents	Hypotension (62%), severe nausea and vomiting, flushing, chills, dizziness, somnolence, hiccups, sneezing, hypocalcemia in susceptible patients (<1%), short- term reversible loss of consciousness (rare), rigors (<1%), mild skin rash
Dexrazoxane	Protective agent for doxorubicin-induced cardiotoxicity	Myelosuppression
Leucovorin	Reduces methotrexate toxicity	Allergic sensitization (rare)
Mesna	Reduces risk of hemorrhagic cystitis	Headache, limb pain, abdominal pain, diarrhea, rash

REFERENCES

1. Kappy MS, Blizzard RM, Migeon CJ, editors. The Diagnosis and treatment of endocrine disorders in childhood and adolescence, 4th ed. Springfield, Ill: Charles C Thomas; 1994.

2. Migeon CJ, Wisniewski AB. Congenital adrenal hyperplasia owing to 21-hydroxylase deficiency: growth, development, and therapeutic considerations. Endocrinol Metab Clin North Am 2001; 30(1):193-206.

3. Geelhoed GC, Turner F, Macdonald WGG: Efficacy of a small dose of oral dexamethasone for outpatient croup: a double blind placebo controlled trial. BMJ 1996; 313:140-142.

4. Rittichier KK, Ledwith CA. Outpatient treatment of moderate croup with dexamethasone: intramuscular versus oral dosing. Pediatrics 2000; 106:1344-1348.

5. Roberts GW. Repeated dose inhaled budesonide versus placebo in the treatment of croup. J Pediatr Child Health 1999; 35(2):170-174.

6. Bracken MB et al. A randomized controlled trial of methylprednisolone or naloxone in the treatment of acute spinal cord injury: results of the Second National Acute Spinal Cord Injury Study. N Engl J Med 1990; 322(20):1405-1411.

7. Bracken MB: Pharmacological treatment of acute spinal cord injury: current status and future projects. J Emerg Med 1993; 11:43.

8. Pickering LK, editor. 2000 Red book: report of the Committee on Infectious Diseases, 24th ed. Elk Grove Village, Ill: American Academy of Pediatrics; 2000.

9. Adams DM et al. High dose oral dexamethasone therapy for chronic childhood idiopathic thrombocytopenic purpura. J Pediatrics 1996; 128.

10. Taketomo CK, Hodding JH, Kraus DM. American Pharmaceutical Association pediatric dosage handbook. Hudson, Ohio: Lexi-Comp; 1998.

28

FORMULARY ADJUNCT

DRUGS IN RENAL FAILURE

Christian Nechyba, MD, and Veronica L. Gunn, MD, MPH

I. DOSE ADJUSTMENT METHODS

A. MAINTENANCE DOSAGE

In patients with renal insufficiency, the dose may be adjusted using the following methods:

1. **Interval extension (I):** Lengthen the intervals between individual doses, keeping the dosage size normal. For this method, the suggested interval is shown.
2. **Dose reduction (D):** Reduce the amount of individual doses, keeping the interval between the doses normal. This method is particularly recommended for drugs in which a relatively constant blood level is desired. For this method the percentage of the usual dose is shown.
3. **Interval and dose reduction (DI):** Lengthen the interval, and reduce the dose.
4. **Interval or dose reduction (D, I):** In some instances, either the dose or the interval can be changed.

Note: These dosage adjustments are for beyond the neonatal period. These dosage modifications are only approximations. Each patient must be monitored closely for signs of drug toxicity, and serum levels must be measured when available. Drug dose and interval should be monitored accordingly.

B. DIALYSIS

The quantitative effects of hemodialysis (He) and peritoneal dialysis (P) on drug removal are shown. "Y" indicates the need for a supplemental dose with dialysis. "N" indicates no need for adjustment. The designation "No" does not preclude the use of dialysis or hemoperfusion for drug overdose.

II. ANTIMICROBIALS REQUIRING ADJUSTMENT IN RENAL FAILURE
(Table 29-1)

III. NONANTIMICROBIALS REQUIRING ADJUSTMENT IN RENAL FAILURE (Table 29-2)

REFERENCES

1. Taketomo C, Hodding JH, Kraus DM. Pediatric dosage handbook, 8th ed. Hudson, Ohio: Lexi-Comp, Inc; 2001-2002.
2. American Society of Health-System Pharmacists. American hospital formulary service. Bethesda, Md: The Society; 1998.
3. Johnson C, Simmons W. Dialysis of drugs. Pharm Practice News Dec 1988, pp 30–33.
4. Micromedex, Inc, Vol. 111, 1974-2002. Expires 3/2002.

TABLE 29-1
ANTIMICROBIALS REQUIRING ADJUSTMENT IN RENAL FAILURE

| | Pharmacokinetics | | | Adjustments in Renal Failure | | | |
| | | | | Creatinine Clearance (mL/min) | | | |
Drug	Route of Excretion[a]	Normal $t_{1/2}$ (hr)	Normal Dose Interval	Method	Mild (>50)	Moderate (10-50)	Severe (<10)	Supplemental Dose for Dialysis
Acyclovir (IV)	Renal	2-4	Q8hr	DI	Q8hr	Q12-24hr	50% and Q24hr	Y (He) N (P)
Amantidine	Renal	10-28	Q12-24hr	I	Q12-24hr	Q48-72hr	Q7 days	N (He) N (P)
Amikacin[b]	Renal	1.5-3	Q8-12hr	I	Q8-12hr	Q12-18hr	Q24-48hr	Y (He) Y (P)
Amoxicillin	Renal	1-3.7	Q8-12hr	I	Q8-12hr	Q12hr	Q24hr	Y (He) N (P)
Amoxicillin-clavulanate	Renal	1	Q8-12hr	I	Q8-12hr	Q12hr	Q24hr	Y (He) Y (P)
Amphotericin B	Renal 40% up to 7 days	Up to 15 days	QD	I	Dosage adjustments are unnecessary with preexisting renal impairment; if decreased renal function is due to amphotericin B, the daily dose can be decreased by 50% or the dose given QOD			N (He) N (P)
Amphotericin B cholesteryl sulfate (Amphotec)	?	28-29	QD	I	No guidelines established			N (He)
Amphotericin B lipid complex (Abelcet)	Renal 1%	170	QD	I	No guidelines established			?

Drug	Excretion	Half-life (hr)	Normal interval	Method				Supplement for dialysis
Amphotericin B liposomal (AmBisome)	Renal ≤10%	100-173	QD	I	No guidelines established			?
Ampicillin	Renal	1-4	Q6hr	I	Q6hr	Q6-12hr	Q12-16hr	Y (He) N (P)
Ampicillin/sulbactam	Renal	1-1.8	Q4-6hr	I	Q4-6hr	Q12hr	Q24hr	Y (He) N (P)
Aztreonam	Renal (hepatic)	1.3-2.2	Q6-12hr	D	75%-100%	50%	25%	Y (He)
Carbenicillin[c]	Renal (hepatic)	0.8-1.8	Q6hr	I	Q8-12hr	Q12-24hr	Q24-48hr	Y (He)
Cefaclor	Renal	0.5-1	Q8-12hr	D	100%	100%	50%	Y (He) Y (P)
Cefadroxil	Renal	1-2	Q12hr	I	Q12hr	Q12-24hr	Q24-48hr	Y (He) N (P)
Cefamandole	Renal	1	Q4-8hr	I	Q6hr	Q6-8hr	Q12hr	Y (He)
Cefazolin	Renal	1.5-2.5	Q8hr	I	Q8hr	Q12hr	Q24hr	Y (He) N (P)
Cefdinir	Renal	1.1-2.3	Q12-24hr	I	Q12-24hr	7 mg/kg/dose Q24hr or 300 mg Q24hr for adults (CrCl <30)		Y (H)

CrCl, Creatinine clearance; He, hemodialysis; P, peritoneal dialysis.

[a]Route in parentheses indicates secondary route of excretion.

[b]Subsequent doses are best determined by measurement of serum levels and assessment of renal insufficiency.

[c]May inactivate aminoglycosides in patients with renal impairment.

cont'd

29

DRUGS IN RENAL FAILURE

TABLE 29-1
ANTIMICROBIALS REQUIRING ADJUSTMENT IN RENAL FAILURE—cont'd

Drug	Route of Excretion[a]	Normal $t_{1/2}$ (hr)	Normal Dose Interval	Method	Mild (>50)	Moderate (10-50)	Severe (<10)	Supplemental Dose for Dialysis
						Adjustments in Renal Failure — Creatinine Clearance (mL/min)		
Cefepime	Renal	1.8-2	Q8-12hr	DI	Q12hr regimens: _Est CrCl (mL/min)_			Y (He)
					30-60	50 mg/kg/dose Q24hr		N (P)
					11-29	25 mg/kg/dose Q24hr		
					≤10	12.5 mg/kg/dose Q24hr		
					Q8hr regimens: _Est CrCl (mL/min)_			
					30-50	50 mg/kg/dose Q12hr		
					10-30	50 mg/kg/dose Q24hr		
					<10	50 mg/kg/dose Q24-48hr		
Cefixime	Renal (hepatic)	3-4	Q12-24hr	D	100%	75% (CrCl 21-60)	50% (CrCl <20)	N (He, P)
Cefotaxime	Renal	1-3.5	Q6-12hr	D	100%	CrCl <20 = ↓ dose by 50%		Y (He)
								N (P)
Cefotetan	Renal (hepatic)	3.5	Q12hr	I	Q12hr	CrCl 10-30 = Q24hr	Q48	Y (He, P)
								N (P)
Cefoxitin	Renal	0.75-1.5	Q4-8hr	I	Normal interval	CrCl 30-50 = Q8-12hr	Q24-48hr	Y (He)
						CrCl 10-30 = Q12-24hr		N (P)

Drug	Route of Elimination	Half-life (hr)	Interval	Method	>50	10–50	<10	Dialysis
Cefpodoxime proxetil	Renal	2.2	Q12hr	I	Q12hr	CrCl <30 = Q24hr	Q24hr	Y (He) N (P)
Cefprozil	Renal	1.3	Q12hr		100%	CrCl <30 = 50%	50%	Y (He)
Ceftazidime	Renal	1-2	Q8-12hr	D	Q8-12hr	CrCl 30-50 = Q12hr / CrCl 10-30 = Q24hr	Q24-48hr	Y (He, P)
Ceftibuten	Renal	1.5-2.5	Q24hr	D	100%	50% (CrCl 30-49)	25% (CrCl 5-29)	Y (He) N (P)
Ceftizoxime	Renal	1.6	Q6-12hr	I	Q8-12hr	Q36-48hr	Q48-72hr	Y (He)
Cefuroxime (IV)	Renal	1.6-2.2	Q8-12hr	I	Q8-12hr	CrCl 10-20 = Q12hr	Q24hr	Y (He) N (P)
Cephalexin	Renal	0.5-1.2	Q6hr	I	Q6hr	Q8-12hr	Q12-24hr	Y (He) N (P)
Cephalothin[d]	Renal (hepatic)	0.5-1	Q4-6hr	I	Q6-8hr	Q6-8hr	Q12hr	Y (He) N (P)
Cephradine	Renal	0.7-2	Q6-12hr	D, I	100%	50% or Q12-24hr	25% or Q36hr	Y (He)
Ciprofloxacin	Renal (hepatic)	1.2-5	Q8-12hr	D, I	100%	50-75% (or Q18-24hr for CrCl <30)	50% (or Q18-24hr for CrCl <30)	Y (He, P)
Clarithromycin	Renal/hepatic	3-7	Q12hr	DI	No change	CrCl <30 = ↓ dose by 50% and administer BID-QD		?

[d]May add to peritoneal dialysate to obtain adequate serum levels.

cont'd

29

DRUGS IN RENAL FAILURE

TABLE 29-1
ANTIMICROBIALS REQUIRING ADJUSTMENT IN RENAL FAILURE—cont'd

Drug	Pharmacokinetics				Adjustments in Renal Failure — Creatinine Clearance (mL/min)				Supplemental Dose for Dialysis
	Route of Excretion[a]	Normal $t_{1/2}$ (hr)	Normal Dose Interval	Method	Mild (>50)	Moderate (10-50)	Severe (<10)		
Co-trimoxazole (sulfa-methoxazole/trimethoprim)	Sulfameth-oxazole: Hepatic (renal) Trimethoprim: Renal (hepatic)	Sulfamethox-azole: 9-11 Trimethoprim: 8-15	Q12hr	D	No change	CrCl 15-30 = 50%	CrCl <15 = not recommended		Y (He) N (P)
Erythromycin	Hepatic (renal)	1.5-2	Q6-8hr	D	100%	100%	50%-75%		N (He, P)
Ethambutol	Renal (hepatic)	2.5-3.6	Q24hr	I	Q24hr	Q24-36hr	Q48hr ± ↓ dose		Y (He) N (P)
Famciclovir	Renal (hepatic)	2-3	500 mg Q8hr	DI	CrCl 40-59 = 500 mg Q12hr CrCl 20-39 = 500 mg Q24hr <20 = 250 mg Q48hr				Y (He)
Fluconazole[d]	Renal	19-25	Q24hr	D	100%	25-50%	25%		Y (He, P)
Flucytosine[b]	Renal	3-8	Q6hr	I	Q6hr	Q12hr	Q24hr		Y (He, P)
Foscarnet	Renal	3-4.5	Q8-12	D	See package insert				Y (He)
Ganciclovir	Renal	2.5-3.6	IV: Q12hr PO: TID	IV: DI PO: DI	IV: 50%-100% and Q12hr PO: 50%-100% and TID	25%-50% and Q24hr 50% and BID-QD	25% and Q24hr 50% and QD		Y (He)

Drug	Elimination	Half-life (hr)	Normal	Method	>50	10-50	<10	Dialysis
Gentamicin[b,d]	Renal	1.5-3	Q8-12hr	I	Q8-12hr	Q12-18hr	Q24-48hr	Y (He, P)
Imipenem/cilastatin	Renal	1-1.4	Q6-8hr	DI	50%-100% and Q6-8hr	25%-50% and Q8hr	25% and Q12hr	Y (He)
Isoniazid	Hepatic (renal)	2-4 (slow)[e] 0.5-1.5 (fast)	Q24hr	D	100%	100%	50%	Y (He, P)
Kanamycin	Renal	2-3	Q8hr	I	Q8-12hr	Q12hr	Q24hr	Y (He, P)
Lamivudine[f]	Renal	1.7-2.5	Q12hr	DI	CrCl 30-49 = 100% and Q24hr; 15-29 = 66% and Q24hr; 5-14 = 33% and Q24hr; <5 = 17% and Q24hr			?
Loracarbef	Renal	0.78-1	Q12hr	D, I	Q12h	Q24hr or 50%	Q72-120hr	Y (He)
Meropenem	Renal	1-1.4	Q8hr	DI	100% and Q8hr	50%-100% and Q12hr	50% and Q24hr	Y (He)
Methicillin	Renal	0.5-1.2	Q4-6hr	I	Q4-6hr	Q6-8hr	Q8-12hr	N (He, P)
Metronidazole	Hepatic (renal)	6-12	Q6-12hr	D	100%	100%	50%	Y (He) N (P)
Mezlocillin	Renal (hepatic)	0.5-1	Q4-6hr	I	Q4-6hr	Q6-8hr (CrCl 10-30)	Q8-12hr	Y (He) N (P)
Norfloxacin	Hepatic (renal)	2-4	BID	I	BID	QD-BID	QD	N (He)
Ofloxacin	Renal	5-7.5	BID	I	BID	QD	QOD	Y (He) N (P)
Oseltamivir	Renal	1-10	Q12-24hr	I	Normal	Q24 hr (CrCl 10-30)	?	Y (He) N (P) ?

[e]Rate of acetylation of isoniazid.
[f]GFR ≥5 mL/min, give full dose as first dose; for GFR <5 mL/min, give 33% of full dose as first dose.

cont'd

29

DRUGS IN RENAL FAILURE

TABLE 29-1
ANTIMICROBIALS REQUIRING ADJUSTMENT IN RENAL FAILURE—cont'd

| Drug | Pharmacokinetics | | | Adjustments in Renal Failure | | | | Supplemental Dose for Dialysis |
| | Route of Excretion[a] | Normal $t_{1/2}$ (hr) | Normal Dose Interval | | Creatinine Clearance (mL/min) | | | |
				Method	Mild (>50)	Moderate (10-50)	Severe (<10)	
Oxacillin	Renal (liver)	0.3-1.8	Q4-12hr	D	100%	100%	Use lower range of normal dose	N (P)
Penicillin G–potassium/ Na⁺ (IV)	Renal (hepatic)	0.5-3.4	Q4-6hr	D	100%	75%	20%-50%	Y (He) N (P)
Penicillin VK (PO)	Renal (hepatic)	30-40min	Q6hr		Q6hr	Q6hr	Q8hr	Y (He) N (P)
Pentamidine	Renal	6.4-9.4	Q24hr	I	Q24hr	CrCl 10-30 = Q36hr	Q48hr	N (He, P)
Piperacillin	Renal (hepatic)	0.39-1	Q4-6hr	I	Q4-6hr	CrCl 20-40 = Q8hr	CrCl <20 = Q12h	Y (He) N (P)
Piperacillin/ tazobactam	Renal	Piperacillin: 0.39-1 Tazobactam: 0.7-0.9	Q6-8hr	DI	100% and Q6-8hr	70% and Q6hr (CrCl 20-40)	70% and Q8hr (CrCl <20)	Y (He) N (P)
Rifabutin	Renal (hepatic)	16-69	Q12-24hr	D	Normal	50% (CrCl <30)		?
Rifampin	Hepatic (renal)	3-4	Q12-24hr	D	100%	50%-100%	50%	N (He, P)
Stavudine	Renal/ hepatic	1.1-1.45	Q12hr	DI	100% and Q12hr	50% and Q12hr (CrCl 26-50) 25%, dosed Q24 hr (CrCl <25)	50% (CrCl <30)	?

Drug	Elimination	Half-life		Method	Normal dose			
Streptomycin sulfate	Renal	2-4.7	Q24hr	I	Q24hr	Q24-72hr	Q72-96hr	Y (He)
Sulfamethoxazole	Renal	7-12	Q12hr	D	100%	50% (CrCl 10-30)	25%	Avoid
Sulfisoxazole	Renal	4-8	Q6hr	I	Q6hr	Q8-12hr	Q12-24hr	Y (He, P)
Tetracycline	Renal (hepatic)	6-12	Q6hr	I	Q8-12hr	Q12-24hr	**AVOID**	?
Ticarcillin[c]	Renal	0.9-1.3	Q4-6hr	I	Q4-6hr	Q8hr (CrCl 10-30)	Q12hr	Y (He) / N (P)
Ticarcillin-clavulanate[c]	Renal	Ticarcillin: 0.9-1.3 / Clavulanate: 1-1.5	Q4-6hr	I	Q4-6hr	Q8hr (CrCl 10-30)	Q12hr (Q24hr if comorbid hepatic impairment)	Y (He) / N (P)
Tobramycin[b,d]	Renal	1.5-3	Q8-12hr	I	Q8-12hr	Q12-18hr	Q24-48hr	Y (He, P)
Valacyclovir	Valacyclovir: Hepatic / Acyclovir: Renal	Valacyclovir: 2.5-3.6 / Acyclovir: 2-4	Q12-24hr	DI	Herpes zoster: 100% and Q8hr	100% and Q12-24hr	50% and Q24hr	Y (He) / N (P)
					Genital herpes (initial): 100% and Q12hr	100% and Q12-24hr	50% and Q24hr	
					Genital herpes (recurrent): 100% and Q12hr	100% and Q12-24hr	100% and Q24hr	
					Genital herpes (suppressive): 100% and Q24hr	50%-100% and Q24hr	50% and Q24hr	

cont'd

29

DRUGS IN RENAL FAILURE

TABLE 29-1
ANTIMICROBIALS REQUIRING ADJUSTMENT IN RENAL FAILURE—cont'd

Drug	Pharmacokinetics			Adjustments in Renal Failure				Supplemental Dose for Dialysis
	Route of Excretion[a]	Normal $t_{1/2}$ (hr)	Normal Dose Interval	Method	Creatinine Clearance (mL/min)			
					Mild (>50)	Moderate (10-50)	Severe (<10)	
Valgancyclovir (see gancyclovir)								
Vancomycin[b]	Renal	2.2-8	Q6-12hr	I	Q6-12hr	Q18-48hr	Q48-96hr	Y/N (He)[g] N (P)
Zalcitabine	Renal	1-3	Q8hr	I	Q8hr	Q12hr	Q24hr	?

[a]If using high-flux hemodialysis (polysulfone polyamide and polyacrylonitrile), give supplemental dose after dialysis.

TABLE 29-2
NONANTIMICROBIALS REQUIRING ADJUSTMENT IN RENAL FAILURE

Drug	Pharmacokinetics			Adjustments in Renal Failure				Supplemental Dose for Dialysis
				Creatinine Clearance (mL/min)				
	Route of Excretion[a]	Normal $t_{1/2}$ (hr)	Normal Dose Interval	Method	Mild (>50)	Moderate (10-50)	Severe (<10)	
Acetaminophen	Hepatic	2-4	Q4hr	I	Q4hr	Q6hr	Q8hr	Y (He) N (P)
Acetazolamide	Renal	2.4-5.8	Q6-24hr	I	Q6-8hr	Q12hr	AVOID	N (He, P)
Allopurinol	Renal	1-3	Q6-12hr	D,I	100% or Q8hr	50% or Q12-24hr	10%-25% or Q48-72hr	?
Amantadine	Renal	10-14	Q12-24hr	I	Q12-24hr	Q48-72hr	Q168hr (7 days)	N (He, P)
Aminocaproic acid	Renal	1-2	Q4-6hr	D	Reduce dose to 15%-25% in patients with renal disease or oliguria. No specific recommendations available.			Y (He)
Aspirin[b]	Hepatic (renal)	2-19	Q4hr	I	Q4hr	Q4-6hr	AVOID	Y (He) Y (P)
Atenolol	Renal (GI)	3.5-7	QD	D,I	100% or Q24hr	50% or Q48hr	25% or Q96hr	Y (He)
Azathioprine[c]	Hepatic (renal)	0.7-3	QD	D,I	100% or Q24hr	75% or Q36hr	50% or Q48hr	Y (He)

He, Hemodialysis; *P*, peritoneal dialysis; *NA*, not applicable.
[a]Route in parentheses indicates secondary route of excretion.
[b]With large doses, the $t_{1/2}$ is prolonged up to 30hr.
[c]Azathioprine rapidly converted to mercaptopurine ($t_{1/2} = 0.5$-4hr).

cont'd

29

DRUGS IN RENAL FAILURE

TABLE 29-2
NONANTIMICROBIALS REQUIRING ADJUSTMENT IN RENAL FAILURE—cont'd

| | Pharmacokinetics | | | | Adjustments in Renal Failure | | | | |
| | | | | | Creatinine Clearance (mL/min) | | | | |
Drug	Route of Excretion[a]	Normal $t_{1/2}$ (hr)	Normal Dose Interval	Method	Mild (>50)	Moderate (10-50)	Severe (<10)	Supplemental Dose for Dialysis
Bismuth subsalicylate	Hepatic (renal)	Salicylate: 2-5 Bismuth: 21-72 days	Q30min-4hr	D	**AVOID**	**AVOID**	**AVOID**	NA
Bretylium	Renal	7-11	Q10-20 min to 6-8hr	D	100%	25%-50%	25%	Y (He)
Captopril	Renal (hepatic)	0.98-2.3	Q6-24hr	D, I	100% or Q8-12hr	75% or Q12-18hr	50% or Q24hr	Y (He) N (P)
Carbamazepine	Hepatic (renal)	Initial: 25-65 Subsequent: 8-17	Q6-24hr	D	100%	100%	75% (monitor serum levels)	N (He, P)
Cetirizine	Renal (hepatic)	6.2-9	BID-QD	D	100%	50%-100%	50%	N (He)
Chloroquine	Renal (hepatic)	3-5 days	Q6hr-7 days	D	100%	100%	50%	?
Cimetidine	Renal (hepatic)	1.4-2	Q6-12hr	D, I	100% or Q6hr	75% or Q8hr	50% or Q12hr	N (He, P)
Codeine	Hepatic (renal)	2.5-3.5	Q6-12hr Q4-6hr	D	100%	75%	50%	?
Digoxin[d]	Renal	35-48	Q12-24hr	D, I	100% or Q24hr	25%-75% or Q36hr	10%-25% or Q48hr	N (He, P)
Diphenhydramine	Hepatic	4-7	Q6-8hr	I	Q6hr	Q6-12hr	Q12-18hr	?

Disopyramide	Renal (GI)	4-10	Q6hr	I	Q6hr	Q8-12hr	Q24hr	Y (He)
Enalapril (IV: Enalaprilat)	Renal (hepatic)	1.3-6	Q8-24hr	D	100%	75%-100%	50%	?
Famotidine	Renal (hepatic)	2.5-4	Q8-12hr	D, I	100% or Q8-12hr	50% or Q24hr	25% or Q36-48hr	N (He, P)
Fentanyl	Renal (hepatic)	2-4	Q30min-1hr	D	100%	75%	50%	N (He)
Flecainide	Renal/ hepatic	8-12	Q8-12hr	D	CrCl <20: 25-50%			N (He, P)
Gabapentin	Renal (hepatic)	5-9	TID	I	TID	BID-QD	QOD	Y (He)
Hydralazine[e]	Hepatic (renal)	2-8	IV: Q4-6hr	I	Normal dosing	Q8hr	Q8-16hr (fast acetylator) Q12-24hr (slow acetylator)	N (He, P)
Insulin (regular)[f]	Hepatic (renal)	5-15min	Variable	D	100%	75%	25%-50%	N (He, P)
Lithium	Renal	18-24	BID-QID	D	100%	50%-75%	25%-50%	Y (He, P)
Loratadine	Renal/ Hepatic	8-15hr	QD	I	Normal	CrCl <30: QOD		N (He, P)

CrCl, Creatinine clearance; He, hemodialysis; P, peritoneal dialysis; NA, not applicable.
[d]Decrease loading dose by 50% in end-stage renal disease because of decreased volume of distribution.
[e]Dose interval varies for rapid and slow acetylators with normal and impaired renal function.
[f]Renal failure may cause hyposensitivity or hypersensitivity to insulin; adjust to clinical response and blood glucose.

cont'd

29

DRUGS IN RENAL FAILURE

TABLE 29-2

NONANTIMICROBIALS REQUIRING ADJUSTMENT IN RENAL FAILURE—cont'd

| Drug | Pharmacokinetics | | | | Adjustments in Renal Failure Creatinine Clearance (mL/min) | | | Supplemental Dose for Dialysis |
	Route of Excretion[a]	Normal $t_{1/2}$ (hr)	Normal Dose Interval	Method	Mild (>50)	Moderate (10-50)	Severe (<10)	
Meperidine	Renal (hepatic) (normeperidine: renal)	2.3-4	Q3-4hr	D	100%	75%	50%	?
Methadone	Hepatic (renal)	4-62	Q3-6hr	D	100%	100%	50%-75%	?
Methyldopa	Hepatic (renal)	1-3	PO: Q6-12hr IV: Q6-8hr	I	Q8hr	Q8-12hr	Q12-24hr	Y (He)
Metoclopramide	Renal	2.5-6	PO: Q6hr IV: Q6-8hr	D	100%	50%-75%	25%-50%	N (He)
Midazolam	Hepatic (renal)	2.9-4.5	Variable	D	100%	100%	50%	?
Morphine	Hepatic (renal)	1-6.2	Variable	D	100%	75%	50%	N (He)
Neostigmine	Hepatic (renal)	0.5-2.1	Single dose	D	100%	50%	25%	?
Phenazopyridine	Renal (hepatic)	?	TID for 2 days	I	Q8-16hr	**AVOID**	**AVOID**	NA

Drug		Half-life		D/I				
Phenobarbital	Hepatic (renal 30%)	65-150	Q8-12hr	I	Q8-12hr	Q8-12hr	Q12-16hr	Y (He, P)
Primidone	Hepatic (renal, 20%)	10-16	Q6-12	I	Q8hr	Q8-12hr	Q12-24hr	Y (He)
Procainamide	Hepatic (renal)	Procainamide: 1.7-4.7 NAPA: 6-8	PO: Q3-6hr IM: Q4-6hr	I	Normal interval	Q6-12hr	Q8-24hr	Y (He) N (P)
Propylthiouracil	Hepatic (renal)	1.5-5	Q8hr	D	100%	75%	50%	?
Ranitidine	Renal (hepatic)	1.8-2.5	Q8-12hr	D	100%	75%	50%	N (He, P)
Spironolactone	Renal (hepatic)	78-84min	Q6-12hr	I	Q6-12hr	Q12-24hr[g]	**AVOID**	?
Terbutaline (IV/PO)	Renal (hepatic)	11-26	Variable	D	100%	50%	**AVOID**	?
Thiopental	Hepatic (renal)	3-11.5	One-time dose	D	100%	100%	75%	?
Triamterene	Hepatic (renal)	1.5-2.5	Q12-24hr	I	Q12hr	Q12hr[g]	**AVOID**	N (He)
Verapamil	Renal (hepatic)	2-8	Variable	D	100%	100%	50-75%	N (He)

[g]Hyperkalemia common with GFR <30 mL/min.

29

DRUGS IN RENAL FAILURE

INDEX

Page numbers followed by f indicate figures; t, tables; b, boxes. References in *italics* indicate color
plates.

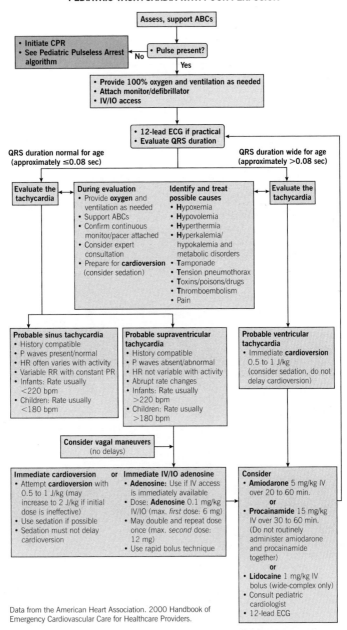

PEDIATRIC TACHYCARDIA WITH POOR PERFUSION

Assess, support ABCs

Pulse present?

No

- Initiate CPR
- See Pediatric Pulseless Arrest algorithm

Yes

- Provide 100% oxygen and ventilation as needed
- Attach monitor/defibrillator
- IV/IO access

- 12-lead ECG if practical
- Evaluate QRS duration

QRS duration normal for age (approximately ≤0.08 sec)

QRS duration wide for age (approximately >0.08 sec)

Evaluate the tachycardia

Evaluate the tachycardia

During evaluation
- Provide **oxygen** and ventilation as needed
- Support ABCs
- Confirm continuous monitor/pacer attached
- Consider expert consultation
- Prepare for **cardioversion** (consider sedation)

Identify and treat possible causes
- **H**ypoxemia
- **H**ypovolemia
- **H**yperthermia
- **H**yperkalemia/ hypokalemia and metabolic disorders
- **T**amponade
- **T**ension pneumothorax
- **T**oxins/poisons/drugs
- **T**hromboembolism
- Pain

Probable sinus tachycardia
- History compatible
- P waves present/normal
- HR often varies with activity
- Variable RR with constant PR
- Infants: Rate usually <220 bpm
- Children: Rate usually <180 bpm

Probable supraventricular tachycardia
- History compatible
- P waves absent/abnormal
- HR not variable with activity
- Abrupt rate changes
- Infants: Rate usually >220 bpm
- Children: Rate usually >180 bpm

Probable ventricular tachycardia
- Immediate **cardioversion** 0.5 to 1 J/kg (consider sedation, do not delay cardioversion)

Consider vagal maneuvers (no delays)

Immediate cardioversion
- Attempt **cardioversion** with 0.5 to 1 J/kg (may increase to 2 J/kg if initial dose is ineffective)
- Use sedation if possible
- Sedation must not delay cardioversion

or

Immediate IV/IO adenosine
- **Adenosine:** Use if IV access is immediately available
- Dose: **Adenosine** 0.1 mg/kg IV/IO (max. *first* dose: 6 mg)
- May double and repeat dose once (max. *second* dose: 12 mg)
- Use rapid bolus technique

Consider
- **Amiodarone** 5 mg/kg IV over 20 to 60 min.

or

- **Procainamide** 15 mg/kg IV over 30 to 60 min. (Do not routinely administer amiodarone and procainamide together)

or

- **Lidocaine** 1 mg/kg IV bolus (wide-complex only)
- Consult pediatric cardiologist
- 12-lead ECG

Data from the American Heart Association. 2000 Handbook of Emergency Cardiovascular Care for Healthcare Providers.